Zuckerman Parker Handbook of Developmental and Behavioral Pediatrics for Primary Care

FOURTH EDITION

Zuckerman Parker Handbook of Developmental and Behavioral Pediatrics for Primary Care

FOURTH EDITION

Marilyn Augustyn, MD
Professor of Pediatrics
Boston University School of Medicine
Division Director, Developmental and Behavioral Pediatrics
Boston Medical Center
Boston, Massachusetts

Barry Zuckerman, MD
Professor and Chair Emeritus of Pediatrics
Boston University School of Medicine
Professor of Public Health
Boston University School of Public Health
Former Chair of Pediatrics
Boston Medical Center
Boston, Massachusetts

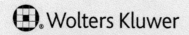. Wolters Kluwer

Philadelphia · Baltimore · New York · London
Buenos Aires · Hong Kong · Sydney · Tokyo

Acquisitions Editor: Kate Heaney
Editorial Coordinator: John Larkin
Marketing Manager: Rachel Mante Leung
Production Project Manager: Kim Cox
Design Coordinator: Joan Wendt
Manufacturing Coordinator: Beth Welsh
Prepress Vendor: TNQ Technologies

Fourth edition

Library of Congress Cataloging-in-Publication Data

Names: Zuckerman, Barry S., editor. | Augustyn, Marilyn.
Title: Zuckerman Parker handbook of developmental and behavioral pediatrics for primary care / [edited by] Marilyn Augustyn, MD Professor of Pediatrics, Boston University School of Medicine, Division Director, Developmental and Behavioral Pediatrics, Boston Medical Center, Boston, Massachusetts, Barry Zuckerman, MD, Professor and Chair Emeritus of Pediatrics, Boston University School of Medicine, Professor of Public Health, Boston University School of Public Health, Former Chair of Pediatrics, Boston Medical Center, Boston, Massachusetts.
Description: Fourth edition. | Philadelphia : Wolters Kluwer, [2019] | Includes bibliographical references and index.
Identifiers: LCCN 2018031835 | ISBN 9781496397393 (paperback)
Subjects: LCSH: Behavior disorders in children—Handbooks, manuals, etc. | Child development deviations—Handbooks, manuals, etc. | Pediatrics—Psychological aspects—Handbooks, manuals, etc. | Primary care (Medicine)—Handbooks, manuals, etc. | BISAC: MEDICAL / Pediatrics.
Classification: LCC RJ47.5 .B37 2019 | DDC 618.92/89—dc23 LC record available at https://lccn.loc.gov/2018031835.

Dedication

—*from Marilyn*
To George, Henry, and Clare for always supporting me to develop to my fullest potential and letting me share in the amazing beings you have become!

To Audrey and Henry Augustyn who embodied the positive parenting I wish for all children.

—*from Barry*
To Berry Brazelton, MD (1918–2018) whose mentorship, inspiration, insights, and warmth are part of all my clinical and academic work including this book.

To Pam, Jake, and Katherine for their love, support, and humor, which makes everything possible, and to Julian Jacob Gilman, a loved and long-awaited grandchild who reminds us daily of the magic and wonder of infancy.

Contributing Authors

Rachel Amgott, MSN, RN, CPNP-PC
Instructor of Pediatrics
Department of Pediatrics
Boston University School of Medicine
Boston Massachusetts

Marilyn Augustyn, MD
Professor of Pediatrics
Boston University School of Medicine
Division Director, Developmental and
    Behavioral Pediatrics
Boston Medical Center
Boston, Massachusetts

Sarah M. Bagley, MD, MSc
Assistant Professor
Department of Medicine and Pediatrics
Boston University School of Medicine
Boston, Massachusetts

Nerissa S. Bauer, MD, MPH
Associate Professor
Department of Pediatrics
Indiana University
Indianapolis, Indiana

Nicole Baumer, MD, MEd
Instructor
Department of Neurology
Harvard Medical School
Boston, Massachusetts

Nicole M. Benson, MD
Clinical Fellow
Child and Adolescent Psychiatry
Massachusetts General Hospital
Boston, Massachusetts

Joseph Biederman, MD
Professor
Department of Psychiatry
Harvard Medical School
Boston, Massachusetts

Peter A. Blasco, MD
Associate Professor
Department of Pediatrics
Oregon Health and Science University
Portland, Oregon

Stephanie Blenner, MD
Assistant Professor
Department of Pediatrics
University of Massachusetts
Worcester, Massachusetts

Natalija Bogdanovic, MD
Clinical Assistant Professor
Department of Psychiatry
Boston University School of Medicine
Boston, Massachusetts

Carolyn Bridgemohan, MD
Assistant Professor
Department of Pediatrics
Harvard Medical School
Boston, Massachusetts

Robert B. Brooks, PhD
Assistant Clinical Professor of Psychology
    (part-time)
Department of Psychiatry
Harvard Medical School
Boston, Massachusetts

Elizabeth B. Caronna, MD
Chief
Department of Developmental and Behavioral
    Pediatrics
Atrius Health/Harvard Vanguard Medical
    Associates
Boston, Massachusetts

Molinda M. Chartrand, MD, FAAP
Associate Professor
Department of Pediatrics
University of Illinois-Urbana Champaign
Champaign, Illinois

Victoria Chen, MD, FAAP
Assistant Professor
Department of Pediatrics
Donald and Barbara Zucker School of
    Medicine at Hofstra/Northwell
Hempstead, New York

**Edward R. Christophersen, PhD,
    ABPP, FAAP (Hon)**
Board Certified Clinical Psychologist
Fellow (Honorary), American Academy of
    Pediatrics
Division of Developmental and Behavioral
    Pediatrics
Emeritus Professor of Pediatrics
UMKC School of Medicine
Children's Mercy Hospital
Kansas City, Missouri

Jayme Congdon, MD, MS
Clinical Fellow
General Pediatrics
University of California
San Francisco, California

Eileen M. Costello, MD
Clinical Professor
Department of Pediatrics
Boston University School of Medicine
Boston, Massachusetts

David L. Coulter, MD
Associate Professor of Neurology
Harvard Medical School
Senior Staff Neurologist
Boston Children's Hospital
Boston, Massachusetts

Howard Dubowitz, MD, MS, FAAP
Professor of Pediatrics
Head, Division of Child Protection;
Director, Center for Families
Department of Pediatrics
University of Maryland School of Medicine
Baltimore, Maryland

Michelle P. Durham, MD, MPH, FAPA
Assistant Professor
Department of Psychiatry
Boston University School of Medicine
Boston, Massachusetts

Mei Elansary, MD, MPhil
Clinical Fellow
Department of Pediatrics
Harvard Medical School
Boston, Massachusetts

Norah Emara, MD
Instructor
Department of Pediatrics
Harvard University
Boston, Massachusetts

Ilgi Ertem, MD
Professor
Department of Pediatrics, Division of
   Developmental-Behavioral Pediatrics
Ankara University School of Medicine
Ankara, Turkey

Heidi M. Feldman, MD, PhD
Professor
Department of Pediatrics
Stanford University
Stanford, California

Angela M. Feraco, MD, MMSc
Instructor
Department of Pediatrics
Harvard Medical School
Boston, Massachusetts

Sara F. Forman, MD
Assistant Professor
Department of Pediatrics
Harvard Medical School
Boston, Massachusetts

Lisa R. Fortuna, MD, MPH
Director
Section of Child and Adolescent Psychiatry
Department of Psychiatry
Boston Medical Center
Boston, Massachusetts

Deborah A. Frank, MD
Professor of Child Health and
   Well-Being
Boston University School of
   Medicine
Boston, Massachusetts

Melissa Beth Freizinger, PhD
Instructor
Department of Psychiatry
Harvard Medical School
Boston, Massachusetts

Tanya Froehlich, MD, MS
Associate Professor
Department of Pediatrics
University of Cincinnati
Cincinnati, Ohio

Arvin Garg, MD, MPH
Associate Professor
Department of Pediatrics
Boston Medical Center
Boston University School
   of Medicine
Boston, Massachusetts

Laurie Glader, MD
Assistant Professor of Pediatrics
Harvard Medical School
Associate in Medicine
Department of Medicine
Boston Children's Hospital
Boston, Massachusetts

Frances Page Glascoe, PhD
Professor of Pediatrics
Division of Child Development
Vanderbilt University Medical Center
Nashville, Tennessee

Laura Goldstein, PsyD
Assistant Professor
Department of Psychiatry
Boston University
Boston, Massachusetts

Richard D. Goldstein, MD
Assistant Professor
Department of Pediatrics
Harvard Medical School
Boston, Massachusetts

Linda M. Grant, MD, MPH
Associate Professor
Department of Pediatrics
Boston University School of
   Medicine
Boston, Massachusetts

Larry Gray, MD
Associate Professor
Department of Pediatrics
Feinberg School of Medicine
Lurie Children's Hospital
   of Chicago
Chicago, Illinois

Jessica Gray, MD
Instructor
Department of Medicine and Pediatrics
Harvard Medical School
Boston, Massachusetts

Ross W. Greene, PhD
Adjunct Associate Professor
Department of Psychology
Virginia Tech
Blacksburg, Virginia;
Adjunct Professor
Faculty of Science
University of Technology Sydney
Sydney, Australia

Betsy McAlister Groves, MSW, LICSW
Lecturer
Human Development & Psychology Program
Harvard Graduate School of Education
Cambridge, Massachusetts

Carly E. Guss, MD, MPH
Instructor
Department of Pediatrics
Harvard Medical School
Boston, Massachusetts

Scott E. Hadland, MD, MPH, MS
Assistant Professor
Department of Pediatrics
Boston University School of Medicine
Boston, Massachusetts

Randi Jenssen Hagerman, MD
Distinguished Professor of Pediatrics and
    Endowed Chair in Fragile X Research
Department of Pediatrics
University of California Davis Medical Center
Sacramento, California

Michael K. Hole, MD, MBA
Assistant Professor
Pediatrics & Population Health
Dell Medical School
The University of Texas at Austin
Austin, Texas

Arda Hotz, MD
Instructor
Department of General Pediatrics
Harvard Medical School
Boston, Massachusetts

Barbara J. Howard, MD
Assistant Professor
Department of Pediatrics
The Johns Hopkins School of Medicine
Baltimore, Maryland

Micaela A. Jett, MD, FAAP
Associate Physician
Developmental Pediatrics
Kaiser Permanente Santa Clara Medical
    Center
Santa Clara, California

Margot Kaplan-Sanoff, EdD
Former Co-Founder and National Executive
    Director
Senior Consultant/Trainer
Healthy Steps for Young Children
Child Development
Department of Pediatrics
Boston University School of Medicine
Boston, Massachusetts

Sabra L. Katz-Wise, PhD
Assistant Professor
Department of Pediatrics
Harvard Medical School
Boston, Massachusetts

Robert D. Keder, MD
Assistant Professor
Department of Pediatrics
University of Connecticut School of Medicine
Farmington, Connecticut

Caroline J. Kistin, MD, MSc
Assistant Professor
Department of Pediatrics
Boston Medical Center/Boston University
    School of Medicine
Boston, Massachusetts

Perri Klass, MD
Professor
Journalism and Pediatrics
New York University
New York, New York

Barbara Korsch, MD *(deceased)*
Professor of Pediatrics
University of Southern California
Keck School of Medicine;
Attending Physician
Department of General Pediatrics
Children's Hospital of Los Angeles
Los Angeles, California

Casey Krueger, PhD
Clinical Assistant Professor (Affiliated)
Developmental-Behavioral Pediatrics
Stanford University School of Medicine
Palo Alto, California

Michele L. Ledesma, MD
Fellow, Developmental-Behavioral Pediatrics
Department of Pediatrics
Yale University
New Haven, Connecticut

Melvin D. Levine, MD *(deceased)*
Director and Chief Executive Officer of
Bringing Up Minds
Rougemont, North Carolina

Yi Hui Liu, MD, MPH
Associate Professor
Department of Pediatrics
University of California San Diego
San Diego, California

Irene M. Loe, MD
Assistant Professor
Department of Pediatrics
Stanford University School of Medicine
Stanford, California

Julie Lumeng, MD
Professor
Department of Pediatrics
University of Michigan
Ann Arbor, Michigan

Tracy Magee, PhD, RN, CPNP
Associate Professor
School of Nursing
Regis College
Weston, Massachusetts

Lucy E. Marcil, MD, MPH
Assistant Professor
Department of Pediatrics
Boston University School of Medicine
Boston, Massachusetts

Jack S. Maypole, MD
Clinical Associate Professor of Pediatrics
Department of Pediatrics
Boston University
Boston, Massachusetts

Neena McConnico, PhD, LMHC
Director
Child Witness to Violence Project
Division of Developmental and Behavioral
Pediatrics
Boston Medical Center
Boston, Massachusetts

Claudio Morera, MD
Assistant Professor
Department of Pediatrics
Boston University
Boston, Massachusetts

Michael E. Msall, MD
Professor of Pediatrics
Kennedy Research Center on Intellectual and
Developmental Disabilities
University of Chicago
Chicago Illinois

Katherine Myers, DO, MPH
Assistant Professor
Department of Pediatrics
Case Western Reserve University School of
Medicine
Cleveland, Ohio

Katherine A. Nash, MD
Instructor
Department of Pediatrics
Boston University
Boston, Massachusetts

Melissa T. Nass, MD, MPH
Clinical Assistant Professor of
Pediatrics
Department of Pediatrics
Boston University School of Medicine
Boston, Massachusetts

Robert Needlman, MD
Professor
Department of Pediatrics
Case Western Reserve University School of
Medicine
Cleveland, Ohio

Caitlin Neri, MD, MPH
Assistant Professor
Department of Pediatrics
Boston University School of Medicine
Boston, Massachusetts

Sarah S. Nyp, MD, FAAP
Associate Professor
Department of Pediatrics
University of Missouri
Kansas City School of Medicine
Kansas City, Missouri

Judith A. Owens, MD, MPH
Professor
Department of Neurology
Harvard Medical School
Boston, Massachusetts

Julie Pajek, PhD
Assistant Professor
Department of Psychiatry
Case Western Reserve University
Cleveland, Ohio

Demetra D. Pappas, MD, MPH
Instructor in Pediatrics
Division of Developmental Medicine
Department of Medicine
Boston Children's Hospital
Harvard Medical School
Boston, Massachusetts

Steven Parker, MD *(deceased)*
Associate Professor of Pediatrics
Division of Developmental and Behavioral
Pediatrics
Boston University School of Medicine
Boston Medical Center
Boston, Massachusetts

**Maureen A. Patterson-Fede, MSW,
LICSW**
Mental Health Clinician
Developmental and Behavioral Pediatrics
Boston Medical Center
Boston, Massachusetts

Elizabeth Peacock-Chambers, MD, MS
Assistant Professor
Department of Pediatrics
University of Massachusetts Medical
School-Baystate
Springfield, Massachusetts

Bahar Bingoler Pekcici, MD
Assistant Professor
Department of Pediatrics
Division of Developmental-Behavioral
Pediatrics
Ankara University School of Medicine
Ankara, Turkey

Ellen C. Perrin, MD, MA
Professor
Department of Pediatrics
Tufts University School of Medicine
Boston, Massachusetts

Megan H. Pesch, MD, MS
Clinical Lecturer
Department of Pediatrics
University of Michigan
Ann Arbor, Michigan

Jaime Wildman Peterson, MD
Academic General Pediatrics Fellow/Clinical
  Instructor
Department of Pediatrics
Stanford University
Palo Alto, California

Genevieve Preer, MD
Assistant Professor
Department of Pediatrics
Boston University
Boston, Massachusetts

Lisa Prock, MD, MPH
Director, Developmental Medicine Center
Associate Chief, Division of Developmental
  Medicine
Department of Pediatrics
Harvard Medical School
Boston, Massachusetts

Jenny S. Radesky, MD
Assistant Professor
Department of Pediatrics
University of Michigan Medical School
Ann Arbor, Michigan

Mandeep Rana, MD
Assistant Professor
Department of Pediatrics
Division of Pediatric Neurology and Sleep
  Medicine
Boston University School of Medicine
Boston, Massachusetts

Leonard A. Rappaport, MD, MS
Chief Emeritus
Division of Developmental Medicine
Boston Children's Hospital
Mary Deming Scott Professor of Pediatrics
Harvard Medical School
Boston, Massachusetts

Nancy Roizen, MD
Professor
Department of Pediatrics
Case Western Reserve University
Cleveland, Ohio

Linda D. Sagor, MD, MPH
Professor
Department of Pediatrics
University of Massachusetts Medical
  School
Worcester, Massachusetts

Ana Carolina Sanchez, MD
Instructor of Medicine
Department of Pediatrics
Boston University School of Medicine
Boston, Massachusetts

Adrian D. Sandler, MD
Adjunct Professor
Department of Pediatrics
UNC Chapel Hill School of Medicine
Chapel Hill, North Carolina

Jodi Santosuosso, NP-C, APRN, BC
Clinical Instructor
Department of Pediatrics
Division of Developmental and Behavioral
  Pediatrics
Boston University School of Medicine
Boston, Massachusetts

Davida M. Schiff, MD, MSc
Instructor in Pediatrics
Department of General Academic Pediatrics
Harvard Medical School and Massachusetts
  General Hospital
Boston, Massachusetts

Kelly Schifsky, DO
Developmental-Behavioral Pediatric Fellow
General Pediatrics
Children's Hospital Los Angeles
Los Angeles, California

David J. Schonfeld, MD
Director, National Center for School Crisis
  and Bereavement
Professor of the Practice
Suzanne Dworak-Peck School of Social Work
  and Pediatrics
University of Southern California
Los Angeles, California

Alison Schonwald, MD
Assistant Professor
Department of Pediatrics
Harvard Medical School
Boston, Massachusetts

Jayna B. Schumacher, MD
Assistant Professor of Clinical Pediatrics
Department of Pediatrics
University of Cincinnati College of Medicine
Cincinnati, Ohio

Kimberly A. Schwartz, MD MPH
Assistant Professor
Department of Pediatrics
Boston University School of Medicine
Boston, Massachusetts

Yasmin Suzanne N. Senturias, MD, FAAP
Professor of Pediatrics
Atrium Health
Adjunct Professor of Pediatrics, UNC
  Chapel Hill
Charlotte, North Carolina

Neelkamal S. Soares, MD
Professor
Pediatric & Adolescent Medicine
Western Michigan University Homer Stryker
    M.D. School of Medicine
Kalamazoo, Michigan

Terry Stancin, PhD, ABPP
Professor
Department of Psychiatry, Pediatrics, &
    Psychological Sciences
Case Western Reserve University
Cleveland, Ohio

Martin T. Stein, MD
Professor of Pediatrics Emeritus
Department of Pediatrics
University of California San Diego
San Diego, California

Naomi Steiner, MD
Associate Professor
Director of Training
Developmental Behavioral Pediatrics
Department of Pediatrics
Boston University
Boston, Massachusetts

Kristine E. Strand, EdD, CCC-SLP
Senior Speech-Language Pathologist
Learning Disabilities Program – Neurology
    Department
Boston Children's Hospital
Boston, Massachusetts

Moira Szilagyi, MD, PhD
Professor
Department of Pediatrics
University of California Los Angeles
Los Angeles, California

Michael H. Tang, MD
Clinical Director of Behavioral Health
    Integration
The Dimock Center
Lecturer, Part-Time, Child Psychiatry
Harvard Medical School
Boston, Massachusetts

Katharine Thomson, PhD
Instructor
Department of Psychiatry
Harvard Medical School
Boston, Massachusetts

Lee A. Trope, MD, MS
Chief Resident
Department of Pediatrics
Stanford University
Palo Alto, California

Stanley Turecki, MD
Attending Psychiatrist
Lenox Hill Hospital;
Associate Attending Psychiatrist
Beth Israel Medical Center
New York City, New York

Amy Turner, MD
Clinical Fellow
Department of Gastroenterology,
    Hepatology, & Nutrition
Harvard Medical School
Boston, Massachusetts

Douglas L. Vanderbilt, MD, MS
Associate Professor of Clinical
    Pediatrics
Department of Pediatrics
Keck School of Medicine University of
    Southern California
Los Angeles, California

Elisha M. Wachman, MD
Assistant Professor
Department of Pediatrics
Boston University School of
    Medicine
Boston, Massachusetts

Laura Weissman, MD
Assistant Professor
Department of Pediatrics
Harvard Medical School
Boston, Massachusetts

Carol C. Weitzman, MD
Professor
Department of Pediatrics
Yale School of Medicine
New Haven, Connecticut

Jodi K. Wenger, MD
Assistant Professor
Department of Developmental and Behavioral
    Pediatrics
Boston University School of Medicine
Boston, Massachusetts

Melora Wiley, MD
Fellow
Developmental Behavioral Pediatrics
Yale University
New Haven, Connecticut

Karen E. Wills, PhD, LP
Pediatric Neuropsychologist
Department of Psychological Services
Children's Minnesota
Minneapolis, Minnesota

Laurel M. Wills, MD
Consultant in Developmental-Behavioral
    Pediatrics
State of Minnesota Mental Health Services
    for Deaf, DeafBlind and Hard of Hearing
    Children & Youth
Vona Center for Mental Health
Department of Pediatrics, University of
    Minnesota
Minneapolis, Minnesota

Maryanne Wolf, EdD
John DiBiaggio Professor of Citizenship and
  Public Service
Director of Center for Reading and Language
  Research.
Tufts University
Medford, Massachusetts;
Visiting Professor
University of California at Los
  Angeles
Los Angeles, California

Janet Wozniak, MD
Associate Professor
Department of Psychiatry
Harvard Medical School
Massachusetts General
  Hospital
Boston, Massachusetts

Julie N. Youssef, DO
Clinical Assistant Professor
Department of Pediatrics
Stanford University
Stanford, California

Barry Zuckerman, MD
Professor and Chair Emeritus of Pediatrics
Boston University School of Medicine
Professor of Public Health
Boston University School of Public Health
Former Chair of Pediatrics
Boston Medical Center
Boston, Massachusetts

Pamela M. Zuckerman, MD
Clinical Assistant Professor
Boston University School of Medicine
Private Practice
Brookline, Massachusetts

Preface

Section I—Reimagining Pediatrics.

We are delighted to have the opportunity with this fourth edition to provide an update on information that has changed over the past thirty years. While children's development remains the same, social transitions have led to changes in parent–child interactions and created new twists on old challenges such as media exposure, difficult behavior, and risk-taking behaviors. Clinicians are being asked to cover more challenges to families in less time. The "new morbidity," which was recognized in the last century, has expanded, and clinicians are now supporting families with behavioral challenges such as autism spectrum disorder and anxiety that are increasing in prevalence. In addition, clinicians continue to be a stabilizing force for families dealing with external stress and the intergenerational implications of parental mental health and adverse childhood experiences, especially trauma.

Because of the changes and challenges mentioned earlier, pediatric care has changed and adapted as well, and we hope to provide insight and direction to that practice in section I, which we consider "Reimagining Pediatrics." In this section, we address child health supervision—honoring the time-tested information such as guidelines on talking to children and parents, promoting early literacy, and teachable moments. In addition, we have added more chapters addressing two generational approaches, because in our experience, the best way to help children is to *help* their parents and the best way to *reach* parents is through their children. Such chapters include parental depression, preventing unplanned pregnancy for parents of our patients, identifying and addressing social determinants of health, and parental self-understanding. We have also added new ideas to improve child health supervision for the 21st century specifically understanding and incorporating growth mindset, implicit bias, financial stress, cultural differences in parenting, and preventing unplanned pregnancy. We hope this new information will enable clinicians to provide the effective and time-efficient care we all strive to deliver to children and families.

Section II—Specific Topics.

In section II of the book, we provide a comprehensive overview of common topics encountered as part of pediatric primary care involving developmental and behavioral pediatrics. These chapters are targeted to the busy clinician and provide an overview for identification, diagnosis, and in some cases treatment or referral.

We hope this book provides a useful resource in caring for the children and youth of the 21st century!

MA
BZ

xiii

Acknowledgments

—*from Barry*
I thank the Center for Advanced Study of Behavioral Sciences at Stanford University for awarding for their support as Fellow for 2016–17, which provided time to think, learn, and write in a beautiful setting with stimulating wonderful colleagues.

—*from Barry and Marilyn*
We also want to thank the Irving Harris Foundation for their support for over 20 years to provide training in Infant Mental Health to pediatric clinicians, nurses, and all front-line clinicians and staff helping children and families.

We would like to acknowledge the prior edition authors for their valuable contribution to the chapters

Chapter 5	Developmental Screening: Kevin P. Marks
Chapter 9	Helping Families Deal with Bad News: Mara Trozzi
Chapter 19	Pain: Neil L. Schechter, William T. Zempsky
Chapter 20	Self-Regulation: Karen Olness
Chapter 21	Using Developmental Themes to Understand Behavior: Gregory F. Hayden
Chapter 26	Anxiety Disorders: Marianne San Antonio, Nili E. Major
Chapter 27	Attention-Deficit/Hyperactivity Disorder: L. Kari Hironaka
Chapter 28	Autism Spectrum Disorders: Celine Saulnier, Fred R. Volkmar
Chapter 34	Cerebral Palsy: Frederick B. Palmer, Alexander H. Hoon
Chapter 35	Child Maltreatment: Physical Abuse and Sexual Abuse: Deborah Madansky, Christine E. Barron, Carole Jenny,
Chapter 36	Chronic Conditions: Ellen C. Perrin
Chapter 40	Depression: Brian Kurtz, Michael Jellinek
Chapter 42	Down Syndrome: Siegfried M. Pueschel
Chapter 43	Eating Disorders in Adolescents: Angela S. Guarda, Alain Joffe
Chapter 52	Lesbian, Gay, Bisexual, Transgender, and Queer Youth: Ellen C. Perrin, Nicola J. Smith
Chapter 53	Grief, Resiliency, and Coping in Children and Families Facing Stressful Circumstances: Ben Siegel, Maria Trozzi
Chapter 57	Intellectual Disability: Evaluation and Management: Theodore A. Kastner, Kevin K. Walsh
Chapter 58	Language Delays: James Coplan
Chapter 59	Learning Disability: Paul H. Dworkin
Chapter 61	Masturbation: John Leventhal
Chapter 62	Digital media: Victor C. Strasburger
Chapter 69	Posttraumatic Stress, Child Victimization, and Exposure to Trauma: Glenn Saxe
Chapter 70	Prematurity: James A Blackman, Robert J. Boyle
Chapter 73	Sensory Processing Difficulties: Marie E. Anzalone
Chapter 76	Sleep Problems: Rebecca McCauley, Barry Guitar
Chapter 78	Substance Use in Adolescence: Anna Maria S. Ocampo, John R. Knight
Chapter 79	Suicide: Heather Walter, Phillip Hernandez, Joanna Cole
Chapter 84	Toilet Training: Laura Sices

Contents

II • Specific Topics

CHAPTER 1

Talking with Parents

Barbara Korsch (deceased)

I. **DESCRIPTION.** It has been documented consistently that the clinician–patient relationship and communication are the strongest predictors of the outcome of a medical visit. The therapeutic alliance is achieved in large measure during the interview. Rapport building, engaging the patient, eliciting psychosocial and personal aspects of the patient's experiences, supporting the parents in their roles as parents, and including the child, grandparent, and significant others are essential to establish a therapeutic relationship.

II. **OPTIMAL COMMUNICATION WITH PARENTS.** Although there are no techniques that work for all patients or all clinicians, there are some basics that virtually always strengthen the therapeutic alliance (Table 1-1), which has become even more important in the era of the electronic health record (EHR) and assistive technology in the examination room.

A. **Listening.** Letting the parent know that you are listening is basic. Body language—sitting down, looking at the parent, leaning forward, and showing appropriate concern—is effective in conveying a listening attitude and does not require extra time in the interview.

Responding to nonverbal expressions of parent affect is also essential. For example, if the mother's face falls when the clinician suggests the use of a pacifier for a colicky baby, the responsive clinician needs to inquire, *"You do not seem to like that idea. Is there any special reason why you do not want your baby to use the pacifier?"* He or she may find out that the mother had difficulty in weaning her firstborn from the pacifier or that she finds pacifiers disgusting. When screening, behavioral checklists have been used (see Chapter 6); also, the parental responses can provide the topics for discussion.

B. **Facilitating the dialogue.** The parent's story should be facilitated by appropriate empathetic responses, such as *"Tell me more about that," "I can see that it did not work out so well for you,"* or *"That must be hard for you."* The clinician should avoid interruptions, subject changes, and judgmental comments and not prematurely pursue other diagnostic hypotheses, which can derail the parent's narrative. Attentive listening during the opening of an interview promotes communication and rarely takes more than a couple of minutes. Yet it has also been shown that, on average, clinicians interrupt the patients within a few seconds or minutes. The reason is conflicting agendas: patients want to tell their story, and clinicians want to pursue their medical task (diagnosis, prescription, or therapeutic recommendation). There are other strategies to facilitate a successful pediatric visit.

C. **Elicit the parent's concerns early in the interview.** *"What worried you especially when you brought John to see us today? Why did that worry you?"*

D. **Elicit the parent's expectations for the visit and acknowledge them.** *"What had you hoped we might be able to do for your child today? What would you like to have us explain to you today?"* These inquiries may reveal unrealistic expectations for specific therapies or magical cures. At other times, such questions make the clinician's job simple if what the family desires is reassurance. Once the parent's expectations have been acknowledged, the clinician, the parents, and the child can set an agenda for the visit, which synthesizes the parent's concerns and biomedical issues. It is only after this opening—after listening attentively to the parent—that the clinician can afford to pursue his or her line of questions and fact-finding. The first phase of the interaction has taken care of urgent concerns, relaxed the parent, and made him or her realize that the clinician is interested. The parent will now be a better historian and partner in the task-oriented portion of the interview. Experience shows that the aforementioned suggestions will make the interview more effective and so lead to earlier closure, which is becoming more and more important these days, with the economic pressures and changes in health care delivery systems.

Table 1-1 • HOW TO ENHANCE THE THERAPEUTIC ALLIANCE

Process Steps	Sample Comments
Greet Introduce self Set agenda jointly	"What concerns do you want to talk about today? Do you have any specific questions?"
Listen Allow pauses Maintain eye contact	Allow there to be silence for a few seconds to give parent time to answer
Facilitate Do not judge Do not interrupt	"Tell me more about that."
Elicit and acknowledge the parent's concern	"You thought the high fever might bring on a seizure?"
Elicit and acknowledge the parent's expectations	"What are you hoping we will do for him/her today?"
Involve the child	"What has this been like for you?"
	"Do you understand why you are here?"
Be family centered	"Do you agree with that proposed plan?"
Guide (not dominate) discourse	"Is that what you expected?"
Elicit the parent's solutions	"What have you tried so far?" "What would you like to try at this time?"
Make treatment decisions jointly	"Do you think you will be able to give him/her the medicine four times a day?"
Make closure and agenda setting explicit	"I have written in our after visit summary the points we will be do after this visit until we see each other again"

E. **Guide but do not dominate the discourse.** General questions allow parents to broach subjects of interest to them. For health supervision visits, clinicians can use simple questions: *"How are things going?" "What are some new things the baby is doing?" "How do things work out at bedtime?" "What is the hardest part of taking care of the baby now?" "What is most enjoyable about taking care of the baby?" "Is the baby's father (or mother) able to give you any help?"* Open-ended, nonjudgmental questions are essential for this phase of the interview. In this context, we are often asked "What do I do when the patient takes up a lot of time in reciting irrelevant information that he or she has obtained from the Internet?" A contemptuous remark such as "Where did you go to medical school" is sure to rupture the therapeutic alliance. Courteous respectful reminders that the time for the visit is limited and he or she needs to focus on the child's problems could be more effective.

F. **Use common courtesy.** All the amenities of human interaction in nonmedical contexts must also be observed. Even clinicians who usually have good manners will, in the task-oriented medical encounter, omit greetings, introductions, and courtesies (such as knocking on the door before entering the examination room or explaining the reasons for keeping someone waiting). These courtesies should include a few appropriate remarks acknowledging the parent as a person, such as *"You sure have your hands full today,"* to the parent who comes with several children and all the attending paraphernalia, or *"I bet you are impatient with us for having kept you waiting so long. I had to deal with another patient emergency."* This is also critically important if one is using an electronic medical record. Acknowledge from the beginning of the visit that at times you will need to type information in the record to ensure patient safety and accuracy.

III. **TALKING WITH THE CHILD.** Early in the visit, an appropriate approach must be made to the child; this is especially important when the social distance between practitioner and family is great or when communication is difficult because of the parent's anxiety, suspicion, or hostility. The awareness of a mutual interest in helping the child creates a bond between the parent and the clinician. Throughout the interview, in spite of the demands of the EHR, the practitioner must try to maintain eye contact frequently with the child and the parent and watch for nonverbal signs of distress or disagreement or of reassurance and relief.

IV. DEALING WITH ACUTE ILLNESSES. During an acute illness, the interview must be focused. As the parent tells the story of the illness, the practitioner can facilitate responsively: *"So the fever has been high for almost 3 days now ... What are some of the other things you have noticed? ... How did you handle that? ... How did that work out? ... What about feeding? ... Sleep? ... Any other changes?"*

- If the parents have used any complementary and alternative therapies, it is essential not to make judgmental statements. If the treatment was harmless and the parent feels it was effective (even when the practitioner would not have chosen it), it is best to support the parent's approach.
- If a parent has attempted an intervention that is potentially harmful (e.g., giving aspirin for a viral infection), the clinician should not use this moment to give alarming warnings (e.g., about Reye syndrome). Yet the family needs to be informed. Our approach is *"I am glad she is feeling better, but I need to give you some new information. Aspirin has been around a long time, and it has provided relief for many patients. However, we have learned that aspirin can have side effects that involve severe liver damage and can be very serious, although rare. Your baby is obviously fine, but I feel strongly that, from now on, you should avoid aspirin and use acetaminophen instead."*
- After the episode is over and the parent is less likely to be overwhelmed by guilt and anxieties, more complete and forceful information can be given. Alternatives and additional treatments can be suggested without undermining the parent's self-confidence and self-esteem.
- To avoid embarrassment and fractures of the clinician–parent alliance, at all times the clinician should ask, *"How have you handled that? What have you been doing or giving him/her so far?,"* before launching into medical advice. Whenever possible, the parent's own solution should be supported. When developing other approaches, it is best to involve the parent. For example, *"Has anyone suggested to you that it is time to start solid foods? Have you yourself contemplated making a change? How ready are you to make the necessary changes?"* Before giving what seems to be appropriate advice, the clinician must assess the families' readiness to change, their conviction that change is necessary, and their confidence that they can, indeed, change. A therapeutic plan has to be a joint venture; rarely should it be imposed without parental input.

V. REDIRECTING THE INTERVIEW. The clinician needs to keep control of the interview, even while being supportive and accepting. When the discussion gets off track, the clinician needs to redirect the discourse—for instance, *"We must sit down and discuss that on another occasion after he/she is over this illness,"* or *"There is some other information I need right now so we can decide about the treatment for this illness."* If the parent makes an unreasonable request, such as *"You will give him/her antibiotics today, won't you?,"* the clinician can back off and state, *"I do not know whether that will be necessary today. We will talk about that after I have examined your son/daughter."*

VI. COUNSELING AND REASSURANCE. Advising and counseling the patient and family can be a continuing process. Some concerns may be addressed at the first mention. For example, if the mother says at 6 months or beyond, *"He/she still wakes up once in the night and calls for me,"* the clinician may reassure promptly that this is not unusual at his/her age: *"He/she misses you in the dark when alone in his/her bedroom. Just comfort him/her, but do not feed him/her again because he/she will get used to being fed to go back to sleep. At this age he/she no longer needs the nutrition at night."* Other concerns may best be allayed during the physical examination: *"The arches of the foot normally do not develop before the child has been weight bearing for a while."* Other topics require a discussion at the end of the visit or even at another scheduled conference time: *"I can see you are having real difficulty in setting limits for his/her behavior at this time"* (see Chapter 3 on teachable moments). *"We need to take some time to see what we can work out to help him/her accept your discipline and to make your life a little easier."*

VII. CLOSURE
  A. Summarize the relevant points the parent has raised and information he or she has given toward the end of the encounter.
  B. Offer other educational materials, such as handouts, and individualize them by underlining certain specific issues or relating them to the parent's concerns.
  C. Invite questions from caregivers, family, and the child. Even when there is no time for full responses, they can be included in jointly setting the agenda for subsequent visits and follow-up health care.

VIII. WORKING WITH AN INTERPRETER. In many communities today, the clinician is faced with cultural and language barriers that complicate the interview. There are no easy solutions for this problem. For language problems, a skilled professional interpreter (preferably not a family member) is the only desirable approach. In the presence of an interpreter, it is essential that the clinician maintain eye contact with the patient, continue to address the patient and family directly, and not discuss problems with the interpreter instead of the patient or caretaker (avoid saying *"tell her that"* or *"ask him what"*). Cultural sensitivities also pose unique challenges to effective health care and require the clinician to employ all his or her skills for assessing not only the individual patient's perceptions, value systems, and health beliefs, but also those that are prevalent in his or her culture. This holds especially true when offering advice and counsel. Awareness of unconscious or implicit bias (see Chapter 13) is especially important for effective communication and to prevent undermining potentially helpful advice.

Bibliography

ACOG Policy Statement on Communication. https://www.acog.org/Clinical-Guidance-and-Publications/Committee-Opinions/Committee-on-Health-Care-for-Underserved-Women/Effective-Patient-Physician-Communication. Accessed January 12, 2018.

Kalet A, Gany F, Senter L. Working with interpreters: an interactive Web-based learning module. *Acad Med.* 2002;77(9):927.

Korsch B, Harding C. *The Intelligent Patient's Guide to the Doctor-Patient Relationship.* New York: Oxford University Press; 1997.

Montague E, Asan O. Physician interactions with electronic health records in primary care. *Health Syst (Basingstoke).* 2012;1(2):96-103.

CHAPTER 2

Talking with Children

Yi Hui Liu | Martin T. Stein

I. THE IMPORTANCE

A. Pediatric clinicians acknowledge the significance of nurturing an independent and trusting relationship with the child.

As a child's primary care provider, the pediatric clinician has the unique opportunity to develop such a bond over time. Even short encounters with children can benefit from the skills required to sustain a longitudinal relationship.

B. The child must be recognized and valued as an equal partner and active participant in his or her care.

This enhances the child's self-esteem as he or she learns about and develops responsibility for his or her own health. The child must view his or her pediatric clinician as a source of not only treatment but also guidance and support. He or she should recognize the pediatric clinician as *his* or *her* clinician, not his or her parent's. These experiences mold the child's view of himself or herself and may contribute to his or her response to health and illness in adulthood.

C. The establishment of a therapeutic alliance with the child allows the pediatric clinician to ascertain important information about the child and his or her environment such as the child's strengths, stressors, developmental status, and place in the family and community. Children may also reveal information that the parent is unaware of or may have omitted. At the same time, the pediatric clinician is able to assess language, speech, and auditory functioning.

D. The pediatric clinician models for parents the art of listening to and respecting the views of their child from as early as infancy.

The pediatric clinician's response to the child's feelings or misbehavior may illustrate to the parent appropriate management techniques (e.g., reflection, limit setting).

II. CREATING THE ENVIRONMENT: PROMOTING EFFECTIVE COMMUNICATION

A. The reception area. A child-friendly environment conveys to the child that this place is for children. If possible, provide separate areas for children of different ages with age-appropriate décor and materials. Toys, a fish tank, books, a drawing board, room to crawl and walk, child-sized furniture, children's drawings, and children's pictures all impart a welcoming environment. Paper and crayons allow the child to draw pictures that may be used to facilitate conversation or to illustrate the child's perception of himself or herself, his or her family, or his or her situation. Consider not having a television in the waiting room as this does not support the message that families should be selective in media use and does not encourage parents to interact with their children. A literacy-rich waiting room is a more positive slant on how children and adults can interact around a book.

B. The examination/interview room. Toys, books, drawing materials, child-sized furniture, and child-friendly décor are useful in making the child feel at ease. A quiet, appealing, and private environment encourages the child to interact with the pediatric clinician. There should be no barriers (such as a large desk) between the pediatric clinician and the child, and the pediatric clinician should place himself or herself at the child's eye level.

C. The greeting. When appropriate, speak to the child first. This promotes the message that the child is the patient. Approach the child in a calm and friendly manner and ask him or her what he or she would like to be called. Commenting on a toy or a book that he or she has brought or the clothes he or she is wearing can be a pleasant icebreaker. If you use a computer-based electronic medical record, acknowledge to the child that sometimes you will need to type during the visit.

III. COMMUNICATION TOOLS

A. Open-ended questions. Start with open-ended questions to allow the child to express his or her thoughts and concerns for the visit. Further questions may elicit the child's personal and culturally influenced perception of his or her situation, helping his or her pediatric clinician understand his or her frame of reference. Closed-ended questions may follow open-ended questions to generate additional specific information.

Members of some cultures will not respond to or be comfortable with an open-ended question if they are expecting the physician to act in a more directive manner.

B. Pauses and silence. Allowing the child time to organize his or her thoughts or regain composure and then to express his or her feelings without pressure shows him or her respect and concern.

C. Reflection (repetition). If the child makes a puzzling or significant comment, repeat the key words or phrases back in a neutral or questioning tone to encourage him or her to clarify or elaborate further.

D. Empathy. Acknowledge and respond to the child's feelings to convey warmth and sympathy. Listen for the message behind his or her words.

E. Active listening. Provide undivided attention and facilitate the conversation through open-ended questions, silences, and repetition to communicate to the child respect and concern. Both body language (leaning forward, eye contact) and verbal expressions (e.g., *"tell me more"*) can convey support and interest, allowing the child to feel comfortable in expressing his or her feelings and thoughts and thus to participate in the visit more fully.

F. Tracking. Allow the child to set the interview's style, pace, and language.

G. Summarizing. After explaining the assessment and plan to the child, review the major points. Avoid using medical jargon. Asking the child to summarize what has been said will ensure that the information has been understood. It is helpful to make the recommendations practical and concrete.

IV. COMMUNICATION TECHNIQUES FOR DIFFERENT AGE GROUPS

A. In general
1. Engage the child early in the visit with talk, play, or other activities to lessen anxiety. Be mindful of the child's temperament and approach the child accordingly.
2. Use age-appropriate words and eye contact. Children younger than 2 years may find eye contact to be threatening and may be comforted by watching their parents respond to the pediatric clinician in a friendly manner. In addition, questions about "when" and "why" may not be useful in young children who do not yet understand time and causality.
3. Start with casual questions about familiar and comfortable subjects in an encouraging manner before moving on to more difficult ones. Talk about a child's interests (sports, music), family, friends, or school to develop rapport with him or her. Use special interests as an opener for subsequent visits.
4. Approach difficult questions in a nonjudgmental and matter-of-fact manner. Indirect statements and questions can be effective in opening discussions about potentially sensitive areas (bullying, fears, school failure, drug use, sex, suicide risk, family conflicts). Starting the discussion about children in general, followed by acquaintances, and then the child is less threatening. *"Some kids tell me that they have a tough time with other kids at school. Do you know anyone with this problem? What has been your experience?"*
5. Humor can dispel anxieties and make the visit enjoyable at all age levels.
6. The **TEACHER** method can enhance communication with children and their parents (Table 2-1).

B. Communicating with children younger than 6 months
1. Developmental stage: Symbiotic. The infant and the primary caregiver have a strong attachment. The child is not significantly fearful of strangers.
2. At this age, the pediatric clinician can model for the parent appropriate ways of speaking to and encouraging language development in babies.

C. Communicating with children 6 months to 3 years of age
1. Developmental stage: Separation–individuation. The child often has stranger awareness and may cling to parents as he or she gradually loosens early attachment and develops a sense of his or her own autonomy.
2. The child should be allowed to stay close to the parent (sitting on the parent's lap) for reassurance.
3. Avoid direct, prolonged eye contact with the child younger than 2 years as this may be perceived as threatening.
4. Approach the child gently and gradually. Watch his or her body language to judge his or her acceptance. Wait until he or she is willing to leave his or her parent's lap.
5. Use play (peekaboo, keys, flashlight, or toy) to capture the child's attention and ease his or her anxiety.
6. Prepare the child for physical contact. Imitation with the parent or a doll/stuffed animal will ease the child's anxiety during the physical examination and any procedures.

Table 2-1 • TEACHER: A METHOD FOR ENHANCING COMMUNICATION WITH PEDIATRIC PATIENTS AND THEIR PARENTS

T	Trust	Build trust and rapport with the child by asking nonthreatening questions not related to illness
E	Elicit	Elicit information from parent(s) and child regarding parental fears and concerns and the child's understanding of the reason for the visit
A	Agenda	Set an agenda early in the visit to help ensure that the parents' concerns are addressed
C	Control	Help the child feel control over the visit (e.g., knowing what will and will not happen) to help decrease fear and increase cooperation
H	Health plan	Establish a health plan with the child and the parent to meet the child's needs and limitations
E	Explain	Explain the health plan to the child in a way he or she can understand
R	Rehearse	Have the child rehearse the health plan as a way of assessing understanding; reinforce the child's jobs related to health care; and explore any potential problems in the plan with the child and the parent

D. Communicating with children 3–6 years of age
   1. Developmental stage: Preschool age—age of initiative. The child has increasing language skills and engages in fantasy play. The child's understanding of illness is mediated by magical thinking.
   2. Use simple language. Expressive and receptive language skills starting at 3 years of age allow the pediatric clinician to begin use of the communication techniques described earlier to elicit the child's concerns and thoughts. Remember, a child's receptive language is more advanced than his or her expressive language.
   3. Encourage the child to ask questions.
   4. Engage the child by explaining procedures and allowing him or her to participate in the examination. Offer choices when possible and talk to him or her about his or her health care.
   5. As these children enter school age, spending some time alone with the pediatric clinician can further the development of an independent relationship.

E. Communicating with children 6–12 years of age
   1. Developmental stage: School age—age of industry. The child has improved cognitive skills and develops the ability to understand cause and effect. Concrete thinking characterizes younger school-aged children, whereas the ability to generalize and begin to understand causes of illness occurs in older preadolescents.
   2. School-aged children enjoy talking about family, friends, school, and other facets of their lives. Their interests and strengths are easily determined.
   3. Explanation of procedures, assessments, and plans becomes important and helpful in eliciting the preadolescent's cooperation.
   4. Spend some time alone with the school-aged child to determine any further concerns and to continue to foster a relationship with the child.

F. Communicating with adolescents
   1. Developmental stage: Age of identity. The adolescent is focused on changing body features and is developing abstract reasoning. He or she is able to understand the general principles of illness and recovery.
   2. Interview the adolescent separate from the parent to respect growing independence, to recognize his or her individuality, and to cultivate the therapeutic alliance.
   3. Elicit and address the adolescent's concerns.
   4. Emphasize and clarify confidentiality issues as adolescents may withhold information that they believe will be relayed to their parents. Obtain the adolescent's permission to share information or discuss certain issues with others.
   5. Do not pressure the adolescent to talk. Be patient and respect the adolescent's privacy. It is better to revisit difficult topics on a later date after trust has been gained.
   6. Address difficult topics (drugs, sex, depression, anxiety, eating disorders) in a nonjudgmental manner after rapport has been developed. Indirect questions and statements as well as asking first about the experience of the adolescent's friends are helpful.

7. Talking about "stress" may be easier than asking directly about depression and anxiety. This is less threatening because "stress" is perceived as a normal part of life.
8. Always be truthful.
9. Acknowledge that the adolescent is responsible for personal health care and advocate for the adolescent with parents.

V. CLINICAL PEARLS AND PITFALLS
A. Cultural sensitivity
1. Respecting a child and family's cultural values, beliefs, and attitudes is essential in facilitating communication and cooperation. Ask about cultural interpretations of medical and social issues. *"What do you call this problem? What do you think caused it? How do you treat it? What do you expect the treatment to do?"*
2. Knowledge about cultures is useful in avoiding unintentional distress. For example, Southeast Asians will show respect to a clinician by avoiding direct eye contact. Being overly complimentary about a child may elicit fears in the Hmong who feel this may bring unwanted attention from malevolent spirits.
B. Nonverbal communication/information. Body language (posture, facial expressions) and quality and tone of speech are important clues to the psychological state of a child. With clinical practice, nonverbal clues may provide crucial information about the veracity or full disclosure of information by a child/adolescent and receptivity to the clinician's assessment and advice. Motor, social, and adaptive skills as well as temperament can be assessed through observation of the child's activity during the encounter.
C. The parent–child interaction. Assess parent–child interactions that may provide insights into attachment, parenting style, parenting skills, and family dynamics. Model appropriate use of language, soothing behaviors, and discipline techniques when a teachable moment presents.
D. Procedures. Developmentally appropriate explanations of procedures (e.g., immunizations, venipuncture, operations) are critical, and rehearsal of the sequence of events helps to ease a child's anxieties. The parent's presence during a procedure usually lessens the stress to the child; separation should generally be avoided. Be truthful if a procedure will cause any pain. Offer choices to the child as possible (which arm to draw blood from, what color cast he or she would like).
E. Illness and hospitalization
1. Anticipatory guidance about diagnostic/therapeutic procedures and an elective hospitalization help both the child and the parent. A preschool child's magical thinking, a school-aged child's concrete thinking, and an older school-aged child's emerging ability to understand causality moderate their response to illness and the clinician's language and content of information.
2. Hospitalization is associated with a sudden environmental change, loss of independence, and separation from primary caretakers. Provide the child with a description of the hospital environment and the procedures encountered. Keep some familiar toys, books, or attachment objects with the child if separation is unavoidable. Engage the assistance of a child life specialist to provide developmentally appropriate support if one is available.
F. Common pitfalls
1. **Communication only with parents.** When the pediatric clinician communicates primarily with the parents, an opportunity to uncover important information and to nurture an independent relationship with the child may be missed. As a preventive measure, start an encounter by greeting the child; the implied message is that the child is the patient.
2. **Simultaneous examination and interview.** This technique does not allow the physician to establish eye contact, communicate effectively, or promote a trusting relationship with the child.
3. **Distractions.** With the increasing use of electronic medical records, the pediatric clinician is cautioned to be aware of how much eye contact is made with the screen rather than with the family. Pagers and cell phones should be set on vibration, and a room-in-use sign can prevent unnecessary interruptions.

Bibliography
Brazelton TB. Your child's doctor. In: Brazelton TB, ed. *Touchpoints: Your Child's Emotional and Behavioral Development*. Reading, MA: Perseus Publishing; 1992:451-461.

WEB SITE
www.kidshealth.org.

FOR PROFESSIONALS

Beresin EV. The doctor–patient relationship in pediatrics. In: Kaye DL, Montgomery ME, Munson SW, eds. *Child and Adolescent Mental Health*. Philadelphia: Lippincott Williams & Wilkins; 2002.

Hagan JF, Shaw JS, Duncan PM, eds. *Bright Futures: Guidelines for Health Supervision of Infants, Children, and Adolescents*. Elk Grove Village, IL: American Academy of Pediatrics; 2017.

Stein MT. Developmentally based office: setting the stage for enhanced practice. In: Dixon SD, Stein MT, eds. *Encounters with Children: Pediatric Behavior and Development*. Philadelphia: Mosby; 2006:73-97.

Stein MT. Encounters with illness: coping and growing. In: Dixon SD, Stein MT, eds. *Encounters with Children: Pediatric Behavior and Development*. Philadelphia: Mosby; 2006:649-673.

Taylor L, Willies-Jacobo L. The culturally competent pediatrician: respecting ethnicity in your practice. *Contemp Pediatr*. 2003;20:83.

Wender EH. Interviewing: a critical skill. In: Carey WB, Crocker AC, Coleman WL, Elias ER, Feldman HM, eds. *Developmental-Behavioral Pediatrics*. Philadelphia: Saunders; 2009:747-755.

CHAPTER **3**

Teachable Moments in Primary Care

Barry Zuckerman | Steven Parker (deceased) | Margot Kaplan-Sanoff

I. DESCRIPTION. Teachable moments (TMs) represent a strategy to help pediatric clinicians engage and educate parents within the time constraints of a typical office visit. By using the basic assessments of the pediatric visit—history taking, physical examinations, and developmental surveillance—as potent TMs, one can exploit the opportunities he or she presents for intervention. The strategy of TMs is to use the behavior of the child and the clinician–parent interactions as compelling, shared experiences that further parents' insights into their child and enhance their sense of competence. Using everyday questions and experiences in the office as a shared context for discussion as the visit progresses is an efficient way to address such issues without appreciably lengthening the visit.

The goals of using TMs:
- To enhance parents' understanding of the child's needs
- To promote "goodness of fit" between the parent and the child
- To model constructive interactions with the child
- To improve the relationship between the pediatric clinician and the parent

A. Using behavior in the office as a TM

1. Observations and discussions of the infant's or child's behavior in the office provide a fruitful context for TMs. Newly emerging and developed skills and behaviors can challenge the equilibrium between the parent and the child. Frequently, a specific behavior that parents find disturbing—for example, mouthing toys at 6 months of age, throwing blocks or food at 8 months of age, refusing to lie down to be diapered at 10 months of age, irrepressible exploration at 18 months of age, playing with his penis at 3 years of age—is developmentally normal and expectable. Parents' concerns about these issues create a special opportunity to promote parental understanding of typical health and development.

   a. Concerns that new parents bring to pediatric visits in the first months of a child's life provide a wealth of TMs (Table 3-1). The infant's behavior creates a special opportunity to promote parental understanding and support. For example, if the infant cries inconsolably during the visit or his or her cues are difficult to read, *the clinician can explore how parents feel and empathize with their frustration* at not being able to calm the baby. The goal of this TM is to blend information about development with the message that the parents are "experts" on their baby and doing a good job caring for their child.

2. When a child's behavior in the office provides a TM, it is up to the clinician to capitalize on it. During these TMs, one might infer or "read" the child's behavior or temperament together with the parents and offer constructive interpretations of its significance. The clinician should then ask parents how they feel about the behavior or use their own reactions to explore parental concerns. If the clinician finds the child's behavior frustrating, chances are so do the parents.

3. If child behaviors do not produce TMs spontaneously, the clinician may employ specific strategies to engage the child and discuss the implications for behavior and development (Table 3-2). Parents tend to watch carefully as the pediatric clinician engages the child in activities—for example, handing the child a toy or a book, rolling a ball back and forth, listening to the heart, or looking into the ears—that demonstrate a particular behavioral or temperamental quality or developmental skill. In some cases, a pediatric clinician can direct his or her comments to the child rather than to the parents: *"You like seeing the pictures of babies in the books, don't you? This book is making you very excited"* as you show parents that even 6-month-olds get fascinated by picture books. If this serves to encourage parents to start sharing books with babies, the first step in learning to love to read has been taken. When children push the clinician's hand away as he or she attempts to listen to the heart, the clinician can talk about other behaviors in which the child is "uncooperative" for the parent.

Table 3-1 • ELICITING TEACHABLE MOMENTS: EXPLORING RELATIONSHIPS

Maneuver	Comment
Birth to 4 mo of age	
Rock a fussy newborn in your arms and speak softly to console him or her. Hold a drowsy newborn in a vertical position on your shoulder to bring him or her to an alert state.	Whether or not your tactics work, explain what you are trying to do and draw the parents' attention to the infant's reactions. If their baby is unresponsive or difficult to arouse or console, they may be feeling rejected. By showing them that this is difficult for you too, you help them understand that they are not to be blamed. Explaining about temperament as an inherent characteristic can encourage them to try new approaches to arousing and consoling their child.
Draw parents' attention to the reciprocal interaction you see going on between parents and the 2- to 3-month-old child as they take turns smiling and cooing at each other.	Tell parents that this playful exchange shows normal emotional development (baby's smiling, happy face), the beginning of language (vowel sounds, ahs and coos), and cognitive ability (taking turns).
Smile at the 3- or 4-month-old child and try to get the baby to smile back and then ask the parents to try.	Point out that parents got a quicker, bigger smile. Explain that although infants at this age smile at everyone, they smile more readily and more fully at the people to whom they feel closest. This can lead to a discussion of who else gets big smiles (grandparents, the babysitter) and help prepare parents for the next stage when the baby's general friendliness will be replaced by stranger anxiety.

Table 3-2 • ELICITING TEACHABLE MOMENTS: EXPLORING THE WORLD

With each maneuver, comment on the child's interest, attention, and excitement. Point out that these attributes will serve the child well in future learning situations.

Maneuver	Comment
Teachable moments 6–12 mo	
1. Put a cheerio in front of the baby within reach. Ask parents to observe how the baby tries to get it.	At 6 mo, the baby will use his or her thumb and all fingers in an uncoordinated, raking movement. Explain to parents that babies at this age do not have the fine motor coordination to pick up a small object. Have them keep watching. At 9 mo, when his or her nervous system is more mature, he or she will pick up a cheerio with a pincer movement of the thumb and forefinger and put it into his or her mouth. Use this behavior as a teachable moment to point out that a baby who can do this with a cheerio can pick up other small objects as well, not all of them edible or safe. Warn about keeping small objects out of reach.
2. Give the child a toy car, about 2 inches long.	What the baby does with the car will change over time. At 5–6 mo, he or she will probably put it in the mouth. Tell parents that mouthing is the first stage in a sequence of learning about the nature of objects. By 7–8 mo, they can expect the child to be into throwing and banging, and at 9 mo he or she will inspect the car intently, turning it over and over in his or her hand and feeling its contours. Each stage yields more information about the car's properties than the one before. At about 1 y of age, he or she will show his or her understanding of the toy's function by running its wheels along the floor.

(continued)

Table 3-2 • ELICITING TEACHABLE MOMENTS: EXPLORING THE WORLD   (CONTINUED)

3. Hide a favorite object under a cloth while the baby is watching.	When the infant takes the cloth away, discuss how this demonstrates his or her beginning understanding of object permanence, the knowledge that objects continue to exist even when the baby cannot see them. This discovery adds to his or her knowledge that the world has some consistency and dependability to it. Infants are beginning to have a mental representation of the object that explains why they can search and find the hidden toy now when they could not do it at 6 mo of age. Compare this ability to understand object permanence with person permanence. Discuss how separation anxiety and protest when the parent leaves the room demonstrates that the baby now has a mental symbol of his or her parent and the discrepancy between that symbol and him or her not being there evokes crying and protest in an attempt to get the parent to return.
4. Engage the child in reaching for a pen that is extended to him or her.	The pediatric clinician can again demonstrate improved visual–motor functioning. The infant will shape his or her fingers midway through the reach, depending on the placement of the pen. This again is a reflection of neuromaturational development and greater efficiency of the visual–motor process.
12 mo (1 y) of age	
1. Again offer the extended pen to the child.	Starting at about 12 mo of age, stranger anxiety often prevents the child from reaching toward a stranger.
2. Give the baby a pop-up toy or busy-box to play with.	Discuss the strategies that the child uses to figure out how to get the toy to perform. The baby who uses various schemes such as banging, shaking, and poking has developed more ways to use objects and to extract meaning from objects. This broadens his or her cognitive understanding of how the world works. Use these exploratory schemes for discovering causality as a teachable moment in response to the classic complaint of most parents that 1-year-olds are "into everything." Emphasize that although this can be annoying to parents and cause for safety concerns, it is the toddler's way of learning about the objects in his or her environment. Discuss ways to amuse busy toddlers while the parents cook, eat, and go about their normal routines.
3. The child's autonomy and stranger anxiety can be seen when the child tries to fend off the physical examination.	This presents an opportunity to discuss with parents the child's temperament, level of persistence and intensity, and autonomy regarding everyday activities.
15 mo of age	
1. In many cases the pediatric clinician need not do anything to provoke an example of the child's growing autonomy. Most children scream as soon as they get into the room with strangers.	The pediatric clinician can model how to anticipate and limit the baby's stranger anxiety by slowly approaching the child using his or her voice as a distraction technique. If that approach is unsuccessful, the pediatric clinician can point to his or her own disappointment and how other family members or friends who see the child infrequently may feel rejected by the child.
2. Give the child a toy telephone and see whether he can demonstrate functional use by putting the phone to his ear. Ask him to let a doll talk on the phone.	Discuss the child's ability to represent the use of a toy phone on a doll. This stage of cognitive development signals the beginning of symbolic representation, when the child can use one object to represent another object that is not present. Children at this age can demonstrate the functional use of cars, dolls, and care-giving activities such as feeding and can imitate housework such as vacuuming and washing dishes.

Table 3-2 • ELICITING TEACHABLE MOMENTS: EXPLORING THE WORLD   (CONTINUED)

18 mo of age	
1. Give the child a container and blocks.	Note the seemingly endless delight that toddlers have in dumping and filling. There is a sense of satisfaction and fulfillment to the activity. There is also a cognitive component. Toddlers are learning about the properties of objects in space, about completing a task (when the bucket is full), and about a parent's reaction to the toddler's goal of filling and dumping. This also gives the pediatric clinician the opportunity to talk about throwing objects and offer suggestions for how to handle limit setting with young toddlers.

24 mo (2 y) of age	
1. Give the child a book.	Talk about the child's attempts at exploring the book, turning pages, looking at all the pictures. Does the child bring the book to the parents to show them or ask them to read it? This activity also offers the opportunity to talk about the importance of reading aloud to young children and the concept of dialogic reading—or asking the child open-ended questions (see Chapter 16). Comment on "joint attention," ways to support the child's attention, and following the child's lead in storytelling.

30 mo of age	
1. Demonstrate the child's receptive language skills by asking the child to complete two- and three-step commands.	Watching their child perform these tasks correctly can be particularly important for parents who are worried about their child's language development. Demonstrating the sophistication with which the child can follow directions often calms the fears of a parent who is worried about a child who is not talking as well as his age-mates.

36 mo (3 y) of age	
1. Use a ball to introduce simple games.	While playing ball games with the child, point out the child's ability to take turns, understand reciprocity, keep the ball within the physical limits set by the game (between your legs and his or hers), and kick it forward.

Adapted from Zuckerman B, Parker S. Teachable moments: assessment as intervention. *Contemp Pediatr*. 1997:103-118.

4. By observing and commenting on the child's behavior, the pediatric clinician encourages the parents to step back and speculate about its meaning. Unrealistic expectations, which can contribute to parental frustration and lead to child abuse or neglect, can be gently corrected. If parents' reactions are negative, the clinician can reframe the child's behavior in a more positive light. The more mobile 12- to 18-month-old child can be described as "exuberant" or "exploratory" rather than "disobedient." The child who is "uncooperative" with the physical examination is really "asserting his or her independence."

   a. For example, parents often describe how their 7- to 8-month-old child throws his or her food off the high chair tray, making a mess for the parents to clean. They then respond by controlling the feeding and not allowing the child to feed himself or herself. The clinician can join with the parents around how messy babies can be and reframe the throwing behavior, explaining how shaking and throwing are the infant's way of exploring objects to discover what the objects can do. This can easily be demonstrated by giving the child a toy in the office and watching him bang, shake, and throw it. The clinician can create a TM by narrating the child's actions, reframing them as acts of exploration rather than as deliberate attempts to make a mess. The clinician can explain how seemingly unimportant tasks, such as using a pincer grasp to pick up a cheerio, are important windows into a baby's development and learning.

b. Another example of reframing behavior involves stranger anxiety. Many children are visibly upset by the 12- to 15-month visit because of their heightened stranger and separation anxiety. They may express this anxiety by actively refusing to cooperate with the examination and by protesting when the pediatric clinician tries to examine them. This behavior, often embarrassing to parents, can be used as a TM to discuss stranger anxiety and its developmental function and to explore its ramifications for the families. Parents are usually relieved to understand why it is a developmental inevitability and a sign of positive emotional and cognitive growth for their baby to become wary of strangers and actively and loudly resist separation. They are also pleased to learn that these behaviors are linked to cognitive growth in object permanence.

c. The 18- to 24-month period is marked by struggles over control, limit testing, and the toddler's ability to get himself or herself into serious trouble as he or she climbs too high or runs away too quickly from a parent. The physical examination and immunizations usually produce enough negative responses from the toddler to bring these issues to the surface. Because the clinician and the parent have both observed these behaviors, they create yet another TM, giving the clinician insight into how the parents understand the behavior and how they respond to it. It is important at moments like these to do the following:

- *Empathize* with the parents. They need assurance that their child's behavior is normal, as is their frustration and embarrassment or anger at their child.
- *Explain* that a toddler's autonomy struggles often feel like the child is "refusing to listen."
- *Model* verbal and behavioral strategies to help the child cope with the experience of being in the office, for example, demonstrating for the parents the importance of setting safe limits for the child while trying to avoid unnecessary power struggles regarding parental control, that is, *"I know that you like jumping off high places, but jumping off the exam table is not safe."*
- *Help* the child feel like he or she has mastered a stressful situation by commenting on his or her attempts, even if relatively unsuccessful, at control: *"I know it was hard for you, but you did a good job when I looked in your ears."* Instead of the child feeling like a failure and the parents feeling embarrassed or angry or both, the family can feel that you understood and accepted their reactions and that you still like their child and respect their parenting efforts.

B. **Using history taking as a TM**

1. **Evocative questions** during history taking, especially in the first year of life, can create special TMs. Such questions might include asking about the parents' own upbringing, the "ghosts/angels in the nursery" that influence their child-rearing practices, and their feelings about themselves as parents (see Chapter 10). Eliciting a family history of depression and alcoholism may help parents understand the impact of these factors on their parenting and their fears about their child's (and their own) vulnerability to these or other mental health problems (see Chapters 7 and 8).

2. Questions about the **child's behavior and development** give parents a chance to discuss concerns in these areas. Especially useful in the early years are questions about the child's temperamental characteristics, developmental milestones, behavioral and family issues, and how the parents feel about these issues.

3. A dialogue about **parental disagreements** is another example of a potential TM during history taking. Asking how a family handles anger or resolves disputes often leads to a discussion of these issues and their impact on child behavior and development. The clinician might say that children benefit when they see their parents come to a peaceful conclusion after an argument, or point out that conflicts are an opportunity to teach children about frustration, anger, and disagreements without fear of the loss of love. Clinicians can advise parents how to "repair" the unpleasant event by saying something like "Mommy and Daddy get angry, we yell at each other but we are ok now."

4. **Clinical judgment** is always required to distinguish when it is appropriate to expand and when to narrow the content of the discussion. Also, it is helpful to remember that although some parents find it helpful to discuss their feelings, others experience personal questions as intrusive. Sensing when not to intrude on the parents' privacy is as important as knowing what, how, and when to probe.

5. Finally, clinicians should be aware that TMs also occur when children who are old enough to understand are asked directly about their health and behavior. Asking 3-year-olds whether they brush their teeth or eat their vegetables conveys the message that they have a responsibility to take good care of their bodies. The opportunity should not be missed.

C. Using the physical examination as a TM

1. The physical examination provides the pediatric clinician with a window into the child's behavior and development. One can comment how *this* child at *this* age responds to the examination, compared to his or her behavior at an earlier age. As the pediatric clinician performs the examination, he or she should narrate a running commentary about the findings: *"Heart sounds great—good, strong heart! Lungs are clear ... No sign of bronchitis. Ears have a little bit of fluid—do you think she is hearing okay?"* This running narrative serves, first and foremost, to reassure mothers and fathers that their child is healthy. In this regard, one should avoid ambiguous statements such as: *"Well, she doesn't sound too bad or I can't find anything wrong."* Such equivocation does little to reassure and may set the anxious parent's mind racing.

2. The examination also serves as a natural springboard to elicit more information or concerns from the observing parent. Neutral, nonjudgmental comments about the child's behavior (e.g., *"He certainly is a busy guy, isn't he?"*) may trigger a host of parental concerns, elicited more easily by focusing ostensibly on the child's physical examination and not on the parental feelings.

3. Finally, the physical examination is a wonderful opportunity for the pediatric clinician to reframe the child's behavior to enhance parent–child interactions. One's demeanor toward the child serves as a model for the parent. Certainly, the physical examination must be approached with respect for the child and sensitivity to issues of power and control. For example, the obstreperous toddler who resists examination offers the opportunity to discuss the child's attempts at autonomy, individuation, and his or her understandable desire to maintain control of his or her body. The child who cries but then consoles himself or herself sets the stage for a discussion of his or her coping skills.

Bibliography

Flocke SA, Clark E, Antognoli E, et al. Teachable moments for health behavior change and intermediate patient outcomes. *Patient Educ Couns*. 2014;96(1):43-49.

Parker S, Zuckerman B. Therapeutic aspects of the assessment process. In: Meisels S, Shonkoff J, eds. *Handbook of Early Childhood Intervention*. New York: Cambridge University Press; 1990;350-371.

Zuckerman B. Family history: a special opportunity for psychosocial intervention. *Pediatrics*. 1991;7:740.

WEB SITES FOR CLINICIANS

http://www.pediatriccareonline.org/pco/ub/view/Bright-Futures-Pocket-Guide/135503/5/core_concepts.

http://www.pediatricsinpractice.org/new/teaching_center/curricular_mod_education.asp.

CHAPTER 4

Parental Self-understanding: Key to Preventing Problems

Barry Zuckerman | Pamela M. Zuckerman

I. **DESCRIPTION OF THE PROBLEM.** Adults are challenged when they become parents first. The tasks are novel and often cause concerns, anxieties, and fears. New parents must also address previously unexplored values and attitudes some originating from their own childhood now brought to the fore by the birth of their baby. New day-to-day activities and routines, new problems needing solutions, and normal struggles and uncertainties at each developmental stage can elicit heightened emotional responses from parents.

Mundane and minor matters can elicit worry (e.g., parents' great anxiety when their infant has not had a bowel movement in 2 days). More serious and threatening experiences also cause internal upset (e.g., a mother's feelings of exhaustion and being literally consumed by her ever-hungry new infant; a father's dismay at his wife's physical and at times emotional unavailability as she completely focuses on the new infant; a parent's visceral response when their toddler defies them).

Universal child-rearing experiences elicit predictable parental concerns and responses:
- How will they protect the child from their own occasional frustration, anger, or irritability?
- How will they avoid being overindulgent and also set limits that are not too harsh or arbitrary?
- How will they balance providing praise appropriately and correcting unwanted behaviors effectively without being either too strict or overly permissive?

II. **PROCESS OF REFECTION AND SELF-UNDERSTANDING.** Child development information and child-rearing strategies are often inadequate to help parents negotiate the myriad feelings and the complex tasks involved in successful parenting. One thing in which parents really need to be successful is to develop an understanding and insight into their own past, especially their relationship to their own parents, and also to understand their own patterns of behavior. Self-understanding for parents develops over time through review of their past upbringing through remembering, retelling, reflecting on, and perhaps reinterpreting past events. This process is catalyzed and assisted through ongoing conversations with spouse, relatives, friends, and other parents and professionals.

Without adequate self-understanding, problems can arise for parents when experiences, attitudes, and fears arising from their own upbringing cause them to respond inconsistently or behave inappropriately toward their child. And when parents do direct excessive anger, withdrawal, sarcasm, harsh criticism, or rigid orders toward their child, it can be upsetting, confusing, and ultimately damaging for the child. To short-circuit inappropriate responses to their child, parents need to be aware of the origins of their attitudes and behaviors. Again, this is achieved through reflection and self-exploration.

Pediatric clinicians can foster self-understanding in parents by asking key questions at critical times and then listening to the answers. Questions that are particularly important address parents' attitudes and values, especially as they relate to their own childhood and how their parents raised them. Growing up in a family that is overly strict or harsh or lacks emotional warmth can program children to recreate the same family style when they become parents. But when parents have reviewed their own upbringing thoughtfully, have considered which aspects were positive and which were not, and have decided how they would like to raise their own children, research shows they are much less likely to repeat maladaptive patterns learned in the past.

A. **Questions for self-understanding.** There are a number of simple, straightforward questions pediatric clinicians can ask that will help parents begin to look at their own personal stories and make connections between their current experiences being a parent now and their past experiences as a child growing up.

General themes to be addressed include experiences of love, nurturing, separation, care when distressed, times of feeling threatened, and experiences of trauma or loss. Other related topics, which may also be helpful, include experiences of being disciplined, the presence of siblings, and changes in the relationship with the parents during adolescence and adulthood. Parents can be relieved when they gain insight into the connections between difficult events in their past and unexpected eruptions in their present life with their children. When these connections are made and parents gain insight into some of the underpinnings of their own behavior, parents are often then able to let go of some struggles or rigidity they are involved in with their children.

The pediatric clinician can begin with gentle questions (Table 4-1) to open the door, invite parents to remember, retell, and rethink the emotional meanings of their past lives in context with their new role as a mother or as a father. Because the pediatric clinician is a trusted professional, the parents can tolerate and respond thoughtfully to these personal questions. The pediatric clinician need not ask all these questions at one visit and should consider this as an ongoing conversation that may vary in need and intensity at different stages in the child's development or parents' life circumstances but especially relevant when parent–child struggles occur.

B. New use of family history—interrupting transgenerational transmission of behavioral health problems.

Family history is traditionally used to identify risk for genetically loaded diseases. Routine family history can be expanded to highlight two common parental health problems affecting children: depression (4% of adult men and 12% of adult women) and alcoholism (12% of adults).

Beyond the potential genetic risk, these disorders convey risk through multigenerational parenting dysfunctions and role modeling starting with grandparents during the childhood of the parents. When the parents were younger, their depressed or alcoholic parents may have had difficulty with emotional regulation and availability to their

---

Table 4-1 • QUESTIONS FOR PARENTAL SELF-REFLECTION

These Questions Can Be Asked Over the Course of Many Visits Over Many Years
Do you plan to raise your child like your mother and father raised you? What was your parents' philosophy in raising children? What was it about it that you liked? What was it about it that you did not like?
How did you get along with your parents? How did the relationship evolve throughout your youth and up until the present time?
How did your relationship with your mother and father differ and how were they similar? Can you describe three characteristics of your childhood relationship to each of your parents?
Why did you choose these adjectives? Are there ways in which you try to be like, or try not to be like, either of your parents?
Do you recall your earliest separations from your parents? What was it like? Did you ever have prolonged separations from your parents?
What kind of discipline did your parent use? Did your mother or father differ? What impact did that have on your childhood, and how do you feel it affects your role as a parent now?
Did you ever feel rejected or threatened by your parents? Were there other experiences you had that felt overwhelming or traumatizing in your life, during childhood or beyond? Do any of these experiences still feel very much alive? Do they continue to influence your life?
Did anyone significant in your life die during your childhood or later in life? What was that like for you at the time, and how does that loss affect you now?
How did your parents communicate with you when you were happy and excited? Did they join with you in your enthusiasm? When you were distressed or unhappy as a child, what would happen? Did your father and mother respond differently to you during these emotional times? How?
Was there anyone else besides your parents in your childhood who took care of you? What was that relationship like for you? What happened to those individuals? What is it like for you when you let others take care of your child now?
If you had difficult times during your childhood, were there positive relationships in or outside of your home that you could depend on during those times? How do you feel those connections benefited you then, and how might they help you now?
How have your childhood experiences influenced your relationships with others as an adult?
How has your childhood shaped the ways in which you relate to your children?

Adapted from Siegel DJ, Kaetzel M. *Parenting from the Inside Out*. New York: Putnam Books; 2003.

children, and inability to set consistent limits. These behaviors are reflected in poignant stories of adult children of alcoholics, whose descriptions of difficulties with self-esteem, nurturing, and relationships suggest problems originating in their childhood. Some alcoholic parents physically and sexually abuse their children. These stories demonstrate how the adult child of an alcoholic may become a dysfunctional parent even though he or she is not alcoholic. Although not yet clearly defined, the parenting of adult children of depressed parents may also be impaired even if they are not depressed. Pediatric clinicians obtaining a family history should therefore ask about the presence of either of these problems in the child's grandparents. If a grandparent suffered from either of these problems, a pediatric clinician should then ask the following questions:

1. Because it runs in families, do the parents or their siblings have any similar problems?
2. If yes, are they being treated?
3. If no, do they think their childhood experiences affect their parenting? For example, are they overprotective, overly strict, or have trouble showing emotions?
4. If the family history of these or related problems is on one side of the family, the parent from the nonaffected side can be asked whether they are concerned about the future? These questions place this important issue on the table.

This type of discussion with the pediatric clinician provides the parents with an opportunity to become aware of their parents' influence on their own parenting. If there is no significant problem at that time, identification of the problem in the family provides the opportunity for parents to talk about their childhood experiences, their concerns regarding their own feelings, and their ability to nurture, support, and promote the self-esteem of their own children. The pediatric clinician should continue to bear this history in mind. There is a high probability that issues will arise during specific stages of the child's development such as adolescence, whether or not parent develop depression or alcoholism throughout the time.

While asking specific listed questions or family history, the clinician needs to spend a little time to listen to the parent's responses. However, you do not have to listen indefinitely or hear it all at once, nor do you have to respond with explanations or advice immediately. If necessary, the appropriate "referral" is to a spouse, friends, or selected family members. The professional can say something like, "*It sounds like you have many memories and feelings. I would encourage you to talk to your spouse, sister, or friends about them to give your insight into what you want to do and don't do as a parent.*"

Outside the pediatric office setting, the issues can be explored in greater depth and complexity in the parents' circle of friends and family, and with other therapeutic professionals if appropriate or desired. Spouses and friends can assist parents in continuing the process of insightful exploration, "making sense" of a parent's personal history with supportive, empathic, emotionally directed conversations.

Both science and clinical experience tell us that parents' reflection and self-understanding can greatly enhance their ability to be good parents and to foster their children's optimal development. The pediatric clinician's role is to raise the issues and support the process of parental self-understanding through reflection and discussion with others. A continuity of care setting allows questions and the unfolding answers and their clarification and import to occur over time.

Bibliography

FOR PARENTS

Siegel DJ, Hartzel M. *Parenting from the Inside Out*. New York: Penguin Putnam; 2003.

FOR PROFESSIONALS

Fraiberg S, Adelson E, Shapiro V. The nursery. *J Am Acad Child Psychiatry*. 1975;14:387-421.

Mav M. Attachment: overview with implications for clinical work. In: Goldberg S, Muir R, Kerr J, eds. *Attachment Theory: Social, Developmental, and Clinical Perspectives*. Hillsdale, NJ: Analytic Press; 1995:407-474.

Zuckerman B. Family history: a special opportunity for psychosocial intervention. *Pediatrics*. 1991;87(5):740-741.

Zuckerman B, Zuckerman P, Siegel DJ. Promoting self-understanding in parents—for the great good of your patients. *Contemp Pediatr*. 2005;22(4):77-90.

CHAPTER 5

Developmental Screening

Victoria Chen | Frances Page Glascoe

I. **PROBLEM OF UNDERDETECTION.** Most children with mental, behavioral, and developmental delays/disorders (MBDDs) have subtle symptoms that are not clear in the absence of measurement. When primary care providers (PCPs) do not use standardized, validated screening tools, 70%–80% of children with disabilities are not detected before school entrance, and vital opportunities for early intervention are missed. As few as 2 years of early intervention before school entrance increases the likelihood of high school graduation, employment, and independent living and reduces the rates of teen pregnancy, criminal activity, and violent crime.

II. **ROLE OF THE PCP.** PCPs have an irreplaceable role in detecting, tracking, and managing children's mental health and behavioral, and developmental issues because of the following characteristics of them:
   - *Frequent, continuous contact*—No other early childhood program or agency can track the development of young children with the same scale and continuity as PCPs (i.e., all young children attend primary care well-visits, but not all young children attend child care/early childhood programs).
   - *A unique perspective*—PCPs have a broad knowledge of the psychosocial and health issues that may affect children's mental health, behavior, and development.
   - *A unique rapport and trust*—PCPs have unique rapport and trust with families through which providers can effectively discuss parental concerns and create treatment plans in a family-centered way.

III. **PEARLS FOR MBDD SCREENING.** When an efficient clinic system is in place, MBDD screening does not necessarily lengthen the well-child visit and yet it simultaneously raises the quality of care via a family-centered approach. The following are pearls for implementing screening in primary care:
   - *Incorporate routine screening into well-visits*—Screen for autism spectrum disorder at 18 and 24 month well-visits. Screen for MBDD at 9, 18, and 30 month well-visits and annually thereafter. Most MBDD problems emerge with time and are not fully detectable in young children (e.g., pragmatic language problems, behavior problems such as attention-deficit/hyperactivity disorder, learning disorders especially reading disabilities, academic deficits due to psychosocial risks). Prevalence studies show that older children have significantly higher rates of MBDD than do younger children.
   - *Use validated screening tools*—Timely, early detection depends on frequent, periodic screening with validated and accurate tools. Informal milestone checklists and untested questions to parents are neither efficient nor effective—the majority of children with MBDD will be missed. (See below for guidance on choosing screening tools.)
   - *Have screening tools completed before the start of the visit*—Screening can be incorporated into office workflows efficiently when tools are completed before the visit begins (e.g., in waiting rooms, through patient portals, or at home and brought in before the visit) so that screening tools can be scored promptly and interpreted in the beginning of the visit. Studies show that screening in the beginning of the visit can reduce the incidence of last-minute issues being brought up at the end of the visit (i.e., the "doorknob phenomenon" or "doorknob question").
   - *Use Web-based screening tools*—Consider using Web-based portals to streamline screening, scoring, report-writing, and referrals. Web sites for specific tools often have useful information on how to apply them in busy practices or incorporate them into electronic health records. Online software with built-in decision support tools has been shown to improve screening accuracy during well-visits (see Table 5-1).
   - *Engage office staff and/or nonphysician health care professionals*—Educating and enlisting office staff and nonphysician health care professionals (e.g., medical assistants, patient care assistants, and nurses) in the processes of MBDD screening, making referrals, and tracking referrals have been shown to be an integral step in successful implementation. This is optimally done through a quality-improvement approach. Office staff and nonphysician health care professionals can take primary responsibility for ensuring that screening tools are complete and/or scored before the family entering the

Table 5-1 • PARENT-REPORT, STANDARDIZED, VALIDATED, AND ACCURATE DEVELOPMENTAL-BEHAVIORAL SCREENS

Parent-Report Developmental and/or Behavioral Screens	Age Range	Description	Scoring	Accuracy
Ages and Stages Questionnaire-3 (ASQ-3) (3rd ed, 2009). Paul H. Brookes Publishing Co., Inc. www.agesandstages.com Electronic/portal options available on website. **Training options:** Presentations and case examples on Web site, webinars, DVDs for purchase, and live training	1–66 mo	Parents indicate children's developmental skills on 30 items plus overall concerns. The ASQ has a different form (5–8 pages) for each age interval. Written at the 4th to 6th grade level. Includes activity handouts for parents that can aid in anticipatory guidance. The ASQ-3 is available in English, Spanish, Arabic, French, or Vietnamese with other translations under way. Can be administered by parents at home or in waiting rooms (with the aid of a materials kit that can be purchased separately [$295.00] or materials assembled from the list proved in the ASQ manual).	Cutoff scores (set at 1 SD or 2 SDs below mean) in five developmental domains. Indicates need for monitoring or referral.	**Across ages:** Sensitivity: 86% Specificity: 85% **By domain:** Sensitivity: 83% Specificity: 91% **In discerning disability types,** i.e., motor, visual, hearing impairments: Sensitivity: 87%
Parents' Evaluations of Developmental Status (PEDS) (2013) PEDSTest.com, LLC www.pedstest.com Electronic/portal options available on website. **Training options:** Offers through its Web site self-training/train-the-trainer support via downloadable slide shows with notes, case examples, FAQs, participant handouts, pre-post-test questions, Web site discussion list (covering all screens), short videos, with some live training available	Birth to 8 y	10 questions eliciting parents' (and providers') concerns in English, Spanish, Vietnamese, Chinese, Somali, and 36 other languages. Items are written at the 5th grade level. Longitudinal Score and Interpretation Forms assign risk levels, track decision-making, and offer specific guidance on how to address concerns. Provides screening, longitudinal surveillance, and triage for developmental as well as behavioral/social–emotional/mental health problems. PEDS is best used in conjunction with the PEDS:DM (below) for compliance with AAP Policy on screening and surveillance.	Identifies levels of risk and provides decision support, i.e., when to: refer; advise parents; monitor vigilantly; screen further; or reassure.	**Across ages:** Sensitivity: 86% Specificity: 83% **In discerning disability types,** i.e., learning, intellectual, language, mental health, autism spectrum and motor disorders: Sensitivity: >80%

PEDS: Developmental Milestones (Screening Version) (PEDS) (2016) PEDSTest.com, LLC www.pedstest.com Electronic/portal options available on website. **Training Options:** Offers through its Web site self-training/train-the-trainer support via videos, downloadable slide shows with notes, case examples, pre-post-test questions, participant handouts, FAQs, with some live training available. The PEDS:DM manual includes extensive suggestions for training medical students, residents, and nurses	Birth to 8 y	PEDS-DM consists of six to eight items at each age level. Each item taps a different domain (fine/gross motor, self-help, academics, expressive/receptive language, social–emotional). The PEDS:DM provides screening, triage, and surveillance via a longitudinal score form for tracking milestones progress. Written at the 2nd to 3rd grade level and can be completed by self-report, interview, or administered directly to children. Forms are laminated and completed with a dry erase marker. At each age level, read-aloud stories about age-appropriate parenting assist in developmental–behavioral promotion. Supplemental measures include the M-CHAT, Family Psychosocial Screen, Pictorial PSC-17, the SWILS, the Vanderbilt ADHD scale, and the Brigance Parent-Child Interactions Scale. Best combined with PEDS to ensure compliance with AAP policy. In English, Spanish, Chinese, Portuguese, Arabic, Serbian, Swahili, with other languages in process.	Met/unmet milestones with cutoffs tied to performance above and below the 16th percentile for each item and its domain. On the assessment level, age-equivalent scores are produced and enable users to compute percentage of delays.	**Across ages:** Sensitivity: 83%; Specificity: 84% **By domain:** Sensitivity: 83%; Specificity: 84% **In discerning disability types,** i.e., autism spectrum disorder: Sensitivity: 79%–82%
Modified Checklist of Autism in Toddlers (M-CHAT-R) (2013) Freely downloadable in multiple languages along with the Follow-up Interview at www. mchatscreen.com. Commercial software vendors must pay a licensing fee. **Training options:** The site contains a guide to the needed follow-up interview for missed items, houses research papers, and reviews on ASD screening	16–48 mo	Parent-report measure with 20 yes-no questions and written at 4th to 6th grade reading level. Screens only for autism spectrum disorder and should not be used without a broadband developmental screening tool. Downloadable scoring template and .xls files for automated scoring. Requires the M-CHAT-R Follow-up Interview if three to seven items are failed and referral if eight or more failed items. Referral sources can be asked to complete the Follow-up Interview. Research is voluminous (and listed/downloadable at www.mchatscreen.com).	Low-, moderate-, high-risk based on the numbers of failed items.	**Across ages** (for autism spectrum disorder): Sensitivity: 91% Specificity: 96%

(continued)

Table 5-1 • PARENT-REPORT, STANDARDIZED, VALIDATED, AND ACCURATE DEVELOPMENTAL–BEHAVIORAL SCREENS (CONTINUED)

Parent-Report Developmental and/or Behavioral Screens	Age Range	Description	Scoring	Accuracy
Communication and Symbolic Behavior Scales–Developmental Profile (CSBS-DP): Infant/Toddler Checklist (ITC) (2008) Paul H. Brookes Publishing Co. www.brookespublishing.com **Training options:** Live training and research support, downloadable slide shows, abstracts, videos, and references at http://firstwords.fsu.edu **Electronic options:** None (apart from CD-ROM offering automated scoring and saving approximately 7 min of time)	6–24 mo	Parents complete the ITC's 24 multiple-choice questions. Examiners verify parents' answers via brief observation and a Caregiver Questionnaire. Reading level is ~5th grade. Can serve as an entry point into the assessment-level, CSBS, and an ongoing monitoring tool. In English, Spanish, Slovenian, Chinese, Swedish, German. The First Words Web site (http://firstwords.fsu.edu) houses research on the ITC and links to the Autism Video Glossary.	Risk categorization (concern/no concern) for three domains—Social, Speech, and Symbolic—and Total Score.	**Across ages:** Sensitivity: N/A Specificity: N/A **By disability types,** i.e., developmental disabilities, autism spectrum disorders: Sensitivity: 78% Specificity: 84%
Safety Word Inventory and Literacy Screener (SWILS) (2012) From PEDSTest.com, LLC with items courtesy of Curriculum Associates, Inc. *The SWILS is included in* PEDS:Developmental Milestones *(PEDS:DM).* Cost: Freely downloadable at: www.pedstest.com/TheBook/Chapter9 **Training options:** None **Electronic options:** None	6–14 y	Children are asked (by parents or professionals) to read 29 common safety words (e.g., High Voltage, Wait, Poison) aloud. The number of correctly read words is compared with a cutoff score. Results predict performance in math, written language, and a range of reading skills. Test content may serve as a springboard to injury prevention counseling and can be used to screen for parental literacy. Because even non-English speakers living in the United States need to read safety words in English, the measure is only available in English.	Single cutoff score by age, indicating the need for a referral.	**Across ages/academic deficits:** Sensitivity: 80% Specificity: 82%

| **Pediatric Symptom Checklist (PSC) and Pictorial PSC (PPSC) (2008)** | PSC/PPSC age range is 4–16 y | Administered by youth/parent self-report or by interview, the PSC/Pictorial PSC are 35 short statements of problem behaviors capturing various mental health challenges. The PSC-17 is a 17-item version producing cutoffs for attention, internalizing (meaning depression or anxiety) and externalizing problems (conduct, impulsivity, etc.) Readability is approximately 2nd grade. In English, Spanish, Portuguese, Chinese, Dutch, Filipino, French, Somali, and several other languages. | For the PSC, a single refer/nonrefer score; for the PSC-17, additional cutoffs for attention, internalizing, and externalizing factors. | **PSC/Pictorial PSC-35 by disability,** i.e., mental problems of any kind, across numerous studies: Sensitivity: 88%–95% Specificity: 68%–100% **PSC-17 by specific disability,** i.e., ADHD, internalizing disorders, externalizing disorders. Psychometric properties vary from low (<70%) to moderate (>80%) depending on subscale or total score cutoff used |

Freely downloadable in multiple languages at http://www.massgeneral.org/psychiatry/services/psc_home.aspx

See electronic options below.

Training options: None

© Glascoe FP, Marks KP, Poon JK, Macias MM, eds. *Identifying and Addressing Developmental-Behavioral Problems: A Practical Guide for Medical and Non-medical Professionals, Trainees, Researchers and Advocates.* Nolensville, Tennessee: PEDStest.com, LLC; 2013. www.pedstest.com (permission is granted for reproduction of this table as long as this copyright notice is shown).

Disclosure: This table was compiled and vetted in collaboration with many researchers, clinicians, and test authors, without regard to the latter's potential financial interests in products mentioned.

examination room, helping with screening by interview, helping with referrals to IDEA (Individuals with Disabilities Education Act) programs or subspecialists, and tracking referrals after families have completed their visit (see section "VIII. Referrals and follow-up" for additional guidance).

- *Assist parents with limited English or limited literacy*—Consider screening by interview for parents who have not graduated from high school, when parents skip items on screens, or when parents fail to write actual comments when prompted with open-ended questions. Obtain official translations of screens from their publishers—these translations are usually vetted and known to work well (i.e., have adequate sensitivity/specificity). Consider telephone-based language translation services such as LanguageLine (www.languageline.com) or in-office interpreters to help with screening by interview with official translations. Parents with limited English or literacy and whose children have problematic performance on screens need referral assistance (i.e., office staff should make follow-up appointments with them). Parent education is often needed and clinicians/staff should make use of websites offering information in other languages.

IV. **CHOOSING MBDD SCREENING TOOLS.** The optimal tools for identifying MBDD in primary care are those that:
- *Have proven levels of accuracy*—At least 70%–80% of children with and without problems should be detected correctly.
- *Have been standardized and validated*—Standardization and validation on a large, national, general (not referred) sample of children is essential.
- *Have been translated in multiple languages and validated in a diverse population.*
- *Are feasible in a primary care setting*—Screening tools that have been successfully implemented in primary care often rely on information from parents. Parent-completed screening questionnaires take little time to administer. Parents, regardless of their level of education or parenting experience, are equally able to provide predictive information about their children.

Several good, quality screening tools that meet the above criteria are presented in Table 5-1.

V. **PITFALLS**
- *Using informal milestone checklists*—Nonstandardized, nonvalidated developmental milestone checklists lack definable scoring/referral criteria and many include items that are far too easy for the age levels given. These informal checklists do not meet the clinical standards set for routine MBDD screening and should not be used in this manner.
- *Not following screening instructions*—Adhering to screening test directions is essential for obtaining correct results, i.e., proven sensitivity, specificity, positive and negative predictive values. Clinicians or office staff should readminister by interview whenever parent-completed screening test protocols have missing answers or when parents fail to write comments. With the *Modified Checklist for Autism in Toddlers, Revised with Follow-up (M-CHAT-R/F)*, asking the associated follow-up questions for children with medium risk scores is recommended and reduces false-positive rates.

VI. **PEARLS FOR MBDD SURVEILLANCE**
- *Definition*—Surveillance is the flexible, longitudinal, continuous, and cumulative process in which knowledgeable health care professionals explore potential causes as well as potential predictors of MBDD. Many aspects of surveillance overlap with screening tests in which case separate measures for surveillance are not needed. Problematic screening results serve as a trigger that enhances surveillance.
- *Incorporating surveillance into the well-visit*—The following list summarizes the steps:
  - Elicit parent/caregiver concerns
  - Screen to measure children's skills
    - Mental, behavioral, and developmental screening
    - Autism screening—if appropriate for age
  - Identify/update psychosocial risk factors
  - Observe/measure parent–child interactions and family resilience factors
  - Identify/update family/child medical history and biological risk factors
  - Conduct physical examination
  - Provide developmental and behavioral promotion
  - Next steps (as needed)
    - Interpret results and discuss findings
    - Document findings/developmental history, order labs, and make referrals
    - Coordinate/facilitate referrals and plan follow-up
    - Communicate findings with outside agencies (e.g., childcare providers, IDEA programs such as Early Intervention)

- *Repeated screening serves as evidence-based surveillance*—Identifying children with child mental health, behavior, and development is best done with validated, standardized screening tools/questions. Although surveillance (meaning clinical observation and judgment) is important, informal methods typically deployed are associated with limited identification rates. Incorporating standardized, validated questions for surveillance of development is preferred. Repeated screening can aid in enhancing surveillance during well-child care.
- *Importance of identifying risk factors*—MBDD surveillance helps identify biologic, genetic, psychosocial, and environmental factors that may adversely affect child development and helps PCPs consider both etiology and treatment plans. For example, a child who is meeting milestones on time but who has health and psychosocial risk factors will benefit from referral to Head Start, quality childcare, and/or parent training programs. Using validated screening questions to identify risk factors is preferred whenever possible. For instance, asking two validated questions to screen for maternal depression is preferred over asking a few informal questions aimed at screening for those issues.
- *For children with multiple risk factors identified on surveillance, direct referral is advised*—Children with concerning developmental delays (e.g., not speaking words at 18 months of age with poor eye contact), psychosocial risk factors (e.g., limited-English-proficient family, inconsistent well-visits, exposure to adverse childhood experience), environmental, genetic, or biologic risk factors (e.g., prematurity) can be directly referred to IDEA and community programs without screening.
- *Importance of identifying and monitoring family/child strengths and protective factors*—Identifying family and child strengths is important for recognizing and supporting positive parenting practices. For example, PCPs should encourage parents who are sharing books, enjoying back-and-forth communication and sound play, using time-out for behavioral problems, etc. Advice to parents whose resilience factors are limited should be monitored for effectiveness (e.g., via a follow-up call in a few weeks). If progress is limited, referrals for parent training and programs such as Head Start or quality day care are needed.

VII. MAKING IT WORK IN PRIMARY CARE. Health care providers can and should document carefully both medical history and physical examination findings to determine whether organic conditions are contributory.
- *Medical history*—It is important to probe for other clinical signs and symptoms that may be related to mental, behavioral, and developmental delays (e.g., get detailed sleep history in cases of social–emotional/behavior delay, rule out constipation or dental caries in children with behavioral problems).
- *Physical examination*—The physical examination should include attention to growth parameters, head shape and circumference, facial and other body dysmorphology, eye findings (e.g., cataracts in various inborn errors of metabolism), vascular markings, signs of neurocutaneous disorders (e.g., café au lait spots in neurofibromatosis, hypopigmented macules in tuberous sclerosis), muscle strength, tone, presence of abnormal reflexes, and disturbance of movement.
- *Further medical evaluation*—A diagnostic evaluation should be done to identify the underlying cause of MBDD findings or concerns. For example, hearing should be screened in cases of language delay, and vision and/or hearing should be screened in cases of attention deficits. Abnormal thyroid function and muscular dystrophy should be ruled out when infants/toddlers are found with low muscle tone by checking thyroid-stimulating hormone and creatine kinase, respectively.

VIII. REFERRALS AND FOLLOW-UP
- *Referrals to IDEA programs*—When screening test results are problematic, referrals should begin with IDEA services, Part C (Early Intervention services for children 0–3 years old) and Part B (Special Education Services for children 3–21 years old through public preschools/schools). Referrals to IDEA Part C or Part B services do not require a confirmation of a diagnosis but can be based on concerns raised by parents or clinicians. It may seem odd to refer for treatment before a diagnosis is finalized, but with young children (who are those who benefit most from early intervention), eligibility criteria are generally only a percentage of delay and do not require a specific diagnosis.
- *Referrals to community programs*—Community-based services are also important partners in treating children with identified MBDD. Quality childcare settings and early education programs such as Head Start may be key allies in helping identify/address psychosocial problems, model positive parenting practices, or provide a stable environment where children's mental, behavioral, or developmental issues can be addressed systematically. Child Care Aware has local Child Care Resource and Referral (CCR&R)

agencies to help families connect to quality childcare services. Other such community-based programs are listed under "Referral and Disability Resources" in Bibliography.

- *Referrals to medical subspecialists*—Referrals to medical specialists are warranted when additional evaluation is needed for diagnosis of delays identified. Developmental behavioral pediatricians, neurologists, geneticists, pulmonologists, and other subspecialists may all play a role in medical workup and treatment plan.
- Key to successful referrals:
  - *Facilitate referrals*—Office practices that facilitate referrals as much as possible have been shown to improve evaluation rates when referred. For examples, faxing Early Intervention referrals directly to agencies rather than giving families phone numbers to call for an evaluation has been shown to improve Early Intervention evaluation rates. Building relationships with local community agencies (e.g., Head Start), Early Intervention referral agencies (as part of IDEA Part C services), preschool referral agencies (as part of IDEA Part B services), and pediatric subspecialists can help practices to better utilize community resources and streamline referral practices to ensure that families face minimal barriers when they are referred. Office staff can also offer to help make subspecialty appointments especially when families face language barriers. Office staff can also designate a "referral expert" (e.g., person or computer database that all office staff can access) in the practice to keep track of what referrals/prescriptions are needed when referrals are made so that these needs are met at the same visit that they are referred.
  - *Track/Follow up on referrals made*—Referrals should be tracked as part of MBDD surveillance so that clinicians can be informed of barriers families face when getting evaluations for or access to IDEA Part C/Part B services, community-based services, or subspecialty services. Families may face cultural barriers to understanding why they need an evaluation through Early Intervention or other IDEA programs. Families may face language barriers or psychosocial barriers to contacting and scheduling an evaluation to IDEA programs or with medical subspecialists. Practices can track referrals through the following:
    - *Maintaining a database with follow-up phone calls*—Practices can create a database of referred families and have follow-up phone calls scheduled with families to find out if evaluation appointments were made and/or if evaluations have occurred.
    - *Prioritizing getting referral reports back*—Practices can streamline how referral reports are sent back to the office by having consent forms in place as needed (e.g., for Early Intervention or school evaluations) or ensuring that subspecialty practices are sending referral reports effectively (e.g., through fax instead of mail).
    - *Making it work through quality improvement*—Creating an office system where tracking and following-up-on referrals are done seamlessly is best achieved using quality-improvement methods. The American Academy of Pediatrics Screening Technical Assistance and Resource (STAR) Center has tools that can help practices change their existing workflow patterns (see "For professionals" in Bibliography). Having these systems in place where office staff are actively involved in screening follow-up can save clinician time at subsequent visits trying to piece together why referral evaluations were not done.
  - *Enlist care coordination services*—Medicaid and other state health programs may have care coordination services available for children with special health care needs to aid in referrals to multiple medical subspecialists.
  - *Additional surveillance*—Children at risk or with known mental, behavioral, or developmental delays should be monitored closely in the office with follow-up visits outside the routine well-visit schedule to track progress of identified concerns or until the appropriate supports are in place to address identified delays.

Bibliography

FOR PARENTS
Child Care Aware. childcareaware.org.
firstwordsproject.com.
www.aacap.org.
www.healthychildren.org.
www.kidshealth.org.
www.text4baby.org.
www.zerotothree.org/resources?type=parenting-resources.

REFERRAL AND DISABILITY RESOURCES
Early Childhood Technical Assistance Center. ectacenter.org.
Early Head Start and Head Start Center Locator. eclkc.ohs.acf.hhs.gov/center-locator.
National Association for the Education of Young Children (NAEYC). families.naeyc.org.

FOR PROFESSIONALS

Council on Children With Disabilities, Section on Developmental Behavioral Pediatrics, Bright Futures Steering Committee, and Medical Home Initiatives for Children With Special Needs Project Advisory Committee. Identifying infants and young children with developmental disorders in the medical home: an algorithm for developmental surveillance and screening. *Pediatrics*. 2006;118(1):405-420.

Harlor ADB, Bower C. Hearing assessment in infants and children: recommendations beyond neonatal screening. *Pediatrics*. 2009;124(4):1252-1263.

Noritz GH, Murphy NA, Neuromotor Screening Expert Panel. Motor delays: early identification and evaluation. *Pediatrics*. 2013;131(6):e2016-e2027.

WEB RESOURCES

American Academy of Pediatrics National Center for Medical Home Implementation. www.medicalhomeinfo.org.

Birth to 5: Watch Me Thrive. www.acf.hhs.gov/ecd/child-health-development/watch-me-thrive.

Bright Futures Tool and Resource Kit. brightfutures.aap.org/materials-and-tools/tool-and-resource-kit/Pages/default.aspx.

Developmental Screening Toolkit. www.childrenshospital.org/developmental-screening.

Learn the Signs. Act Early. www.cdc.gov/ncbddd/actearly/index.html.

Screening Technical Assistance and Resource Center (STAR Center). www.aap.org/en-us/advocacy-and-policy/aap-health-initiatives/Screening/Pages/default.aspx.

BOOKS

Dixon SD, Stein MT. *Encounters with Children: Pediatric Behavior and Development*. 4th ed. Philadelphia, PA: Mosby Elsevier; 2006.

Glascoe FP, Marks KP, Poon JK, Macias MM, eds. *Identifying and Addressing Developmental Behavioral Problems: A Practical Guide for Medical and non-medical Professionals, Trainees, Researchers, and Advocates*. Nolensville, TN: PEDStest.com, LLC; 2013.

Hagan JF, Shaw JS, Duncan PM, eds. *Bright Futures: Guidelines for Health Supervision of Infants, Children, and Adolescents*. 4th ed. Elk Grove Village, IL: American Academy of Pediatrics; 2017.

CHAPTER 6

Behavioral and Emotional Screening

Terry Stancin | Ellen C. Perrin | Julie Pajek

I. **DESCRIPTION OF THE PROBLEM.** Regular developmental screening in pediatric settings is important because effective interventions lead to more positive impact if children are identified and referred for appropriate services as early as possible. Systematic screening protocols should include indications of cognitive, language, motor, and emotional/behavioral difficulties. In this chapter we will address screening for emotional/behavioral symptoms.

Studies in primary care settings have shown that close to 25% of children have significant emotional/behavioral problems. Recent research has shown that many emotional and behavioral disorders manifest recognizable symptoms as early as the first 3–5 years of life—thus providing an opportunity for prevention and early intervention. However, pediatric clinicians fail to identify many of these early symptoms, and effective programs to help parents manage early signs of difficulties and prevent their escalation are rarely available in pediatric settings. Clinicians refer successfully only a minority of children to mental health professionals for further evaluation and treatment.

Effective monitoring for emotional/behavioral difficulties consists of repeated observations and periodic *screening* using validated instruments at regular intervals in the context of routine pediatric care. This surveillance of a child's emotional and behavioral health status should be a part of every health supervision visit. Following positive screening results, further evaluation may be performed by pediatric clinicians and/or a mental health consultant. Growing numbers of pediatric practices are employing psychologists and/or social workers to be on-site partners to assist with screening, further evaluation, preventive strategies, and short-term treatments, and to facilitate effective referrals for longer therapy.

II. **SELECTION AND UTILIZATION OF EMOTIONAL/BEHAVIORAL SCREENING INSTRUMENTS.** Most viable screening methods available for emotional/behavioral problems rely on caregiver reports, often via questionnaires or rating scales. For youth 11 years and older, several self-report measures are available. Standardized screening instruments may allow comparisons to normative standards, analogous to showing parents a child's weight on a standardized growth chart. Most can be administered in advance of clinical encounters and scored easily by clerical staff and thus are efficient and inexpensive methods for collecting information. As electronic web-based methods of administering and scoring such questionnaires become more widespread and accepted, the efficiency and utility of their use will increase further. Rating scales can be an excellent way to collect and compare the opinions of multiple observers as well, e.g., from both parents and from teachers.

The use of standardized screening instruments and other systematic procedures have been shown to increase identification of child behavior problems in primary care settings. Formal screening procedures should be psychometrically sound, acceptable to parents, accurate, cost-effective, and fit into the practice setting. Monitoring of behavioral/emotional status using standardized instruments should occur within the context of a clinical evaluation of every child, combining information from the checklist with the history, direct observation, physical examination, and diagnostic tests.

A. **Factors to be considered for selection of instruments.** Selection of instruments depends on the particular goals of screening but should take into consideration the following factors:
   - Age of the child to be screened
   - Informants (parent, teacher, and child)
   - Characteristics of available screening tools (sensitivity, specificity, acceptability, efficiency, and cost)
   - Training and supervision of staff necessary for implementation and maintenance of screening procedures
   - Cost and reimbursement issues

- Procedures for implementing and tracking further evaluation and interventions of children who screen positive
- Mental health resources available
- Possible adverse consequences of screening

Table 6-1 contains a list of some behavioral screening instruments that have been recommended because of their acceptable psychometric characteristics and utility in primary care settings. Ongoing comparative studies are important to assist with decisions about selecting one instrument over others.

B. **Types of emotional/behavioral screening instruments**
- Tools intended for regular screening in primary care contexts are generally short and appropriate to administer routinely to parents of all children, either at home before the pediatric visit or while in the waiting room. These are "**first-level**" screening instruments that can be completed and scored in less than 10 minutes. Increasingly such instruments can be made available electronically. First-level screening measures typically address *global/general functioning* across many domains of emotional and behavioral and family functioning.
- Specific high-frequency *targeted conditions* (e.g., attention problems, depression, anxiety) may merit routine, first-level screening among children of specific ages or populations. For example, clinicians may elect to screen all adolescents for depression and substance abuse. Likewise targeted screening for ADHD or anxiety disorders may be implemented with children based on parental concerns or for children with known developmental challenges or strong family history. First-level targeted screening methods should be used with caution to be sure not to overlook other co-occurring problems not addressed by narrow measures.
- A "**second-level**" assessment instrument may follow positive results of a first-level screening or whenever a clinician suspects or identifies a specific emotional/behavioral problem. These longer questionnaires or checklists are completed by a parent and/or an older child or administered by the pediatrician or a mental health consultant. They are often available in formats for completion by multiple observers including teachers. *Second-level targeted screening tests* elicit more details about the nature and severity of specific suspected concerns (e.g., ADHD, depression, anxiety).
- For concerns about a child's overall well-being and functioning across multiple domains, a broad *multidimensional behavioral checklist* may be appropriate as a second-level follow-up to screening. These measures have normative standards for comparison of severity of problems across different domains.

C. **Cautions regarding the use of standardized screening questionnaires**
- Screening is intended to identify those in need of further evaluation and assessment, not to provide a diagnosis. Clinicians should never base a diagnosis on screening test results only.
- Screening is not a goal in and of itself, but rather an entry into a system of care. In developing a screening program in a primary care setting, it is important to have in place a system for follow-up actions and tracking of positive screening results.
- Interpretation of screening test results must consider the fact that caregiver's perceptions are subject to biases. Procedures that rely on parent report may yield false-negative results when the parent does not perceive behaviors as problematic or false-positive results if the caregiver has reason to be excessively worried about certain behaviors. Use of multiple informants (including teachers) is ideal.
- Screening procedures carry costs for implementation (e.g., purchase of materials, implementation costs, scoring, and subsequent care).
- Screening places administrative demands on office staff to administer questionnaires properly. Training, supervision, and expertise are necessary to ensure proper scoring and valid interpretation of results. To properly interpret results, the clinician must be familiar with and understand the meaning of a test's psychometric properties and norms. Because of the complexities described earlier, pediatric clinicians may benefit from consultation from a knowledgeable pediatric psychologist when selecting and incorporating formal rating scales into practice.

D. **Beyond screening**
- Most pediatric clinicians will benefit from help with the *management* of children with behavioral problems even more than with their *identification*. Follow-up actions after a positive screening test may be taken by the clinician, members of the office team (including a psychologist or a social worker, if available), and/or referral to a community-based mental health clinician.

Table 6-1 • SELECTED BEHAVIORAL SCREENING TOOLS

Title of Instrument	Screening Focus	Informant*	Ages (Years)	Free in Public Domain	Comments	Link
First-Level Global Screening Measures						
Ages and Stages Questionnaire (ASQ)—Social Emotional, 2nd ed (SE-2)	Social-emotional/behavior	Parent	0.5–5		8 questionnaires for different ages. Assesses domains of communication, gross motor, fine motor, problem-solving, and personal-social. Used alone or in conjunction with the ASQ-3.	http://www.agesandstages.com
Baby Pediatric Symptom Checklist	Social-emotional/behavior	Parent	0–1½	X	12 items comprise 3 subscales assessing infant behaviors. Component of the Survey of Wellbeing of Young Children. Scores of 3+ on any subscale suggest a child is "at risk" and needs further evaluation.	https://www.floatinghospital.org/The-Survey-of-Wellbeing-of-Young-Children/Parts-of-the-SWYC/BPSC.aspx
Brief Infant-Toddler Social-Emotional Assessment Scale (BITSEA)	Emotional competencies and problems	Parent	1–4		42 items drawn from the longer version (ITSEA) yield Problems and Competence scores that suggest "possible problem" or "possible delay."	http://www.pearsonclinical.com/childhood/products/100000150/brief-infant-toddler-social-emotional-assessment-bitsea.html
Early Childhood Screening Assessment (ECSA)	Emotional and behavioral functioning	Parent	1½–5	X	36 items assessing child emotional functioning + 4 items assessing parental distress. Cutoff score of 18+ warrants additional assessment.	http://www.infantinstitute.org/wp-content/uploads/2013/07/ECSA-Manual-0509.pdf
Parents' Evaluation of Developmental Status (PEDS)	Development, behavior, social-emotional/mental health	Parent	0–8		10 items assessing whether parent concerns about child's cognitive, language, and motor development indicate possible developmental problems.	www.pedstest.com
Pediatric Symptom Checklist (PSC)	General psychological functioning	Parent	4–16	X	35-item and shorter 17-item versions available. Cutoff scores depend on age.	http://www.massgeneral.org/psychiatry/services/psc_forms.aspx

Measure	Domain	Respondent	Age		Description	URL
Pediatric Symptom Checklist—Youth Report (Y-PSC)	Social-emotional/behavior	Adolescent	11–16	X	35-item, self-report measure. Cutoff scores depending on age suggest impairment in need of further evaluation.	http://psc.partners.org/psc_english_Y.pdf
Preschool Pediatric Symptom Checklist (P-PSC)	Social-emotional/behavior	Parent	1½–5	X	18-item component of the Survey of Wellbeing of Young Children. Scores of 9+ suggest a child is "at risk" and needs further evaluation.	https://www.floatinghospital.org/The-Survey-of-Wellbeing-of-Young-Children/Parts-of-the-SWYC/PPSC.aspx
Strengths and Difficulties Questionnaire (SDQ)	General behavioral functioning	Parent, teacher, adolescent	3–16	X	25 items of positive and negative attributes. Scores interpretable as normal, borderline, or abnormal.	http://www.sdqinfo.com
First-Level Targeted Symptom Screening Measures						
CAGE – AID	Substance abuse	Adolescent	12–17	X	4-item questionnaire. 1+ positive response indicates positive screen for substance abuse.	https://www.integration.samhsa.gov/images/res/CAGEAID.pdf
Center of Epidemiologic Studies Depression Scale (CESD)	Depression	Child/adolescent	6–17	X	20 items. Cutoff score of 15+ suggests symptoms of depression.	http://cesd-r.com/
CRAFT (Car, Relax, Alone, Forget, Friends, Trouble)	Substance abuse	Adolescent	11–21	X	Interview format. 3 or 9 items, depending on responses to initial questions. Scores suggest "low" or "high" risk of substance use disorders.	http://www.ceasar-boston.org/CRAFFT/pdf/CRAFFT_English.pdf
Generalized Anxiety Disorder – 7 (GAD – 7)	Anxiety	Child/adolescent	13+	X	7 items. Cutoff scores suggest mild, moderate, and severe levels of anxiety.	http://www.phqscreeners.com/sites/g/files/g1001626 1/f/201412/GAD-7_English.pdf

(continued)

Table 6-1 • SELECTED BEHAVIORAL SCREENING TOOLS   (CONTINUED)

Title of Instrument	Screening Focus	Informant*	Ages (Years)	Free in Public Domain	Comments	Link
Patient Health Questionnaire modified for Adolescents (PHQ-A)—2 and 9	Depression	Parent, adolescent	12+	X	2-item and 9-item versions available. Rates severity of symptoms of depression, including suicidal ideation.	http://www.phqscreeners.com/sites/g/files/g1001626 1/f/201412/PHQ-9_English.pdf
NICHQ Vanderbilt Assessment Scales	ADHD	Parent, teacher	4–12	X	Initial and briefer follow-up versions available. Gathers impressions of child's behavior parallel to DSM-5 symptoms. Additional items screen for oppositional defiant disorder (ODD), conduct problems, anxiety/depression.	https://www.nichq.org/resource/nichq-vanderbilt-assessment-scales
Second-Level Targeted Screening Measures						
Children's Depression Inventory (CDI)	Depression	Child/adolescent	7–17		27 items grouped into 5 factors. Raw scores converted to T-scores and suggest severity of depressive symptoms.	http://www.pearsonclinical.com/psychology/products/100000636/childrens-depression-inventory-2-cdi-2.html
Conners Comprehensive Behavior Rating Scales	ADHD and other mental health concerns	Parent, teacher, child/adolescent	3–17		Short (e.g., 45 items) and long (e.g., 110 items) versions available. Includes items relevant to ADHD common comorbid disorders. Scores are compared with normative sample to indicate the level of concern.	https://www.wpspublish.com/store/p/2713/conners-3-conners-third-edition
Mood and Feelings Questionnaire (MFQ)	Depression	Parent, child/adolescent	7+	X	Short (13 items) and long (33 items) versions available. Scoring 12+ on short version and 27+ on long version may indicate depression.	http://devepi.duhs.duke.edu/mfq.html
Screen for Child Anxiety Related Disorder (SCARED)	Anxiety	Parent, child/adolescent	8–18	X	41 items, 5 factors that mirror DSM classifications. Total and subscale cutoff scores suggest heightened anxiety.	http://www.psychiatry.pitt.edu/sites/default/files/Documents/assessments/SCARED%20Child.pdf

Instrument	Construct	Reporter	Age range		Description	Web site
SNAP – IV	ADHD, ODD	Parent, teacher	6–18	X	90- and 18-item versions available. Scales are summed and cutoff scores suggest ADHD/ODD.	https://www.addrc.org/child-adolescent-screening-tests/
Spence Children's Anxiety Scale (SCAS)	Anxiety	Parent, child/adolescent	6–18 3–5 for preschool	X	38 items, 6 subscales designed to broadly map on to DSM classifications.	https://www.scaswebsite.com/
Strengths and Weaknesses of ADHD Symptoms (SWAN)	ADHD	Parent, teacher	6–18	X	30- and 18-item versions available. Designed to help identify ADHD and distinguish between subtypes.	https://www.attention-point.com/x_upload/media/images/swan-description-questions.pdf
Second-Level, Multidimensional Assessment Measures						
Behavior Assessment System for Children (BASC-3)	Emotional and behavioral functioning	Parent, teacher, child/adolescent	2–22		Broad-based measure of pathology. Provides a profile of internalizing and externalizing problems; other problems (atypicality, withdrawal); and adaptive skills. Standard T-scores provide norm-based comparisons by age and gender.	http://www.pearsonclinical.com/education/products/100001402/behavior-assessment-system-for-children-third-edition-basc-3.html
Child Behavior Checklists (CBCL, TRF, C-TRF, YSR)	Emotional and behavioral functioning	Parent, teacher, child/adolescent	1½–18		Broad-based measure of pathology. Provides a profile of internalizing and externalizing problems. Standard T-scores provide norm-based comparisons by age and gender, with DSM-compatible scales.	http://www.aseba.org/
Infant-Toddler Social-Emotional Assessment Scale (ITSEA)	Emotional competencies and problems of infants and toddlers	Parent, child-care provider	1–4		166 items comprising 17 subscales address 4 domains that focus on strengths and weaknesses. Three clusters can be calculated: maladaptive, social relatedness, and atypical.	http://www.pearsonclinical.com/childhood/products/100000652/infant-toddler-social-emotional-assessment-itsea.html

Portions adapted from Perrin E, Stancin T. A continuing dilemma: whether and how to screen for concerns about children's behavior in primary care settings. *Pediatr Rev.* 2002;23:264-282 and From Stancin T, Aylward GP. Screening instruments: behavioral and developmental. In: Ollendick T, Schroeder C, eds, *Encyclopedia of Pediatric and Child Psychology.* New York: Kluwer Academic/Plenum Publishers; 2003:574-577. Test author information available upon request and at most test Web sites. Parent = parent or a primary caregiver.

- Communication between mental health professionals and primary care clinicians is often cumbersome and frequently inadequate. Therefore, a collaborative relationship with one or more mental health professionals integrated into the practice or in the community is advisable.
- Models of colocated, collaborative, and integrated care offer important opportunities to create increased access to behavioral health services to extend the capacity for pediatricians to manage care in their practices. However, improved payment mechanisms are urgently needed to create a fully responsive system for regular and comprehensive child health supervision and care.

Bibliography

Briggs-Gowan MJ, Carter AS. Social-emotional screening status in early childhood predicts elementary school outcomes. *Pediatrics*. 2008;121(5):957-962.

Godoy L, Carter AS. Identifying and addressing mental health risks and problems in primary care pediatric settings. *Am J Orthopsychiatry*. 2013;83:73-88.

Perrin E, Stancin T. A continuing dilemma: whether and how to screen for concerns about children's behavior in primary care settings. *Pediatr Rev*. 2002;23:264-282.

Vogels AGC, Crone MR, Hoekstra F, et al. Comparing three short questionnaires to detect psychosocial dysfunction among primary school children: a randomized method. *BMC Public Health*. 2009;9:489.

Weitzman W, The Section on Developmental and Behavioral Pediatrics, Committee on Psychosocial Aspects of Child and Family Health, Council on Early Childhood, Society for Developmental and Behavioral Pediatrics. Promoting optimal development: screening for behavioral and emotional problems. *Pediatrics*. 2015;135(2):384-395.

CHAPTER 7

Parental Depression: Implications for Pediatrics

Barry Zuckerman

I. DESCRIPTION OF THE PROBLEM. Parental depression is a risk factor for children's health, social–emotional and cognitive development, and behavior. Because mothers are commonly the primary caregivers and their depression likely has a more direct effect on children, most studies focus on mothers' depression. Potential adverse outcomes for a child include low birth weight, behavior problems, somatic complaints, learning difficulties, poor growth, accidents, and mental health problems especially depression.

The term "depression" may refer to:
- Depressive symptoms/mood that consists of feelings of sadness, hopelessness, and gloom.
- Major depressive disorder. In the *Diagnostic and Statistical Manual of Mental Disorders, Fifth Edition* (DSM-5), diagnosis of depression is more than just sadness; it involves a loss of interest or pleasure, an emotional emptiness, and a feeling of "flatness." A diagnosable condition is more likely when these feelings are intense, persistent, and interfere with everyday living consistent with specific DSM-5 criteria.

Child-rearing itself appears to be an important factor associated with an increased risk of depression among women.

II. EPIDEMIOLOGY

A. Mothers. Approximately 12% of mothers will have a diagnosis of depression during their child-rearing years, including 1%–7% with a major depressive disorder. Depressive symptoms are twice as common and can occur among 20%–50% of mothers with highest rates (40%–60%) among poor mothers. Other risk factors for depression are isolated and stressed mothers, minority mothers, and mothers with children with chronic disease or disability and family history of depression.

B. Fathers. Approximately 4% of fathers will be depressed in child's first year and by age 12 years, almost 20% of father's will have had an episode of depression.

C. Postpartum depression. Up to 1 in 7 women may experience postpartum depression days or even months after delivering a baby; it can last for many weeks or months if left untreated. The DSM-5 does not recognize postpartum depression as a separate diagnosis; rather, patients must meet the criteria for a major depressive episode and the criteria for the peripartum-onset specifier. The definition is therefore a major depressive episode with an onset in pregnancy or within 4 weeks of delivery. Postpartum depression disproportionately affects low-income and minority women.

Postpartum blues, on the other hand, occur in about 40% of mothers and consist of daily or less episodes of sadness and crying following delivery for 1–2 weeks.

Very severe sometimes called "psychotic" depression occurs in about one to three of a thousand women who are severely impaired with symptoms including paranoia, delusions, and suicidal and homicidal thoughts. These mothers need timely identification and help, including medication, because they are unable to care for their babies and in rare instances harm them.

III. IDENTIFICATION. For most parents, child health supervision visits may be the only consistent ongoing contact they may have with a health care clinician. This affords a special opportunity for the child health clinician to identify a depressed parent by their affect and/or concerns about their child's behavior or child-rearing problems. A rule of thumb is that when a child is having trouble, there is a high likelihood that one parent is depressed as a cause and/or consequence of child's difficulty. The clinician can help the parents understand how their mood might affect parenting and contribute to the child's symptoms. It is important to keep a high level of suspicion of parental depression when child's behavior problems such as sleep, social isolation, out-of-control behavior, and family stress are discussed during the young child health visit. In school-age children and adolescents, difficulties in child behavior and impaired functioning at home, school, or with peers should alert the clinician to the possibility of parental depression as well. Children from families with a history of depression are especially at risk to become depressed or display other mental health problems especially during adolescence.

IV. CLINICAL ROLE

A. Screening. Clinicians should use a structured screening instrument followed by additional information or referral for further evaluation or treatment if needed. Both the American Academy of Pediatrics and US Public Health Task force recommend routine screening for mothers at pediatric visits at 1, 2, 4, and 6 months. Fathers should also be screened if they are present at the visit as well. Screening or specific questions listed below should be used at any visit when there is suspicion of depression due to parents affect or children's behavior problem as described earlier.

Options include the following:
- Edinburgh Postnatal Depression Scale
- Center for Epidemiological Studies Depression—Revised (CESD-R)
- Patient Health Questionnaire 9 (PHQ 9)
- Patient Health Questionnaire 2 (PHQ 2)

In 2016, emphasizing the importance of screening for maternal depression, the Center for Medicare and Medicaid Services (CMS) issued a statement that states Medicaid programs should pay for such screening. Many but not all states developed payment policies.

B. Interview. When mothers or fathers exhibit a depressed affect or express hopelessness or lack of energy, clinicians can revise some of the screening questions above by stating empathically: *"you seem depressed, sad or irritable, are you?"* If they answer no, the clinician can then administer the PHQ 2: Over the past 2 weeks:

1. Have you ever felt down, depressed, or hopeless?

2. Have you felt little interest or pleasure in doing things?

One yes answer is a positive screening result. This screen is suitable to indicate risk of depression for adults in general and is not specific to postpartum depression.

Depression involves dysfunction of the body's regulatory system, so individuals with depression can have dysregulated sleeping, eating, affect, and motor activity. Clinicians can ask *"How is your sleeping? are you sleeping more or less than usual? How is your appetite? are you eating more or less than usual and are you more lethargic or restless than usual?"* The clinician should be more concerned if parents express one of these changes along with feeling sad. Follow-up questions can include *"it's hard work being a parent, and many parents in my practice go through ups and downs. Are you worried about how you feel? Do you think you can feel better? Would you like to?"* Although parents do not usually expect pediatric clinicians to inquire about their health, it is usually accepted and appreciated when done in the context of a trusting and caring clinician–parent relationship. In fact, parents who demonstrate a depressed affect or verbalize depressed feelings may often be asking for help. The parents who hide their feelings and affect will probably not be identified by a pediatric clinician.

V. PEDIATRIC MANAGEMENT.

If a parent has depressive symptoms—feeling sad or angry—clinicians can help them identify the social origin of these feelings, including marital discord, isolation, and material stressors such as financial resources, as a helpful first step. The next step is to help them develop a plan to address these problems. This might include referral to a social service agency, marital counseling, or a community-based parent support group. Because behavior problems in young children are associated with maternal depression, helping the mother manage the child's behavior problem may also help relieve her feelings of helplessness. Examples include basic instruction or behavior management to help resolve a child's sleep problems or out-of-control behavior. This is not a substitute for addressing the mother's depressive symptoms.

The needs of the children will depend on the range of other supports in the family and neighborhood and the severity of the parents' condition. For school-age children it is important to assess how children cognitively understand their parents' symptoms. As part of children's egocentric thinking, they may feel responsible for the parents' episodes of sadness, withdrawal, and anger. At times they may even be accused of causing the symptoms by the other parent.

If a screening or interview seems to indicate the presence of a diagnosable depression, especially if depressed affect is obvious and/or somatic symptoms are present, then the clinician should present the assessment to the parents and ask whether they would like help. Open discussion should lead to mental health referral for further assessment and treatment.

One way to help encourage parents to seek help is by appealing to their basic concern for their children. Mothers can be asked how their feelings of sadness are expressed at home (e.g., crying, yelling, withdrawal) and what impact they believe this has on their children. Any implications that the mother is being blamed for poor mothering should be avoided. Depressed mothers will be especially vulnerable to both feeling guilty and blaming themselves for everything. To facilitate referral, clinicians can ask: "would you like me to refer you to someone who may help you feel better?" The clinician can refer to any insight the mother may have expressed and say *your ability to express insight into your feelings mean you will likely be helped by a therapist.*

If a parent is resistant to seeking help, the clinician should schedule a follow-up in a few weeks to check the status. This expression of concern also prevents the parent from feeling rejected by the clinician. If, on a follow-up visit, the pediatric clinician believes the parents' depression is preventing them from seeking help and there is concern for child safety, protective services may need to be consulted although this is very rare. Practices who have integrated mental health clinicians available are often more successful in making the link to mental health referrals.

Bibliography

FOR PARENTS

POEM: Perinatal Outreach and Encouragement for Moms. http://www.poemon.ine.org.
Postpartum Support International. http://www.postpartum.net.

FOR PROFESSIONAL

AAP. https://www.aap.org/en-us/advocacy-and-policy/aap-health-initiatives/Screening/Pages/Maternal-Depression.aspx.
Earls MF. The Committee on Psychosocial Aspects of Child and Family Health. Incorporating recognition and management of perinatal and postpartum depression into pediatric practice. *Pediatrics.* 2010;126(5):1032-1039.
https:/mchb.hrsa.gov/sites/default/files/mchb/MaternalChildHealthTopics/maternal-woman's-health/Depression_During_and_After_Pregnancy_ENGLISH.pdf.
US Department of Health and Human Resources, Health Resources and Services Administration (HRSA).
US Preventive Services Task Force. Screening for depression: recommendations and rationale. *Ann Intern Med.* 2002;136(10):760-764.

CHAPTER 8

Parental Substance Use and Opioid-Exposed Newborns

Elisha M. Wachman | Eileen M. Costello | Davida M. Schiff

I. OVERVIEW

- The lasting impact of in utero exposure to maternal opioids and the effect of ongoing parental substance use have received renewed attention in the midst of the current epidemic of opioid use in the United States.
- Children growing up in households affected by parental substance use may experience a number of medical, behavioral, and psychosocial problems.
- Pediatric clinicians have a unique opportunity to assess substance use in families and stability of recovery for parents, particularly during the frequently scheduled well-child visits during the first 2 years of life.
  This chapter will focus on the impact of in utero exposure to opioids including the immediate management of neonatal opioid withdrawal syndrome (NOWS), the treatment of the families affected by parental substance use, and what is known about the short- and long-term developmental outcomes of opioid-exposed infants.

II. EPIDEMIOLOGY.
The rate of infants who experience withdrawal symptoms from in utero opioid exposure increased by more than fivefold between 2000 and 2012, increasing from about 1.2 infants per 1000 live births to more than 6.0 infants per 1000 live births, with higher rates in the eastern portion of the United States.

Infants who develop withdrawal symptoms may be exposed in utero to prescribed opioids for chronic pain or chronic diseases such as sickle cell disease, methadone or buprenorphine for the treatment for opioid use disorder, or illicit/nonmedical use of opioids. The severity of symptoms of opioid withdrawal in newborns vary, depending on several poorly understand factors including the type of in utero opioid exposure, type of infant nonpharmacologic and pharmacologic treatment for withdrawal symptoms, genetics, and exposure to additional maternal psychiatric medications.

Data from 2009 to 2014 National Survey on Drug Use and Health estimates that 1 in 8 children (8.7 million) aged 17 years or younger live with a parent who had a substance use disorder in the past year and 1 in 35 children (2.1 million) with a parent with an illicit drug use disorder. Approximately 3% of adults in the United States report past month prescription opioid or heroin use.

III. NEONATAL OPIOID WITHDRAWAL SYNDROME—HOSPITAL MANAGEMENT

- **Monitoring**: It is recommended that all opioid-exposed newborns be monitored in the hospital for 4–7 days for signs and symptoms of opioid withdrawal that could warrant medication treatment.
- **Testing**: Toxicology testing (urine, meconium, and/or cord blood) from the infant and/or mother should be sent around the time of delivery to determine evidence of recent maternal use.
- **NOWS symptoms**: Symptoms typically develop 2–3 days after birth for infants exposed to long-acting opioids (e.g., methadone, buprenorphine) but may occur sooner with exposures to short-acting opioids (e.g., heroin, oxycodone). Signs and symptoms are listed in Table 8-1.
- **NOWS assessment tools**: A NOWS assessment tool should be used every 3–4 hours to assess infants for signs and symptoms of withdrawal. The mostly used tool is the Finnegan Scale, with commonly accepted cutoffs of three consecutive scores >8 or two scores >12 to initiate and titrate pharmacotherapy. An alternative approach is the function-based "Eat, Sleep, Console" assessment approach, which is associated with lower rates of pharmacotherapy.
- **Nonpharmacologic care**: Nonpharmacologic care measures are first-line treatment. This includes rooming-in, skin-to-skin contact, swaddling, calm quiet environment, breastfeeding, and on-demand feeding. These measures have been associated with 30%–50% reduction in need for pharmacologic treatment.
- **Breastfeeding**: Breastfeeding should be promoted in mothers who have sought out treatment for their addiction (i.e., methadone or buprenorphine), with adequate

Table 8-1 • NOWS SIGNS AND SYMPTOMS

Neurologic	Autonomic	Gastrointestinal
Altered sleep	Fever	Poor feeding
Irritability/crying	Tachypnea	Vomiting
High muscle tone	Sweating	Diarrhea
Tremors	Yawning	
Hyperactive startle	Sneezing	
Myoclonic jerks	Skin excoriations	

prenatal care, and no illicit drug use around the time of delivery. Breastfeeding recommendations for oral short-acting licit opioids are dependent on total daily dose. (Recommend following current guidelines in Hale and Rowe, *Medications in Mothers' Milk.*) Codeine (given risk of higher concentrations in high metabolizers) should be used with caution. Hepatitis C infection in the mother is not a contraindication to breastfeeding, unless a mother has cracked, bleeding nipples.
- **Pharmacologic treatment**: Infants who meet criteria to initiate pharmacologic treatment should be treated with replacement opioids. First-line agents may include the following:
  - Morphine
  - Methadone
  - Buprenorphine

  Opioids are typically titrated until symptoms are improved, as measured by standardized scoring tools such as the Finnegan Scale or Eat, Sleep, Console approaches described earlier, and then weaned by 10%–20% daily. Infants should be monitored for 24–48 hours off opioids before discharging home. Second-line agents include phenobarbital or clonidine. There is insufficient evidence to support one pharmacologic agent over another for either first- or second-line agents.
- **Inpatient outcomes**: NOWS inpatient outcomes vary significantly according to treatment protocol and hospital setting, as well as coexposures such as maternal psychiatric medications, tobacco, and other drugs/alcohol exposure. Overall, 30%–80% of opioid-exposed infants are treated pharmacologically, with an average length of hospitalization of 18–22 days.
- **Safe discharge evaluation**: Before discharge, all families should be evaluated by social work, and state-specific policies should be followed regarding reporting to child welfare agencies to determine safety of discharge home with the parents.

IV. ISSUES OF PARENTAL ADDICTION AND IMPACT ON PRIMARY CARE. Primary care for the substance-exposed newborn (SEN) is best achieved with a multigenerational lens and team approach, as many parents in recovery have comorbid medical or mental health conditions that can have an impact on the child's health through caregiving environment. Parents are often highly motivated in their recovery early in the postpartum period. Supporting parents in their recovery can be critical to promoting the health and well-being of their infants and children.
- An ideal medical home for substance-exposed families includes primary care and selected others, e.g., developmental pediatricians, social work, nursing, and case management to help parents keep track of their own care as well as the many appointments that SENs require in the first months of life.
- Referral to community agencies that support parenting, including a home visiting program if available, will optimize outcomes for infants and parents and promote likelihood of success.
- Parents with opioid use disorders may have other children not currently in their care, which can increase the anxiety concerning the role of Child Protective Services.
- Open communication with parents about the pediatric clinician's role as child and family advocate with safety as a primary consideration is critical. Clear expectations about a clinician's response to disclosure of parental relapse will strengthen the relationship with a primary care provider.

  Parents, particularly mothers, with substance use disorders often have a history of trauma, contributing to the development of their substance use disorder or a consequence of their substance use. In the primary care setting this may translate into heightened anxiety about typical issues of infants and children surrounding sleeping and eating, crying, arching, diaper rashes, etc. A trusting, therapeutic relationship is critical to be able to provide reassurance. All parents should receive mental health services after the birth as part of their ongoing substance use disorder treatment plan.

Signed releases of information early in the primary care relationship will help team members communicate with community agencies, Child Protective Services, childcare programs, and others working to promote wellness in the mother/infant dyad. Clear communication with families over the sharing of information across agencies and providers is important to an open dialogue among members of the care team of the family.

V. PEARLS FOR CARING FOR THE CHILD IN PRIMARY CARE

- **Fussy babies**: Once discharged from the inpatient setting, infants may continue to exhibit milder symptoms of withdrawal such as crying, fussiness, increased tone, loose stools, and sneezing. These symptoms typically do not warrant medication treatment, and mothers should be reassured that they are doing the right caregiving to prevent them from believing they are doing something wrong. Educating caretakers about swaddling and holding to console infants is important and will relieve anxiety about these symptoms. Weekly visits for the first 4 weeks after discharge can allay anxiety and provide opportunity for anticipatory guidance and relationship building.
- **Hepatitis C**: Many women with a history of injection drug use will also be infected with hepatitis C. Maternal hepatitis C antibodies will be present at birth and can remain positive for up to 18 months, yet transmission of hepatitis C virus (HCV) itself is uncommon. Infants should be monitored with screening of HCV antibody and RNA and LFTs every 6 months, starting between 2 and 6 months of age and until Ab test is negative. Additionally, parents should be encouraged to seek curative treatment once they are stable in their recovery.
- **Growth**: Elevated rates of low birth weight, prematurity, and increased metabolic needs due to opioid withdrawal contribute to the increased caloric requirements for infants with in utero opioid exposure to maintain adequate weight gain. The low birth weight is multifactorial and often related to coexposure to nicotine in 80% (a primary care opportunity for maternal intervention to improve the health of the family). Microcephaly is not uncommon and places child at significant risk for developmental delay. 22–24 calories per ounce is the typical caloric supplementation until catch-up growth is achieved.
- **Ocular comorbidities**: Ophthalmic abnormalities in infants and children with a history of in utero opioid exposure (particularly methadone) include reduced acuity, nystagmus, delayed visual maturation, strabismus, refractive errors, and cerebral visual impairment. For this reason it is recommended that all infants be referred for ophthalmologic evaluation between 4 and 6 months of age.
- **Diaper rashes**: SENs have higher rates of diaper rash with skin breakdown due to increased frequency of stools. Keeping clean and dry and exposing to air before application of barrier creams is an effective strategy.
- **Compassionate care**: Mothers with opioid use disorders are vulnerable. They may have trauma history and/or history of incarceration, report feeling judged and treated with scorn, and may feel guilt and shame about their child's prenatal exposure. Open communication and understanding about the stress of early recovery while caring for an infant goes a long way toward building trust and developing a team to foster the best possible outcome for the child.

VI. NEURODEVELOPMENTAL OUTCOMES.
Children born to women with substance use disorders are at higher risk for poor developmental outcomes and difficulties with attachment, behavior, and learning. Unstable living arrangements, high levels of stress, and insufficient stimulation further contribute to poor outcomes. All such infants and toddlers with NOWS should be referred for an Early Intervention evaluation upon discharge from the hospital. Regular developmental surveillance with primary care is critical with referral to a developmental specialist as indicated. Of note, studies examining the neurodevelopmental outcomes of children with in utero opioid exposure are primarily based on retrospective data or large population-based studies and are largely inconclusive and conflicting. Studies often fail to account for important differences in prenatal exposures, maternal and neonatal treatment regimens, and postnatal environmental factors. The findings of these preliminary studies are summarized below.

A. Short term (<12 months)
- Ocular abnormalities (see above).
- Infants who have been pharmacologically treated for NOWS are at higher risk for poor regulation and quality of movements in the first few months of life.
- Developmental outcomes in the first year of life are often within normal limits with little differences found based on neonatal pharmacologic treatment regimens.

B. Long term (1–15 years)
- Research is ongoing on the long term developmental impact.
- Children with a history of a NOWS diagnosis are at higher risk of not meeting educational standards at 8–15 years.
- Children with in utero opioid exposure are at higher risk for worse executive function and lower IQ scores compared with controls, however, still performing within the normal range for IQ.
- Children are at increased risk for attentional and behavioral problems.
- Children of parents with opioid use disorders are 10 times more likely to develop an opioid addiction than controls due to a combination of genetic, epigenetic, and environmental factors. This is an opportunity for primary care intervention and counseling in the adolescent years.

Bibliography

FOR PROFESSIONALS

Baldacchino A, Arbuckle K, Petrie DJ, McCowan C. Neurobehavioral consequences of chronic intrauterine opioid exposure in infants and preschool children: a systematic review and meta-analysis. *BMC Psychiatry*. 2015;14:104. doi:10.1186/1471-244X-14-104.

Grossman MR, Berkwitt AK, Osborn RR, et al. An initiative to improve the quality of care of infants with neonatal abstinence syndrome. *Pediatrics*. 2017;139(6). doi:10.1542/peds.2016-3360.

Hudak ML, Tan RC, Committee on Drugs, Committee on Fetus and Newborn, American Academy of Pediatrics. Neonatal drug withdrawal. *Pediatrics*. 2012;129(2):e540-e560. doi:10.1542/peds.2011-3212.

Ko JY, Patrick SW, Tong VT, Patel R, Lind JN, Barfield WD. Incidence of neonatal abstinence syndrome - 28 States, 1999-2013. *MMWR Morb Mortal Wkly Rep*. 2016;65(31):799-802.

Nygaard E, Moe V, Slinning K, Walhovd KB. Longitudinal cognitive development of children born to mothers with opioid and polysubstance use. *Pediatr Res*. 2015;78(3):330-335.

Reece-Stremtan S, Marinelli KA. ABM clinical protocol #21: guidelines for breastfeeding and substance use or substance use disorder, revised 2015. *Breastfeed Med*. 2015;10(3):135-141.

Smith VC, Wilson CR, Committee on Substance Use and Prevention. Families affected by parental substance use. *Pediatrics*. 2016;138(2):e20161575. doi:10.1542/peds.2016-1575.

Wachman EM, Schiff DM, Silverstein M. Neonatal abstinence syndrome: advances in diagnosis and treatment. *JAMA*. 2018;319(13):1362-1374.

CHAPTER 9

Helping Families Deal with Bad News

Angela M. Feraco | Richard D. Goldstein

I. ISSUES IN DELIVERING BAD NEWS. The task of sharing bad news is among a clinician's most solemn responsibilities and a special human encounter. In addition to competently understanding the medical facts to be shared, it demands presence and authenticity on the part of the clinician. Balancing honesty with encouragement and, fundamentally, some hope requires focus, practice, and reflection. Clinicians may struggle to find this balance and often enter these conversations with discomfort and feelings of incomplete preparation.

A. What is bad news?. Sharing bad news involves complex medical communication during critical life events. In pediatrics, disclosing bad news may include initial discussions of a life-altering diagnosis, such as a chronic or life-threatening illness or a developmental disability. But bad news is not simply a function of the severity of the disease process. It also refers to the impact of the shared information on the recipients' sense of quality and meaning in life, their expectations, and their goals. As such, identifying the many complex reactions aroused in patients and their parents is crucial to providing meaningful family-centered care.

B. More than a communication of facts. Cassell has written that "the imperative to tell the truth seems an insufficient guide to what you should tell patients." A more complete perspective requires that the sharing of information reduces uncertainty, provides a basis for action, and strengthens the patient–clinician relationship. This becomes possible when the clinician looks beyond stating facts and prognosis and attempts to appreciate *how* the receiver of the information will understand the matters being addressed. This patient-centered approach involves attempting to grasp how the new reality and options might seem to the patient and family and helping them with first steps in its integration. Information and the way it is conveyed can be important therapeutic tools with direct implications for later management.

Studies document long-lasting consequences of poorly perceived disclosure, including impaired patient–doctor alliance and negative parent perceptions of the clinician's attitude toward the child. Conversely, successfully conveyed bad news can establish helpful themes and foci for the parents to use in their efforts to clarify the goals of their child's care.

C. The clinician's role. Six prototypes of the physician sharing bad news have been described: the inexperienced messenger, the emotionally burdened, the rough and ready, the benevolent but tactless, the distanced doctor, and the empathic professional. These reflect different approaches to navigating patient boundaries, with the emotionally burdened doctor perhaps employing insufficient boundaries while the distanced doctor veers too far. Imparting complex medical information requires identification and acknowledgment of the patient/parent's emotions upon hearing life-altering news while also maintaining the role of guiding expert. This is best exemplified in the approach of the empathic professional. While this approach may be more likely to impart hope, each approach may have some strengths.

It is important for the clinician to understand his or her personal feelings before attempting to communicate bad news. Commonly expressed fears include being at fault and blamed, unleashing a disagreeable reaction, or not knowing all the answers during a critical conversation. Understanding that these apprehensions exist and working to minimize their impact helps increase the potential for meaningful communication. Many clinicians feel that the skills involved in this communication are untaught or unknown and worry about performing at the level the situation demands. Clinicians may also experience personal discomfort with illness and death, which can exhibit itself as discomfort with hopelessness.

Minimizing clinician-based impediments to communication is not simply a matter of acting in the way the clinician believes the recipient desires, but rather one of assuring that this communication does not undermine a parent or dissolve hope. It is important to reinforce the goals the family has for their child. Most of the time, there will be opportunities for further refinements in the future and the sharing of news is the beginning of the process.

D. Difficulties with prognosis. Foreseeing the future course of an illness is often challenging, but providing meaningful anticipatory guidance to the family is a central responsibility of the clinician. When considering how to approach prognosis discussions, clinicians must consider the degree of certainty based on existing medical evidence, the parent and patient's perspectives and contexts, and their own beliefs and tendencies. Studies investigating prognosis have found that clinicians are accurate only 20% of the time and tend to be overly optimistic. Although studies have shown that more experienced clinicians tend to have less error, there is also a correlation between the length of a relationship with a patient and a lowered likelihood that the shared prognosis will be correct. Despite this tendency toward error on the part of clinicians, patients nonetheless seek clear disclosure. They interpret hidden or minimal information as their doctor withholding frightening information. Patients who receive more elements of prognostic disclosure are more likely to report communication-related hope, even when the likelihood of cure is low. Equally important is to tell parents the concrete ways their child's condition will change and be monitored over time. Foretelling the quality and likely burdens in the patient's and family's life through this predicted course is a separate set of considerations beyond timelines and is worthy of its own attention.

II. THE PROCESS OF DELIVERING BAD NEWS. Different circumstances present different constraints. It would be simplistic and inaccurate to portray the successful giving of bad news as following a formula. It relies not only on technique, but also on experience and instinct. There are, however, certain helpful keys to a successful encounter.

A. Tell the family as soon as possible and in person. Studies of parents' reactions to bad news about their children have demonstrated that most families prefer to be told as soon as the health care provider suspects there is a problem. Sensitive clinicians must feel comfortable sharing available information, even if it is incomplete or uncertain, if the clinician spells out the steps and duration of time to obtain a firm diagnosis. Critical conversations are best not conducted by telephone. When possible, planning an in-person meeting allows the family time to make arrangements for the right people to attend.

B. Prepare a roadmap. Preparation for the sharing of bad news begins with an understanding of the facts and the clinician's emotional response to them. The communication of those facts should be organized and well-paced. This is most likely when thought has been given to the manageable number of points that the family can hear. In emotionally overwhelming encounters, parents may understand and retain relatively little. Conversely, the clinician's phrasing and word choices may be recalled years later. Before entering into this conversation, it may be helpful to rehearse the language to be used, consciously trying to speak accurately without overreliance on medical terminology. Consider whether a decision must be made during the discussion in which bad news is shared. If so, what information must be gathered to assist and prepare for this decision?

C. Prepare a space. When circumstances permit, critical information should be shared in a private and safe environment that will minimize distractions and allow for safe emotional expression by the patient/family. Except in cases of older children and adolescents (who should be involved), this is best done away from the bedside for hospitalized patients or at an arranged time for outpatients. The key decision-makers should be present, generally parents and guardians. Some thought should be given to seating arrangements, assuring that the people giving and those receiving the news are proximate. The numbers of health care personnel and family members should be restricted to the minimum necessary to assure a less distracted and more emotionally attentive interaction. Depending on the practice setting and resources available, it may be helpful to include a professional with expertise in psychosocial and spiritual care, for example, social work or clergy. The room should be supplied with tissues.

D. Make the space feel secure. Allow for all participants to come in and be seated before beginning. If possible, pagers and phones should be silenced. Once the door closes, every effort should be made for all involved to remain in the room until the interaction concludes. Everyone in the room should introduce themselves. The names of the child and the parents should be known before the conversation begins as well as how they would prefer to be addressed. It must be clear that the family has the clinician's undivided and unrushed attention.

Attention to body language can be helpful. Sitting at the same level, facing the parents and establishing eye contact, promotes directness and connection, provided it does not seem threatening. It is just as important to read the body cues of the receivers, respecting their defenses and looking for opportunities to reassuringly meet their gaze.

E. Diagnose the recipients of information. Different parents have different needs for information and details. The success of the encounter relies in part on understanding those needs and addressing them appropriately. As the meeting begins and an agenda is set out, a helpful opening can be asking parents what they understand of the situation and what they want to know. As they speak, the appropriate level of detail needed may be deduced to inform the clinician's sharing of medical information. The terminology they use can be employed, and their priorities can be reflected in the ensuing discussion. The requirement for being socially and culturally attuned cannot be overstated. All who will share bad news must be mindful of the variable implications and interpretations of language, whether spoken or through body language.

F. Communicate for them. Receiving bad news represents a major life event. Part of that experience is certain to be a high degree of emotion. Such emotion will influence the encounter and may cloud the communication.

Speak about essential facts in small manageable amounts and wait for their questions to elaborate on details. Watch for their saturation point and stop the flow of words when it is sensed. Acknowledge all parent responses. It is powerful to absolve parents of responsibility for misfortunes if that is possible. When appropriate, let them know that this is only the first of many discussions and be clear about what is required of them at this point.

When the answer to a parent's question is unclear, it is important to distinguish between responses that cannot be answered due to the clinician's knowledge (e.g., "*I don't know the answer to that question, but I will help you find out*") and responses to questions that are essentially unanswerable (e.g., "*It is difficult to say what your child will be like 5 years from now*"). In the latter case, it is helpful to explain why the question cannot be answered, and how the illness will be monitored over time to help answer the question.

G. Monitor and maneuver through emotional density. The emotions experienced during the sharing of bad news are an essential part of the communication. The clinician must model permission to express emotions during the exchange. There are technical aspects to show that feeling is permitted during the exchange of information. Draw it out with silence, with affirmation followed by a pause, or with body cues. Silence will invite response. A response with affect reflects fuller communication than one that asks only for clinical details. Regardless of the response, focus on it and address it, while keeping in mind the larger goals for the conversation. The common desire to soothe distress with reassurance should be controlled, as it can sometimes cut off the development of the parent's perspective, although this should not be done without feeling. Nonetheless, feelings expressed deserve an empathic response.

Parents often have concerns related to the impact of the situation on siblings. When conditions permit, it can be helpful to explore whether they have concerns about disclosure to siblings or worries about their coping. It is productive to explore this area with them, affirming its importance.

Some parents have complained about hearing the phrase "I'm sorry" too much from health professionals. While they appreciate the sympathy, and it is important to express it, they want to know, for example, that although the situation is dire, everything is being done so that it does not hurt their child, or that although there is great uncertainty, strong efforts will be made to understand as much as possible and work toward their expressed goals of care. Fundamentally, parents want to know that their clinician is a strong, committed advocate who will focus his or her efforts and intellect on promoting what is in the best interest of their child.

H. Answer their questions. It is important to elicit parents' questions and answer them. Parents are sometimes too overwhelmed to know what, if anything, to ask. If they feel unable to ask questions, it can be helpful to ask them to summarize what they have heard, or to ask them to share what's going through their minds as they hear your words. As they do so, the clinician may need to gently shift focus to address essential concerns or, sympathetically, reiterate basic facts.

I. Finish in alliance. When it is clear that the essential points have been communicated, that there is a sense of how the family is managing the information, and critical and timely decisions have been made, it is time to end the meeting. The last words generally belong to the clinician and can have a lingering impact. One useful sequence is to offer an empathic statement balanced by a pledge to work toward the expressed goals of care. Any decisions made should be reiterated, available supports reviewed, and the timing of the next occasion to meet should be stated. Closing the meeting with a statement of ongoing commitment to the care of the child and family affirms the clinician–family relationship.

Bibliography

Buckman R. Breaking bad news: why is it still so difficult? *BMJ*. 1984;288:1597-1599.

Cassell EJ. Talking with patients. In: *Clinical Technique*. Vol 2. Cambridge, MA: MIT Press; 1985:148-193.

Christakis NA, Lamont EB. Extent and determinants of error in doctor's prognoses in terminally ill patients: prospective cohort study. *West J Med*. 2000;172:310-313.

Fallowfield L, Jenkins V. Communicating sad, bad, and difficult news in medicine. *Lancet*. 2004;363:312-319.

Friedrichsen MJ, Strang PM, Carlsson ME. Breaking bad news in the transition from curative to palliative cancer care: patient's view of the doctor giving the information. *Support Care Cancer*. 2000;8:472-478.

Levetown M, American Academy of Pediatrics Committee on Bioethics. Communicating with children and families: from everyday interactions to skill in conveying distressing information. *Pediatrics*. 2008;121:e1441-e1460.

Mack JW, Wolfe J, Cook EF, et al. Hope and prognostic disclosure. *J Clin Oncol*. 2007;25: 5636-5642.

Miller SZ, Schmidt HJ. The habit of humanism: a framework for making humanistic care a reflexive clinical skill. *Acad Med*. 1999;74:800-803.

Skotko BG, Capone GT, Kishnani PS, Down Syndrome Diagnosis Study Group. Postnatal diagnosis of Down syndrome: synthesis of the evidence on how best to deliver the news. *Pediatrics*. 2009;124:e751-e758.

CHAPTER **10**

Cultural Aspects of Parenting

Elizabeth Peacock-Chambers | Mei Elansary | Barry Zuckerman

I. **DESCRIPTION OF THE ISSUE.** A cultural group is **a collective of individuals who share a system of meaning**, which includes values, beliefs, and assumptions expressed in daily interaction through a definite pattern of language, behavior, attitudes, and practices. Individuals may have more than one identity that shape their beliefs including ethnic heritage, geographic region, occupation, gender, sexual orientation, or lifestyle. Cultural and group identity are fluid and may change with time and context. Clinicians enter into the clinician–patient relationship with their own set of values, beliefs, and assumptions acquired from their culture as well as the "culture of medicine." When beliefs and practices of a family are discordant with a pediatric clinician's personal or biomedical view, it becomes crucial to find ways to bridge the gap between the two belief systems.

II. **CULTURAL CONCEPTS**

   A. **Culture versus class and minority status.** In many industrialized countries, individuals from minority cultural groups are overrepresented in low-socioeconomic strata of society. This socioeconomic disadvantage results in differential access to services and frequently greater exposure to toxic levels of stress. The effects of (1) traditional cultural beliefs, (2) poverty and access to material goods, and (3) being a part of a racial or ethnic minority are distinct but often interlinked. The clinician needs to be aware of these distinctions and try to tease out whether parenting issues are related to any or all of these three separate but interrelated issues. This chapter will focus on the role that culture plays in guiding parenting practices and ultimately a child's health and development.

   B. **Intracultural variability.** *There is as much variability in beliefs and practices within cultural groups as between cultural groups.* Any one individual's approach to parenting and child development is an amalgamation of personal beliefs, past experiences, perceptions of personal control, *and* traditional cultural beliefs (as well as other factors). Nonetheless, it is important to have a general understanding of traditional beliefs and practices as a starting point for discussion and communication with families.

   C. **Cultural change.** One source of intracultural variability is the effect of **acculturation**, defined as *the changes in cultural beliefs that take place over time in individuals or groups due to continuous contact with other cultures and living environments.* Acculturation is not a unidirectional process; individuals do not acculturate from a traditional culture to the majority culture. Instead, the process is "bicultural" or "multicultural." Individuals retain certain aspects of their traditional culture while incorporating beliefs and values of other groups, including the majority culture, into their personal beliefs. In addition, the majority culture may incorporate customs and practices from minority cultures into its identity as well. Cultural change occurs in a variety of areas that influence parenting, including language, food, ethnic pride, and self-identity.

III. **EPIDEMIOLOGY.** By approximately 2020, more than half of US children are expected to be identified as part of a minority race or ethnic group. People who identify with two or more races are projected to be the fastest-growing population in the next several decades. Parents of different cultures need to negotiate their child rearing attitudes and practices to adapt to these shifting demographics in addition to adjusting to the majority culture.

IV. **FACTORS CONTRIBUTING TO PARENTING IN DIFFERENT CULTURES.** Parenting and culture intersect because parents intend to raise children to succeed according to their society's values and norms.

   A. **Family composition/structure.** Family structures impact many aspects of raising children and vary among different cultures. Families may include cohabitation with or living near extended family, grandparents, or fictive kin (e.g., godparents or nonrelated cousins).

   B. **Cultural norms: autonomy and interdependence.** A useful framework to understand cultural parenting practices is related to child behaviors along the continuum from autonomy/independence to interdependence. This framework is rooted in the values and traits needed for individual success and community survival for different societies and cultures. For example, US or European "Western" culture tends to stress independence, autonomy, and social assertiveness; self-esteem for individual success based on the societal self-image of rugged individualism; frontiersman; etc. As part of the thrust toward autonomy, infants not only sleep in their own bed but often in their own room. Young children are encouraged to make individual decisions in everyday situations (e.g., "Which shirt do you want to wear?" and "What do you want for breakfast?") and are praised for their everyday personal accomplishments such as eating vegetables and toilet training. Parents encourage behaviors that promote autonomy, such as feeding themselves, sleeping in their own room, having their own toys, choosing their own activities, and controlling their emotions (self-regulation).

In interdependent cultures, such as those commonly found in Asian, African, and Latin American countries and throughout most of history, children typically are socialized to be responsible for their families, and their families in turn are responsible for them. The family unit generally includes extended family members, and optimal development is rooted in the ability to sacrifice personal goals for the good of the group. Parenting behaviors in interdependent cultures originated in agrarian societies in which survival of the community required pooling limited resources and distributing them equitably. The focus on connection and collaboration over personal self-interest is thought to be promoted by family routines such as cosleeping, weaning at older ages, emphasizing obedience and respect toward adults, caring for sick relatives playing collectively, and sharing household responsibilities.

Parents in agrarian societies are attentive to their infants' safety and nutritional needs but may not regularly engage in social interaction or direct speech with children before they start to talk. For example, in many cultures, early communication does not involve much verbal or face-to-face interactions but rather physical gestures. Mothers respond with touch and rarely with language to comfort and feed a crying infant. Contingent verbal communication, including verbal turn taking and scaffolding, are not frequently used. For older children, most speech by parents involves commands for the child to do something, rather than using language to expand on a children's interest (e.g., label vegetables in the market, talk about objects in the environment, or give praise). In most societies parents do not get down on the floor and play with children or talk in an animated way. As the child grows, parents help the child develop skills that make them an integral member of the family, taking on important responsibilities such as watching younger siblings or preparing food.

These concepts are not mutually exclusive or static; however, they serve as a useful lens for understanding different parental aspirations and values that may differ from majority.

C. **Perceptions of normal child behavior and development.** Parenting responses to normal child behavior and development are strongly influenced by the perceptions of the positive and negative consequences that child behavior may have on the future adult the child will grow to become. In different cultures and societies, for example, a physically active child may be seen as "hyperactive" or "disobedient" by some while others may perceive the child as "naturally inquisitive" or "strong" or "creative." Similarly, a quiet child may be seen as "slow" or "unmotivated" in one context but "quiet" or "respectful" in another. Culture also influences perceptions of developmental abilities. For example, in some contexts a "smart child" contributes to household tasks and is obedient and cooperative. This is in contrast to emphasis on language abilities such as telling stories or asking questions. Individual children may spend time in settings with different expectations (e.g., school, home, church) and must learn to navigate different rules.

D. Parenting practices and parent perceptions of children are based on what the society needs and values: obedience, respect, hard work, individual drive, or verbal and cognitive skills. Currently economically with the increase in service and other business-related jobs requiring verbal, reading, and cognitive skills, parental values and practices are starting to change to emphasize these skills and longer duration of school attendance, especially in urban areas globally.

V. **CLINICAL APPROACHES**
A. **Clinician training**
   Cultural competency. "Cultural competency" is not simply a technical skill obtained through training but rather requires that a clinician be curious and inquire into the individual values behind the parenting practices of a particular family.

Screening. Most questionnaires and instruments used to assess development and behavior were created and tested on white, middle class children. Although they may have been translated to other languages, they may not reflect differences in cultural beliefs, practices, and perceptions of normal and abnormal behavior that need to be taken into account when evaluating responses. Clinicians should try to choose instruments that have validity and reliability testing for the demographic populations they serve.

B. Communication

Explore expectations of "success." Based on cultural differences and to build trust with parents, clinicians should explore what parents perceive as "success" for their child in the present time and for the future. In addition, clinicians can encourage the parents early on to think about how they plan to achieve these goals and how their actions early in the life of their child may be connected to those long-term goals.

Parent beliefs. Clinicians should inquire into the parent's "ethnotheories" about their children's behavior to ascertain whether or not the behavior is being viewed by the parent as problematic. What might be considered a problem from the clinical standpoint may not be a problem from the perspective of the parent, or vice versa. One way to begin this conversation is to ask the parent about their own parents' rules and expectations, and how they hope to provide similar or different experiences for their own children.

C. Key clinical questions. Examples of questions eliciting the patient's or family's perspective include the following:

Prevention

- *When do you think a child should sleep in her own bed? Own room* (if there is a separate bed room)?
- *When do you think a child should feed himself/herself?*
- *How did you decide on this practice? Who/what influenced your decision? What would you do when your child misbehaves or talks back? Or does something you don't like?*
- *Tell me about the way you were raised as a child with respect to (sleep, food, behavior)?*
- *How do you think a __-year-old act should act?* (This may also uncover attitudes and knowledge about child behavior and development expectations for further discussion.)

Parent perceptions of a behavior problem

- *Do you think this behavior is a problem? Why or why not?*
- *Did you have a similar problem when you were a child?*
- *How did your parents handle your behavior as a child?*
- *Why do you think she/he has this problem?* (Elicit beliefs about causation that may need to be addressed before intervention.)
- *What have you tried to deal with this problem?*
- *Have friends or family given you opinions and ideas about it? Have you tried any of their suggestions?* (Inquire about alternative treatments and practices in a nonjudgemental way.)

D. Supporting families. By inquiring about the family's goals and expectations for their child, a clinician communicates a ***strength-based approach*** to providing guidance. The clinician expresses understanding that there are different approaches to parenting influenced by culture and that she/he can provide better guidance by becoming more familiar with the families' beliefs. For example, when discussing cosleeping, a clinician can comment "*I know having your baby close to you at night is very important to you. Can you think of any ways to help your baby sleep safely (on their back, in their own crib) while still making sure you are close together and happy?*" In this way, clinicians can help parents weigh pros and cons of cosleeping and think about ways of *reducing risks*. The same can be applied to feeding practices, verbal communication, discipline, playing games, etc. This approach empowers the parent as the decision-maker and helps them decide how best to integrate medical recommendations into their own cultural and parenting norms. Ultimately, they may or may not follow clinician recommendations as is common in all of medicine. The goal is for families to have safety and trust in their relationship with you to tell you what they are doing even when it is not consistent with your recommendations.

Bibliography

Greenfield PM, Cocking RR. *Cross-cultural Roots of Minority Child Development*. 1994/2014.

Johnson L, Radesky J, Zuckerman B. Cross-cultural parenting: reflections on autonomy and interdependence. *Pediatrics*. 2013;131(4):631-633.

LeVine RA. Human parental care: universal goals, cultural strategies, individual behavior. *New Dir Child Adolesc Dev.* 1988;1988(40):3-12.

LeVine RA, LeVine S. *Do parents Matter? Why Japanese Babies Sleep Soundly, Mexican siblings Don't Fight, and American Families Should Just Relax.* Public Affairs; 2016.

WEBSITES FOR CLINICIANS

https://www.hrsa.gov/cultural-competence/index.html.

https://npin.cdc.gov/pages/cultural-competence.

CHAPTER **11**

Social Determinants of Health

Arvin Garg

I. **DESCRIPTION OF THE PROBLEM.** The World Health Organization (WHO) defines social determinants of health as the conditions in which people are born, grow, work, live, and age and the wider set of forces and systems shaping the conditions of daily life. In the United States, poverty, unfortunately, is a prevalent and harmful social determinant of health for children. Currently, 18% of children live below the federal poverty level (FPL), and 39% are in low-income group, defined as income <200% FPL. Unmet material needs such as housing stability and food security are more common for low-income children than their counterparts. Such needs, both individually and cumulatively, are associated with detrimental child outcomes, including worse health and higher rates of hospitalizations.

II. **PEDIATRIC CLINICIAN'S ROLE IN ADDRESSING SOCIAL DETERMINANTS AT PEDIATRIC VISITS.** Pediatric clinician have struggled to identify and address the social needs of their patients and their families during the delivery of care. Determining such needs has been enhanced by the IHELLP mnemonic developed for medical–legal partnerships as a strategy for clinician to remember critical social domains (i.e., income, housing, utilities, education, legal status, literacy, personal safety) to discuss with parents and caregivers. However, studies suggest that few pediatric clinicians routinely ask and identify unmet social needs at pediatric visits because of lack of time, training, and knowledge of community resources.

III. **PROFESSIONAL GUIDELINES ON SCREENING FOR SOCIAL DETERMINANTS OF HEALTH.** There is growing evidence that screening for unmet social needs at pediatric visits coupled with providing resource information and/or navigation can increase the identification of needs, discussion of needs with their pediatric clinician, and receipt of community-based services and improve the parental reporting of children's health status. In response to the emerging evidence of the positive impact that screening may have on families and children, the American Academy of Pediatrics (AAP) recently recommended that pediatric clinicians screen for risk factors within social determinants of health at patient encounters.

A. **Screening methods.** Screening for social determinants can be conducted via various methods such as verbally (face-to-face, telephone) or via a written screener given either in paper form or electronically (e.g., iPad). Some evidence suggests that screeners that are not administered face-to-face may increase the disclosure rates for social needs. Screening instruments may be given to families by the front desk, other office support staff, or health care providers.

B. **Screening instruments.** There is currently a plethora of screening instruments available that screen globally for material need, multiple unmet social needs, or a specific social determinant (e.g., food insecurity, housing instability, utilities). The global screening question *"Do you have difficulty making ends meet at the end of the month?"* has been demonstrated to have 98% sensitivity for alerting a pediatric clinician to the need for linking families to community resources. The WE CARE survey is an example of a screening instrument that screens for multiple unmet material needs (e.g., parental education, employment, childcare, homelessness risk, food insecurity, utility need) as well as a family's desire for assistance. It is written at the third-grade level, has high reliability, and has been shown to increase parental enrollment in community resources when used with a Family Resource book. For employment, the screening question is *"Do you have a job?"* If a parent indicates no, the follow-up question is *"Would you like help with finding employment?"* Answer choices include yes, no, and maybe later. For childcare need, the screening question is *"Do you need childcare for your child?"* If a parent indicates yes, the follow-up question is *"Would you like help finding it?"* In this care model, if a parent indicates desire for assistance on the screener, the pediatric clinician would discuss this need, provide resource information sheets from the Resource book, and/or refer the parent to a clinic staff member who can assist the parent in navigating community agencies.

Examples of other screening instruments aimed at identifying multiple needs include the Centers for Medicare & Medicaid Services (CMS) health-related social needs survey, Pediatric Intake Form, and the SEEK parent screening questionnaire.

The Hunger Vital Sign is a published two-question scale that the AAP recommends pediatric clinicians use to screen children for food insecurity. The questions are (1) *"Within the past 12 months, have you worried that your food would run out before you got money to buy more?"* (2) *"Within the past 12 months, the food you bought just didn't last and you didn't have money to get more?"* A parent would screen positive for food insecurity if he or she selects "often true" or "sometimes true" for either question.

IV. **GUIDING PRINCIPLE FOR SCREENING FOR SOCIAL DETERMINANTS OF HEALTH.** Currently, there is great interest in implementing screening for social determinants of health into routine pediatric care. However, this type of novel screening could lead to unintended consequences such as unfilled expectations for both families and clinicians, which may harm the clinician–patient relationship. Screening should therefore occur in a family-centered manner, respecting a family's desire or not for assistance, and involve shared decision-making. Screening should also be performed only when an actionable plan in assisting families with needs is in place. This may include providing families with community resource information listings or referring to office staff who can assist families in identifying and navigating community services. Screening for social determinants has the potential to lead to greater understanding of our patients' social circumstances and mitigate social determinants that threaten children's well-being.

Bibliography

FOR PROFESSIONALS

American Academy of Pediatrics, Council on Community Pediatrics. Poverty and child health in the United States. *Pediatrics*. 2016;137.

Billioux A, Verlander K, Anthony S, Alley D. *Standardized screening for health-related social needs in clinical settings: the Accountable Health Communities screening tool. Discussion paper*. Washington, DC: National Academy of Medicine. https://nam.edu/wp-content/uploads/2017/05/Standardized-Screening-for-Health-Related-Social-Needs-in-Clinical-Settings.pdf.

Chung EK, Siegel BS, Garg A, et al. Screening for social determinants of health among children and families living in poverty: a guide for clinicians. *Curr Probl Pediatr Adolesc Health Care*. 2016;46:135-153.

Hager ER, Quigg AM, Black MM, et al. Development and validity of a 2-item screen to identify families at risk for food insecurity. *Pediatrics*. 2010;126:e26-e32.

CHAPTER 12

Promoting Growth Mind-set to Improve Health, Learning, and Parenting

Barry Zuckerman

I. **MIND-SET.** Mind-set is a set of beliefs or frames of mind held by individuals that guide attention and motivation and shape behavior. Sometimes grounded in facts and sometimes not, mind-sets are simplified versions of what is right, natural, or possible (e.g., "girls are not good in math," "it doesn't matter what I do my child will end up poor like me," "diabetes runs in my family so losing weight will not matter"). Although mind-set can occur along a spectrum, the two ends—fixed and growth—have important implications for behavior.

Individuals with a fixed or unchangeable mind-set think there is nothing they can do to effect change in a certain area that is reinforced by poor performance or failure. On the opposite end of the spectrum are individuals with a growth mind-set who believe success is based on effort or hard work. Family, media, or social values create and reinforce such mind-sets.

A. **Fixed mind-set.** Children with a fixed mind-set about intelligence show less persistence and even worse performance even after minor failure, whereas those with growth mind-set about intelligence try harder and perform better at similar learning tasks. A fixed mind-set about their health may underlie adolescents failing to effectively manage their chronic disease through lack of adherence to medication and/or lifestyle changes. Similarly, parents with a fixed mind-set may perceive they have a lack of efficacy to help their children learn and be successful.

B. **Growth mind-set.** Growth mind-set, on the other hand, appears to stem from an underlying belief that success comes with challenges, including failure, and that performance whether its grades, learning, managing a chronic disease, or parenting can be improved through hard work.

C. **Mixed mind-set.** It is also important to realize that individuals do not have either fixed or growth mind-set for all areas of functioning but rather some topics may be fixed and others not. Similarly, an individual can have a growth mind-set and eat healthy and a fixed mind-set about exercise.

II. **IMPLICATIONS FOR LEARNING**

A. **Promoting growth mind-set for learning.** Research shows that parents who believe that children's ability to learn is innate as a fixed mind-set interact with their children in less stimulating and more controlling way, focusing on their performance rather than on effort. Parents who praise performance can inadvertently induce a fixed mind-set in their child. On the other hand, parents who praise children for their effort are more likely to have children who have a growth mind-set for intelligence years later and learn more. When accomplishing a difficult task, parents should say "Wow you worked really hard at that" rather than "you are so smart." When children believe, in part because of parent praise, that they are really smart, they may shy away from difficult tasks because if they do not do well, they are afraid they will be "found out" to themselves and others that they are not that smart.

B. **Promoting growth mind-set for intelligence.** Studies show that students do better if they have a growth mind-set for intelligence, and intellectual abilities can be developed. These students tend to see difficult tasks as a way to increase their abilities and often will seek out challenging learning experiences that help them do so. As a consequence, they get better grades than children with a fixed mind-set who believe intelligence is not changeable and therefore tend to avoid situations in which they may struggle or fail because these experiences undermine their sense of intelligence. A related aspect is that low-income students are more likely to have a fixed mind-set but among the low-income students; those with growth mind-set do much better than those with fixed mind-set and can decrease the achievement gap between high- and low-income students. Interventions with simple verbal or visual prompts that describe the brain as a muscle that can be strengthened lead to a growth mind-set and improved grades based on extensive evidence. Many schools nationally have implemented strategies to promote growth mind-set for students. Online interventions have been shown to be effective and should be recommended to parents and adolescents especially if they are not implemented in their school.

III. **SUPPORTING PARENTS.** Parents' mind-sets shape their interactions with their children. Parents with a growth mind-set report more engagement in reading and math activities compared with parents with a fixed mind-set who interact in less constructive ways with their children. A number of studies show that changing parent mind-sets promotes parent activities that lead to better child learning. It is hypothesized that low-income parents disproportionately are more likely to have fixed mind-set because they have or believe they have little control of their life, e.g., "It doesn't matter what I do, my child will end up like me." For all parents, especially low-income parents, it would be important to communicate that they can make a difference in their child's life and learning. It is worth emphasizing that it will not be easy and there will be challenges and failures but the pediatric clinician needs to emphasize that youth can learn from their failure and work harder because parents make an important difference in their child's life. The best analogy might be an athletic coach or music teacher who communicates his or her belief that success comes only with hard work and practice. Parents need to have that mind-set about themselves and communicate it to children.

IV. **IMPLICATIONS FOR HEALTH MIND-SET.** Research shows that mind-sets or expectations to heal, like placebos, can trigger specific neurobiologic changes including immune functioning. In fact, placebos are driven in large part by the mind-set that the pill is effective. Unlike placebos, which involve deception, mind-sets can be changed nondeceptively to improve effectiveness of active medications and behavioral treatments. Explicit comments by clinicians reinforcing the power of the medication are known to increase efficacy in multiple studies. Statements such as *"this medicine will make you feel much better"* probably will affect symptoms more than *"I am going to give you a prescription for a medicine."*

Similarly, adolescents with type 1 diabetes and a growth mind-set tested their blood glucose level more frequently and had lower A1C levels over a 2-year period compared with adolescents with a fixed mind-set. Losing weight or changing eating habits are important and difficult challenges for adolescents who say or think "well everyone in my family is fat so I guess there is little I can do" (fixed mind-set). Helping adolescents believe they have the capacity to change and improve is important. Although there are not yet evidence-based strategies to promote a growth mind-set for behavioral changes such as weight loss, clinicians should take a page from what effective coaches do for adolescent athletes and encourage effort and expect to learn from failure.

Bibliography
Claro S, Paunesku D, Dweck C. Growth mindset tempers the effects of poverty on academic achievement. *Proc Natl Acad Sci U S A.* 2016;113(31):8664-8668.
Crum A, Zuckerman B. Changing mindset to enhance treatment effectiveness. *JAMA.* 2017;317(20):2063-2064.
Mueller CM, Dweck CS. Praise for intelligence can undermine children's motivation and performance. *J Pers Soc Psychol.* 1998;75(1):32-52.
Mueller C, Rowe ML, Zuckerman B. Mindset matters for parents and adolescents. *JAMA Pediatr.* 2017;171(5):415-416.
Paunesku D, Walton GM, Romero C, Smith EN, Yeager DS, Dweck CS. Mindset interventions are a scalable treatment for academic underachievement. *Psychol Sci.* 2015;26(2):784-793.

FOR PARENTS
Dweck C. *Mindset: The New Psychology of Success.* New York: Random House; 2006.
www.mindsetkit/growthmindset for parents.com.

CHAPTER **13**

Addressing the Challenge of Implicit Bias

Katherine A. Nash

I. **DESCRIPTION OF THE PROBLEM.** Health disparities based on race and ethnicity are well documented and well known. In its landmark 2002 report, *Unequal Treatment*, the National Academy of Medicine identified the critical role of provider bias in perpetuating these inequities. We now have substantial evidence that health care providers hold biases based on patient race, class, sex and other patient characteristics and that these biases affect their clinical decision-making and ability to communicate effectively with patients.

II. **WHAT IS BIAS?** Bias, prejudice in favor of or against one thing, person, or group, can come in multiple forms and is universal to human behavior. *Explicit* biases are conscious—we know that we possess them, and because of this awareness, they can weaken over time with education and social desirability bias. In fact, overt demonstrations of prejudice related to racial stereotypes have declined substantially over time because of evolving societal norms. In contrast, *implicit* biases are unconscious and involuntary but nonetheless affect behavior and human interaction. Although implicit biases are subtle cognitive processes, their impact on behavior and decision-making can be mitigated.

III. **EVIDENCE DEMONSTRATING THE PRESENCE OF IMPLICIT BIAS IN MEDICINE**
   - For the purposes of research, the Implicit Association Test (IAT) is the most widely accepted and used tool to evaluate individuals' implicit biases. The IAT is an online tool that can be used to test bias of various forms including racial, gender, religious, and obesity bias.
   - A recent literature review examining racial bias in health care providers with the IAT found that the majority of health care providers tested had some level of pro-white/anti-black bias. An additional study found moderate implicit bias against black children in contrast to white children, demonstrating that these biases are relevant for pediatric clinicians in addition to adult providers.
   - Comparing care delivered to white and black patients, studies have demonstrated that providers hold implicit associations between "medical compliance, cooperativeness and patients race".
   - Additional studies showed provider bias against Hispanic patients, American Indian patients, darker-skinned patients, and obese patients.

IV. **EVIDENCE DEMONSTRATING THE IMPACT OF BIAS IN CLINICAL CARE**
   - Several studies have examined the association between implicit bias and clinical decision-making including the use of thrombolysis in cardiac arrest, pain management, antibiotic use in urinary tract infection, and treatment of attention-deficit/hyperactivity disorder.
   - Additional studies have demonstrated an association between provider implicit bias and patient's perspective of their ability to communicate and connect with their providers, with people of color more likely to believe that there is bias in healthcare than white patients.

V. **MITIGATING THE IMPACT OF BIAS.** We can assume that the majority of pediatric clinicians want to treat any patient who walks into their office equally. If implicit biases are unconscious, how do we prevent them from affecting our interactions?
   - **Develop awareness of your personal implicit biases.** Take the online IAT, reflect on your answers, and consider how they might affect your care of patients. Discuss cases with your colleagues and how bias might affect care in individual cases.
   - **Slow down your thought process.** Dual process theory describes a framework for how people integrate information when they make judgments or solve problems, providing a distinction between fast thinking (rapid autonomous processes/System 1) and slow thinking (higher-order reasoning/System 2). Fast thinking is more susceptible to implicit bias. When you are taking care of patients where you know you are biased, try to slow down and use slow thinking and consider how your biases come into play.

- **Perspective taking and individuation to improve empathy.** Individuation (in contrast to categorization) is to focus on an individual's unique characteristics as opposed to those of the group to which they belong. Perspective taking is a cognitive process associated with empathy that involves considering a situation from the position of another. Both individuation and perspective taking help providers arouse empathy and reduce bias.
- **Interact with people who are different than you. Diversify your practice.** Talk to other providers of different races, ethnicities, and backgrounds about the issue of implicit bias. Explore other perspectives and challenge your own.
- **Practice self-care and mindfulness.** Stress and fatigue decreases our capacity for System 2 thinking and empathy and therefore increases the likelihood that we act on our unconscious biases.
- **Ask your patients about their experiences with discrimination.** Ask your patients if they have ever experienced discrimination or racism in the health care system in the past. Asking this question acknowledges that there can be racism and bias in health care, validates your patient's or the parent's experiences, and shows that you care. You might gain insight into the context of how your patient or the parent interacts with or experiences the health care system.

Bibliography

Burgess D, van Ryn M, Dovidio J, Saha S. Reducing racial bias among health care providers: lessons learned from social-cognitive psychology. *J Gen Intern Med*. 2007;22:882-887.

http://www.ihi.org/resources/Pages/Tools/Liberation-in-the-Exam-Room-Racial-Justice-Equity-in-Health-Care.aspx.

https://implicit.harvard.edu/implicit/.

Johnson TI, Winger DG, Hickey RW, et al. Comparison of physician implicit racial bias towards adults versus children. *Acad Pediatr*. 2017;17(2):120-126.

Maina IW, Belton TD, Ginzberg S, Singh A, Johnson TJ. A decade of studying implicit racial/ethnic bias in healthcare providers using the implicit association test. *Soc Sci Med*. 2018;199:219-229.

CHAPTER 14

Helping Families Reduce Financial Stress

Lucy E. Marcil and Michael Hole

I. **DESCRIPTION OF THE PROBLEM.** Poverty, affecting one in five children in the United States, undermines children's health and development including brain development. Children growing up in poverty experience a double jeopardy: they more likely experience poor health and development and suffer greater consequences from the same problem compared with their more well-to-do peers. For example, a premature child with low birthweight born to a poor woman will likely have more developmental problems than the same child born to affluent parents. As a result, the American Academy of Pediatrics has committed to "reducing and ultimately eliminating child poverty in the United States." This goal is crucial to improving child health, but economic and policy trends have impeded progress. Although screening for other social needs (i.e., food, housing) has become more common (see Chapter 11), clinicians do not routinely discuss financial problems with patients.

II. **WHAT ARE POVERTY AND FINANCIAL STRESS?** Poverty in the United States is defined by the federal poverty level (FPL), calculated based on the assumption families spend 33% of their budget on food as they did in the 1960s and allowing for the cheapest, nutritionally adequate USDA-approved food plan. The FLP for a family of three is $20,420 in 2017. Some argue the FPL is too low, given budgetary shifts away from food (10% of the average family budget in 2017). Thus, programs vary in eligibility thresholds (i.e., Medicaid is 138% of FPL or $28,180 for a family of three; the health care tax subsidy is 400% of the FLP or $81,680 for a family of three).

Financial stress arises from a broader array of financial problems than absolute poverty, including financial instability (e.g., fluctuations in income from unpredictable and seasonal jobs), inadequate wages relative to cost of living, debt, poor credit scores, and inadequate access to fair loans. Financial stress like other sources of stress is an important target of inquiry for pediatric clinicians; it may affect parents' ability to be empathic, protective, positive, and responsive to their child leading to poorer health and development.

III. **EVIDENCE ON THE POSITIVE IMPACT OF REDUCING FINANCIAL STRESS**
   - The Earned Income Tax Credit, a federal refundable tax credit designed to bring low-income, working families out of poverty, is the largest antipoverty program in the United States. It has been associated with many health benefits including decreased preterm births, increased infant birthweight, decreased child abusive head trauma, decreased maternal depression, decreased maternal smoking, and decreased food insecurity.
   - A recent randomized study found individuals who were prompted to save during tax time reported less material and health hardship 6 months later.
   - Randomized trials have found that financial coaching can reduce debt (including medical debt) and financial stress and increase savings.
   - Studies have found associations between financial stress and hostile parenting as well as increased child behavioral problems.

IV. **IDENTIFY FINANCIAL STRESS AND REFER FOR HELP.** We recommend providers ask patients directly about financial stress in their lives.
   - **Make sure to explain to patients why you're asking.** *"We know financial stress can negatively affect health, so we want to make sure we help you with this stress if we can."*
   - **This approach may uncover more underlying problems for child health** than asking conventional questions about sleep, elimination, and other bodily functions when growth and vital signs are within normal limits.
   "Do you ever have difficulty making ends meet at the end of the month? What impact does this have on your family? What do you do about it?"
   "Have you ever used free tax preparation services? Do you know if you get the Earned Income Tax Credit?"

V. MITIGATING THE IMPACT OF FINANCIAL STRESS AND POVERTY

- **Consider systematic screening** as with other routine screening questions patients receive (see Chapter 11).
- **Make sure an intervention follows screening.** Counseling, including emotional support and concrete resources, helps families materially and encourages hope about their child's future. Many programs offer resources and may be national, community-based, or integrated into the clinical setting.
  - *National*:
    IRS VITA: Free tax preparation exists in most communities; this service saves families money and ensures they get their Earned Income Tax Credit and Child Tax Credit (https://www.irs.gov/individuals/free-tax-return-preparation-for-you-by-volunteers).

    Prosperity NOW: A general financial empowerment and stability organization; hosts a Medical–Financial Partnership Learning Collaborative bringing doctors and financial organizations together to break silos and help families (https://prosperitynow.org/resources/medical-financial-partnership-learning-community-webinar-recording).

    Financial Coaching: Most programs are local. Prosperity NOW (https://prosperitynow.org/issues/financial-coaching) and Asset Funders (https://assetfunders.org/wp-content/uploads/Fin_Coaching_Census_2016_Brief.pdf) are centralized information sources.

    Job Training: Many programs are local; the Urban League is one national organization running job training programs (http://nul.iamempowered.com/what-we-do/our-programs/workforce-development-division).

    Medical–Legal Partnership is for families with complex financial problems in need of legal help (http://medical-legalpartnership.org/).

    SaveYourRefund incentivizes tax time savings through cash prize drawings (https://saveyourrefund.com/home/).

    StreetCred partners with local hospitals and tax help coalitions to bring free tax preparation to low-income families (www.mystreetcred.org).
  - *Community-based*: Many communities have their own efforts to promote financial well-being. Identifying such programs in your community to refer families is an important step. An Internet search for "financial capability program," "financial coaching," "credit building," or "incentivized savings program" may be a good first step.
  - *Integrated*: Some programs are integrated into clinical settings. Examples include **WE-CARE** (http://pediatrics.aappublications.org/content/135/2/e296), **Medical-Legal Partnership** (http://medical-legalpartnership.org/), and **StreetCred** (www.mystreetcred.org).
- **Develop awareness of poverty and low-income in your clinical population.** *"Do you feel financially stressed? Tell me more about that."*
- **Explore a poverty simulation:** https://www.myunitedway.ca/poverty-simulation/or http://makethemonth.ca/.
- **Variation in financial stress.** Families not living in poverty may still face significant stress including child education costs, high rent costs, and debt. Making more money decreases eligibility for government programs like food stamps (SNAP). Patients are the experts on their own lives and may have a specific need you would not have predicted. If they endorse feeling financially stressed, follow up with, *"What can we do to help?"*

Bibliography

AAP Council on Community Pediatrics. Poverty and child health in the United States. *Pediatrics*. 2016;137(4):e20160339. PMID:26962238.

Brcic V, Eberdt C, Kaczorowski J. Corrigendum to development of a tool to identify poverty in a family practice setting: a pilot study. *Int J Family Med*. 2015;2015:418125.

Conger RD, Ge X, Elder GH, Lorenz FO, Simons RL. Economic stress, coercive family process, and developmental problems of adolescents. *Child Dev*. 1994;65(2):541-561.

Despard MR, Taylor SH, Ren C, Russell BD, Grinstein-Weiss M, Raghavan R. Effects of a tax-time savings experiment on material and health care hardship among low-income filers. *J Poverty*. 2017. Advance online publication. doi:10.1080/10875549.2017.1348431.

Jones MK, Bloch G, Pinto AD. A novel income security intervention to address poverty in a primary care setting: a retrospective chart review. *BMJ Open*. 2017;7:e014270.

CHAPTER 15

Pediatric Role in Family Planning

Lee A. Trope | Jayme Congdon

I. **DESCRIPTION OF THE PROBLEM.** More than half of pregnancies in the United States are unplanned. Mothers often obtain contraception at a single postpartum visit, although postpartum appointments are attended by only about half of women. There are additional barriers to family planning services due to insurance coverage and the fragmented nature of adult care. In contrast, well-child checks are frequent and well attended, presenting many opportunities to help parents plan the number of children they want and the best timing for a subsequent pregnancy.
   A. **Effects on existing children.** Unplanned pregnancy may negatively affect existing children by limiting financial resources available to the family. Parental time, nurturing, and material resources might also be diminished with an unplanned pregnancy.
   B. **Effects on future children.** Children resulting from unintended pregnancies at a birth interval less than 18 months are at higher risk of low birthweight, preterm birth, perinatal death, abuse, and neglect.
   C. **Effects on parents.** Women who have an unplanned pregnancy have higher rates of depression and intimate partner violence. Lower parental educational attainment and lower income are also common.

II. **HISTORY: SCREEN FOR PREGNANCY INTENTION USING ONE KEY QUESTION®**
   A. *"Would you like to become pregnant in the next year?"* Ask all mothers regardless of age. Possible answers include *Yes, No, Ok either way,* or *Unsure* (Fig. 15-1).

III. **MANAGEMENT.** Like screening for postpartum depression or intimate partner violence, parental family planning promotes a two-generation model of care that acknowledges the interconnection of children's health with that of their parents. Although family planning discussions are currently uncommon in child health care, they can be helpful to families because of the special trust and relationship parents have with their child's clinician.
   A. **For mothers who intend to become pregnant or are unsure about intentions.** Review birth spacing guidelines that recommend a minimum interval of 18 months. Inquire about access to obstetric care. Recommend preconception care, early prenatal care, daily folic acid, and healthy behaviors.
   B. **For mothers who do not intend to become pregnant or are unsure about intentions.** Inquire about the current method of contraception and satisfaction with the current method. If she is not currently using contraception, using a method with lower efficacy, or unsatisfied with the current method, counsel about contraceptive options (Table 15-1).
      1. **Emphasis on highly effective methods.** When counseling or offering resources on contraceptive options, emphasize the effectiveness of long-acting reversible contraceptive (LARC) methods. The new generation of LARCs is the safest, most effective, and most cost-effective reversible option.
      2. **Provision.** To improve timely access to preventive reproductive care, consider provision (same day if possible) of contraception to mothers who reasonably fall within the scope of a pediatric practice. Clinicians can easily be trained to insert implantables and can bill for it in addition to the pediatric visit.
      3. **Referrals.** For women who fall outside the scope of your practice because of medical complexity, age, or training in intrauterine device (IUD) placement, we encourage forming relationships with local family planning providers and making closed-loop referrals.
      4. **Considerations for breastfeeding mothers**
         a. Breastfeeding women should avoid combined oral contraceptives, patches, and rings. All other methods, including hormonal IUDs and progestin-only pills, are considered safe and have not been shown to affect milk supply or infant growth (Table 15-1).

b. Breastfeeding is about 98% effective against pregnancy only if all the following conditions are met: (1) less than 6 months postpartum, (2) exclusive breastfeeding at least every 4–6 hours, and (3) amenorrhea. The duration of amenorrhea is typically several months longer than the duration of postpartum anovulation and should not be used alone as a marker of infertility.

C. For pregnant mothers. Inquire about access to prenatal care and plans for postpartum contraception. Counsel about postpartum LARCs.

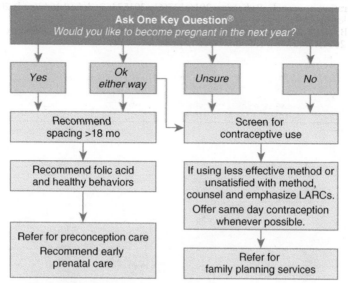

Figure 15-1   Maternal family planning algorithm.

Table 15-1 • EFFECTIVENESS OF CONTRACEPTIVE METHODS

	Contraceptive Method	Pregnancy Rate in 1 y of Typical Use (%)	Safe While Breastfeeding
Highly effective	IUD	<1	✓
	Implant	<1	✓
	Injectable	<1	✓
Effective	Pill (progestin-only)	6	✓
	Pill (combined)	6	
	Patch	9	
	Ring	9	
	Diaphragm	12	✓
Less effective	Male condom	18	✓
	Female condom	21	✓
	Withdrawal	22	✓
	Fertility awareness	24	✓
	Spermicide	28	✓

Adapted from Trussell J. Contraceptive failure in the United States. *Contraception.* 2011;83:397-404.
IUD, intrauterine device.

Bibliography

FOR PARENTS

https://www.bedsider.org.

https://www.marchofdimes.org/pregnancy/before-pregnancy.aspx.

https://www.plannedparenthood.org/learn/birth-control/breastfeeding/whats-best-birth-control-option-while-breastfeeding.

FOR PROFESSIONALS

https://www.cdc.gov/reproductivehealth/contraception/index.htm.

Cheng TL, Johnson SB, Goodman E. Breaking the intergenerational cycle of disadvantage: the three generation approach. *Pediatrics*. 2016;137(6):e20152467. doi:10.1542/peds.2015-2467.

https://providers.bedsider.org.

Zuckerman B, Nathan S, Mate K. Preventing unintended pregnancy: a pediatric opportunity. *Pediatrics*. 2014;133(2):181-183. doi:10.1542/peds.2013-1147.

CHAPTER 16

Promoting Early Literacy

Perri Klass

I. **DESCRIPTION OF THE PROBLEM.** Language exposure in the first years of life is vital for brain development, and both spoken and written language are important, right from the beginning. Children who grow up with little exposure to books and to printed language, in "print-poor" homes where they are not read to and do not see adults using written language during the first 5 years of life, are unlikely to acquire the essential early literacy skills, which will help them learn to decipher print once they get to school. In addition, those same home environments may lack spoken language exposure and the kind of positive back-and-forth interactions with parents which support brain development. Reading aloud and looking at books with young children offers parents an opportunity for language-rich interactions, which also help children develop specific early literacy skills. Early picture book reading has been linked to patterns of brain activation, which incorporate both language and visual processes. Books also offer parents a way to build routines, which can help children feel secure and comfort, even in families under stress. Children with more limited language exposure, spoken and written, are likely to reach the age of school entry with poorer language skills, poorer school readiness, as measured in essential early literacy skills such as letter recognition, and poorer motivation. They may be unskilled in handling books, lacking the positive associations that develop early in infants and toddlers who associate picture books with physical contact with a parent and the sound of the parent's voice, along with the sense of security that develops around bedtime rituals. By the time they start school, and begin learning to decipher print, they are already at risk for reading problems. Children who are not able to develop reading skills on grade level by third grade are at increased risk to continue through elementary school and even high school reading below the grade level, which puts them at risk for school failure and its concomitant risks, from low self-esteem to early pregnancy and substance abuse to dropping out.

II. **EPIDEMIOLOGY.** Fewer than half the poor children in the United States have the skills they need to start school and learn to read, and even among those children who grow up in moderate- and high-income families, one in four is still not ready for school. In particular, almost a third of poor children score very low on reading skills. Reading difficulties in the early years of school may reflect the child's home environment and experience—or lack of it—in preschool, as well as language issues and learning disabilities. Low socioeconomic status and poor parental literacy skills significantly increase children's risk of reading problems.

III. **ETIOLOGY/CONTRIBUTING FACTORS.** There are many reasons why children may not be read to or may grow up in print-poor environments, and these same factors may put them at risk for generally reduced language exposure.
- Parents who were not themselves read to as children may not understand the importance of reading aloud especially to very young children. Parents who have limited literacy skills may not be in the habit of using written language (newspapers, magazines, books, written messages) either for entertainment or to convey or receive information.
- Adults who struggled in school, or who still struggle with written language, may look on reading aloud as a difficult task, or a reminder of failure and defeat.
- Parents may doubt their own abilities to introduce children to written language and may feel that "educational" apps or devices that have been heavily marketed can do a better job.
- Families may lack resources to buy books or live in areas where appropriate children's books are not easily available.
- Minority families may not see themselves reflected in the children's books that are available and may feel marginalized or excluded when a diverse array of books is not provided.
- Non–English-speaking parents may not have books available in their languages, may be intimidated by books in English, or may deliberately refrain from reading (or even speaking) to their children in their native language in the hope that the children will grow up speaking English.

61

- Families may be under significant time stress and have trouble building regular routines; this may be true for families anywhere on the socioeconomic spectrum.
- Parents who are themselves educated may not be directly caring for their own young children or may feel unsure about what books and reading techniques are suitable for infants and toddlers.
- Screen time continues to loom large in the lives of families in the 21st century, and parent–child interactions may be replaced by many competing modes of "entertaining" young children, including touchpads, smartphones, television, video, and other electronic media.
- These same electronic alternatives are available to parents and may work against "face time" and "lap time" with young children or "family time" centered around books.

IV. **WHICH FAMILIES NEED LITERACY PROMOTION?** The American Academy of Pediatrics recommends that pediatric primary care should include early literacy promotion and an emphasis on the importance of using books to foster parent–child interactions, for all families, regardless of socioeconomic status and parents' educational level. Special attention should be paid to families whose economic circumstances or educational background make reading aloud more challenging for parents or place their children at additional risk, to parents who have not completed high school, to parents whose English language skills are limited, to adolescent parents, and to families under extreme social and/ or financial stress. Because one goal of reading aloud is to link books with pleasure in the child's mind, literacy promotion should take place on a highly positive note, encouraging parents to help their children learn and achieve and to use books to build loving routines into their children's days, which will help families navigate bedtime, build security and comfort for children, and provide enjoyment to parents and children.

A. **Taking the history.** *"How are your child's language skills? Do you read aloud to your child? What books do your children enjoy? Tell me about your bedtime routine. Are books a part of your daily routines with your child? Does anyone in the family have a library card?"* Ask children directly: *"What is your favorite book?"*

B. **Identifying families at risk.** It is important to try and identify parents who may be at increased risk and may need extra help because they themselves have limited literacy skills. Their children are at risk for reading difficulties and school problems, and these are often parents who are intimidated by dealing with schools and teachers and therefore have trouble advocating for their children when they need extra help. Limited literacy can affect the health of both adults and children in a variety of ways; these families may also be at additional health risk because of the parent's limited ability to understand other written materials, including prescriptions, handouts, and pamphlets. Asking about parental literacy level may feel uncomfortable and intrusive, but parents are usually receptive to being asked about their own educational experiences, and it can be an important part of the background to know if a parent was in special education or has been diagnosed with learning problems. It is possible to ask for objective information (i.e., how far a parent went in school) as a routine part of patient intake; asking all parents for this information also removes the risks of making assumptions about literacy level. A parent history of reading delay, learning problems, or school retention may offer important information for counseling parents and screening children. One study has shown that the number of children's books in the home can be a good indicator of parental literacy level, with parents who claim less than 10 children's books in the home more likely to perform poorly on a test of health literacy. For families of concern, one possible approach is to ask parents whether they are interested in improving their own reading skills and to offer a referral to local adult or family literacy services.

V. **MANAGEMENT: LITERACY PROMOTION IN PRIMARY CARE**

A. **Model for effective literacy promotion.** Reach Out and Read (ROR) was founded in 1989 by pediatric clinicians and early childhood educators, and now reaches over 4.7 million children every year. ROR advocates a three-component model of literacy promotion in pediatric primary care.

1. Primary care providers are trained to counsel parents at the health supervision visit about looking at books together and reading aloud, starting at the newborn visit.
2. Providers give each child a new, age-appropriate children's book at health supervision visits, with at least one book given in the first months of life and with a developmentally appropriate book at each visit from 6 to 60 months, so that the child acquires a home library of 9–10 books by school entry age.
3. Literacy-rich waiting rooms reinforce the message with displays about reading aloud, family literacy, libraries; with gently used books that children can take home; and, whenever possible, with volunteers in the waiting room who read aloud to

children and thereby model reading-aloud techniques for parents are an option for some practices.

In multiple published studies, ROR has been shown to result in significantly higher rates of parents reading to children, significantly more positive attitudes toward books and reading on the part of parents and children, and significantly improved receptive and expressive language skills in high-risk children as young as 18 months.

B. Anticipatory guidance

  1. Brief and age appropriate

   a. Parents need to understand what to expect from young children with respect to books and reading (e.g., that a newborn already recognizes a parent's voice, that it is normal for a 6-month-old immediately to put a board book in his mouth, or that a 2-year-old may not sit still for an entire story).

   b. Encourage age-appropriate parent–child interaction, using the book as a prompt or a script, as in holding an infant face to face for reading, talking, or singing, asking a toddler to name a picture, a 2-year-old to provide an animal noise, a 3-year-old to point out colors, or a 4-year-old to tell you what he or she thinks will happen next in the story.

   c. Model pointing and questions that let a child demonstrate vocabulary, color knowledge, spatial concepts such as over and under, and early math skills such as counting.

  2. Linked to other issues of behavior and development discussed in the health supervision visit

   a. Discuss reading at bedtime in the context of discussing sleep issues and bedtime routines and in the context of keeping screens out of children's bedrooms and turning all screens off well before bedtime to help children sleep.

   b. Offer suggestions for how to incorporate books into other aspects of the child's routines, including waiting times (such as the doctor's waiting room), times the child needs to calm down and relax, and trips to the library.

   c. Encourage parents to follow the child's cues—let the baby turn over several board pages at once, let the toddler choose the book and hold it—and to respond positively when the child brings over a book as a way of asking for a story.

   d. Encourage parents who are looking at childcare and preschool programs to look for situations where books are available and reading aloud is built into the schedule.

   e. When talking about watching television or videos or electronic games and young children, offer reading aloud as an alternative entertainment; emphasize to parents that their participation in looking at books with their child makes this both meaningful and educational for the child.

   f. Discuss the importance of reading aloud in the context of language exposure and acquisition for infants and toddlers and emphasize that young children do not learn language from screens.

   g. Discuss the relationship of reading aloud and school readiness for preschoolers.

   h. Introduce the concept of "dialogic reading," in which parents encourage toddlers and preschool-aged children to comment on pictures and the story, to engage the child and promote a conversation about the book or story.

  3. Positive and reinforcing for the parents

   a. Give parents positive feedback if they are already reading; point out the child's book-handling and page-turning skills.

   b. Emphasize the importance of the parent's voice in the child's development, starting at birth (and even before).

   c. Encourage physical contact between parent and child, cuddling, "face time," "lap time," all of which will make the books and reading more desirable and important to a young child.

   d. Present reading with the child as something that should be fun; acknowledge the parent's wish to see the child learn and succeed, and, especially with preschool children, look ahead to the child successfully learning to read in school.

   e. Talk about reading routines as ways a parent can help a child calm down, focus, and feel secure, while learning language and coming to love books.

   f. If you are concerned that the idea of reading seems intimidating to parents, talk about looking at books together, about describing pictures, and about looking at pictures and telling a story.

   g. Encourage bilingual and non–English-speaking parents to read in whatever language is most comfortable; acknowledge the importance of storytelling and oral traditions.

C. Using books in the examination room. If books are available to be given to the child at the visit
- Bring the book early in the visit.
- Offer the book to the child and observe the child's behavior with the book while you speak with the parent.
- Use the book as part of your observation of the child's developmental skills and also as a way to watch the parent–child interaction.
- Link the book to the anticipatory guidance that you give about bedtime, positive parenting, school readiness, screen time, and other relevant subjects—and help parents see that the book is a tool with which they can apply this advice starting today.

D. Choosing age-appropriate books for children
1. For **newborn and very young infants**, choose books that encourage parents to hold them, talk, read, and sing to them.
2. For **6–12 months of age**, choose small board books, with pictures of faces and only a few words per page.
3. For **1–2 years of age**, choose board books with pictures of familiar objects, family life, and animals; choose simple stories and books with rhyme and repetition.
4. Some **2-year-olds** still need board books; many can handle paper pages and enjoy books with more complex stories; rhyme and repetition remain important.
5. For **3–5 years of age**, it is often helpful to offer the child a choice of books. Fantasy stories are popular, as are funny stories and family stories; also consider alphabet books and counting books.
6. Many clinicians offer books to school-age children as well, usually donated gently used books—these need to be screened and sorted by approximate reading level, and children can then select their own choices.

E. Books as developmental observation tools
1. Observe fine motor development as the child handles book, looking for pincer grasp in turning pages and pointing with one finger (at 9 months of age), for increasing skill in handling paper pages (by 2 years of age).
2. Assess speech and language as the child responds to book: infants should vocalize, 1- to 2-year-olds should label with single words, and older children may be asked to name objects or colors.
3. Discuss the child's language with parents in the context of the book: by 15–18 months, children begin filling in words at the ends of familiar sentences; by 2 years, they can "read" familiar books to themselves or their stuffed animals.
4. Assess parent–child interaction and whether parent is able to pick up child's cues, answer child's questions, and respond to child's interests.
5. At the 4- or 5-year-old visit, use the book as a tool to look at the child's school readiness skills, asking the child to name colors, count objects, identify letters on the page, and describe what is happening in illustrations.

VI. CLINICAL PEARLS AND PITFALLS
- Hand the book to the child early in the visit, and observe the child's handling of the book and the parent's response.
- Be sure to have the book in the room during the visit and not to use it as a "give-away" (such as a sticker or a lollipop) at the end of the visit.
- Model simple dialogic book-reading strategies in the examination room—pointing at pictures and naming them with infants and toddlers (*"That's a baby, where's the baby's nose?"*), asking more complicated questions with older children (*"What do you think will happen if he gives that cookie to the mouse?"*).
- Compliment parents when children take pleasure in the books, or manifest book-handling skills (*"He [or she] really seems to like books—that's because you read to him [or her] at home."*).
- If there are any concerns about the parent's own literacy skills, encourage the parent to enjoy the book with the child without emphasizing the word "read," by talking about looking at books together, naming the pictures, and telling a story.
- Help parents use the book as a prompt to build home routines; emphasize the value of bedtime reading and the importance of keeping screens out of the child's bedroom.
- Include questions about parents' experience in school in your history, and be alert for parental history which may suggest struggles with written language and literacy.
- Be prepared to offer referrals to adult and/or family literacy programs to parents who express a desire to improve their own literacy skills.
- With non–English-speaking families, it is of course very helpful to have books available in the appropriate language; but when this is not possible, parents should be encouraged to look at pictures and discuss books with their children, even when they cannot read the words.

- Mothers with new babies can read aloud to an older child while nursing the baby, and this is meaningful for both children.
- It's fine to read the same picture book to children of different ages.
- Older siblings can be encouraged to read aloud to younger children and should be celebrated for their reading skills.
- Do not let this become a drill or a way of pressuring children to read early. Reading aloud should be about enjoying books together. Older children will certainly begin to pick up information about print and letters, and parents can encourage this, but hearing a story should not be a test!
- Encourage parents to go on reading with older children, even after they have started learning to read in school.
- Recommend that families explore the local library; consider providing information in the office or the waiting room about library programs and story hours.
- Help parents understand the link between a younger child who enjoys being read to—in part, because it means parental attention and "face time"–and an older child who likes books and feels eager and ready to learn to read.

Bibliography

FOR PARENTS

WEBSITES

http://www.reachoutandread.org/parents/.
http://www.readingrockets.org/.
http://www.bankstreet.edu/literacyguide/main.html.
https://www.nap.edu/read/6014/chapter/3.

BOOKS

Fox M. *Reading Magic: Why Reading Aloud to Our Children Will Change Their Lives Forever.* Boston: Mariner Books; 2008.

Lipson ER. *The New York Times Parent's Guide to the Best Books for Children.* 3rd ed. New York: Three Rivers Press; 2000.

Silvey A. *Everything I Know I Learned From A Children's Book.* New York: Roaring Book Press; 2009.

Trelease J. *The Read-Aloud Handbook.* 7th ed. New York: Penguin; 2013.

FOR PROFESSIONALS

Council on Early Childhood. Literacy promotion: an essential component of primary care pediatric practice. *Pediatrics.* 2014;134:1-6.

Duursma E, Augustyn M, Zuckerman B. Reading aloud to children: the evidence. *Arch Dis Child.* 2008;93(7):554-557.

High PC, LaGasse L, Becker S, et al. Literacy promotion in primary care pediatrics: can we make a difference? *Pediatrics.* 2000;104:927-934.

Hutton JS, Horowitz-Kraus T, Mendelsohn AL, et al. Home reading environment and brain activation in preschool children listening to stories. *Pediatrics.* 2015;136:466-478.

Klass P, Dreyer BP, Mendelsohn AL. Reach out and read: literacy promotion in pediatric primary care. *Adv Pediatr.* 2009;56:11.

Mendelsohn AL, Mogilner LN, Dreyer BP, et al. The impact of a clinic-based literacy intervention on language development in inner-city preschool children. *Pediatrics.* 2001;107:130-134.

WEBSITES

https://littoolkit.aap.org/Pages/home.aspx.

CHAPTER 17

Behavioral Management: Theory and Practice

Edward R. Christophersen | Sarah S. Nyp

Traditional behavioral management techniques can be very useful to the primary care clinician. This chapter describes the concepts and techniques that the primary care clinician can routinely recommend to parents to use when interacting with their children.

I. TECHNIQUES TO TEACH OR IMPROVE BEHAVIORS

A. Time-in and verbal praise

1. *Time-in* refers to brief, nonverbal, physical contact provided to a child when a parent notices that the child is displaying appropriate or acceptable behavior. Examples include a pat on the back or a tussle of the hair. Time-in can be described to parents as a two-handed approach. One hand is on the child and the other hand is over the parent's mouth. This description illustrates to parents the importance of providing physical contact as an encouragement to the child to continue the current behavior. The nonverbal nature of the communication decreases the chances of distracting the child from the behavior that is being praised. If a child is sitting quietly while working on puzzles with her sibling and her mother "interrupts" the appropriate play and interaction by providing a verbal comment, even verbal praise, the child is less likely to continue the activity. The physical contact of time-in provides the child with knowledge that the behavior was noticed and appreciated, without distracting the child from the acceptable activity. Parents should be encouraged and educated to provide their children with time-in whenever their children are engaging in acceptable behavior. They should not wait for "good behavior."

2. *Verbal praise* is provided when a child has done something "good." The best time to use verbal praise is during natural breaks in an activity. For example, when a child is engaged in a coloring activity, the parent should provide lots of brief, nonverbal, physical contact (time-in). Once the child has finished coloring or stops coloring to show it to a parent, verbal praise is appropriate. Note: When the parent is actively working to eliminate an undesired behavior, verbal praise for even minimally acceptable behavior should be utilized and maximized. Example: A child typically hits her younger sibling when the younger sibling takes a toy from her. The parent will provide time-in when the child "uses his or her words" to express displeasure in the sibling's actions, even if the words used at a volume considered to be yelling. At this stage, it is best to avoid "backhanded compliments" such as "I like the way you used your words, but don't yell." A simple verbal praise "I like the way you used your words" is ideal.

   Advantages. Time-in and verbal praise encourage children to continue to engage in acceptable behaviors. When applied correctly, these techniques take no additional parent time and do not distract children.

B. Incidental learning.
Children learn behaviors by being around individuals who engage in those behaviors. This is called *incidental learning*. For example, if both parents smoke cigarettes, their child is significantly more likely to become a smoker than if neither parent smokes. A surprising number and variety of children's behaviors appear to have been learned incidentally, including language, gestures, and anger management strategies.

   Advantages and disadvantages. Incidental learning can be achieved without any additional effort on the part of the parents. They need only be aware that such learning occurs naturally and be cognizant of incidental learning during the time they spend with their children. The negative side is that children also learn behaviors the parents never intended for them to learn (e.g., swearing).

C. Modeling

1. Two basic modeling techniques exist: live and video recordings. Most modeling procedures work best if the model is approximately the same age as the target child. For example, a 6-year-old boy who has previously had his teeth cleaned by a dentist and who behaved appropriately during the procedure could be observed live or on

video recordings while being examined. A second child who observes the dental procedures being performed on this model can learn both what to expect of dental procedures and how to react to those procedures.

Advantages and disadvantages. Children are more likely to believe what they see a peer doing than what their parents *tell* them, particularly if the two messages are contradictory (e.g., one a verbal message that the child should relax and the other the anxiety that a child feels in the dental chair). However, modeling can teach maladaptive behaviors as well as adaptive behaviors. For example, if a child is observing a peer model in the dentist's office and the peer model becomes very upset, the target child will probably have a more difficult time when it is his or her turn for the procedure. For this reason, the potential peer models should always be observed at least once to determine their appropriateness as peer models.

D. Reinforcement. Few topics in the behavioral literature have been more misunderstood than reinforcement. An item or activity can be said to have reinforcing properties for an individual child if and only if that child has previously worked to obtain access to that item or activity.

It is important to understand the differences between reinforcement and punishment. Effective reinforcement will increase a behavior. For example, a child who receives an extra story at bedtime after finishing his or her vegetables is more likely to eat the vegetables at the next meal. The bedtime story serves as "positive reinforcement" because the child is likely to increase a preferred behavior to receive the reinforcer. A child who is required to rewash the dishes after doing a poor job the first time is more likely to wash the dishes correctly at the next opportunity. The repeat of the chore serves as a "negative reinforcement" because the child is likely to increase a preferred behavior to avoid the consequence. Punishment is meant to decrease a behavior. For example, a child who is aggressive at a birthday party and is sent to time-out is more likely to avoid aggressive behavior when allowed to return to play. The loss of fun at the party serves as a "punishment" for the undesired behavior because the child is likely to decrease an undesired behavior in order to avoid the punishment.

1. **Choosing rewards.** Under the right circumstances, reinforcement, by definition, will work with virtually any age group and with many different behaviors. However, no item or activity can be accurately described as a reinforcer unless and until it has produced a change in behavior. For example, although candy is reinforcing for the vast majority of children, it cannot be referred to as a reinforcer until it has been demonstrated that the child will work to obtain the candy.

2. **Principles of reinforcement,** or the way the reinforcer is made accessible to a child, are extremely important.
   a. **Small rewards offered frequently are better than large rewards offered infrequently.** A physical hug offered several times during a household chore will usually be more effective than a big reward at the end of the chore. Small rewards during the chore and a reward at the end will also work nicely.
   b. **Repetition, with feedback, enhances a child's learning.** A child will learn more from performing the same task repeatedly, with help from his or her parent, than from performing it once. Although parents will often expect their child to perform a task correctly the first time, the child will actually learn the task better if he has many opportunities to practice. For example, a child who helps one of his or her parents to do the laundry several times each week for 2 years will probably be able to do the laundry for the rest of his or her life.
   c. Making the choice to participate in acceptable behavior is a learning process. Like many adults, children learn more quickly and retain the learning better if they are **relaxed while they are learning.** While helping children to acquire the skills to make appropriate choices can be very frustrating, the parent who becomes angry or impatient only exacerbates the situation. Similarly, an upset child does not learn as rapidly or permanently as a calm child. Parents should be reminded that children learn a significant amount about what behaviors are "appropriate" by watching how their parents respond when presented with frustrating or otherwise challenging situations.
   d. **Warnings only make behavior worse.** Parents have a natural tendency to warn their children. It is far more effective to discipline the child (provide a consequence), for not performing the task after the first time the request is ignored and then give the child another opportunity to fulfill the command, than it is to provide frequent warnings that the tasks must be done. In fact, children who receive warnings before consequences often learn that they may continue to disobey their parents several times before they will either be forced to complete

the request or receive a consequence. This "planned ignoring" on the part of the child often becomes increasingly frustrating to the parent and may even lead to "incidental learning" from inappropriate parental behavior that was not anticipated by the parent.

e. **A behavior must already be learned before it can be reinforced.** If the child does not know how to perform the expected behavior, offering a reward, in lieu of teaching the child how to perform the behavior, is ineffective. For example, if a child has never tied his own shoes, offering him a new bicycle if he ties his shoes is not likely to be effective.

Advantages and disadvantages. Reinforcing items and activities frequently can become part of normal, everyday life without substantial planning on the parents' part. Examples may include 10 minutes of one-on-one time playing catch with a parent or an extra story at bedtime. It should also be noted that reinforcing items and activities may sometimes be inadvertent. For example, when a parent waits until his or her child has been crying for several minutes in the morning, the parent may be reinforcing that child for crying. If the same parent had picked the child up BEFORE he or she started crying, however, the parent would be reinforcing the child for playing quietly in the crib instead of waiting until he or she was crying. In addition, the child's behavior may return to its prereinforcement level as soon as the reinforcers are no longer available. Procedures that have been shown to be successful in maintaining desired behaviors after reinforcement ceases include gradually making the reinforcer available less often (e.g., on the average, every second behavior is reinforced, then every third behavior, then every fourth behavior). Once a behavior becomes habitual, many individuals will engage in it whether it is reinforced or not.

E. **Conditioned reinforcers.** Many items and activities that have no intrinsic reinforcing properties can take on reinforcing properties. Money, for example, is not usually a reinforcer to a small child. When the child learns what he can purchase with money, it begins to take on reinforcing properties. As another example, a child can be offered small tokens (poker chips) that can later be exchanged for a reinforcing item or activity. In time, the small tokens will likely take on reinforcing properties.

Advantages. Conditioned reinforcers are usually more readily available than the actual reinforcer, and most children will work just as hard for a conditioned reinforcer as they will for the actual one. Conditioned reinforcers, such as money or tokens, also have the advantage that they can be traded for a wide variety of items or activities, as the child's tastes and preferences change. Conditioned reinforcers are often much more flexible than tangible reinforcers.

F. **The token economy.** Conditioned reinforcers work best if there is a consistent method of exchange. In the case of money, the exchange system is already in place, and the money becomes a "token" of what can be purchased. Entire "token economies" have been devised as treatment programs for children from age 4 years to adulthood. The term "token economy" refers to the organized manner in which tokens are gained and lost, as well as what can be purchased with them. The success or failure of a token economy depends almost entirely on how it is implemented and on how many reinforcing activities are realistically available to the individual who must earn, lose, and spend tokens. The mere use of tokens does not make a token economy successful.

Token economies are most effective when they are used as motivational systems to encourage children to engage in socially appropriate behaviors. Three different types of token economies are widely used to modify common behavioral problems:

1. A **simple exchange system** provides a means of keeping track of the child's appropriate and inappropriate behaviors. A list of behaviors can be posted on the door of the refrigerator. (Depending on the child's age/developmental level, the "list" may actually be a pictorial representation.) As the child completes assigned or volunteered tasks or chores, he or she marks these on the "positive side" of the exchange chart. Similarly, as the child engages in inappropriate behaviors, he or she marks these on the "negative side." When the child wants a special privilege or activity, there must be more positive marks than negative marks to "afford" the special privilege. The simple exchange system is appropriate for children aged 5–12 years.

2. In **chip systems,** the child earns a token, such as a poker chip, for positive behaviors. Each time poker chips are earned, the parent verbally acknowledges the child's appropriate behavior while offering chips. The child is then expected to take the chips from the parent's hand, look the parent in the eye, and say, "thank you." In this way, the child not only receives the tokens for the appropriate behavior but also practices appropriate social behaviors. Similarly, when the child engages in a

behavior that loses chips, he or she is expected to hand the chips to the parent politely and may receive one chip back for "accepting the fine so nicely." The chip system is useful for children aged 3–7 years.

3. The **point system** is like the chip system but can be much more sophisticated. Points can be used to motivate children and teenagers to practice the behaviors they are lacking, such as taking feedback well and sharing their feelings appropriately. Each time they engage in these types of behaviors, they earn points that can be used to purchase items and activities they want. The point system is useful for children aged 6–16 years.

4. Variations of these systems are available as "apps" for use on smartphones/tablets. Parents should be cautioned that for the system to be effective in this format, the child must be immediately aware that he or she is either earning or losing a chip or point.

G. **Fading.** Fading refers to changing a behavior gradually instead of abruptly changing it. For example:

• For a toddler who is drinking too much juice, a cup can be provided with juice, which is gradually diluted from 100% juice to 90% juice:10% water, then 80% juice:20% water, and so on, until the toddler is drinking 100% water from the cup.

• Raising training wheels on a bicycle 1/8 inch every 2 weeks until they are about 3 inches off the ground and no longer necessary is usually far more effective than simply removing the training wheels.

• Changing a child's bedtime by 15 minutes each night at daylight savings time instead of abruptly changing it the entire hour in one night is less likely to be noticed by the child and therefore result in easier transition.

• Teaching a child how to swallow pills by starting out with very small cake sprinkles to wash down with a favorite beverage and then gradually moving to larger candies is likely to allow the child to feel success without as much anxiety. The use of candies/preferred beverages may also serve as a reinforcer. Note: Typically using six to eight steps (sizes) is very effective in teaching pill swallowing.

Advantages and disadvantages. Fading often helps to avoid confrontations with a child. It can be used to accomplish something without incident that otherwise may have been difficult to accomplish. The disadvantage of fading is that these procedures typically take more time than if their child could abruptly make the desired changes.

II. PROCEDURES TO DECREASE OR DISCOURAGE BEHAVIORS

A. **Time-out.** Probably the most frequently recommended disciplinary technique is time-out. As initially used, time-out was actually referred to as "time-out from positive reinforcement." Over the past three decades or so, the term has been shortened to "time-out," and, in doing so, the idea of removing a pleasant interaction has been ignored or forgotten. Time-in and time-out are effective from infancy to early adolescence. **It is very important for parents to realize that in absence of good "time-in," there really is no such thing as "time-out."** There is often confusion regarding how long a time-out should last. This question can be answered by discussing with parents the purpose of time-out. The purpose is twofold. The first is to stop the undesired behavior (noncompliance, tantrum, etc.). The second is to encourage the development of self-quieting (calming) skills. Once a child is able to sit silently with quiet hands and feet, the child has accomplished both of these goals.

The following variables have the most impact on the effectiveness of time-out:

• It must be presented immediately after an inappropriate behavior. Warnings about using time-out should be eliminated.

• It must be presented every time the inappropriate behavior occurs.

• The time-out must remove or make unavailable an otherwise pleasant state of affairs (i.e., time-in), in most cases ALL interaction with the parent must cease.

• The time-out should not be considered "over" or "finished" until the child has quieted down.

• The child should be completely ignored during the time-out, regardless of how outrageous the behavior might become. One study demonstrated that time-out becomes more effective when the time-in is "enriched" (more fun, more enjoyable) and becomes less effective when the time-in is "impoverished."

Time-out can be implemented in any environment and should remain "portable." It should not be restricted to only one chair or corner of the room. Establishing a "strict" location for time-out can lead to difficulty using time-out when outside of the home. For example, time-out could be used on a bench outside a restaurant or store.

Advantages. Time-in and time-out provide parents with an effective alternative to nagging, yelling, or spanking. Their consistent use also encourages children to develop self-quieting skills (a child's ability to calm himself without the assistance of a parent).

It encourages these skills because the parents are modeling the ability to cope with an unpleasant situation and because the child is learning how to cope with feelings he or she experiences when he or she does not like something the parents have done.

B. Extinction. Extinction is defined as the withdrawal of all attention after a child engages in undesirable behaviors. One of the most common examples of extinction is not paying attention to a child's whining. When used properly, extinction involves completely ignoring a child's whining.

A major problem with using extinction is an initial sharp increase in the child's inappropriate behavior, called an *extinction burst*. For example, when a child is ignored during a temper tantrum or when whining, these behaviors usually increase in intensity and duration at first, perhaps leading parents to feel that the procedure is actually making the behavior worse and thus discouraging the parents from continuing the extinction procedure. If the parents continue with the extinction procedure, however, the change in the child's behavior will usually be forthcoming.

Although extinction procedures are often successful, parents may not be able to tolerate the technique. Several modifications have been made to make extinction techniques more acceptable to parents. For example, the "day correction of bedtime problems technique" involves teaching the parents to use extinction for whining and fussing during the day. The parents then gain confidence in their ability to use it properly, and the child learns that the parents will follow through with the use of extinction once they start it. Only after the parents and the child are familiar with the use of extinction during the day are the parents encouraged to use it at bedtime. The day correction technique is actually more effective than using extinction only at bedtime.

Advantages and disadvantages. Extinction procedures have been effective with many different childhood problems. The time necessary to educate parents on the use of these procedures is reasonable, given the constraints of primary care practices. The main disadvantage is the extinction burst and the parents' potential inability to tolerate their child's initial distress at being ignored.

C. Planned ignoring. The parents gradually ignore their child's behavior for longer and longer periods of time (as opposed to introducing complete extinction abruptly). Planned ignoring may result in less of an extinction burst, but it takes longer to be effective. Probably the most common use of planned ignoring is for bedtime resistance.

D. Spanking. With spanking, caregivers can vent their own frustration at the same time they are hoping to discourage a child from engaging in the behavior that resulted in the spanking. In addition, spanking will often produce an immediate, yet often temporary, decrease in the child's behavior.

Advantages and disadvantages. Spanking can teach a child that hitting is an acceptable way to express frustration or anger. The child, after being spanked, is likely to avoid or try to escape from the caregiver who administered the spanking. To maintain its effect, the magnitude of spanking often must increase over time (harder spanking). This may lead to injury or abuse. Spanking can also result in other discipline methods losing their effectiveness. Thus, a child who is frequently spanked at home is less likely to be responsive to the use of extinction at childcare. Since time-in and time-out can produce virtually the same effects as spanking but without the side effects, spanking should not be recommended for parents.

E. Job grounding. This is a form of grounding whereby the child has control over how long the grounding is in effect. When a child has broken a major rule (e.g., gone to a shopping center on his or her bike without telling parents), he or she is "grounded." The child loses all privileges (including television, telephone, having a friend over, playing with games, snacks, and desserts) until he or she has completed one job properly. The jobs, which can each be written on a 3 inches × 5 inches card, should be agreed upon by both the parent and child during a quiet, peaceful time, should not be one of the child's typical household chores, and should take 5–10 minutes to complete (washing the windows of the family car, picking up pet waste from the yard). The child, upon being grounded, is asked to pick from a stack of cards that are held face down by the parent. Once the job is chosen, the child is restricted from all activities, with the exception of family meals and homework, until the job is completed. The parents are instructed to refrain from nagging, prodding, and reminding. As soon as the child has completed the job (most jobs should take only 5–10 minutes to complete and be tasks that the child has done many times before), he or she is "off grounding." Job grounding differs from traditional time-based grounding in that the child determines how long the grounding lasts and, under most circumstances, the child has the option of getting the job done without missing valued social activities.

Advantages and disadvantages. Job grounding is usually effective; it lets the child practice a job that he or she probably did not want to do in the first place, and it gives him the opportunity to avoid losing a valued activity. The disadvantage is that if the child has no planned activities, he or she may stall on completing the job until some external motivation is present.

F. Positive practice. Positive practice is the procedure of having a child practice an appropriate behavior after each inappropriate behavior. For example, when a previously toilet-trained child wets his or her pants, he or she is required to practice "going to the bathroom" 10 times; 5 times from the place where the incident was discovered and 5 times from alternative sites such as the front yard, the backyard, the kitchen, and the bedroom. When used correctly, with no nagging or unpleasant behavior on the part of the caregivers, positive practice can produce dramatic results.

Advantages and disadvantages. Positive practice gives a child many opportunities to practice appropriate behaviors. This technique is typically effective quickly. The disadvantages include the length of time necessary to implement the practice, as well as the fact that the practice should be done immediately after the inappropriate behavior, which is not always convenient.

G. Practice, praise, point out, and prompt. Several of these procedures can be combined into a very effective teaching tool. For example, when a child's interruption is a problem, they can be taught an alternative to interrupting. Encourage the parents to practice having their child gently place his or her hand on the parent's forearm, and the parent immediately place his or her hand on the child's hand and ask his or her what they would like to say. This should be practiced daily with a reward for practicing. The parents should "point out" to their child when the parents wait instead of interrupting or when a character in a book is seen to be waiting. The parents can also "prompt" their child to place his or her hand, for example, on Daddy's arm when he or she wants to get his attention. This strategy combines incidental learning, modeling, reinforcement, and praise.

H. Habit reversal training or comprehensive behavioral intervention for tics. Habit reversal training (HRT) and comprehensive behavioral intervention for tics (CBIT) procedures were developed for use with habit disorders and motor or vocal tics. Habit reversal training requires a level of cognition not reached before a mental age of about 4–5 years.

1. Components of HRT/CBIT are the following:
   - Increase the child's awareness of the habit on a daily basis.
   - On a daily basis, the child should look into a mirror while performing the habit on purpose.
   - Parents help the child to become aware of how his or her body moves and what muscles are being used when he or she performs the habit.
   - The child identifies each time he or she engages in the habit by either raising the hand when the habit occurs or by stating something like, "that was one," when the habit occurs.
   - If parents see the habit occur but the child does not appear to be aware that it occurred, parents use a prearranged signal, gesture, or expression to help make the child aware.
   - Keeping track of how often the habit occurs is the only way that the parent and child can tell when progress is being made. Depending on the child's age, the child may be able to participate in self-monitoring by recording each occurrence of the habit on a 3 × 5 card. If the child is not able to do this independently, the parent and child can complete the card together.
   - A competing response is a movement or posture, which renders completing the action of the habit impossible. For example, placing hands in one's pants pockets renders nail biting impossible.
   - The competing response should be practiced daily. Have the child practice his or her competing response in the mirror. This helps the child become comfortable with the response and assures him that the competing response is not noticeable socially. For example, a child who is blinking his or her eyes excessively can practice blinking the eyes very gently and the child who is pulling his or her hair can practice holding the thumbs on the waist of the pants.
   - The child is encouraged to use the competing response when he or she feels the urge to engage in the habit or in situations where the child has a history of engaging in the habit.
   - The child is encouraged to use the competing response for 1 minute following the occurrence of the habit.

- Stress anxiety reduction procedures (all should be practiced daily):
  - Progressive muscle relaxation training
  - Visual imagery
  - Breathing exercises
2. Parent involvement
   Although many children and adolescents will notice a decrease in their habit within a couple of days, the greatest change from using these procedures occurs during the second and third months.
   Advantages and disadvantages. HRT/CBIT is effective and has no physical side effects. The overall reduction in habit disorders and tics is also far greater with this technique than with medication. The disadvantage is the time it takes to teach and monitor, as well as the time it takes to reduce the habit (usually days).
   - **Feedback.** Parents work with the child to increase awareness of his or her habit by helping him or her identify the habit when it occurs.
   - **Support and encouragement.** Parents encourage their child to use the competing response and praise the child for doing so. Parents also praise any noted decrease in rates of the habits.

III. **GENERAL REMARKS AND CONCLUSIONS**
   - Although the term "behavior management" frequently has been used to refer to coercive action taken in an effort to discourage a child from engaging in inappropriate behavior, many positive alternatives are available. Generally, the emphasis should be on teaching children appropriate behaviors, rather than concentrating on reducing inappropriate behaviors.
   - The single most important consideration in implementing such behavior management strategies is taking a history that can help to identify precisely what strategy should be offered to the caregiver and how to offer that strategy. The clinician now has a variety of evidence-based behavior management strategies available for dealing with situations encountered in the provision of care to typically developing children with minor behavior problems.
   - As with many of the "medical interventions" offered to parents from the clinician, the use of written handouts summarizing the treatment recommendations can be very helpful to the parent who is trying to follow the clinician's recommendations.

Bibliography

FOR PARENTS

Christophersen ER. *Little People: Guidelines for Commonsense Child Rearing.* 4th ed. Shawnee Mission, KS: Overland Press; 1998.

Christophersen ER, Mortweet SL. *Parenting that Works: Building Skills that Last a Lifetime.* Washington, DC: American Psychological Association; 2003.

Schmitt BD. *Your Child's Health.* 2nd ed. New York: Bantam Books; 1991.

WEB SITES

http://www.patienteducation.com/.

http://www.disciplinehelp.com/.

FOR PROFESSIONALS

Christophersen ER, McConahay KH. Day correction of pediatric bedtime resistance. In: Perlis ML, Aloia M, Kuhn BR, eds. *Behavioral Treatments for Sleep Disorders: A Comprehensive Primer of Behavioral Sleep Medicine Interventions:* Elsevier/Academic Press; 2010:311-317.

Christophersen ER, Mortweet SL. *Treatments that Work with Children: Empirically Supported Strategies for Managing Childhood Problems.* 2nd ed. Washington, DC: American Psychological Association; 2013.

Christophersen ER, VanScoyoc SM. What Makes Time-Out Work (and Fail)? AAP Section of Developmental and Behavioral Pediatrics Newsletter; 2007.

Mortweet SL, Christophersen ER. Coping skills for the angry/impatient/clamorous child: a home and office practicum. *Contemp Pediatr.* 2004;21(6):43-55.

Piacentini J, Woods DW, Scahill L, et al. Behavior therapy for children with Tourette Disorder: a randomized controlled trial. *J Am Med Assoc.* 2010;303:1929-1937.

Schmitt BD, ed. *Pediatric Advisor.* Englewood, CO: Clinical Reference Systems. Computer software; 2003.

Schriver MD, Allen KD. *Working with Parents of Noncompliant Children: A Guide to Evidence-Based Parent Training for Practitioners and Students.* Washington, DC: American Psychological Association; 2008. http://www.aap.org/ConnectedKids/.

CHAPTER 18

Managing Behavior in Primary Care

Barbara J. Howard

I. **DESCRIPTION OF THE PROBLEM.** Behavioral and emotional issues comprise an estimated 25%–50% of all presenting problems raised by parents in primary care visits. Pediatric primary care clinicians are in an ideal position to deal with such concerns: They are well known to the family, generally respected, viewed as supportive by both the parent and child, and already know much about the child and the family. In addition, the office setting is seen as friendly, nonstigmatizing territory.

II. **IDENTIFYING PROBLEMS**

A. **Open-ended questions.** The first requirement for addressing behavioral problems is their identification. This is not always easy because children rarely ask for help and the parents may not realize that the clinician has either the interest or the expertise to help. Discussing behavior and development at each visit, using screening questionnaires online or on paper, and educating oneself to have practical advice will all encourage parents to discuss behavioral concerns. Open-ended questions (ones that cannot be answered by one word) such as *"How are things going?"* allow the parent and child to express their own agenda for the visit. For children aged 3 years and older, an interview of the children first can convey their centrality to the visit and elicits their point of view before they have heard (and potentially clammed up from) parental complaints. In other families, the clinician may need to ask specifically about *behavior at home, at school, or in child care.* Another approach that broadens the agenda is to ask routinely, *"What is the hardest part of taking care of your X-month-old?"*

B. **Observations in the office.** Observations of behavior in the office and waiting room can be revealing. Toys in the examination room are an invaluable way to observe the child's behavior and development (as well as to enhance the enjoyment of the visit). These observations can then be used to start the discussion (e.g., *"I noticed that he is very active. How is that for you at home?"*). Such comments should be asked in a non-judgmental way so that the parents' responses can reveal if they view the behavior as problematic. The clinician's own feelings and intuitions about the child and family should be compared with parental and child reports and used to raise questions or to formulate clinical hypotheses about the child's behavior. Asking the child to *"draw a picture of a boy or a girl"* and relate a story about that child or a Family Kinetic Drawing (*"Everyone in your family doing something."*) can be very informative about the child's perceptions as well as about the cognitive and fine motor skills.

C. **Screening questionnaires.** Questionnaires can be a valuable time-saver and tool for identifying behavioral problems and providing documentation. Use of validated screening tools for behavior are now recommended by the American Academy of Pediatrics as standard care annually from age 4 years and when there are concerns because informal methods have low sensitivity (see Chapters 5 and 6).

D. **Collecting additional information.** The next task is to collect additional information by questions, observations, direct physical examination or testing, and often requesting information from other sources such as notes from childcare or school report cards. Depending on the acuity of the problem and time available, this may be deferred to a scheduled follow-up visit.

III. **MANAGING BEHAVIORAL PROBLEMS**

A. **Defining the problem and setting goals.** The first step to successful problem resolution occurs during the initial discussion in defining the problem. After initial open-ended questions, it is crucial to elicit details of specific examples including about the onset and attempted solutions, as well as times when the problem was not present (e.g., when alone with father) to look for relevant causal factors. A survey of the areas of daily functioning (including bedtime, meals, toileting, peer interaction, separation abilities, family relationships, and school adjustment) is all needed to detect patterns that suggest gaps in skills or dysfunctional management.

It is important for the clinician to summarize the parents' (or his or her own if the parent has none) concerns to demonstrate that their worries have been heard. The clinician should formulate and explain his or her clinical hypotheses about the underlying child, family, and environmental factors contributing to the child's behavior. The problem should be discussed nonjudgmentally and reframed in a positive light of what skills need to be developed rather than the less actionable goal of ending a behavior (e.g., *"You would like him to listen to instructions [rather than to not act up]"*).

The initial discussion should set the stage for treatment by clarifying the problem, interpreting the meaning of the behavior, setting a positive tone, engaging other family members by determining how it affects them, and not blaming or insulting the child (who may be listening).

The next step is to convey some *hope and confidence* that a solution is possible and *collaboratively design an initial plan* or "homework" that addresses relevant goals for behavior change and also the meanings attributed to the behavior. It is important to guide family members in selecting homework tasks that apply to the family dynamic that seems causative, include tasks for each family member that are doable and measurable, and are of a scope that is not overwhelming and also not trivial. Additional diagnostic information comes from seeing how the family acted on this advice (or not) when they come for a follow-up.

B. **Levels of intervention in primary care.** There are different levels of behavior management suitable for different practitioners depending on their amount of interest, skill, time available for this work, and acceptability as advisors to the family who may prefer a referral.

1. **Education.** The simplest level of behavioral intervention is caregiver's education. This usually entails discussing with the family what the behavior may mean to them and to the child, what behavior is normal for age, and how temperament may be involved. This level of intervention should also include teaching families how to set up the environment to reduce the child's frustration and stress (e.g., put away remotes, assure enough sleep) and how the caregivers should model managing emotions themselves, for example, through self-control, verbalizing feelings, or walking away. Education about what can unintentionally reinforce a behavior is also important including giving attention, backing off requests, or scolding.

2. **Advice.** The second level of intervention involves all of the abovementioned plus giving specific advice for the problem behavior. Obtaining details about the A, B, C, and G of a specific incident: Antecedent (including the meaning); Behavior that occurs or Belief evoked; Consequence (including emotions); and any Gap in skills that set the child up to act in the undesired way is essential and will generally reveal patterns of family interaction. Often children act up at times when they are being asked to make a transition to a new activity or other repeated situations such as the morning rush. In other cases, the meaning of the behavior is revealed in examples such as opposition sparking when parents argue. Clarifying these patterns may be all that is needed for a family to solve the problem for themselves. Further coaching may be needed on how to anticipate these scenarios and how to verbalize about, praise, and give marks or points for even small improvements in emotion control, flexibility, or cooperation.

3. **Dealing with underlying issues.** Higher-level interventions involve dealing with underlying issues in the child, adult, family interaction, or the environment. To successfully work on this level, the clinician needs to understand and make hypotheses based on a transactional model that takes into account mutual influences among these factors.

   a. **Child issues.** Child issues that result in frustration such as functional weaknesses in motor skills, language, emotional regulation, or attention control may need further evaluation. Treatment for weaknesses and bypass strategies can be advised including things such as special education support, therapy for strengthening skills, reducing demands, altered placement, and medication for attention-deficit/hyperactivity disorder (ADHD).

      The behavior itself or the situations eliciting the problem may have meaning to the child that must be addressed directly or symbolically. Clinicians may efficiently hypothesize these meanings on the basis of an understanding of developmental stages and commonly associated family issues, for example, sibling jealousy that emerges when infants begin to crawl and get into the other's toys. Other ways of determining the meaning of a behavior include asking directly, *"What does it make you think when he does that?"* or telling the child or family *"Any kid who ..."* (e.g., wonders if a divorce is his fault might act up to elicit punishment)" while watching the person's emotions. Sometimes the meaning can be inferred from a reaction to "homework" that addresses the issue, for example, infantilizing activities during special time for the child who seems to act up due to seeking more nurturance.

There are common patterns of family dynamics associated with child behavior problems at different ages. For example, young children may be out of control when a laissez-faire style has resulted from a reaction against a parent's own history of being punished harshly as a child. Sleeping problems in a child may result when there is marital discord causing ambivalence about the parents' sleeping together. Biting may occur when parents cannot agree on whether or not to use corporal punishment. School underachievement may occur when a sibling is glorified for academics. Promiscuity may signal incest or sexual abuse. Substance abuse may result from depression. After gathering data for a hypothesis about meaning the clinician shares this with the child and/or family and works with both to help the family members clarify and communicate their feelings and to establish new adaptive ways of interacting that are no longer based on reactions to these issues but fill the needs of all parties.

b. **Parent issues.** It may become clear after simple advice has failed that interfering parent issues need to be addressed such as the parent viewing the child as special or vulnerable, inability to tolerate angry emotions from the child due to their own past exposure to violence, inability to prevent interfering with the other parent's management, covert satisfaction in a child's misbehavior, or lack of energy or motivation to do the hard work of behavior management.

Eliciting past experiences that are reawakened during child management is often the key. Engaging cooperation from all relevant adults is always helpful and may be essential. When the adults understand how their own issue is affecting the child's behavior, they are better able to change their interaction patterns. Writing down the costs and benefits to maintaining the interaction patterns is a useful intervention as is done in motivational interviewing. Referral for further individual work or therapy for the adult may also be needed.

c. **Interactional issues.** A parent with reasonable overall parenting skills may still be susceptible to maladaptive practices with an individual child. This may be due to a mismatch in temperament with the child, an unreasonable expectation in light of this child's attributes, or a change in circumstances or different energy from that available at other periods of parenting for providing adequate attention to the child's positive behaviors. Education and clarification may be sufficient, but providing alternative nurturers for the child is sometimes the only solution.

d. **Environmental issues.** It is not unusual for a child's behavior to be due to outside conditions, especially with the current culture of extensive time in childcare. Toxins such as lead, poor-quality care by others, and models or stress from observing dysfunctional adult behaviors should all be considered when kindly, reasonable parents are unable to resolve child behavior in a previously well-adjusted child. The mediating factors may also be sleep debt, hunger, sibling, or peer influence or abuse. These factors often occur in combination with the abovementioned so that all need to be addressed.

C. **Special "problem visits".** Once a problem has been identified, one or more visits of longer duration than usual are generally needed. To arrange an effective "problem visit," the vitally important people in the child's life should be invited to attend, if possible. Mother's boyfriend, neighbors, or babysitters, for example, may be crucial to the solution of the problem if parents give consent for them to attend.

1. **Visit duration.** Frequently, a longer (e.g., 30–60 minutes) problem visit can be scheduled at the beginning or the end of the workday, when no sick children are waiting to be seen and telephone calls can be postponed. (It is often advantageous to schedule the problem visit at the beginning of the day, when clinician energy is high.) Sometimes the most delicate or powerful issue is not raised until the last moments of the visit in a "parting shot." Such important statements at the end of the hour need to be acknowledged with appropriate empathy, recorded in the chart, and promised as first agenda items at the next visit (which may need to be scheduled sooner, depending on the information revealed).

Another problem occurs when families or key family members arrive late for an appointment. This may be an important statement of that person's ambivalence about the issues being discussed. The emotional difficulty can be acknowledged directly and with empathy, but the visit should be kept on schedule.

2. **Space considerations.** Many offices lack an examination room large enough to seat all the family members. A conference room or even the waiting room may better serve and can be private enough before or after regular office hours.
3. **Documentation of the visit.** Because details of the session are critical to understanding and managing the problem and documenting complexity for billing, the clinician should leave adequate time to record the salient aspects of the visit. Note-taking is possible during the session for some clinicians but should be interrupted when it interferes with the therapeutic alliance with the family and the patient.
4. **Billing for the visit.** It is important that the extended problem visit be adequately billed with a higher level of care usually based on time spent. Patients should be informed of the fee *before* the first extended visit. Offering to accept payment over time may decrease the burden of the extra fee for some families. Third-party reimbursement may be available depending on the diagnosis, the clinician's experience and training, and state insurance regulations. Clinicians generally cannot refer their own patients to themselves and then record the visit as a consultation. Experience suggests that most patients *are* willing to pay for counseling if they are able. Many of the barriers to adequate billing are in the mind of the clinician, who is insecure about whether she or he really has something valuable to offer.

D. Expanding counseling skills. Books, journals, lectures, videotapes of master therapists, workshops, courses, and fellowships in behavior and development, child psychiatry, or family therapy are available to help clinicians strengthen their behavioral counseling skills. The ultimate method, however, is through experience. For example, working as cotherapist with a more experienced clinician in the session with the family is a very valuable format. Case discussions with another clinician or in a group provide support and often help clarify the family's and clinician's emotional reactions, as well as providing input into the content and process of management. This process is called *supervision* and can be either direct (another professional attends the counseling session or observes through a one-way mirror) or indirect (the other professional reviews cases later from audiotape, videotape, verbatim process notes, standard notes, or clinician presentation, and makes suggestions to be incorporated into future patient visits). The Bureau of Maternal and Child Health has funded a number of Collaborative Office Rounds demonstration projects to provide such case discussion for groups of 8–10 practicing pediatric clinicians, or a similar group can be assembled with an agreement to pay the supervisor for his or her time.

E. Communicating with schools. Some behavioral problems are situationally specific and occur only in school or day care. In such cases, it may be essential to obtain an objective description of the problem from the school. Have parents sign a note of consent for two-way communication at the first visit that can be faxed to the other relevant sites. A behavioral questionnaire can be sent to the teacher via the child, mail, fax, or an online system or a written note requested. Ideally, direct telephone contact between clinician and teacher is the most revealing. (It is easiest to reach teachers at 7:30 AM or noon.) Teachers are generally very grateful for the clinician's interest and can be extremely helpful in providing more information about the family and the child. A single clinician visit to a school to meet one child's teachers, principal, and guidance counselor can facilitate communication for years to come about many children.

F. Making effective referrals. One of the most important (and underrated) skills of the primary care clinician lies in making effective referrals. An estimated 68% of mental health referrals made for children are unsuccessful because the family has been poorly prepared, important members do not perceive the problem as significant or treatment as valuable, the family has negative perceptions of mental health professionals, or there is a poor fit between the specialist's therapeutic style and the family's or child's expectations.
1. **Help the family to identify their distress.** The first steps in making an effective referral are to ensure that each member of the family feels that his or her voice has been heard and to identify the distress that will motivate the family and child to accept counseling. It is always better for a clinician to refer the family for a problem that bothers *them*, even if it is not the one that appears primary to the clinician (e.g., a referral for the child's truancy rather than the father's alcoholism). The therapist taking on the case may need to do further work before the family is able to face the central issue.
2. **Discuss issues in a constructive way.** Behavioral and family issues should be discussed in nonjudgmental terms, citing their strengths and using issues from the family's current (rather than past) situation to suggest further work. In the case of a separation from an abusive spouse, for example, one might say, "*It took so much*

courage to make this break that I can see that you really want what is best for your son. Now you can focus on improving your relationship with him and seeing him as a different kind of male from your ex-husband."

3. Find the appropriate referral. The next step in making an effective referral is to identify an appropriate consultant for the family. There is often no choice, given the limitations of insurance or family ability to pay. The clinician should inquire about the family's past experiences with counseling and demystify the process of counseling (e.g., by pointing out that therapy is just like the talking that has been going on in the exploratory sessions).

It is ideal to have ready the names and telephone numbers of several therapists who are available and have interest and skills in the type of problem at hand. This takes some preparation in getting to know the counseling style of a cadre of therapists: for example, what kinds of cases they prefer; whether they practice cognitive behavioral therapy, family therapy, or psychodynamic therapy; and whether they offer groups. Determine their fees and accepted insurance and how best to exchange information with them.

Consider introductory face-to-face meetings with local therapists. This provides some basis for discussing the therapists with families and will facilitate future communications between the physician and therapist. The clinician should ideally provide the family and patient with details about the therapists so that they can make an informed choice. The gender of the therapist is not usually central to the success of treatment, although some family members may have a strong preference, which should be respected. The relationship of the family with this professional is vital to the treatment, so they should be actively involved in the initial referral. In addition, they should be told that they can always change counselors, should the need arise. This is important so that their problems do not go unresolved simply because of an initial mismatch.

4. Follow-up. Finally, it is important for the family to know that the primary care clinician will stay involved and will continue to manage other problems as before. This reassures them that they are not being rejected, especially if they have revealed information about themselves that could be perceived as undesirable. The clinician should be clear in defining exactly what problems will be handled by which professional, obtain written consent to communicate, and stay in touch with the referral therapist to assist or back up the therapist's plans and to facilitate ongoing communication with the family.

G. Alternative counseling strategies in the office

1. Groups for families. Group sessions for a number of families concerning common behavioral problems (e.g., temper tantrums, toilet training, discipline issues, choosing a day care provider, homework strategies) can be an effective way to address those issues and to provide parents with a support system of other parents in similar circumstances. Other groups can be made available for parents of children with a specific problem, such as ADHD, oppositional defiant disorder, or developmental disabilities. Local branches of national diagnosis-specific organizations may already offer these or may arrange them when sufficient interest is shown. It has been shown that noncategorical groups, for example, for parents of children with a variety of chronic illnesses, can be as effective as diagnosis-specific groups. One-time sessions may be arranged to deal with crises, such as a publicized suicide, disaster, abuse in a local childcare center, or death of a public figure. For families, the existence of others with similar problems can be a tremendous relief in itself.

These groups can be led by a primary care clinician in the practice or by an outside consultant, or coled by both. They may be offered in the office or elsewhere, sponsored by the practice, or simply made known to patients in the practice. It is important to remember that the needs of the individual child or family are frequently not entirely met by these groups, so the leaders must carefully monitor the participants and ensure that supplemental support, guidance, or management is available if needed.

2. Group checkups. There are some advantages to offering health supervision visits in groups. By seeing eight 18-month-old babies together over 1 hour, the clinician can spend much more time providing teaching, anticipatory guidance, and discussion of behavioral issues. It is important to also offer some private time for each family, however, as there may be issues that they do not care to share in a group.

3. Call hour. Many offices have a designated call-in hour for health and behavior questions conducted by either the physician or an experienced nurse or nurse practitioner. Although telephone consultations have obvious major disadvantages, when supervised carefully they can be part of a spectrum of office services for dealing with behavioral problems and help motivate families for behavior counseling if the call line information alone does not suffice.

4. **Housing other professional disciplines within the practice.** Many practices are choosing to provide office space for specialists from other disciplines to deal with specific behavioral and emotional problems. In private practices, the specialist may receive the space free, share in the costs and income of the group, have payment leveraged with an insurer, be paid a salary by the group, or be a totally independent colocated contractor renting space and billing independently. The practice benefits by having a known, trusted, and readily available person to whom to refer their patients. The entire practice can be strengthened by the comprehensive care that ends up being delivered within its walls.

Bibliography

Allmond BW, Tanner JL, Gofman HF. *The Family Is the Patient*. Baltimore: Williams & Wilkins; 1999.

Coleman WL, Howard BJ. Family-focused behavioral pediatrics: clinical techniques for primary care. *Pediatr Rev*. 1995;16:448-455.

Greene R. *The Explosive Child*. 2nd ed. New York: HarperCollins; 2001.

Shepard SA, Dickstein S. Preventive intervention for early childhood behavioral problems: an ecological perspective. *Child Adolesc Psychiatr Clin N Am*. 2009;18(3):687-706.

Stein MT, Coleman WL, Epstein RM. We've tried everything and nothing works: family-centered pediatrics and clinical problem-solving. *J Dev Behav Pediatr*. 2001;22:S55-S60.

CHAPTER 19

Pain

Caitlin Neri | Laura Goldstein

I. **DEFINITION AND BACKGROUND.** Pain is defined by the International Association for the Study of Pain as "an unpleasant sensory and emotional experience associated with actual or potential tissue damage or described in terms of such damage." This definition implies that pain has two components—a neurophysiologically determined sensation that results from stimulation of nociceptors and the interpretation of that stimulus, which is impacted by a host of genetic, personality, cognitive, developmental, experiential, environmental, and emotional factors. These factors may ease or magnify the amount of pain and suffering that the stimulus causes to the individual. Research suggests that previous repeated exposure to painful stimuli or significant focus on pain sensations can worsen the pain experience. Current understanding of pain, therefore, implies that because the experience of pain is so individualized, providers must tailor their care to meet the needs of each child. This chapter will focus on acute pain; we will touch on some aspects of chronic pain, as some of the general principles including a multimodal and interdisciplinary approach are relevant to the treatment of both acute and chronic pain.

Historically, pain has been undertreated in children for a variety of complex reasons. Owing to difficulties with pain assessment in children, social attitudes, and ethical and financial constraints on research, there was little emphasis on the importance of pain in children. In addition, up until 30 years ago, it was widely believed that infants and young children did not experience pain in the same way as older children or adults due to having an immature neurologic system. It is now clearly established that by the end of the second trimester, fetuses have in place the anatomical and chemical capabilities to experience discomfort. Preterm and newborn infants may, in fact, be hyperalgesic because they have the same number of nociceptors in a smaller surface area and because they lack descending modulation of pain through psychological means.

Inadequate pain management clearly has short- and long-term negative consequences. Untreated pain may inhibit immune function, induce stress hormone release, increase blood pressure, inhibit healing due to immobility, and decrease the pain threshold, which subsequently results in hyperalgesia and allodynia. Inadequately addressed pain in young and school-aged children with illness may cause worsening procedure anxiety during routine health care maintenance. It can also lead to elevated negative emotional states during visits and unpleasant or even traumatic experiences for the child and family. For many children with chronic conditions who have frequent doctors' appointments, inadequately treated procedure pain may result in increased anxiety about subsequent medical encounters and reluctance to attend of medical visits.

II. **DIAGNOSIS.** Adequate assessment is the cornerstone of pain treatment, and the individual's self-report of his or her discomfort is the gold standard for assessment. Pain assessment typically focuses on measures of pain intensity. In adults and children older than 8 years, the visual analog scale that quantifies pain intensity from 0 to 10 is traditionally used. Because of developmental immaturity in children aged 3–8 years, modification of the visual analog scale is necessary. The Wong Baker Faces Scale is the most commonly used and allows children 3 years and older to score pain for young children on the widely accepted 0–10 scale. Research is now exploring simplified scales (Simplified Faces Pain Scale [S-FPS] and Simplified Concrete Ordinal Scale [S-COS]) for use with preschool-aged children. For children younger than 3 years, physiologic parameters (increased heart rate, increased respiratory rate, decreased SaO_2) and behavioral measures such as facial expression, body position, and crying have all been used as nonspecific indicators of pain. Attempts have been made to cluster together these parameters into clinically usable scales (examples of these include the Faces, Legs, Activity, Cry, and Consolability [FLACC] for use in children 2 months–7 years, and the Children's Hospital of Eastern Ontario Pain Scale [CHEOPS], for use in children 1–7 years. Scales for term infants include the Neonatal Infant Pain Scale [NIPS] and the Neonatal Pain, Agitation and Sedation Scale [N-PASS] and for preterm infants (Premature Infant Pain Profile [PIPP]) as well as for children with significant developmental disabilities (Non-communicating Children's Pain Checklist—Revised [NCCPC-R]). When an intervention occurs to address an elevated pain intensity rating, a repeat assessment should typically occur within an hour to ascertain the efficacy of the intervention. Pain intensity rating scales are often inappropriate for children with chronic pain who should not be queried repeatedly about their level of discomfort. Functional scales such as the functional disability inventory (FDI) and the Child Activity Limitations Interview-21 (CALI-21), and quality of life measures such as Pediatric Quality of Life Inventory™ (PedsQL™) and Patient Reported Outcomes Measurement Information System® (PROMIS), and psychological measures to assess pain catastrophizing (Pain Catastrophizing Scale [PCS]) should be considered instead.

III. TREATMENT

A. General principles. The primary goal of treatment of children with acute pain is to make them as comfortable as possible, recognizing that it may not be possible to eliminate all discomfort. There needs to be a balance between pain relief and the side effects associated with treatment. However, a number of general principles have emerged:

1. It should be generally assumed that whatever hurts an adult will hurt a child and appropriate pain relief should be planned.

2. A preventative approach is key. Where pain is predictable, it makes much more sense to prevent pain from occurring than to ablate it once it has occurred. This suggests that around-the-clock dosing as compared with as needed dosing is preferable.

3. An interdisciplinary approach that includes pharmacologic, cognitive–behavioral, physical, and integrative approaches should be considered for all pain problems—both acute and chronic.

4. Preferred routes of administration for medications are oral, sublingual, subcutaneous or intravenous, as opposed to the more noxious intramuscular, rectal, or intranasal (IN) routes.

5. Needlesticks are extremely troubling for children and parents, and needle pain should be addressed in all inpatient and outpatient settings. Evidence-based approaches include comfort positioning, use of topical anesthetics, distraction and other mind–body strategies, and breastfeeding or use of sucrose for infants.

6. Prolonged pain may lead to sleep problems and immobilization, and both these problems can increase pain. Both should be considered when addressing pain.

B. Behavioral/cognitive approaches. Nonpharmacologic approaches vary depending on the type of pain and the age of the child. Minor alterations to the environment or basic calming techniques may be the only approaches necessary in situations where limited pain may be magnified by anxiety. However, these approaches are often most effective when used in conjunction with pharmacologic treatments.

1. **Parental presence and demeanor.** Parental presence during painful procedures and parental involvement in treatment decisions often have a significant impact on the amount of pain the child experiences. During procedures, parents can function as a "coach" and often their presence can be comforting or soothing to the child. It is essential, however, that parents be instructed on age-appropriate pain-relieving techniques. Practitioners should include parents in treatment decisions to reduce their own anxiety. When parents are anxious themselves, they may model anxious behaviors for their children and parental attempts at soothing the child may inadvertently exacerbate the child's anxiety. For example, parents should be instructed to avoid statements such as "it won't hurt" or "it won't hurt that bad," as they can appear dishonest and discount the child's feelings. Research has shown that children whose parents are overly apologetic or overly solicitous report more pain and display more pain behaviors than children whose parents are matter of fact, use distraction, and encourage coping techniques.

2. **Preparation.** Children are more successful when they are given age-appropriate information regarding upcoming procedures. Research has found that children who are not prepared (e.g., surprise injection) experience more distress. Preparation for procedures should include only necessary information about what will happen before, during, and after the procedure. It is important to only share information that will help prepare the child, as too many details can also be overwhelming to younger children and lead to increased anticipatory anxiety. When preparing a child for a painful procedure, the timing of the preparation should be determined by the child's developmental age and temperamental style. In general, younger children and children with high anxiety should be informed and prepared closer to the procedure.

3. **Visual imagery/distraction/hypnosis.** Relaxation and distraction techniques help children cope with painful illnesses or procedures by focusing their attention away from their discomfort and promoting relaxation. Relaxation will calm their anxiety and, in turn, their pain experience. Deep breathing strategies are easy for children to learn and may be taught through play (e.g., blowing pinwheels or bubbles). Children can also use guided imagery, a technique that involves imagining a more desirable or

calming place. In addition, body scan or progressive muscle relaxation techniques help the child to be more aware of his or her body while tensing and relaxing different muscle groups. Hypnosis also actively involves the child in a fantasy and uses suggestion to reframe the experience. Distraction techniques include playing with a preferred toy, looking at pictures, reading books, listening to music, asking the child unrelated questions, or watching videos. Parents may want to come prepared with a child's favorite toy or book to use for distraction. There are also numerous distraction and relaxation apps that can be easily accessed during the procedures.

C. Physical approaches. Massage, heat, cold, pressure, and vibration in the form of transcutaneous electrical nerve stimulation all work by flooding the nervous system with nonnoxious stimuli, thereby serving as a natural pain blocker. Research has shown that using these nonpharmacologic techniques can be very helpful in pain reduction.

D. Pharmacologic approaches. A number of categories of pharmacologic agents are helpful in pain relief. They may have direct pain-relieving properties, anxiety-reducing properties, or potentiate analgesia.

1. **Local anesthetics.** A number of topical anesthetics are presently available, which should be used during pain associated with needle insertion or other painful procedures involving the skin. It should be noted that, to achieve maximum benefit from these topical anesthetics for procedural pain management, they should be used in combination with other evidence-based therapies including proper positioning, distraction, and sucrose or breastfeeding for infants.

   • **Eutectic Mixture of Local Anesthetics (EMLA), lidocaine 2.5% and prilocaine 2.5%,** a topically administered cream, is extremely effective for venous cannulation, phlebotomy, and reservoir access and has some efficacy on the pain associated with injections as well. 1–2 g should be applied to skin for 60 minutes and covered with an occlusive dressing; duration of analgesia is 1–2 hours.

   • **LMX4, 4% liposomal lidocaine (formally Ela-Max),** 1–2.5 g should be applied to skin for 30 minutes, does not require an occlusive dressing, is available without prescription, and provides 1 hour of analgesia.

   • **LET gel, lidocaine 4%, epinephrine 0.18%, and tetracaine 0.5%,** is ideal for superficial laceration treatment and repair. 1–3 mL is applied to an open wound for 20–30 minutes; duration of action is 45–60 minutes.

   • **J-tip, needle-free injection system,** sterile, single use, jet injector that uses CO_2 gas to create a stream of liquid analgesia using 1% buffered lidocaine or standard preservative-free lidocaine.

   • **Vapocoolant sprays** are sprayed on skin for approximately 10 seconds, until the skin blanches and produces immediate anesthesia for a few seconds, which can be helpful for injection or immunization pain.

2. **Drugs for mild to moderate pain.** Acetaminophen and nonsteroidal anti-inflammatory drugs (NSAIDs) (Table 19-1) are the first-line pharmacologic therapy for childhood pain and are typically adequate for mild to moderate pain.

These categories of drugs act peripherally and inhibit cyclooxygenase, which has a role in prostaglandin synthesis. All of the drugs in this category have a "ceiling" effect, beyond which no further analgesia is achieved.

   • **Acetaminophen,** the most commonly used drug in this category, provides analgesia but has no anti-inflammatory effect.

   • Unfortunately, all available over-the-counter **NSAIDs,** which have anti-inflammatory activity, also have associated bleeding and gastrointestinal side effects. These agents are preferable to acetaminophen for pain associated with inflammation such as the pain of otitis media, pharyngitis, and muscular aches.

   • **COX-2 inhibitors** were developed to reduce the side effects often associated with NSAIDs and initially held great promise. Unfortunately, they have been associated with increased cardiovascular events in older adults, although a select few are available for use in children.

3. **Drugs for moderate to severe pain.** Opioids (Table 19-2) are the drugs of choice for moderate to severe pain. There are known predictable side effects associated with these drugs, such as constipation, somnolence, respiratory depression, and itching, and these should be anticipated and treated. In the current climate of the opioid epidemic, clinicians must pay attention to responsible prescribing guidelines and regulations, which can vary from state to state. This may include an assessment of risk factors for addiction, counseling on the addictive potential of opioids, a single prescriber agreement for opioid prescriptions, limits on amount of opioid dispensed, and requirements to review electronic prescription drug monitoring systems before prescribing opioids. As a general rule, opioids should not be used for chronic pain, aside

Table 19-1 • DOSING DATA FOR ACETAMINOPHEN AND NONSTEROIDAL ANTI-INFLAMMATORY DRUGS (NSAIDS)

Drug	Usual Adult Dose	Usual Pediatric Dose	Comments
Oral NSAIDs			
Acetaminophen	650–1000 mg q 4 h	10–15 mg/kg q 4 h	Acetaminophen lacks the peripheral anti-inflammatory activity of other NSAIDs; available as oral suspension.
Ibuprofen	400–600 mg q 4–6 h	10 mg/kg q 4–6 h	Available as several brand names and as generic; available as oral suspension.
Naproxen	500 mg initial dose followed by 250 mg q 6–8 h or 500 mg q 12 h	For patients >2 y of age 5 mg/kg q 12 h	Dose is expressed as naproxen base; 200 mg naproxen is equivalent to 220 mg naproxen sodium. Available as oral suspension.
Celecoxib	100–200 mg q 12 h	For patients >2 y of age ≥10 kg to ≤25 kg, 50 mg q 12 h >25 kg 100 mg q 12 h	COX-2 inhibitor may cause less bleeding and gastritis. Useful for children with thrombocytopenia.

Table 19-2 • DOSING DATA FOR OPIOID ANALGESICS

Drug	Route	Initial Pediatric Dose	Initial Adult Dose
Morphine	IV/SC PO/SL/PR	0.05–0.1 mg/kg q 2–4 h 0.15–0.3 mg/kg q 2–4 h	5–10 mg q 2–4 h 10–15 mg q 2–4 h
Hydromorphone	IV PO/SL	0.015 mg/kg q 3–4 h 0.05 mg/kg q 3–4 h	0.2–0.6 mg q 2–4 h 1–2 mg q 3–4 h
Fentanyl	IV/IN	1–2 µg/kg q 10–60 min	25–75 µg q 10–60 min
Oxycodone	PO/SL	0.1–0.2 mg/kg q 4–6 h	5–10 mg q 4–6 h
Tramadol	PO/SL		50–100 mg q 6 h

from specific situations such as end of life, when a pain management or palliative care specialist should ideally be consulted. Clinicians should be using the appropriate term "opioid" when discussing this class of drugs and their therapeutic use in the management of pain. The term "narcotic" should be avoided when discussing these medications owing to its negative associations with the legal system and addiction.

• **Codeine** is no longer recommended for use in children younger than 12 years and is not recommended for any pediatric patient undergoing tonsillectomy or adenoidectomy owing to its risk for (potentially fatal) breathing problems. These safety concerns, as well as the understanding that 10%–15% of persons cannot metabolize codeine into morphine, which is required for its action, have caused this drug to be removed from the formulary at many children's hospitals.

• **Tramadol** is an analgesic that has the features of both a µ-receptor agonist and a selective serotonin reuptake inhibitor (SSRI) and has been thought to be a less sedating and weaker opioid. However, safety concerns similar to those around codeine led to warning about its use in any child younger than 12 years and in postoperative pediatric patients <18 years. This is related to variability in metabolism to the active component of the drug. Additionally, reports have indicated an increased risk for serotonin syndrome with concurrent use of tramadol and SSRIs or selective serotonin/norepinephrine reuptake inhibitors (SNRIs). Thus, this combination of drugs should be avoided.

- Oral agents such as **oxycodone, hydrocodone,** and **oxymorphone** are alternatives, which are effective for pain. When these drugs are used in fixed drug preparation with an NSAID (i.e., acetaminophen and oxycodone [Tylox, Percocet]), care should be taken to avoid excessive NSAID ingestion.
- For severe pain, **morphine** remains the drug of choice. It can be administered through a number of routes, and its pharmacokinetics are well-established in children. When morphine is contraindicated or there are excessive unwanted side effects, then **hydromorphone** or **fentanyl** can be used. These agents can be used safely in children but should be used with caution in a carefully monitored setting, particularly with infants. Fentanyl has been successfully used by IN administration in cases of severe pain such as orthopedic injury and sickle cell crises in pediatric patients, always in a carefully monitored setting such as the emergency department.
- For severe pain that persists, **long-acting opioids** (morphine [MSContin], oxycodone [OxyContin]) are available and generally should be used in consult with an expert in pain management. When using a long-acting opioid, a short-acting opioid should always be prescribed simultaneously for breakthrough pain.
- **Methadone** is a useful drug for in the hands of an experienced prescriber, given its unique activity as both a μ-receptor agonist and an N-methyl-D-aspartic acid antagonist. Owing to its drug interactions and long half-life, consultation with an expert in pediatric pain management is recommended.

4. **Adjunctive drugs.** Drugs in this category include anticonvulsants (**pregabalin** and **gabapentin**) and antidepressants (**amitriptyline** and **duloxetine**), which have efficacy against the pain of nerve injury and neuropathic pain. This type of pain, which is often opioid resistant, has unique characteristics and is often described as burning, shooting, or electric. Treatment of comorbid anxiety should be considered using medications such as **benzodiazepines** and SSRIs. **Benzodiazepines** can also be useful to treat muscular spasms associated with pain. Management of sleep disorders using **melatonin, amitriptyline, trazodone,** or **zolpidem** may also be necessary.

IV. **CHRONIC PAIN.** Chronic pain is increasingly recognized as a significant problem of childhood, and its prevalence is increasing. The most common presentations to pediatric clinician's offices include chronic headaches, chronic abdominal pain, and musculoskeletal pain. These complaints ought to first prompt a medical evaluation for known causes. Once all typical causes have been reasonably ruled out, it may be appropriate to begin to focus on treatment of the pain itself. Chronic pain in childhood is often associated with school avoidance, sleep disturbances, anxiety, and mood symptoms. Children may withdraw from social interactions and previously enjoyed activities due to the pain. An interdisciplinary approach is most appropriate in management of chronic pain and may include some medication management, attention to sleep, school reentry, addressing the role of parents, psychotherapy, and psychoeducation about chronic pain. Furthermore, addition of nonpharmacologic therapies including integrative medicine techniques (such as acupuncture, massage, aromatherapy, and mind–body strategies), dietary interventions, and physical therapy can be helpful adjuvants. There are a number of interdisciplinary pediatric chronic pain clinics around the country that accept referrals for children with complex chronic pain presentations.

V. **SUMMARY.** Most acute pain problems are treatable using relatively simple, safe approaches. A systematic approach to assessment is the cornerstone of adequate treatment. Unless pain is documented, it cannot be adequately treated nor can the success of interventions be monitored. An individualized or tailored approach is often required, taking into account the origin of the pain, age and developmental stage of the child, and past pain experiences. Multimodal treatment (such as pharmacologic, cognitive–behavioral, and physical approaches) is essential in any comprehensive plan for pain relief.

Bibliography

BOOKS AND JOURNALS

Berde CB, Sethna NF. Analgesics for the treatment of pain in children. *N Engl J Med.* 2002;347:1094-1103.

Chambers C, Taddio A, Uman L, et al. Psychological interventions for reducing pain and distress during routine childhood immunizations: a systematic review. *Clin Ther.* 2009;31:77-103.

Finley GA, McGrath PJ, Chambers CT. *Bringing Pain Relief to Children: Treatment Approaches.* Totowa, NJ: Humana Press; 2006.

Friedrichsdorf SJ. Four steps to eliminate or reduce pain in children caused by needles (part 1). *Pain Manag.* 2017;7(2):89-94. doi:10.2217/pmt-2016-0050.

McGrath PJ, Walco GA, Turk DC, et al. Core outcome domains and measures for pediatric acute and chronic/recurrent pain clinical trials: PedIMMPACT recommendations. *J Pain.* 2008;9:771-783.

Slifer K. *Clinician's Guide to Helping Children Cope and Cooperate with Medical Care.* Baltimore: The Johns Hopkins University Press; 2014.

WEBSITES
https://www.iasp-pain.org/.
http://pediatric-pain.ca/.
https://online.lexi.com/.
http://jtip.com/.
https://buzzyhelps.com/.

CHAPTER 20

Self-Regulation

Jodi Santosuosso | Naomi Steiner

I. **SELF-REGULATION.** Self-regulation can be defined as the ability to control one's thinking, attention, feelings, and behavior appropriately with the demands of the situation, for example, being able to resist highly emotional reactions to upsetting stimuli, to calm down when disappointed, to adjust to a change in expectations, and to handle frustration without an outburst.

Self-regulation involves many neurologic messengers in the brain, including the brain stem, reticular formation, hypothalamus, thalamus, autonomic nervous system, cerebellum, limbic system, all sensory systems, such as from the cortex, and the vestibular system.

As children mature, they develop a set of skills to direct their behavior toward a goal, even in the face of insecurity. This self-regulatory competence is important in young children, as they enter school to promote school achievement and social competence with peers and adults.

Self-regulation therapy is a mind body approach aimed to return the autonomic nervous system back to a homeostatic balance by developing the ability to modulate emotional and behavioral responses and the capacity to self soothe.

A. **Background of the autonomic nervous system.** This system regulates homeostasis between the sympathetic and parasympathetic nervous systems.

The **sympathetic autonomic nervous system's** main function is to activate the physiological changes that occur during the **fight-or-flight** response. It prepares the body for stressful situations. A simple analogy would be stepping on the gas pedal. Effects of this system are vast but generally include increasing heart rate, constricting blood vessels to the skin and viscera (thereby increasing blood flow to muscles), and decreasing salivation. These responses all promote survival in a dangerous situation.

The **parasympathetic autonomic nervous system** prepares the body for restful situations and is often called the "**rest and digest**" system. A simple analogy would be putting on the brakes. Effects of the parasympathetic nervous system include slowing heart rate, increasing gastric motility, and increasing salivation. These responses help the body recover as well as prepare for stressful situations by storing nutrients.

The parasympathetic and sympathetic systems work at the same time, often in opposition to one another working to keep the body in balance. When one of the systems is working harder, or is stimulated more frequently, some dysfunction may happen.

For example, in today's world, many children are faced with toxic stress, always on the go, with inadequate sleep, and overly stressed on a daily basis. This activates the sympathetic nervous system putting the body in a sympathetic overload. When this happens, heart rate and blood pressure increase, and the child may experience an overall feeling of being "stressed," unable to regulate his or her behavior and emotions. At the same time, this overwhelms the parasympathetic system, which cannot function well resulting in poor digestion of food, inability to rest or sleep as well, leaving the child tired throughout the day placing the body in an imbalance.

One way to help regain the body's balance is though self-regulation therapy. There are many therapeutic ways to restore the body back into balance and lowering the body's stress response.

B. **Therapeutic approaches to self-regulation**
   1. **Mindfulness.** Mindfulness-based stress reduction (MBSR) is based on a program created by Jon Kabit-Zinn, PhD, who established the Stress Reduction Clinic. Initial research studies of patients with chronic pain and illness showed that participating in an MBSR course significantly decreased stress, anxiety, pain, depression, anger, physical symptoms, and use of medication. Participants in MBSR courses showed an increased ability to cope with pain and felt that their lives were more meaningful and fulfilling.
   MBSR has become a standard clinical intervention and community offering for adults, and research is emerging for MBSR in children and adolescents.

Mindfulness is not a therapy but rather a daily practice though which one develops the awareness of the working of the mind and the influence of thoughts and feelings on reactions. It is not about thinking or doing at all but rather paying attention to cues from the body.

Mindfulness practice is a way of teaching children to focus their attention, become less reactive, and be more compassionate with themselves and others to promote a more fulfilling and healthier way of being. Mindfulness practices include skills for children to deal with ordinary daily stressors of life.

Mindfulness practices include breathing exercises to activate the parasympathetic nervous system to help slow down the mind and body.

Four steps of mindfulness practice:
   a. Stop—habitual reactions.
   b. Observe—what is going on at this moment.
   c. Relax and notice the breath that shifts thoughts out of the head and into the body.
   d. Choose—to address the situation consciously instead of reacting impulsively and involuntarily.

Mindfulness enables the child to recognize reactive behavior, such as "stepping on the gas pedal." When a child becomes mindful, he or she becomes aware when there is a need to draw in a relaxation or meditation technique to calm himself or herself down. Practicing these exercises will provide an opportunity for children to calm and sooth their body, mind, and nervous system.

2. **Yoga.** The purpose of yoga poses is to increase strength, flexibility, and balance. When yoga poses are paired with yoga breathing techniques, students learn how to use breathing to relieve stress and tension. Mindfulness in the yoga pose helps with centering one's self in the present moment.

   Yoga is an effective tool to balance both the sympathetic and parasympathetic systems.

   Yoga promotes self-confidence and builds self-esteem. It helps children with attention-deficit/hyperactivity disorder and autism improve their ability to self-calm, focus, and build social skills. Studies have shown that yoga practices decrease the level of cortisol in the body, thus bringing the body into balance.

3. **Occupational therapy.** Occupational therapy addresses a child's cognitive, emotional, and physical needs through functional, activity-based treatment.

   An occupational therapist works with children to bring them back to an optimal state of alertness or calming effect by providing proprioceptive input to regulate the brain function.

4. **Heart rate variability biofeedback.** Heart rate variability (HRV) is the beat-to-beat changes in heart rate. Heart rate physiologically increases during inspiration and decreases during expiration, so that this variation essentially reflects a person's respirations. The HRV device leads the practitioner to breathe slowly and easily, for an adult at around 5–6 breaths per minute (the so-called coherence). Children breathe at a faster rate. This leads to an increase in parasympathetic activation and relaxation. HRV training leads to faster and easier shift toward this relaxed state with positive outcomes for the desired concern (see Table 20-1).

5. **Hypnosis.** Images carefully laid out by a highly trained therapist lead the child into a state of highly focused attention frequently associated with relaxation. Children achieve this state more easily than adults. Hypnotherapy uses this induced state for therapeutic purposes using therapeutic suggestions. These suggestions might use an image decided upon with the child and related to the therapeutic goal at hand, such as decreasing pain related to headaches.

6. **Guided imagery.** As the child becomes relaxed, a sequence of imagery suggests a solution to a specific concern. For instance, a child might be prompted to visualize letting go their worries into a train that drives away. Guided imagery training can be as simple as downloading an app with audio to listen to and practice at home. These protocols do not require a highly trained therapist and they are inexpensive and easy to use. The imagery can also be combined with other approaches such as progressive muscle relaxation.

The physiological effects of these approaches overlap, as they decrease sympathetic nervous system activity and increase that of the parasympathetic. Personal preferences are important, for instance, not all children have the same level of hypnotic suggestibility. Some children enjoy and benefit from the practice from multiple approaches, for instance, yoga and guided imagery. Others show clear preference for one specific approach. This is

Table 20-1 • SELF-REGULATION APPROACHES

	Mindfulness	Yoga	Sensory Approaches OT	Biofeedback HRV	Hypnosis	Guided Imagery
Stress anxiety	X	X	X	X	X	X
Depression	X		X		X	–
ADHD	X	X	X	X		
Sleep insomnia	X	X	X	X	X	
Headaches	X		X		X	X
Chronic abdominal pain	X		X		X	X
Asthma				X		X
Medical procedures	X	X			X	X

ADHD, attention-deficit/hyperactivity disorder; HRV, heart rate variability; OT, occupational therapy.

an active field of research with little evidence of the superiority of one approach over another. On the other hand, emerging research with follow-up studies shows that, once skills are learned, they can be applied long-term and in various settings.

Bibliography

Thompson R. Doing what doesn't come naturally: the development of self-regulation. *Zero to Three*. 2009;30(2):33-38.

Dr. Susan LaCombe Psychologist. 4536 Willingdon Avenue Suite 101 Powell River, BC V8A 2M8 (website).

BOOKS/PROGRAMS

Barbara Neiman, OTR. *Yoga and Mindfulness: Brain Body Tools for Children and Adolescents*. Eau Claire, WI: PESI Publishing & Media; 2014.

Saltzman A. *A Still Quiet Place: A Mindfulness Program for Teaching Children and Adolescents to Ease Stress and Difficult Emotions*. Oakland, CA: New Harbinger Publications, Inc.; 2014.

Snel E.. *Sitting Still Like a Frog: Mindfulness Exercises for Kids (And Their Parents)*. Boston, MA: Shambhala Publications, Inc.; 2013.

Williams MS, Shellenberger S. *"How Does Your Engine Run"? A Leader's Guide to the Alert Program for Self Regulation*. Albuquerque, NM: TherapyWorks, Inc.; 1996.

WEBSITES

Center for Mindfulness in Medicine, Health Care, and Society.
Center on the Developing Child at Harvard University
Child Mind institute.
Radiant Child Yoga (www.childrensyoga.com).
Yogajournal.com.
www.zensationalkids.com.
www.AlertProgram.com.

CHAPTER 21

Using Developmental Themes to Understand Behavior

Barry Zuckerman | Marilyn Augustyn

I. **INTRODUCTION.** During a well-child visit, there are several potentially competing agendas: the parent's, the child's, and the clinician's. A useful question at the start of any encounter is to ask the family what they hope to accomplish during the visit. Suggested ways to open include: *"Since I last saw you, are there specific concerns you have that we need to discuss?"* or *"Do you have any questions for me we need to get to before we conclude today so I can note them?"* After the toddler period, it also useful to ask the child at some point during the visit, *"Do you have any questions for me?"*

The clinician's agenda is equally complex. Bright Futures 4th edition from the AAP is a useful guide containing questionnaires, parent handouts, and other tools for each visit that can help set the clinician's agenda.

II. **FOUR KEY DEVELOPMENTAL PROCESSES.** An alternative to a formal mechanism such as Bright Futures is an understanding of four key developmental processes to note or directly address at every encounter.

Social–emotional development and interactive patterns are based on how all children and youth of all ages form relationships and interact with their caregivers and later peers and others. Clinicians can best help parents deal with everyday universal struggles and challenges by understanding the components of social–emotional development: attachment, separation, autonomy, and mastery. Although struggles within these stages are predictable and universal, the behaviors vary depending on the child's temperament.

A. **Attachment.** Attachment describes the enduring specific emotional bond that develops over time between children and caregivers. Although parent–child attachment behaviors differ at different ages, the goal of attachment remains constant, maintaining the child's internal security. Parents who are emotionally available, sensitive, and effective at meeting the needs of the child are likely to have securely attached infants and children. The process of parent–child attachment, however, is not instantaneous. Most families require several months of trial and error before they feel they know and understand their infant's needs and can respond accordingly. Through trial and error, parents gradually learn effective responses to the infant's need for food, rest, or social interaction. Throughout childhood, a child with secure attachment possesses a foundation on which to build positive relationships with peers and unrelated adults. Such a child also has more effective coping with stress, resiliency, and better performance at school. The internal security associated with secure attachment continues from infancy to early adulthood; when in the face of stress, an illness, hospitalization, or a bad week at college, hearing a parent's voice on the phone rekindles the security embedded by attachment that helps to cope with adversity.

Not all children develop secure parent–child attachment. Parents burdened by illness, psychiatric impairment including trauma, substance abuse, or other crises may find it particularly difficult to respond warmly and consistently to their child's frequent demands. Young children who have experienced chronically inconsistent nurturing may appear less interested in exploring their surrounding world even in the caregivers' presence. Other children appear actively angry and distrustful of their caretakers. A serious disturbance of attachment should be suspected when children between 9 months and 2 years fail to demonstrate behavioral preference for their parents in response to stress. If such behaviors persist, mental health referral for the family is indicated. Likewise, throughout development, children may display difficulty with relationships, risk-taking behavior, ambivalent relationship with their parents, and less resilience in the face of stress.

B. **Separation.** Negotiation of separation, both psychological and physical, poses a continuous challenge to the parent and child. Physical separation from an attachment figure/significant parent/caregiver rarely happens anymore in the United States except in cases of military deployment and foster care (see Chapters 49 and 63). On the other hand, children and parents are confronted with everyday experiences of short duration that can be both physically and, at times, emotionally challenging such as bedtime, childcare, or parental travel. Face time on iPhones is a new and helpful strategy for parents when they are traveling away from home. Appropriate management of a physical separation depends on its duration, context, and the developmental readiness of both parents and the child. Brief predictable physical separation from the parents, especially if the child is cared for by someone they know, facilitates successful psychological separation for young children.

When parents express disproportionate anxiety about their child's well-being during routine separations, they are often expressing ambivalence about the child's evolution of independence. Explicit discussion of the parents' feelings about separation can be more effective than reassurance that their child will be fine. For example, the clinician might suggest that it is not easy for parents to be away from their babies. Initial difficulties with separation subside only to become acute again at 7–9 months of age when children begin to show separation protest, e.g., crying when their parents especially mother leaves their presence. Clinicians can help parents recognize that the separation protest results from normal cognitive phenomena of object permanence and will diminish as a child learns from multiple brief separations and reunions that parents reliably return. Sometimes parents intentionally sabotage their child's establishment of independence when they perceive their child is unusually "vulnerable" because of past illness or other factors that make the child special (see Chapter 87). In this case, parents can become overprotective, which involves their difficulty in supporting age-appropriate separation by allowing the child his or her independence. Difficulty with separation can return as an issue around starting childcare, kindergarten or general "homesickness."

C. **Autonomy and mastery.** The infant's intrinsic need for autonomy and mastery drives developmental progress. Autonomy refers to the achievement of behaviors associated with independence. Mastery describes the child's quest for ever-increasing competence. These complementary processes require that caregivers and children continually renegotiate control of the child's bodily functions and social interactions. Parental concerns about thumb-sucking, temper tantrums, lack of adherence to parent requests to not climb furniture or play with special objects, to cooperate with putting clothes on, and toilet training provide for the common clinical examples of autonomy issues. Basically, from a child's perspective it's my way or the highway. The label "terrible twos" reflects an imbalance of the child's expression of autonomy with maturation of the frontal lobe, which controls acting on impulses related to desires. Distracting the child and permitting success in a more manageable activity can be a helpful maneuver to alleviate this type of tantrum. Parental responses to such tantrums should encourage self-control. Inappropriate balance between necessary limits and support for independence requires frequent negotiation throughout a child's life. In general, successful limits are firm, consistent, and selective. Children thrive on routine instruction. Breaking a child's will should never become an end.

Attachment, separation, autonomy, and mastery form the basis of most behavioral discussions throughout childhood and into young adulthood. An attempt to understand how specific parental concerns fit into one or more of these developmental themes can help parents address the problem. Observation and discussion of these themes at all encounters can provide the basis for parental reflection and solving problems when they occur.

III. **HOW BEHAVIORAL ISSUES APPEAR IN THE EXAM ROOM.** A range of positive and negative parent and child behavior happens in examination rooms. Children are uncertain and stressed and parents may feel under pressure in the spotlight to ensure their child is cooperative with the clinician. Under these circumstances, some children will impulsively climb furniture, whine and yell at mother, or display other problematic behaviors that elicit anger, frustration, or excessive concern in the parent. At the other extreme is the parent who does not intervene, suggesting that the parent feels defeated and hopeless to manage his or her child's behavior, which should suggest parental depression (see Chapter 7).

A. **The child's perspective.** This is a special moment for children. They may be upset or anxious for a variety of understandable reasons. They have to separate from the parent and let a stranger touch them and they cannot express their autonomy and escape the clinician "controlling" them all the while trying, with variable success, to master the situation. Additionally, they may have gotten up earlier than usual, breakfast was rushed or even omitted in the hurry, maybe the bus was late, maybe finding a parking space was difficult, maybe the wait in the waiting room was long. These issues are coupled with recollections of what happened to them the last time they were in this room—maybe immunizations, maybe a finger stick or venipuncture, or maybe a forced and painful ear examination. Doubtless, the examination room offers many interesting possibilities for exploration, expressing autonomy—a door with a knob, drawers with handles, a wastebasket, a sharps disposal unit, a sink with running water and a paper towel dispenser, boxes of latex gloves that make interesting balloons, and much more. Although children do not want to get into trouble as their mother is preoccupied talking with the clinician, some children will engage in a behavior for their own amusement and/or to get the mother's attention: autonomy and mastery again.

B. The parent's perspective. This is also a difficult moment for the parent, especially if having other important or acute stresses at home or work. Many thoughts and emotions may fly through the parent's head as he or she tries to concentrate on what you are saying about fluoride and the temperature of his or her hot water heater. Maybe he or she felt embarrassed last visit because his or her child was very uncooperative. When the child misbehaves while you are in the examination room, the parent is unsure what to do. At some level the parent is aware that threats ("Stop that or else ... ") do not seem to work very well. Spanking seems sometimes to work, but he or she does not think you would approve. A bribe is another possibility ("Behave and I'll take you to ... on the way home"). Anything he or she does, however, will call the behavior to your attention and he or she is hoping that you are either too preoccupied to notice or too hurried to talk to him or her about it.

C. The clinician's perspective. When your patient misbehaves, you have to decide whether or not to intervene. If you intervene, you do not want to offend the child's parent nor do you want the child to hurt himself or herself and you want to decrease the noise level in the office and return focus to your history taking, physical examination, and anticipatory guidance. The challenge is the child's attachment (in face of stress) and autonomy to do what he or she wants, or not do what the doctor or the parent wants him or her to do. These simple ongoing themes can be reflected back to parent, "*When children are stressed like he/she is now, they only want you; this shows you are their source of security. It won't undermine attachment if I have to exam him/her in spite of wanting to hold on to you.*"

IV. OBTAINING MORE HISTORY—AGAIN USING OPPORTUNITY TO REFRAME USING THE FOUR DEVELOPMENTAL THEMES
  A. *Why do you think your child is behaving this way today? Does he/she act like this at home? Does he/she behave the same way with other adults (other parent/grandparent, teacher, etc.)? Does this behavior bother you?*
  B. *What do you do at home? Does it work? Do you sometimes feel overwhelmed?*
  C. *Would you like some help with this? What kind? Would you be willing to talk to a child psychologist (or other professional) about this?*

V. CLINICAL PEARLS
  A. Cultural sensitivity. It is critically important to recognize cultural differences between your own values and the family's values. Opening with a question such as "*Is this behavior OK with you?*" may give you a small window into the family's expectations. Respect to parents and other authority figures (such as clinicians) is important in many cultures, and parents will often respond with speed and directness at signs of disrespect. Nuances of developmental themes may vary in non-US cultures and is important to identify.
  B. Make a note about this episode in the chart so that the next time you see the parent you can ask him or her about ongoing occurrences and whether any interventions have been helpful.
  C. If the parent hits the child in front of you, it is important to acknowledge what just happened. Ignoring it will implicitly tell the parent it is "OK." You can respond that your office is a "no-hitting" zone followed by a discussion about what a child learns by being spanked: hitting is OK. Children love to imitate, especially people whom they love and respect. Spanking demonstrates that it is all right for people to hit people, especially for big people to hit little people, and stronger people to hit weaker people.
  D. Tell the parent that spanking a child when angry makes it very difficult to maintain control and the child could be injured. It also teaches the child to hit when frustrated or angry. As the child's clinician, you need to ensure his or her safety. If the spanking seems excessive (e.g., hitting with an object) or has resulted in injuries (e.g., bruises or welts), tell the parent that you will need to involve protective services for a more thorough investigation of the home. Acknowledge that you know the parents love the child and reassure them that you will support them through the process but that for the child's safety, an investigation needs to occur. Never contact protective services without telling the family or your chances to maintain the relationship will be severed.

Bibliography

FOR PARENTS

https://www.healthychildren.org/English/Pages/default.aspx.

FOR PROFESSIONALS

Flocke SA, Clark E, Antognoli E, et al. Teachable moments for health behavior change and intermediate patient outcomes. *Patient Educ Couns*. 2014;96(1):43-49.

Hooper LM, Tomek S, Newman CR. Using attachment theory in medical settings: implications for primary care physicians. *J Ment Health*. 2012;21(1):23-37.

CHAPTER 22

Neuropsychological Testing: What Clinicians Need to Know

Casey Krueger | Irene M. Loe

I. **WHAT IS PEDIATRIC NEUROPSYCHOLOGY?** Pediatric neuropsychology is the study and understanding of brain–behavior relationships in children with difficulties learning due to known or suspected brain injury, neurodevelopmental disorders, or other congenital or acquired disorders. It is a specialty within the field of clinical psychology. A pediatric neuropsychologist is a licensed, doctoral-level psychologist with specialized training in the assessment of children. Neuropsychological tests are specifically designed to measure one or more underlying neurocognitive functions usually associated with specific brain structures or pathways. A set of neuropsychological test results build a detailed understanding of how these functions cumulate to explain complex cognitive, language, literacy, and memory skills or social–emotional behaviors. Batteries of standardized tests vary, are tailored to answer specific referral questions, and focus on cognition, behavior, and functional capacities (Table 22-1).

II. **WHY ARE CHILDREN REFERRED FOR NEUROPSYCHOLOGICAL TESTING?** Neuropsychological assessments are useful for delineating complex abilities or behaviors into component skills to focus interventions. Referral reasons may include the following.

   A. Brain injury such as following a stroke, brain tumor, epilepsy, or traumatic brain injury, or various treatments that compromise brain structure or function, such as cranial irradiation. Brain injuries may be a result of premature birth, fetal alcohol, or other in utero exposures.

   B. Poor response to intervention in learning, attention, socialization, or emotional control. In such cases, specific neuropsychological processes may be deficient, thereby interfering with recovery or rehabilitation.

   C. Defining the phenotype associated with specific conditions, such as genetic or chromosomal disorders.

   D. Clarification of diagnosis and treatment planning in children with significant learning, behavior, social, adaptive, or emotional control problems.

III. **WHAT DOMAINS MAY BE ASSESSED?** Various mental functions are evaluated, which may include but are not limited to the following:

   * Intellectual functioning—global measurement of ability to think and solve problems
   * Academic achievement—performance in reading, mathematics, and written expression
   * Language—reception, comprehension, and/or production of symbolic communication
   * Memory—short- and long-term recollection and recall
   * Visuospatial skills—ability to recognize, manipulate, or create visual information
   * Attention and concentration
   * Executive function (e.g., working memory, organization, planning, inhibition, and flexibility)
   * Fine motor control—ability to control the hands for writing, drawing, and manipulating small objects
   * Behavioral and emotional functioning—ability to express and regulate strong emotions, including anger
   * Social skills—ability to understand, explain, and demonstrate skills essential to build and maintain relationships
   * Adaptive functioning—performance in everyday life outside of the clinical setting, including daily living skills, social abilities, and communication

   A. **What is the process?**
   * Clinicians interview parent/caregiver to obtain detailed developmental, behavioral, and social history.
   * Caregivers complete questionnaires about the child's development and behavior.
   * Teachers may provide additional data.
   * Clinicians observe the child's play and/or interview the child.

Table 22-1 • TYPICAL TESTS IN NEUROPSYCHOLOGICAL REPORTS

Type of Test	Specific Name	Comments
Intelligence testing	Wechsler Intelligence Scale for Children—Fifth Edition (WISC-V)	Standardized in English and Spanish, ages 6–16 y
	Wechsler Preschool and Primary Scale of Intelligence—Fourth Edition (WPPSI-IV)	Ages 2.6–7.7 y
	Differential Ability Scales—Second Edition (DAS-II)	Often used in schools, ages 2.6–17.11 y
Achievement testing	Woodcock–Johnson Tests of Achievement—Fourth Edition (WJ-IV)	Ages 2–90+ y
	Wechsler Individual Achievement Test, Third Edition (WIAT-III)	Ages 4–19.11 y
Executive functioning (EF)	Delis–Kaplan Executive Function System (D-KEFS)	Ages 8–89 y
	NEPSY-II: A Developmental Neuropsychological Assessment, Second Edition	Evaluates six domains (EF, language, memory, sensorimotor, visuospatial, and social perception), Ages 3–16.11 y
Memory	Wide Range Assessment of Memory and Learning, Second Edition (WRAML-2)	Ages 5–90 y
	Children's Memory Scale (CMS)	Ages 5–16 y
Language	Preschool Language Scales, Fifth Edition (PLS-5)	Standardized in English and Spanish, ages 0–7.11 y
	Clinical Evaluation of Language Fundamentals, Fifth Edition (CELF-5)	Ages 5–21.11 y
Visuospatial skills	Beery–Buktenica Developmental Test of Visual–Motor Integration, Sixth edition (VMI)	Ages 2–100 y
	Wide Range Assessment of Visual Motor Abilities (WRAVMA)	Ages 3–17 y
Projective testing	Rorschach Test	Ages 5 years to adult
	Children's Apperception Test (CAT), Thematic Apperception Test (TAT)	CAT: Ages 3–10 y
		TAT: Children and adults
Social communication	Autism Diagnostic Observation Scale, Second Edition (ADOS-2)	Five modules depending on age and language level, 12 months to adult
Behavior inventories	Child Behavior Checklist (CBCL)	Ages 1.5–90+ y
	Behavior Assessment Scale for Children, Third Edition (BASC-3)	Ages 2–21 y
Adaptive functioning	Vineland Adaptive Behavior Scales, Third Edition (Vineland-3)	Ages 0–90+ y
	Adaptive Behavior Assessment System, Third Edition (ABAS-3)	Ages 0–89 y

- Clinicians spend 3–6 hours of testing in 1 day or over multiple days, depending on the age of the child and referral question. Assessments include hands-on activities, responses to questions, paper and pencil tasks, and/or computer tasks.
- Clinicians provide feedback to referral sources, the patient, and family: review test results, provide diagnosis if appropriate, supply written report, most importantly offer recommendations for home and school.

B. How do the results of the evaluation contribute to the clinical process?
Evaluations provide a comprehensive understanding of a child's neuropsychological strengths and weaknesses for diagnostic and treatment planning purposes. A treatment plan is designed to help a child achieve his or her full potential in school, home, and the community. That plan may include interventions to strengthen areas of weakness and opportunities to cultivate areas of strength. The evaluation also serves as a baseline against which to measure the outcome of treatment or the child's development over time.

C. Terms used in measures of performance. Tests of knowledge or performance compare a child's abilities to what would be expected for someone of the same age, and results typically are reported in one or more of the following ways.

1. **Standard score**
   This approach converts a child's performance to a scale on which the expected or "average" child of that age will achieve a test score of 10, 50, or 100, depending on the test. Because individual performance is not that exact, these tests also define a "normal" range of performance, called a standard deviation.

2. **Percentile rank**
   Knowledge-based tests often report a child's performance as a ranking. The scale is 1–99, with 99 the highest.

3. **Age equivalent**
   This approach is less rigorous than a standard score but may seem more "real life." It estimates how old an **average** child would need to be to achieve a specific score.

4. **Grade equivalent**
   Some tests report performance on the basis of the grade at which an **average** child would be expected to achieve the same result.

D. How should clinicians interpret results and explain results to parents?
Standard scores of assessment may be plotted on the bell curve. Most scores fall in the middle of the graph, reflecting expected or average performance (see Fig. 22-1). Scores falling outside the expected range may represent areas of strength or weakness. See Table 22-2 for examples and descriptions of standard scores. It is usually best to talk to parents in terms of percentiles or age/grade equivalents because they are more readily understandable. If a child received an IQ score at the 75th percentile, then we know that the child performed better than 75% of children of same age who took the same test.

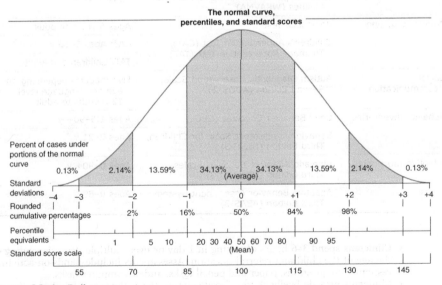

Figure 22-1 Bell curve.

Table 22-2 • STANDARDIZED SCORE INTERPRETATION

Descriptor	Scaled Score	Standard Score	T Score	Percentile (%)
Extremely low	1–3	<70	<30	1
Borderline	4–5	70–79	30–36	2–8
Low average	6–7	80–89	37–42	9–24
Average	8–12	90–110	43–57	25–75
High average	13–14	111–120	58–63	76–91
Superior	15	121–129	64–69	92–97
Very superior	16+	130+	70+	98+

Publishers vary slightly on the classification descriptor of standard scores. For example, Wechsler tests consider a standard score of 110 (75th percentile) to be high average.

Bibliography

FOR CLINICIANS

Lezak MD, Howieson DB, Bigler ED, Tranel D. *Neuropsychological Assessment*. 5th ed. Oxford: Oxford University Press; 2012.

Miller E. Some basic principles of neuropsychological assessment. In: Crawford JR, Parker DM, McKinlay WM, eds. *A Handbook of Neuropsychological Assessment*. Hove: Laurence Erlbaum Associates; 1992.

Semrud-Clikeman M, Ellison PAT. *Child Neuropsychology: Assessment and Interventions for Neurodevelopmental Disorders*. 2nd ed. New York: Springer; 2009.

The Houston Conference on Specialty Education and Training in Clinical Neuropsychology (PDF). *American Academy of Clinical Neuropsychology*; 1998. http://www.uh.edu/hns/hc.html.

FOR PARENTS

Braaten E, Felopoulos G. *Straight Talk about Psychological Testing for Kids*. 1st ed. Guilford Press; 2003.

Flink D. *Thinking Differently: An Inspiring Guide for Parents of Children with Learning Disabilities*. William Morrow Paperbacks; 2014.

Wilmshurst L, Brue A. *A Parent's Guide to Special Education: Insider Advice on How to Navigate the System and Help Your Child Succeed*. 1st ed. Amacom; 2005.

CHAPTER 23

Psychopharmacology

Demetra D. Pappas | Alison Schonwald

I. DESCRIPTION OF THE PROBLEM. In the United States, 20% of children and adolescents have a diagnosable mental health disorder that requires intervention or monitoring and interferes with daily functioning. Primary care providers currently assume all mental health care for the majority of the affected children. With the increased recognition of childhood psychiatric disorders, ease of obtaining information on the Internet, and ongoing marketing of psychotropic medications, the need for primary care providers to stay current with treatment options remains clinically imperative.

The use of psychopharmacologic agents in children most commonly occurs in the treatment of attention-deficit/hyperactivity disorder (ADHD)/impulse control problems, aggression and irritability associated with autism spectrum disorder, disruptive behavior, tic disorders, mood and anxiety symptoms, and psychosis.

Although many studies demonstrate highly effective and safe treatment of pediatric ADHD, data for efficacy with most other symptom complexes remain limited. Because of the paucity of research on children, most uses of medications for non-ADHD symptoms remain "off-label."

II. EPIDEMIOLOGY BY THE (APPROXIMATE) NUMBERS
- 20% of US children and adolescents are affected by mental health disorders.
- 14% of US children aged 2–8 years have been diagnosed with a mental, behavioral, or developmental disorder.
- 11% of US children aged 4–17 years have been diagnosed with ADHD.
- 3.5% of individuals aged 3–17 years have behavioral or conduct problems.
- There is a 31.9% lifetime prevalence of an anxiety disorder in US youth older than 13 years.
- There is an 11.7% lifetime prevalence of depression in US youth older than 13 years.
- Roughly, 2.1% of children and adolescents are affected by depression.
- There is a 2.9% lifetime prevalence of bipolar disorder in adolescents.

III. DECISION TO TREAT WITH MEDICATION. Determining a child's need for psychopharmacology requires the following:
- Identification of target symptoms
- Review of appropriate home and school supports and interventions
- Assessment of the degree to which symptoms cause functional impairment
- Informed consent

These decisions can be complicated by difficulties in clearly diagnosing the pediatric population, as well as concerns about potential long-term effects of psychotropics on brain development.

Children with depression, anxiety, severe aggression, or psychotic thinking ideally should work with a therapist, who can help identify contributing stressors and teach the child strategies to cope with or reframe tension, worries, fears, and negative thoughts. For many, individual psychotherapy will be augmented by psychopharmacologic intervention.

When medication is deemed necessary, it is critical to use validated rating scales to monitor progress. Examples of such scales are the Clinical Global Impression Scale, Aberrant Behavior Checklist, Self-report for Childhood Anxiety Related Emotional Disorder (SCARED), and Multidimensional Anxiety Scale for Children (MASC). See bibliography for information regarding these tools.

IV. MEDICAL AND PHILOSOPHICAL CONTROVERSIES. Clinicians frequently extrapolate findings from adult psychopharmacology to children, as there is less research documenting the efficacy and safety of psychotropic medications in the pediatric population. Many of the medications used have potentially serious side effects, which must be weighed against the adverse effects of not treating difficult or dangerous behaviors. With the increasing prevalence of mental health disorders recognized in children, there is a rising need to understand and provide safe, effective treatment. Debate remains over which clinicians are best suited to oversee both behavioral and medication management and, in some areas, a paucity of clinicians limits options.

V. HISTORY: KEY CLINICAL QUESTIONS
- *"What are your greatest concerns at this time? How impairing are these behaviors or feelings?"*
  Medication may be helpful to the child whose depression, anxiety, or aggression prevents adequate learning, participation in the classroom, or social success. Setting realistic expectations to improve sleep, brighten affect, or improve school behavior comes from clear discussion of what the problems are and how the medication will help.
- *"What interventions or medications have been tried in the past?"*
  Confirming that therapeutic and behavioral support has been appropriately offered is often the first step. Positive and negative responses to previous medication trials and doses help in deciding what medications to consider or avoid.

VI. TREATMENT.
Dosing of psychopharmacologic agents in children is often not established. Although taking the adult dose and dividing it by 75 yields an approximate mg/kg per day dosing target, this can underestimate the dose required. It is always important to consult the package insert and the clinical trial literature for more specific dosing guidelines. When dosing guidelines for psychiatric indications are not available, there may be some guidance from dosing of other indications. When a medication is used "off-label," it is important to document in the medical record that a discussion with family recognized this off-label use and family was in agreement with plan and risks/benefits.

A. Psychopharmacologic medication classes
1. **Selective serotonin reuptake inhibitors and serotonin norepinephrine reuptake inhibitors.** Selective serotonin reuptake inhibitors (SSRIs), and more recently serotonin norepinephrine reuptake inhibitors (SNRIs), are often chosen to treat depression and anxiety in children and adolescents (Table 23-1). These medications require no laboratory monitoring and the majority come in liquid and pill forms. Side effects are usually minimal; however, there is a risk of manic activation and suicidal ideation, which families must closely monitor.

   The Food and Drug Administration (FDA) black box warning regarding an increased risk of suicide associated with these agents must be discussed and weighed against the adverse effects and possible risk of suicide associated with untreated depression.

   SSRIs/SNRIs generally require several weeks to reach full efficacy and should be weaned over weeks to minimize withdrawal symptoms. Cytochrome P450 interactions are common with fluoxetine, fluvoxamine, and paroxetine. Common medication interactions include dextromethorphan, theophylline, phenytoin, tricyclic antidepressants, and atomoxetine.

   The SSRIs/SNRIs are not as toxic in overdose as tricyclic antidepressants.
2. **Atypical and tricyclic antidepressants.** Several antidepressants that work via mechanisms other than selective serotonin reuptake inhibition are also widely used, although few are approved in the pediatric population (Table 23-2). Several atypical antidepressants have side effect profiles that must be carefully considered when prescribing (Table 23-3).
3. **Antiepileptics and mood stabilizers.** This group of medications has played an increasing role in treating childhood bipolar and impulse/aggression disorders (Table 23-4). They are often well tolerated but may require combined pharmacotherapy and sometimes blood tests for monitoring (Table 23-5). Many interact with commonly used medications, such as antidepressants.
4. **Atypical neuroleptics.** Atypical neuroleptics are used with increasing frequency in children with psychosis; bipolar and disruptive behavior disorders; medication-resistant ADHD; eating disorders; tic disorders; and aggression, irritability, and or/dysfunctional behavior in the setting of autism spectrum disorder (Table 23-6). They have less risk for extrapyramidal side effects than the first generation of antipsychotics; however, they can have significant short- and long-term side effects, and only modest data indicate efficacy and safety.

   The only medications in this class with FDA approval in children include risperidone, aripiprazole, and olanzapine (Table 23-6). Quetiapine and asenapine are approved for use in children older than 10 years. Paliperidone is approved for use in adolescents.

   Risperidone, olanzapine, quetiapine, and paliperidone are linked to weight gain, and possibly to diabetes and hyperglycemia. Electrocardiographic (ECG) changes may be seen with Ziprasidone, and prolactin elevation occurs most prominently with risperidone. Clozapine (i.e., Clozaril) has a significant risk of agranulocytosis and has been associated with seizures and myocarditis; it is rarely prescribed for children.

Table 23-1 • SELECTIVE SEROTONIN REUPTAKE INHIBITORS (SSRIs) AND SEROTONIN NOREPINEPHRINE REUPTAKE INHIBITORS (SNRIs)

Brand Name (Generic Name)	Age and Approved Indications	Off-Label Clinical Indications	Metabolism	Preparation	Start Dose per Day (mg)	Target Dose per Day (mg)
SSRIs						
Celexa (citalopram)	No pediatric approval	Depression, anxiety, OCD	Weak IID6, IIIA4, IIC19	10, 20, 40 mg; 10 mg/5 mL	10–20	10–40
Lexapro (escitalopram)	≥12 y: MDD	GAD	Weak IID6, IIIA4, IIC19	5, 10, 20 mg; 5 mg/5 mL	5	5–20
Luvox (fluvoxamine)	≥8 y: OCD	Depression, anxiety	IA2, IIIA3–4, IIC19	25, 50, 100 mg; 100, 150 mg ER	25	25–200 (<12 y); 25–300 (≥12 y)
Paxil (paroxetine)	No pediatric approval; not recommended for depression under 18 y	Anxiety, OCD, social anxiety	IID6, IIIA4	10, 20, 30, 40 mg; 12.5, 25, 37.5 mg CR, 10 mg/5 mL	10	10–60
Prozac (fluoxetine)	≥8 y: MDD ≥7 y: OCD ≥10 y: depression associated in bipolar disorder (with olanzapine)	Anxiety, selective mutism	IID6, IIIA3–4, IIC19	10, 20, 40 mg; 20 mg/5 mL; Delayed release (weekly): 90 mg	5–10	5–20 MDD; 20–60 OCD
Zoloft (sertraline)	≥6 y: OCD	Depression, anxiety	Weak IID6, IIC19	25, 50, 100 mg; 20 mg/mL	12.5–25	25–200
SNRIs						
Effexor (venlafaxine)	Over 18 y	Depression, anxiety, ADHD	IId6, IIIa4	25, 37.5, 50, 75, 100 mg; 37.5, 75, 150 mg ER capsule; 37.5, 75, 150, 225 ER tablet	37.5 mg XR	150–225 mg XR
Cymbalta (duloxetine)	≥7 y: GAD	Depression, anxiety	IId6, Ia2	20, 30, 40, 60 mg	30 mg	60–120 mg

OCD, obsessive compulsive disorder; MDD, major depressive disorder; GAD, generalized anxiety disorder; ER or XR, extended release; CR, controlled release.

Table 23-2 • ATYPICAL AND TRICYCLIC ANTIDEPRESSANTS

Brand Name (Generic Name)	Age and Approved Pediatric Indications	Off-Label Clinical Indications	Metabolism	Preparation	Start Dose per Day	Target Dose per Day
Atypical antidepressants						
Buspar (buspirone)	No pediatric approval	Anxiety, depression	IIIa4	5, 7.5, 10, 15, 30 mg	2.5 mg	20–60 mg divided tid
Desyrel (trazodone)	No pediatric approval	Depression, insomnia	IIIa4/5	50, 100, 150, 300 mg; 150, 300 mg ER	25 mg	25–150 mg qhs
Remeron (mirtazapine)	No pediatric approval	Insomnia, depression, anxiety, weight loss	IId6, IA2, IIIa4	7.5 (generic), 15, 30, 45 mg	15 mg qhs	15–45 mg
Wellbutrin SR, Zyban, Aplenzin (bupropion)	No pediatric approval	Depression, ADHD	IIb6, IIIa4	75, 100 mg; 100, 150, 200, 300 mg ER	50 mg SR	50–200 SR bid, 150–450 XL qd
Tricyclic antidepressants						
Anafranil (clomipramine)	Over 10 y for OCD	ADHD	IId6, Ia2, IIa4/5	25, 50, 75 mg	25 mg	Up to 200 mg (2–5 mg/kg)
Norpramin (desipramine)	No pediatric approval	ADHD, chronic pain, depression	IId6	10, 25, 50, 75, 100, 150 mg	10–25 mg	100–200 mg (2–5 mg/kg)
Pamelor (nortriptyline)	No pediatric approval	ADHD	IId6	10, 25, 50, 75 mg 10 mg/5 mL	10–25 mg	0.5–4 mg/kg, plasma level 50–175 ng/mL
Tofranil (imipramine)	Childhood enuresis in children older than 5 y	ADHD, depression	IId6, IIc9, 11c18/19, IIa4/5	10, 25, 50, 75, 100, 125, 150 mg	10–25 mg	75 mg
Elavil (amitriptyline)	≥12 y for depression	ADHD, depression, chronic pain	IId6	10, 25, 50, 75, 100, 150 mg	10 mg tid, 20 mg qhs	50–100 mg

ER, extended release; OCD, obsessive compulsive disorder; ADHD, attention-deficit/hyperactivity disorder; SR, sustained release.

Table 23-3 • ATYPICAL ANTIDEPRESSANT SIDE EFFECTS

Medication	Notable Side Effects	Management Considerations
Buspar (buspirone)	Dizziness, drowsiness, headache, nausea, vomiting	Use with caution in patients with renal of hepatic disease
Desyrel (trazodone)	Sedation, priapism	Use for insomnia
Effexor (venlafaxine)	Sustained hypertension	Avoid in patients with high BP
Remeron (mirtazapine)	Sedation, increased appetite, rare agranulocytosis	Use for insomnia and poor appetite, consider monitoring CBC count
Wellbutrin (bupropion)	Weight loss, tics, activation, lower seizure threshold	Avoid in patients with bulimia or anorexia, uncontrolled seizures, risk for seizures
All tricyclics	Increase PR, QRS, QTc; tremor, sedation, dry mouth, constipation, blurry vision, dizzy	Monitor vital signs, plasma levels and ECG; do not provide more than 1 wk supply to patients at risk for overdose

BP, blood pressure; CBC, complete blood count; QTc, corrected QT; ECG, electrocardiogram.

Chapter 23 • Psychopharmacology 101

Table 23-4 • ANTIEPILEPTICS AND MOOD STABILIZERS

Brand Name (Generic Name)	Age and Approved Pediatric Indications	Off-Label Clinical Indications	Metabolism	Preparation	Start Dose per Day	Target Dose per Day or Plasma Level
Depakote (divalproex sodium)	≥10 y: epilepsy	Manic episode, mixed mania, behavioral disorders; prophylaxis of major depression	Glucuronidation, mitochondrial oxidation	125 mg sprinkles; 125, 250, 500 mg tablets; 250, 500 mg ER; 250 mg/5 mL	10–15 mg/kg divided tid, or qd with ER	Plasma level: 50–125 mg/mL
Keppra (levetiracetam)	≥4 y: seizures	Bipolar disorder	Not extensively metabolized	250, 500, 750, 1000 mg tablets; 500, 750 mg ER tablets; 100 mg/mL solution	5–10 mg/kg per day divided bid or tid	60 mg/kg per day
Klonopin (clonazepam)	Panic disorder over 18 y, seizure disorders in children	Anxiety with insomnia	IIIa, nitroreduction in liver then excreted in urine	0.5, 1, 2 mg tablets: 0.125, 0.25, 0.5, 1, 2 mg wafers	0.01–0.03 mg/ kg divided bid—tid	0.02–0.2 mg/kg
Lamictal (lamotrigine)	Adjunct for partial seizures, Lennox-Gastaut, or tonic-clonic seizures in children, bipolar disorder in adults	Mood stabilization, depression	Glucuronidation	25, 100, 150, 200 mg tablets; 2, 5, 25 mg chewable; 25, 50, 100, 200, 250, 300 mg ER; 25, 50, 100, 200 mg orally disintegrating tablets	Dosing depends on weight, age, and concomitant medications	Consult package insert for titration schedules
Lithium (lithium carbonate)	≥12 y: bipolar disorder	Explosive or extreme aggression, major depression with predictors of bipolar disorder	100% bioavailability, mostly excreted by kidneys	150, 300, 600 mg capsule, 300, 450 mg ER tablets; 8 mEq/5 mL,	900 mg/d divided bid or qid	Plasma level: 0.6–1.2 mEq/L

(continued)

Table 23-4 • ANTIEPILEPTICS AND MOOD STABILIZERS (CONTINUED)

Brand Name (Generic Name)	Age and Approved Pediatric Indications	Off-Label Clinical Indications	Metabolism	Preparation	Start Dose per Day	Target Dose per Day or Plasma Level
Neurontin (gabapentin)	Adjunct for partial seizures in children older than 3 y	Anxiety, posttraumatic stress disorder	Not metabolized	100, 300, 400 mg capsule; 600, 800 mg tablets; 250 mg/5 mL, 300 mg/6 mL solution	100–300 mg divided tid	400–2400 mg divided tid
Tegretol (carbamazepine)	Childhood epilepsy, adults with bipolar disorder	Mania, intermittent explosive disorder, rage	IIIa4	100 mg chewable; 200 mg tablet; 100, 200, 400 mg ER tablets; 100, 200, 300 mg ER capsule; 100 mg/5 mL suspension	200 mg/d	Plasma level: 8–12 µg/mL
Topamax (topiramate)	Partial onset seizures, or primary generalized tonic-clonic seizures and Lennox–Gastaut syndrome in children older than 2 y; migraine prophylaxis ≥12 y	Mood stabilization	Not extensively metabolized	25, 50, 100, 200 mg tablets; 15, 25 mg sprinkles; 25, 50, 100, 200 mg ER capsule; 25, 50, 100, 150, 200 mg ER sprinkle	1–3 mg/kg or 25–50 mg/d	5–9 mg/kg up to 200–400 mg
Trileptal (oxcarbazepine)	Childhood epilepsy	Mania, intermittent explosive disorder, rage	Reduced by cytosolic liver enzymes, IIC19, IIIA4/5	150, 300, 600 mg tablets; 300 mg/5 mL suspension; 150, 300, 600 mg ER tablet	8–10 mg/kg, up to 600 mg divided bid	Target dose based on weight

ER, extended release.

Table 23-5 • SIDE EFFECTS OF ANTIEPILEPTICS AND MOOD STABILIZERS

Medication	Side Effects	Management Considerations
Depakote (divalproex sodium)	Nausea, vomiting, pancreatitis, hepatitis, weight gain, thrombocytopenia, tremor, rash	Baseline CBC count, LFTs, BUN/Cr, ECG, follow-up CBC count, LFTs, plasma level; take with meals
Keppra (levetiracetam)	Drowsiness, aggression, irritability, leukopenia, neutropenia	Serum creatinine, BUN, CBC count
Klonopin (clonazepam)	Headache, drowsiness, ataxia, dizziness, confusion, hepatic dysfunction, paradoxical CNS stimulation can occur	Monitor CBC count, LFTs; tolerance may develop; risk of dependence increases with duration of treatment and in those with a history of drug or alcohol abuse
Lamictal (lamotrigine)	Rash, nausea, vomiting, dizziness, ataxia, drowsiness, headaches	Monitor CBC count; discontinue if rash appears at any time given concern for SJS or TEN
Lithium (lithium carbonate)	Weight gain, kidney and thyroid dysfunction; low therapeutic index	Baseline ECG, baseline and follow-up thyroid and kidney function, plasma level q 1–3 mo
Neurontin (gabapentin)	Disinhibition in 10%–15%	Few medication interactions, no serum monitoring
Tegretol (carbamazepine)	Neutropenia, agranulocytosis, hepatitis, rash, sedation	Baseline CBC count, LFTs, TSH, ECG and follow-up CBC count, LFTs, plasma level; consider HLA-B*1502 genotype screening in patients of Asian descent before initiating medication as it increases risk of SJS and/or TEN
Topamax (topiramate)	Weight loss	May be used to minimize weight gain
Trileptal (oxcarbazepine)	Sedation, dizziness, headache, nausea, impaired concentration	Consider monitoring sodium levels; many CNS effects are dose related

CBC, complete blood count; LFTs, liver function tests; BUN/Cr, blood urea nitrogen/creatinine; ECG, electrocardiogram; CNS, central nervous system; SJS, Stevens–Johnson syndrome; TEN, toxic epidermal necrolysis; TSH, thyroid stimulating hormone.

B. Monitoring. Regular monitoring, including blood work, is recommended for all atypical neuroleptics (Table 23-7). Patients should be monitored routinely for abnormal involuntary movements. The Abnormal Involuntary Movement Scale (AIMS; see Bibliography section) is often useful. Weight should be documented before treatment; at 1, 2, and 3 months; and then at quarterly intervals. Practitioners should consider switching to a different antipsychotic agent for weight gain ≥5% of the initial weight or other signs of metabolic syndrome. Atypical neuroleptics may interact with antidepressants and antiepileptics.

VII. CLINICAL PEARLS AND PITFALLS
- "Start low, go slow": Start at the lowest possible dose and increase slowly. Children may respond well to a lower dose of medication than an adult and may have more side effects as the dose increases.
- Consider the rest of the picture: if the medication "stops working" or seems to be associated with side effects, ask if there are other contributors to the child's presentation, such as classroom changes, stressors at home, concomitant illness, new medications, or puberty.

Table 23-6 • ATYPICAL NEUROLEPTICS

Brand Name (Generic)	FDA Approval in Children	Off-Label Clinical Indications	Metabolism	Preparation	Start Dose per Day	Target Dose per Day
Abilify (aripiprazole)	≥13 y: schizophrenia ≥10 y: bipolar disorder ≥6 y: irritability/agitation associated with autism ≥6 y: Tourette syndrome	Psychosis, manic, and aggressive symptoms	IId6, IIIa4	2, 5, 10, 15, 20, 30 mg; 10, 15 mg disintegrating tablet; 1 mg/mL	2–5 mg	10–30 mg/d
Clozaril (clozapine)	No pediatric approval	Severe psychosis not responsive to other neuroleptics, treatment-resistant autism, treatment-resistant PTSD	Ia2, IId6, IIIa4, IIA6, IIC9, IIC19	25, 50, 100, 200 mg tablets; 12.5, 25, 100, 150, 200 mg disintegrating tablet; 50 mg/mL	12.5 mg	up to 300 mg/d
Geodon (ziprasidone)	No pediatric approval	Psychosis, manic and aggressive symptoms, bipolar disorder, schizophrenia, Tourette syndrome, major depressive disorder	IIIa4, Ia2, IID6	20, 40, 60, 80 mg capsule	20 mg bid	1–3 mg/kg up to 160 mg divided bid
Risperdal (risperidone)	≥5 y: irritability/agitation in autism ≥13 y: schizophrenia ≥10 y: bipolar mania	Psychosis, manic, and aggressive symptoms; Tourette syndrome, aggression in ADHD (not responsive to stimulants), anorexia	IId6, IIIA4	0.25, 0.5, 1,2,3, 4 mg tablets; 0.25, 0.5, 1, 2, 3, 4 mg orally disintegrating tablets; 1 mg/mL suspension; long-acting form via injection	0.25–0.5 mg/d	0.5–6 mg/d (0.5–3 mg for autism; 0.5–2.5 mg for bipolar disorder; 0.5–3 mg for schizophrenia); may divide dose bid if somnolence

Seroquel (quetiapine)	≥10 y: bipolar disorder ≥13 y: schizophrenia	Psychosis, manic, and aggressive symptoms, OCD, tics	IIIa4, IID6	25, 50, 100, 200, 300, 400 mg tablets; 50, 150, 200, 300, 400 mg ER tablets	25–50 mg	400–800 mg divided bid or tid
Zyprexa (olanzapine)	≥13 y: bipolar disorder ≥13 y: schizophrenia ≥6 y: Tourette syndrome ≥10 y: depression associated with bipolar disorder (in conjunction with fluoxetine)	Psychosis, manic, and aggressive symptoms, Tourette syndrome, anorexia	Ia2, IIIa4, IID6, IIC9	2.5, 5, 7.5, 10, 15, 20 mg tablets; 5, 10, 15, 20 mg orally disintegrating tablets	2.5–5 mg	2.5–20 mg/d
Invega (paliperidone)	≥12 y: schizophrenia		IId6, IIIa4	1, 5, 3, 6, 9 mg ER tablet	3 mg	3–12 mg/d
Saphris (asenapine)	≥10 y: bipolar disorder	Schizophrenia	IId6	2.5, 5, 10 mg sublingual tablet	2.5 mg bid	5–10 mg bid

ER, extended release.

Table 23-7 • MONITORING PARAMETERS FOR ATYPICAL NEUROLEPTICS

Timeline in Months	Baseline	1	2	3	6	9	12	Ongoing
BMI	BMI	BMI	BMI	BMI	BMI	BMI	BMI	BMI (Q 3 months)
Blood pressure and pulse	Blood pressure and pulse			Blood pressure and pulse	Blood pressure and pulse	Blood pressure and pulse	Blood pressure and pulse	Blood pressure and pulse (Q 3 months)
Neuromotor signs and symptoms	Neuromotor signs and symptoms			Neuromotor signs and symptoms	Neuromotor signs and symptoms	Neuromotor signs and symptoms	Neuromotor signs and symptoms	Neuromotor signs and symptoms (Q 3 months)
Fasting blood glucose and lipids	Fasting blood glucose and lipids			Fasting blood glucose and lipids	Fasting blood glucose and lipids	Fasting blood glucose and lipids		Fasting blood glucose and lipids (Q 6 months)
Electrolytes, full blood count,[a] renal and liver function	Electrolytes, full blood count,[a] renal and liver function						Electrolytes, full blood count,[a] renal and liver function	Electrolytes, full blood count,[a] renal and liver function (Q 12 months)
Consider ECG[b]	Consider ECG[b]							
Consider prolactin[c]	Consider prolactin[c]							
Eye examination[d]	Eye examination[d]				Eye examination		Eye examination	Eye examination (Q 6 months)

[a]Clozapine may require more frequent evaluation of complete blood cell count with differential.
[b]An **ECG** should be checked for patients on ziprasidone or clozapine at baseline, and if taking ziprasidone, during titration and at maximum dose.
[c]Morning **prolactin** should be checked at baseline if abnormal sexual signs or symptoms are present or at any time in which they appear.
[d]Ophthalmologic examination is recommended at 6 month intervals when using quetiapine or olanzapine secondary to concern for cataracts.

- Choose medications with side effects in mind: for children who have trouble sleeping, you may opt for a sedating drug, whereas in overweight children you may avoid medications that tend to cause weight gain.
- Read newspapers and journals: pediatric psychopharmacology is a hot topic in the media, where parents often learn both valid and invalid information. New medications and new potential side effects of older medications are often well publicized, so keep on top of the field to provide top care.

Bibliography

FOR PARENTS

American Psychiatric Association and American Academy of Child and Adolescent Psychiatry. *Parents Med Guide: The Use of Medication in Treating Childhood and Adolescent Depression: Information for Patients and Families.* Available from: www.parentsmedguide.org/pmg_depression.html.

FOR PROFESSIONALS

American Academy of Child and Adolescent Psychiatry. *Practice Parameter for the Use of Atypical Antipsychotic Medications in Children and Adolescents.* This practice parameter is available on the Internet (www.aacap.org).

Bostic JQ, Prince J, Frazier J, et al. Pediatric Psychopharmacology Update. Available from: http://www.psychiatrictimes.com/p030988.html.

Kutcher SP, ed. *Practical Child and Adolescent Psychopharmacology.* New York: Cambridge University Press; 2002.

Southammakosane C, Schmitz K. Pediatric psychopharmacology for treatment of ADHD, depression, and anxiety. *Pediatrics.* 2015;136(2):351-359.

Strawn JR, Dobson ET, Giles LL. Primary pediatric care psychopharmacology: focus on medications for ADHD, depression, and anxiety. *Curr Probl Pediatr Adolesc Health Care.* 2017;47(1):3-14.

WEBSITES FOR CLINICIANS

The Abnormal Movement Scale (AIMS) is available from: http://www.cqaimh.org/pdf/tool_aims.pdf.

Information regarding access to many monitoring and/or screening scales can be found from: www.schoolpsychiatry.org.

CHAPTER 24

Resilience

Robert B. Brooks

I. **DESCRIPTION OF THE PROBLEM.** Many children in today's world have trouble managing the daily tasks they face. Lacking resilience, they experience a high level of stress and anxiety that affects negatively on all aspects of their lives, including the quality of peer relationships, success at school, the ease and effectiveness of dealing with mistakes and failure, the motivation to persevere at tasks, and the ability to be more empathic.

Resilience may be understood as the capacity of a child to deal effectively with stress and pressure; cope with everyday challenges; rebound from disappointments, mistakes, trauma, and adversity; develop clear and realistic goals; solve problems; interact comfortably with others, and treat oneself and others with respect and dignity. Given the *importance of resilience throughout the lifespan and the number of children who lack this quality*, it is a worthwhile goal of the primary care clinician to become knowledgeable about effective strategies to foster a child's sense of competence, hope, and resilience.

A. **Etiology/contributing factors**
1. **Parent–child "goodness of fit".** The development of resilience is a complex process that can best be understood as occurring within the dynamic interaction between a child's inborn temperament and the environmental forces that affect the child. "Mismatches" between the style and temperament of caregivers and children may trigger anger and disappointment in both parties. In such a situation, children may come to believe that they have disappointed others, they are failures, or others are unfair and unkind. A lack of confidence and a sense of pessimism are common outcomes unless parents can lessen the impact of these mismatches by understanding and appreciating their child's unique makeup and by modifying their own expectations and reactions so that they are more in concert with their child's temperament. An important role of the primary care clinician is to educate parents about the impact of temperament on a child's emotions, thinking, and behavior.
2. **Attribution theory.** Attribution theory is one framework for understanding the thought processes that affect resilience. It is a theory that examines the reasons that people offer for why they think they succeeded or failed at a task or situation. The explanations given are directly linked to an individual's feeling of competence and resilience. Children who are better able to handle challenges perceive their successes as determined in large part by their own efforts, resources, and abilities. These children assume realistic credit for their achievements and possess a sense of personal control over what is occurring in their lives. This feeling of personal control is one of the foundations of a resilient mind-set and lifestyle.

   In contrast, children with low self-esteem often believe that their successes are the result of luck or chance and factors outside their control. Such a view weakens their optimism about being successful in the future.

   Attribution theory also helps us to understand the different ways in which children perceive mistakes and failures in their lives. Children who are more resilient typically believe that mistakes are experiences to learn from rather than to feel defeated by. The occurrence of mistakes is attributed to factors within their power to change, such as a lack of effort on a realistically attainable goal. Children who possess this view are better equipped to deal with setbacks and, thus, are more resilient.

   On the other hand, children who lack confidence, when faced with failure, tend to believe that they cannot remedy the situation. They believe that mistakes result from situations that are not modifiable, such as a lack of ability, and this belief generates feelings of helplessness and hopelessness. This profound sense of inadequacy makes future success less likely because these children expect to fail and begin to retreat from age-expected demands, relying instead on self-defeating coping strategies. Resilience is noticeably absent when a child's life is dominated by feelings of resignation and hopelessness.

Table 24-1 • COUNTERPRODUCTIVE COPING STRATEGIES: SIGNS OF LOW SELF-ESTEEM

Behavior	Example
Quitting	Ending a game before it is over to avoid losing
Avoiding	Not even trying something for fear of failure
Cheating	Copying answers from someone else on a test
Clowning around	Acting silly to minimize feeling like a failure
Controlling	Telling others what to do
Bullying	Putting others down to hide feelings of inadequacy
Denying	Minimizing the importance of a task
Rationalizing or making excuses	Blaming the teacher for failing a test

Attribution theory has significant implications for designing interventions for reinforcing self-esteem, optimism, and resilience in children. It serves as a blueprint for asking the following questions:
- "How do we create an environment in homes and schools that maximizes the opportunity for children not only to succeed but also to believe that their accomplishments are predicated in great measure on their own abilities and efforts?"
- "How do we create an environment that reinforces the belief in children that mistakes and failure often form the very foundation for learning and growth—that mistakes are not only *accepted* but *expected*?"

These are important questions to address because a feeling of being in control of and taking responsibility for one's life and coping effectively with mistakes and setbacks are significant features of resilience.

II. MAKING THE DIAGNOSIS. The signs of a lack of resilience may vary considerably within the same child. Children may display limited perseverance and resilience in situations in which they feel less than competent but not in those in which they are more successful. For instance, children with a learning disability may feel "dumb" in the classroom but may engage in sports with confidence. For some children, a sense of inadequacy is so pervasive that there are few, if any, situations in which they feel confident.

For some children there is little question that they are not very resilient. They say things such as "I'm dumb," "I hate how I look," "I never do anything right," "I always fail," "I'm a born loser," and "I'll always be stupid."

Other children do not directly express their lack of confidence and resilience. Rather, it can be inferred from the coping strategies they use to handle stress and pressure. Resilient youngsters use strategies for coping that are adaptive and promote growth (such as a child having difficulty mastering long division who asks for additional help from a teacher or a child striking out several times in a Little League game who seeks assistance from his coach). They demonstrate a feeling of hope, a belief that they can strengthen skills.

In contrast, children who are not very resilient often rely on coping behaviors that are counterproductive and intensify the child's difficulties. These self-defeating behaviors typically signal that the child is feeling vulnerable and is desperately attempting to escape from the problematic situations. Commonly used self-defeating coping behaviors are listed in Table 24-1. Although all children at some time engage in some of these behaviors, it is when these behaviors appear with regularity that a significant problem with self-confidence and resilience is strongly suggested.

III. MANAGEMENT
A. Primary goals. The strategies that follow have the greatest chance of being effective if adults convey to the child a sense of hope, caring, and support. It is well established that a foundation of resilience in children is the **presence of at least one adult (hopefully, several) who believes in the worth and goodness of the child**. The late psychologist Julius Segal referred to that person as a "charismatic adult," an adult from whom a child "gathers strength." Primary care clinicians, even in brief encounters with a child, can become charismatic adults for that child as well as for the child's parents.

Strategies to nurture resilience should always define the child's *islands of competence*, that is, areas that are (or have the potential to be) sources of pride and accomplishment. Caregivers have the responsibility to identify and build on these islands of competence, and, in so doing, a ripple effect may occur that prompts children to be more willing to venture forth and confront the tasks that have been problematic for them. Interviews with parents (as well as with children) should include a question such as "*What do you see as your child's interests, strengths, islands of competence?*" This kind of question immediately establishes a more positive, strength-based approach.

If children say they cannot think of any strengths that they have, primary care clinicians can reply, "*That's okay. Maybe together we can figure out what things you do very well since all kids have certain strengths.*" Such a comment introduces a path toward identifying each youngster's islands of competence and sets a more positive, hopeful tone during the clinician's interview with the child and/or parents.

B. **Selected strategies for fostering resilience**

1. **Developing responsibility and contributing.** If children are to develop a sense of ownership and commitment, it is important to provide them with opportunities for assuming responsibilities, especially those that involve helping them to feel that they are capable and are contributing in some way to their world and that they are truly making a difference. For example:
   - Asking an 8-year-old to set the table at dinner or a 4-year-old to place his clothes in the laundry bag at the end of each day—requests framed as ways of helping the family.
   - Encouraging and helping a child to write a story about his learning disability to be used to increase the understanding of others about the challenges faced by children with learning problems.
   - Asking a sixth grader with low self-esteem who enjoyed interacting with younger children to tutor first and second graders in the school or to be a babysitter.
   - Enlisting children to participate in a "Walk for Hunger" charity drive.

2. **Providing opportunities for making choices and decisions and solving problems.** An essential ingredient of a resilient mind-set is the belief that although there are events in our lives over which we have little, if any, control, what we have more influence over than we may realize are our attitude and response to those events. To reinforce this viewpoint, children must also believe that they possess skills to solve problems. From an early age, caregivers must provide children with opportunities to make choices and decisions, and to solve problems that have an impact on their lives. These kinds of choices promote a sense of personal control and ownership. For example:
   - A clinician allowing a fearful child the choice of having his eyes or ears examined first so that the child is provided a sense of control.
   - Parents permitting a finicky eater to select (and eventually help prepare) the dinner meal at least once a week.
   - Having a group of elementary school students interview a town selectman, a police officer, and a lawyer as part of the process to decide whether skateboards should be allowed on school grounds, especially given the possible liability issues.
   - Parents asking their children whether they wanted to be reminded 10 or 15 minutes before bedtime that soon it will be time to get ready to go to bed.
   - A 9-year-old boy asking a clinician, "Why did God chose me to be the one with ADHD?" To promote a sense of personal control and to enlist problem-solving skills, the clinician in an empathic way replied that one doesn't know why some kids are born with attention-deficit/hyperactivity disorder (ADHD) and others are not, but now that the boy knew he had ADHD, there were strategies he could learn to confront the problem. The discussion led the boy to recognize that although he did not have control over being born with ADHD, he could have an impact in terms of how he responded.
   - A teenager deciding at what time parents may remind him to take medication, should he or she forget to do so.

3. **Offering encouragement and positive feedback and helping children to feel appreciated.** Resilience and self-worth are reinforced when adults communicate appreciation and encouragement to children. Words and actions conveying encouragement and thanks are always welcoming and energizing. They are especially important for children burdened by self-doubt. Even a seemingly small gesture of appreciation can trigger a long-lasting, positive effect. For example:
   - Parents setting up a "special" 15-minute time in the evening with each of their two young children. The time can occur before each child goes to bed. The parents can highlight the importance of this time by calling it "special" and by saying that

even if the telephone rings they will not respond to the call but instead will let the answering machine do so.

- A primary care clinician sending a postcard to a child after an examination, saying how much he or she enjoyed seeing the child (if this is an honest sentiment).
- Parents writing a brief note to their child commending the child for an accomplishment.
- A recognition assembly in school in which student achievements and contributions are highlighted.

4. **Establishing self-discipline.** If children are to develop resilience, they must also possess a comfortable sense of self-discipline, which involves the ability **to reason and to reflect on one's behavior and its impact on others**. The goal of discipline is to teach children, not to ridicule or humiliate them. If children are to take ownership for their actions and become resilient, they must be increasingly involved in the process of understanding and even contributing to the rules, guidelines, limits, and consequences that are established. Adults must maintain a delicate balance between being too rigid and too permissive. They must strive to blend warmth, nurturance, and acceptance with realistic expectations, clear-cut rules, and logical consequences. In addition, if children are continuously misbehaving, the adults in their lives should attempt to understand why and focus on ways to prevent misbehavior from occurring in the first place. Examples of the effective use of discipline—including those that emphasize a preventive approach—are as follows:

- Parents having difficulty getting a preschool child to bed. They yelled, but this only made matters worse. A consultation with a clinician revealed that the child was having nightmares and was frightened about going to bed. Greater empathy on the part of the parents and the use of a night-light, as well as placing a photo of the parents next to the child's bed, significantly lessened his anxiety and misbehavior.
- Parents not permitting their child to use the bike for several days after he had taken a bike ride on a dangerous street that he was not allowed to ride on (an example of the use of logical consequences).
- Parents asking a child who bounced a ball that broke a window in the house to help pay for the repairs.

5. **Teaching children to deal with mistakes and failure.** The fear of making mistakes and feeling embarrassed is a potent obstacle to meeting challenges, taking appropriate risks, and therefore, to the achievement of self-confidence and resilience. Caregivers should find ways to communicate to children that mistakes go hand in glove with growing and learning. Examples of helping children to deal more effectively with mistakes include the following:

- Parents who avoid overreacting to their children's mistakes and who avoid remarks such as "Why don't you use your brain?" or "What a stupid thing to do!"
- Adults who share what they personally learned from mistakes and failures during their own childhood.
- A teacher who on the first day of the new school year asks students, "Who thinks they will probably make a mistake or not understand something in class this year?" Then, before any of the children can respond, the teacher raises his own hand. Acknowledging openly the fear of failure renders it less potent and less destructive and increases the child's courage to face new tasks. This courage is a major characteristic of resilient children.

Bibliography

FOR PARENTS

BOOKS

Brooks R, Goldstein S. *Raising Resilient Children: Fostering Strength, Hope, and Optimism in Your Child*. New York: McGraw-Hill; 2001.

Brooks R, Goldstein S. *Raising a Self-Disciplined Child: Help Your Child Become More Confident, Responsible, and Resilient*. New York: McGraw-Hill; 2009.

Lahey J. *The Gift of Failure: How the Best Parents Learn to Let Go So Their Children Will Succeed*. New York: Harper; 2016.

WEBSITES FOR PARENTS AND PROFESSIONALS

www.kidsinthehouse.com.
www.drrobertbrooks.com.
www.parenting.com.

FOR PROFESSIONALS
Brooks R. *The Self-Esteem Teacher*. Circle Pines, MN: American Guidance Service; 1991.
Goldstein S, Brooks R, eds. *Handbook of Resilience in Children*. New York: Springer; 2012.
Shure M. *Raising a Thinking Child*. New York: Holt; 1994.

CHAPTER **25**

Adoption

Lisa Prock

I. DESCRIPTION

A. Epidemiology and nomenclature
- Approximately 2% of the US population is adopted with more than 120,000 children been adopted annually since the early 1990s.
- Federal reporting in the United States classifies adoption into three categories:
  - domestic private agency, kinship (including step-parent), and tribal adoption (greater than 50% of annual adoptions);
  - domestic public (child welfare agency) adoption (greater than 40%); and
  - international adoption (<5% of US adoptions in recent years).
- The legal process of adoption is widely variable between each of the 50 states with respect to waiting time for adoptive parents because of voluntary termination of parental rights by birth mothers and notification of birth fathers. Internationally, adoption to the United States and other member countries is governed by the Hague Convention on Intercountry Adoption, which establishes ethical practices for intercountry adoption.
- Although the exact numbers are not known, families may elect to "disrupt" an adoption, estimated to occur in less than 3% of adoptions.
  - Placement with one or two parents is equally successful.
  - In general, the younger the child is at the time of adoption, the less likely an adoption will disrupt.
- A child's history of adoption should be considered a risk factor for later developmental and emotional disorders, given preadoptive experiences and genetic risk factors.
- Preferred terminology when discussing members of the **adoption triad** includes **birth parents, adoptive parents,** and **adopted child/person.** Terms to avoid include "real" or "natural" parents.

II. PRIMARY CARE CLINICIAN'S ROLE: INFORMATION GATHERING

A. Preadoption. If involved during the preadoption process, a clinician should encourage families to attempt to obtain information from birth parents and medical records via the adoption agency. Children with a history of adoption are somewhat more likely than the general population to later be diagnosed with attention-deficit/hyperactivity disorder, fetal alcohol spectrum disorder, intellectual disability, or congenital malformations. The clinician should specifically ask about known family history and consider the relevance for the adoptive parents and their child. The clinician should also try to obtain details about the birth parents' appearance, interests and talents, education and work, and their reason for placing the child for adoption—all information that an adopted child may be interested in learning later in life.

B. Postadoption. Studies indicate that **adoptive families may struggle with transitional problems but that adequate preadoptive preparation can decrease this risk.** All parents may have idealized expectations about their child's behaviors that may not be realized, and adoptive parents may additionally be dealing with the loss of their fantasized birth child. As a result, a clinician should plan a follow-up visit sooner after a newly adopted child joins his or her family rather than later, and keep close and frequent contact with the adoptive parents to understand parental expectations and child behavior. Especially after international adoption, children should be screened for a range of possible infections as well as having routine vision, hearing, and developmental/behavioral surveillance.

C. Older child adoption. For children adopted beyond the newborn period, the clinician should seek additional information on the history and quality of the child's social attachments, history of adverse experiences (such as abuse, deprivation, neglect, rejections, and separations), and educational experience (including quantity, quality, and potential special needs). Parents should be encouraged to take time away from their work to assist in the transition to a family/school when adopting older children as they would with a newborn child.

III. MANAGEMENT

A. When to tell the child he or she is adopted. Most experts suggest that families begin discussing adoptive and birth history as soon as a child joins the family. For newborns, this allows parents to become comfortable discussing the topic of adoption without worrying about a child's response. It is imperative that all children learn the important points of their adoptive history from their adoptive parents rather than from someone else. For children adopted in toddlerhood and beyond, memories of their preadoptive experiences will need to be integrated with their story of adoption. Many adoptive children find creating a "life book," which details their history before and after joining their adoptive family to be a positive experience.

B. How to tell the child he or she is adopted. A discussion of a child's "history of adoption" can be expected to happen many times over the years rather than in a single "disclosure conversation." A child's adoption story should be explained at an appropriate developmental level and with enough, but not too much, information. The following elements are helpful to convey to a child or adolescent about being adopted during conversation:

1. Acknowledge the important role of the birth parents in the creation of the child.
2. Discuss adoptive parents' motivation for adoption.
3. Explain that the child was conceived, grew inside the birth mother, and was born just like all other children.
4. Emphasize that the decision of the birth parents to place him or her for adoption was in no way the fault of the child.
5. Acknowledge that there are happy (especially for adoptive parents) and sad feelings (for birth and adoptive parents as well as adopted individuals) associated with the history of adoption.
6. A statement of the adoptive parents' love for the child and how happy they are that he or she joined their family.
7. The specifics of each adoption story will vary according to the circumstances.
   - The adoption story might be something like, "We could not make a baby ourselves so we decided to adopt. You were made by another man and woman, your birth parents, and born to your mother, just like all other children. But, your birth parents could not take care of a baby, so we adopted you. We're sure that they were sad that you were separated from them. You came to live with us, and we're happy we're a family."

C. Sequence of developmental issues. A child's understanding of adoption changes as he or she develops. At different ages, children will focus on different issues and need access to different information (Table 25-1).

1. During the **preschool** age, children are interested in the facts of how they were born and came to be part of their families. A picture book that depicts the story can be very helpful. Children at this time are also increasingly aware of how "same" and "different" they are when compared with their adoptive parents and siblings.

Table 25-1 • ADOPTION TOPICS FOR CHILDREN AT DIFFERENT AGES

Preschool
"Where did I come from?"
Questions about life and death issues
Adoption as a concrete fact (similar to eye color)

School age (7–11 y)
"Why was I adopted when most people aren't?"
May worry about their value as a person because they are adopted
Increasing concerns about being different
Aware that they have lost someone who played an extremely important role in their life
Fantasize that birth parents are rich, famous, and more attractive than adoptive parents

Adolescence
Identity development: discovering how they are different and how they are connected to birth and adoptive families
Wondering about birth, family history of health or mental health concerns, appearance, and aptitude
Emerging or continued interest in meeting birth parents

2. Around **age 7–11 years,** children begin to appreciate the uniqueness and implications of his or her adoptive status. Children's questions about the birth family may be viewed by adoptive parents as a potential rejection. Clinicians can prepare parents for this experience and reassure them that the emergence of the child's questioning is part of the normal development sequence and should be responded to in a factual and developmentally appropriate manner to maintain open communication about this important topic. Children at this age may imagine their birth parents to be richer, more famous, and otherwise more attractive than their adoptive parents. Many adoptive parents share letters from and pictures of the birth parents with children at this age to begin to introduce facts that they know about the child's history. If birth parents are known to the child (but not as his or her birth parents), the elementary school years are an opportune time to share this information with the child.

3. In the **early adolescent phase of identity development,** adopted children may begin to seek more specific information about their birth parents. Teenagers embark on the task of identity development by discovering how they are different from every other human being and how connected they are to their birth and adoptive families. Having more than two parents adds an additional dimension to this task. If little is known about birth parents, adolescents may continue to idealize them and may seek to understand more about their birth parents.

4. In the **late adolescent period,** topics of sex, marriage, and children may lead to an increased interest in birth family history. Concerns about medical and mental health concerns may increase. By adolescence, individuals should have all available information about their birth family available to help them to facilitate their making sense of their entire life story. Disclosure of difficult topics, including rape and incest, may best be facilitated by working with a therapist.

D. **Questions about birth parents.** As a child or adolescent asks more probing questions about his or her birth mother and why she was not able to parent him or her, adoptive parents should endeavor to provide optimistic yet realistic answers to support the child's creation of his or her own life history. In a discussion of this issue, a parent could say, "Your mother chose adoption for you because she felt unprepared to raise a child, any child, at that time. She probably thinks about you and wonders about how you are doing." An adoptive parent could explain that their child's birth mother felt unprepared for reasons related to a lack of money, maturity, and resources or illness. Adoptive parents should emphasize that adoption was not related to something the child did, but related to birth parent circumstances.

Often there is little information available about birth fathers at the time of adoption. As children realize that there, most certainly, was a father involved, he or she recognizes abandonment by a birth father as well. An adoptive parent could say: "Your birth father may have been overwhelmed by the situation and thought that he was not entitled to be more involved. He probably thinks about you and wonders about how you are doing." As with discussions about birth mothers, optimistic yet honest comments about birth fathers are best.

If birth parents were known or suspected to have had challenges such as alcoholism, drug abuse, child abuse, domestic violence, or mental illness, which contributed to child's adoption history, these circumstances need to be discussed and explained in a supportive and realistic way. For example: "Your parents needed help, but were not getting the help that they needed. As a result, they needed someone else to care for their child."

E. **Outsiders and adoption.** People may ask personal and at times intrusive questions about adoptive families out of curiosity or because the child looks different from the adoptive parents. Parents should never hide the fact that a child is adopted but should always respect their child's right to privacy with regard to details about birth parents and their child's adoptive circumstances. Private details might include genetic and social history or details that have not yet been shared with the child. Parents may respond by stating: "I prefer not to discuss the details of my child's history because I think it should be his or her choice at an older age as to what information will be shared and with whom."

Parents should also be aware that, especially in preschool years, children may "overshare" their adoptive story. As a result, details of their adoptive history that might better not be shared with peers and strangers may best be saved until children better understand the concept of privacy. In the early elementary school years, children with a history of adoption may be teased about being adopted. Parents should prepare their children for that when this happens; it is fine to have a response that puts a positive spin on adoption. For example, children can be coached to say, "Yeah, I'm adopted, so what? So were Presidents Ford and Reagan and Steve Jobs!"

F. Searching for birth parents. Some children and adolescents express an interest in meeting their birth parents, whereas others may only be interested in knowing certain information (such as what they look like). More than 40% of adopted adults report seeking for the identity of their birth parents (known as "adoption search") or seek to locate and meet them (known as "adoption reunion"). In contrast to the fears of many adoptive parents, studies show that following reunions with birth parents, the majority of adopted children/adults report similar or more positive relationships with their adoptive parents. The best time to search for or reunite with birth families is quite controversial, little researched, and may be very different for different children/families. Some experts suggest that searching and meeting with birth family members during childhood or adolescence while residing with adoptive parents can provide a safe environment to make sense of one's adoption story. Others advocate waiting until a young adult is living independently and can process information about their birth family after having become physically independent from their adoptive families.

G. Special-needs adoptions. Children categorized as "special-needs adoptions" in the United States may have known chronic medical challenges or significant developmental challenges or may be demographically "harder to place," including children from certain minorities, older children, or part of a sibling group. It is imperative that preadoptive counseling for parents adopting older children or sibling groups explores potential challenges and provides resources to family. Adoption agencies and "adoption medicine clinicians" (see AAP Section on Adoption and Foster Care in Bibliography) may be particularly helpful in these situations.

H. Transracial or mixed racial adoption. In concert with international consensus and children's right advocates, the American Academy of Pediatrics supports children being placed with a family of the same racial and cultural background whenever possible. However, as minorities are overrepresented in the group of children available for adoption, clearly this is not necessarily realistic. With respect to identity development, between 3 and 7 years of age, children are becoming aware of difference in skin color and racial groupings. Because every child needs a positive sense of racial and ethnic identity, adoptive parents have a responsibility to acquaint a child with his or her heritage and to integrate aspects of the child's heritage into the family's life (e.g., celebrating the holidays of the child's ethnic origin, making foods from the child's country of origin). Positive role models and family friends who share an adopted child's racial and ethnic identity are very helpful in supporting healthy racial identity development for all children including those with a history of transracial adoption.

I. Open adoption. "Openness in adoption" occurs along a continuum of information sharing between and in-person meetings with birth and adoptive families before and after the adoption of a child. One advantage of openness in adoption is immediate access to information as the child feels a need for it. In some cases, such as significant parental mental illness or active substance use, current research suggests that openness in adoption is associated with long-term positive experiences for adopted individuals as well as their birth and adoptive families.

J. International adoption. For several decades before 2004, international adoptions to the United States included more than 20,000 children per year. Ninety percent of these children were born in Asia, South America, and Eastern Europe. Since 2007, the number of internationally adopted children has declined annually with just over 5000 children being adopted internationally in 2016 because of increased domestic adoption of the healthier children in many birth countries. As a result, the medical conditions of children routinely being adopted in 2017 are generally identified as a "special need," including developmental delays, older child, or an identified surgical need such as a cleft lip/palate. Given the poor health and economic conditions in most birth countries, many children joined their families following international adoption with treatable or chronic disease, developmental delays, and growth retardation; the American Academy of Pediatrics provides extensive guidance regarding postadoptive screening (see Healthychildren.org in the Bibliography). All medical records must be scrutinized and laboratory tests should be performed in the United States in most situations.

Bibliography

FOR PARENTS AND PROFESSIONALS

BOOKS

Eldridge S. *Twenty Things Adopted Kids Wish their Adoptive Parents Knew*. New York, NY: Dell Publishing; 1999. (Explores common emotions that adoptees experience through vignettes and case examples. Gives practical advice for helping children to understand and resolve their feelings.).

Pavao JM. *The Family of Adoption*. Boston, MA: Beacon Press; 1998. (An adult adoptee and life-long therapist working with birth families, adoptive families, and adult adoptees discusses her model of adoption, with the use of anecdotes from her own life and practice. A MUST read for anyone—family, friend, or professional—touched by adoption.).

MAGAZINE

Adoptive Families. http://www.adoptivefamilies.com/.

WEB SITES

Healthy Children.org. International Adoption. https://www.healthychildren.org/English/family-life/family-dynamics/adoption-and-foster-care/Pages/Internationally-Adopted-Children-Important-Information-for-Parents.aspx.

American Academy of Pediatrics Council on Foster Care, Adoption and Kinship Care. https://www.aap.org/en-us/about-the-aap/Committees-Councils-Sections/Council-on-Foster-Care-Adoption-Kinship/Pages/Foster-Care-Adoption-Kinship.aspx.

U.S. Department of State Office of Children's Issues. http://adoption.state.gov/.

Evan B. Donaldson Adoption Institute. https://www.adoptioninstitute.org/ Organizations.

North American Council on Adoptable Children. http://www.nacac.org/about/about.html.

National Adoption Center. http://www.adopt.org/assembled/home.html.

FOR PROFESSIONALS

American Academy of Pediatrics. Clinical report: comprehensive health evaluation of the newly adopted child. *Pediatrics*. 2012;129(1).

Mason PW, Johnson DE, Albers Prock L, eds. *Adoption Medicine: Caring for Children and Families*. American Academy of Pediatrics; 2014.

CHAPTER **26**

Anxiety Disorders

Michele L. Ledesma | Carol C. Weitzman |
Carolyn Bridgemohan

I. DESCRIPTION OF THE PROBLEM. The occurrence of anxiety is a normal part of child development. Stranger anxiety, in the first year of life, can be an example of developmentally appropriate behavior. Stranger anxiety and separation awareness, in the first year of life, can be examples of developmentally appropriate behavior as young children begin to develop a sense of object permanence. Fears about monsters and the dark are common in preschool-aged children, whereas school-aged children typically worry about injury and natural events, such as storms. Older children and adolescents often have worries about school performance and social competence. Distinguishing between normal fears and worries, temperamental variations, and clinically significant anxiety may be challenging.

Anxiety becomes clinically significant when fear or worry is excessive and developmentally inappropriate and results in behavioral disturbances as well as functional impairment. It is important to identify children with anxiety because effective, evidence-based treatments are available.

The context in which the anxiety symptoms are primarily produced or manifested differentiates the specific anxiety disorders. However, many children will present with symptoms of more than one type of anxiety. Below are commonly encountered specific disorders. Other anxiety-related disorders, including posttraumatic stress disorder, selective mutism, and specific phobias, are also discussed elsewhere in this book.

A. Anxiety disorders

1. **Generalized anxiety disorder (GAD)** is characterized by chronic and excessive worry in a number of areas (e.g., schoolwork, social interactions, family, health/safety, world events) that is difficult to control.

2. **Separation anxiety disorder (SAD)** refers to excessive and developmentally inappropriate distress experienced when separated from home or from major attachment figures.

3. **Social anxiety disorder (social phobia)** is characterized by feeling scared or uncomfortable in social and performance situations due to fear of embarrassment.

4. **Specific phobias** refer to a repeated pattern of excessive fear and anxiety about a specific object or situation that is out of proportion to the actual risk.

5. **Selective mutism** is the persistent inability to speak in specific situations while being able to speak at other times and is not due to a speech/language deficit or disturbance.

6. **Panic disorder (PD)** refers to repeated unexpected panic attacks. Panic attacks are episodes of sudden intense fear. Panic attacks can also occur in the context of other anxiety disorders.

7. **Obsessive–compulsive disorder (OCD)** is defined by the presence of recurrent, intrusive, unwanted and preoccupying thoughts (obsessions), and repetitive physical or mental acts (compulsions) that are often aimed at neutralizing these thoughts. These obsessions and compulsions cause marked distress, are time-consuming, and/or significantly interfere with the child's normal functioning. Although OCD is no longer classified in the *Diagnostic and Statistical Manual of Mental Disorders, Fifth Edition* (*DSM-5*) as an anxiety disorder but is now in a separate category called obsessive–compulsive disorders, it shares many similar features with anxiety disorders. In addition, individuals with OCD may also have other anxiety disorders.

B. Epidemiology. Anxiety disorders are among the most common behavioral and emotional disorders affecting children and adolescents. The estimated lifetime prevalence for having any anxiety disorder ranges from 25% to 31.9% among several large-scale studies. Anxiety disorders are typically more frequent in girls than in boys, with ratios of 2:1 to 3:1 by adolescence. Anxiety disorders may begin at any time, but more than 70% of adults diagnosed with an anxiety disorder report that their symptoms started in childhood. Although the average age of onset for specific anxiety disorders varies, they tend to be enduring and may either persist or change to another form of anxiety later on. In general, the more severe and impairing the disorder, the more likely it is to persist. There is also an increased risk for the later development of other disorders, such as depression and substance abuse. Anxiety disorders are highly comorbid with other anxiety disorders, and the triad of GAD, social anxiety, and separation anxiety is recognized as the "pediatric anxiety triad." Other psychiatric disorders commonly co-occur, such as attention-deficit/hyperactivity disorder (ADHD), mood disorders, oppositional disorders, somatoform disorders, substance abuse, and learning and language disorders.

1. **GAD.** Reported prevalence rates are estimated to be from 1% to 2.2%. Children with comorbid depression often have a poorer prognosis and longer duration of symptoms.
2. **SAD.** Prevalence rates are estimated to be as high as 7.6%. Although SAD typically has the highest remission rate of all the anxiety disorders, it remains a risk factor for the later development of other anxiety and depressive disorders.
3. **Social phobia.** The estimated lifetime prevalence of social phobia is 9.1%. There is evidence that social phobia in adolescents is a unique risk factor for the development of subsequent substance dependence disorders.
4. **Specific phobias.** The estimated 12-month prevalence for specific phobias is 7%–9%, typically lower in younger children (5%) compared with adolescents (16%), and is more common in females. Most children with specific phobias have more than one phobia.
5. **Selective mutism.** Selective mutism is a relatively rare childhood disorder and has an estimated point prevalence of 0.3%–1%. It is more likely to manifest in young children, usually before the age of 5 years, although it may not come to attention until school entry.
6. **PD.** Although children and adolescents may experience panic attacks, PD is rare, occurring in <0.4% of children and 2%–3% of adolescents. It is more common in females with a ratio of 2:1.
7. **OCD.** Prevalence of OCD ranges from 1% to 4% in children and adolescents. In childhood, OCD is more common in boys with a ratio of 3:2. This changes to a slight female predominance in adulthood. Tic disorders are a common comorbid condition in children with OCD.

   Of note, in the emergence of anxiety disorders, separation anxiety and specific phobias tend to manifest earlier in life, with performance anxiety and social anxiety emerging later in childhood. PDs and OCDs are more common in adolescence.

C. **Etiology**
   1. **Genetic and biological factors.** Although there are no specifically identified genes in humans associated with anxiety disorders, there is high heritability, and children who have a first-degree relative with an anxiety disorder are more likely to develop one themselves. Neuroimaging studies have shown that anxiety disorders are related to atypical activity of the prefrontal cortex–amygdala circuitry. Abnormalities in neurotransmitters such as serotonin, dopamine, gamma-aminobutyric acid (GABA), and glutamate have been postulated to be associated with anxiety disorders, although the exact mechanisms remain unclear. Asthma or respiratory distress may be risk factors for PD.
   2. **Environmental factors.** Family behavior patterns may play a large role in childhood anxiety. Parents and family members who model anxious behavior can contribute to the development of an anxiety disorder in a child. Importantly, parents may also reinforce or accommodate a child's anxiety, often inadvertently, by allowing their child to avoid a situation or object or by providing excessive reassurance, rather than affirming confidence in the child's coping abilities. By doing this, the child's fears are legitimized, and the accommodation maintains and facilitates further avoidant behavior. Parents who are overinvolved, controlling, highly critical, or have excessively high expectations of their children may also contribute to their anxiety. Transitions and losses, such as moving, the death of a relative, or a parent who loses a job, can also trigger anxiety in children. It is important to keep in mind that anxiety in a child can be a red flag for significant stress or violence in the home. Individuals with PD, compared with other anxiety disorders, have higher rates of reported childhood sexual and physical abuse.
   3. **Temperamental factors.** Children with a temperamental style known as *behavioral inhibition* are at increased risk for the development of anxiety disorders, particularly social phobia. These children typically exhibit fearfulness and withdrawal when faced with new people and situations.

II. MAKING THE DIAGNOSIS

A. Signs and symptoms. The presentation of anxiety disorders can vary, as many children may not recognize that their fear and worry are excessive. They will frequently report somatic complaints such as headaches, stomachaches, or nausea. Anger, oppositionality, irritability, and crying are often present, when the child is confronted with the fearful stimuli, and may be misconstrued as oppositional behavior. Critically, anxiety symptoms interfere with the child's normal functioning in school, with friends, and at home. Common clinical presentations of the individual anxiety disorders are presented below, along with specific information regarding *DSM-5* diagnostic criteria (with special attention paid to differences in criteria that pertain to diagnosis in children).

1. **GAD.** Children with GAD have anxiety and worries about a variety of topics, events, and/or activities that are difficult for them to control. They are often conforming perfectionists who regularly seek approval and reassurance. Anxieties may take different forms at different ages:
   - Preschool: imaginary creatures
   - 5–6 years: threats to physical well-being of themselves and their family members
   - 7–14 years: school performance, health, personal harm, extreme weather, and world events (with geographical proximity being a factor)
   - Adolescent: social issues

   Symptoms must be present for at least 6 months. *In children, only one associated symptom listed in the DSM-5 is required for diagnosis.*

2. **SAD.** Children with SAD exhibit distress when faced with separation from major attachment figures. Parents often note that their children with SAD:
   - Follow them around the house
   - Refuse to be alone to sleep or to use the bathroom
   - Often worry excessively about their parents' safety and health
   - Experience nightmares with themes of separation
   - When away from home, are extremely homesick and fear being lost
   - Refuse to go to school or to camp
   - Experience stomachaches and headaches on weekdays but not weekends

   According to *DSM-5* criteria, symptoms must be present for at least 4 weeks in children and adolescents. Under the *DSM-5*, onset of symptoms may occur at any time across the life span.

3. **Social phobia.** Children with social phobia experience fear associated with social scrutiny in social settings such as classrooms, restaurants, and extracurricular activities. These children may have difficulty reading aloud or answering questions in class, initiating conversations, eating at restaurants, using public restrooms, and attending social events. The duration of symptoms must be at least 6 months. There are a number of clarifications in the *DSM-5* pertaining to making this diagnosis in children:
   - Children must have the ability to develop age-appropriate friendships, and the anxiety must occur in peer settings as well as with adults.
   - The anxiety may be expressed by crying, tantrums, freezing, or shrinking from social situations.

4. **Specific phobias.** Children with specific phobias experience marked fear and anxiety when confronted with or in anticipation of a particular object or situation that is out of proportion to the actual danger. They will actively avoid or endure with intense distress the phobic object or situation. The duration of symptoms must be at least 6 months.

5. **Selective mutism.** Children with selective mutism present with a consistent failure to speak in specific social situations at which they are expected to speak (e.g., school), yet they are able to speak in other situations (e.g., home). This failure to speak is not due to speech/language or cognitive deficits or unfamiliarity with the spoken language. The symptoms must last at least 1 month (see Chapter 72).

6. **PD.** Youth with PD present with repeated panic attacks that are *unexpected*—not attributed to an identified trigger—and are characterized by *four or more* of the following as per the *DSM-5*:
   - Palpitations, rapid heart rate
   - Sweating
   - Trembling, shaking
   - Feeling short of breath or smothered
   - Feeling of choking
   - Chest pain

- Nausea or GI pain
- Dizziness or light-headedness
- Chills or hot spells
- Numbness or tingling
- Feeling detached or unreal
- Fear of going "crazy" or losing control
- Fear of dying

Symptoms must be accompanied by avoidant or other maladaptive behavior related to the attacks and at least 1 month of worries about future attacks. PD is not diagnosed when the youth only has panic attacks related to an *expected* trigger (such as in an individual with a phobia). However, individuals with PD can have both expected and unexpected attacks.

7. **OCD.** Children with OCD have obsessions (recurrent and intrusive thoughts, impulses or images that cause marked distress) and compulsions (repetitive behaviors or mental acts that the person feels driven to perform in response to an obsession) that take up large parts of their day and interfere with how they function both at home and at school. When these rituals are confronted or broken, tantrums frequently occur. *Children do not need to recognize that the obsessions and compulsions are excessive or unreasonable for the diagnosis to be made.*

- Common **obsessions** seen in childhood are concerns about getting dirty or sharing germs, danger to self or family, and the need to keep things in a particular order.
- Common **compulsions** include excessive hand washing, checking things (e.g., seeing if a door is locked), putting things in order, and counting things.
- Diagnosis can be delayed, as children may attempt to hide their symptoms for as long as possible, and parents may inadvertently compensate for their atypical behaviors. For example, parents may tolerate increasingly frequent bathroom breaks, not realizing that their children are using these times to compulsively wash their hands.
- Children may come to medical attention because of sequelae from their ritualistic behaviors, such as eczematous changes from repeated hand washing or encopresis resulting from refusal to use public restrooms.
- As with all of the anxiety disorders, it is necessary to distinguish developmentally appropriate behaviors (e.g., wearing a "lucky" cap for sporting events), which rarely interfere with the child's life, from more serious and impairing symptoms of OCD.

B. **Differential diagnosis.** Developmentally appropriate anxiety should always be considered in the differential diagnosis.

- **Neurodevelopmental disorders.** A number of other neurodevelopmental disorders may present with symptoms similar to those seen in anxiety disorders and should be considered in the differential. It is important to keep in mind that these disorders often also exist as comorbidities with an anxiety disorder. Likewise, it is important to assess for comorbid anxiety when considering any of these disorders as a primary diagnosis.
  - *ADHD*—hyperactivity, inattention, and impulsive behaviors
  - *Depression*—social withdrawal, sleep difficulty, somatic complaints, irritability
  - *Autism spectrum disorders*—social withdrawal or atypical social interactions, repetitive language and behaviors, adherence to routines, preoccupying thoughts, overfocused interests, atypical sensory sensitivities or interests
  - *Learning disabilities*—persistent worry about school, school avoidance, poor school performance particularly in specific subjects
  - *Psychotic disorders*—restlessness, social withdrawal, unusual or delusional thoughts, hallucinations
- **Physical conditions and drug effects.** The clinician should consider physical conditions that may present with anxiety-like symptoms such as hyperthyroidism, asthma, migraines, seizure disorders, hypoglycemia, cardiac arrhythmias, pheochromocytoma, or central nervous system disorders. Substance use or withdrawal (e.g., cocaine, amphetamines, caffeine, alcohol, cannabis, nicotine) may result in symptoms that mimic somatic manifestations of anxiety such as palpitations or nausea, as might side effects from prescription (e.g., stimulants, antipsychotics, steroids) and nonprescription (e.g., cold medicines, antihistamines, diet pills) medications.
- **Psychosocial problems.** Children with symptoms of anxiety should always undergo a thorough assessment that includes screening for possible psychosocial stressors including abuse, neglect, parental mental illness, and violence in the home.

C. **Key questions and useful questionnaires.** When assessing a child for the presence of an anxiety disorder, it is beneficial to obtain information from multiple sources (e.g., parents, child, teachers). Children may be more aware of their own symptoms and inner distress, whereas parents may be more perceptive of the impact the anxiety has on the child's functioning. A combination of directed interviewing and the use of standardized screening tools can be helpful in revealing types and sources of anxiety.

1. **Interview questions for children**
   - *What kinds of things do you worry about?*
   - *Do you think you worry more than other children?*
   - *Does worrying about things get in the way of sleeping, going to school, or having friends?*
   - *Do the things you worry about stop you from going anywhere or doing anything?*
   - *For how long have these worries been bothering you?*
   - *Are you afraid that something bad will happen to your mom or dad?*
   - *Do you have nightmares about getting lost or kidnapped?*
   - *Are you scared around large groups of children, such as at birthday parties?*
   - *Are there thoughts you cannot get out of your head?*
   - *Are there things that you do repeatedly to make another worry go away?*

2. **Interview questions for parents**
   - *Would you describe your child as nervous or a worrier?*
   - *What things does she/he worry about?*
   - *How does your child's worry interfere with daily activities such as school, friendships, or fun?*
   - *Is there anything you do to ease your child's worry? Do you have to go out of your way to ease your child's worry? How much time does this take?*
   - *Does anyone in the family have a history of anxiety or depression?*
   - *Does your child have any difficulty falling asleep alone? Does he or she need the lights on or need to sleep in your bed with you?*
   - *Have you ever had to pick up your child early from school or from a social event such a sleepover?*
   - *Does your child complain of headaches and stomachaches on weekdays but not on weekends?*
   - *Does your child worry that he or she will do something embarrassing in front of other people?*
   - *Is your child afraid of meeting or talking to new people?*
   - *Have you ever had to get your child out of a social obligation or a performance?*
   - *Does your child have bad or unrealistic thoughts or images that he or she cannot get out of his or her head?*
   - *Does your child have certain habits, rituals, or routines that he or she performs over and over (e.g., washing hands, counting objects, checking the door is closed)? How much time does this take?*

3. **Questionnaires.** There are two broad categories of questionnaires that clinicians can use to screen for anxiety disorders.
   - General behavioral/emotional screens assess for symptoms of a wide range of disorders. Some general screens are the *Pediatric Symptom Checklist* (PSC) and the *Behavior Assessment System for Children* (BASC). The *NICHQ Vanderbilt Assessment Scales* are designed primarily to assess for symptoms of ADHD but include a screen for anxiety and depression as well.
   - Screening tools that specifically assess for symptoms of anxiety disorders are also available. Examples of anxiety-specific screens are the *Screen for Child Anxiety Related Disorders* (SCARED) and the *Multidimensional Anxiety Scale for Children* (MASC). Both are available in parent and child (self-report) versions. More recently, scales have been developed to assess for anxiety in younger children, such as the *Spence Preschool Anxiety Scale*.

III. **MANAGEMENT.** For children with mild symptoms of anxiety and limited impairment in functioning, supportive counseling and psychoeducation can be offered in the office, both for the parent and the child. Parents should be counseled to provide support and encouragement, promote "brave behaviors," and help their child develop coping skills, rather than accommodate and reinforce their child's anxiety and avoidance. Visual supports (such as a Faces Scale or Feelings Thermometer) and use of journals or symptom diaries can help children recognize and quantify their symptoms. For children with social anxiety, previewing new situations, use of scripts, and role-playing can reduce avoidance. Activities that provide a holding place for worries such as making a dream catcher to hang in the child's bedroom or creating a box of calming activities can build coping skills. For children with moderate symptoms of anxiety and OCD, psychotherapy, specifically cognitive behavioral therapy (CBT), is the first line of treatment; there is growing evidence that CBT can be adapted for children younger than 7 years. For children and adolescents with more severe symptoms, a multimodal treatment approach with psychotherapy, medication, and family therapy is often needed.

A. Parent education and guidance. The first step in management is to educate both parents and children about the disorder. The discussion should include information about the symptoms of the disorder, course, treatment options, risks of treatment, and consequences of not seeking treatment. Parents and children should be given concrete suggestions and techniques for how to deal with symptoms at home and at school. Parents should try to attend to their children's concerns, recognize their children's distress, and help them identify their feelings. They can model positive coping styles and "brave behavior," as well as help the child prepare for anxiety-producing transitions by practicing new routines and exploring new environments. Parents may, as a protective instinct, try to ease a child's worries by providing excessive reassurance or allow anxiety-related avoidance of a specific object or situation; however, in doing so, they often inadvertently reinforce the anxiety, leading to further avoidant behaviors. When avoidance happens too often, it teaches a child to steer away from anxiety-producing situations and gets in the way of the child discovering his or her own courage, strength, and resilience.

B. Psychotherapy

1. **Cognitive behavioral therapy.** Substantial evidence supports the use of CBT in the treatment of pediatric anxiety disorders and OCD. CBT is a time-limited, goal-directed therapy in which children learn to react in a different way to situations that are anxiety-producing. Children learn to manage their somatic symptoms, restructure how they think about anxiety-provoking situations, face their fears via exposure and desensitization techniques, and make plans for what to do if anxiety returns. A widely utilized CBT protocol known as the Coping Cat Program consists of 14–18 sessions over 3–4 months. Given the significant role that parents and families may play in the development and maintenance of anxiety symptoms, parents are frequently involved in the CBT treatment process. There have been a number of studies that have shown added benefit when a parent component is added to child CBT, particularly if the parent also has symptoms of anxiety.

2. **Play therapy.** Play therapy may work well for young children as well as older children with language or cognitive impairments who may have difficulty participating in CBT. Therapists use toys such as animals, dolls, blocks, and puppets to help the child express their feelings and experiences through play. Most of the existing literature regarding the use of play therapy focuses on trauma-related anxiety disorders.

3. **Group psychotherapy.** For children with social phobia, group therapy may help them to confront their fears and facilitate positive interaction with others in an accepting group of people with shared problems.

C. Medication. Selective serotonin reuptake inhibitors (SSRIs), such as sertraline, fluoxetine, and fluvoxamine, are the first-line medications used in children with anxiety disorders. There is no evidence that a particular SSRI is more effective than another in treating pediatric anxiety disorders. It may take up to 4–8 weeks to see an effect; if no or only a partial effect is seen at that time, consider slowly increasing the dose or switching to a different SSRI. If a child has been stable for at least a year, a trial off of medication can be attempted (best done during a low-stress period such as summer vacation) (see Chapter 23). Selective serotonin/norepinephrine reuptake inhibitors (SSNRIs) such as duloxetine (the only Food and Drug Administration [FDA]–approved drug for GAD for ages 7 years and older) and venlafaxine have also been shown to be efficacious in treating anxiety and are similar to SSRIs in terms of side effect profile. Of note, in February 2004 the FDA issued a black box warning on the use of SSRIs along with SSNRIs in pediatric patients owing to studies that showed a small increased risk of suicidal ideation and behavior in patients with depression taking these medications. This has not been studied specifically in patients with anxiety. It is important to monitor closely for these symptoms in the first 4 weeks of treatment. Multiple randomized, controlled trials conducted in children with SAD, GAD, and social phobia have shown that both SSRIs and CBT are equally effective in reducing symptoms of anxiety compared with placebo, while a combination of CBT and medication was superior to either therapy alone. There is also strong evidence for efficacy and FDA approval for SSRIs to treat OCD in children. Other medications used in the treatment of pediatric anxiety disorders include tricyclic antidepressants, buspirone, and benzodiazepines. Limited studies of the safety and efficacy of these medications are available.

D. School. A student may need a 504 Plan for school that details accommodations for anxiety, but care should be taken that these school accommodations do not become a means of further avoiding a child's anxiety triggers. For more severe anxiety, a student may require an Individualized Education Plan (IEP) under the educational classification of emotional disturbance with intensive behavioral support that is tailored to the individual student. Teachers and other school staff should be educated about the disorder and provided with strategies for how to best help the child with anxiety in the classroom.

IV. PEARLS AND PITFALLS

- Anxiety is a part of the universal human experience; however, once it becomes excessive and developmentally inappropriate and causes behavioral disturbances or functional impairment, it becomes clinically significant.
- Anxiety often differs in presentation based on a child's developmental age and can often present with somatic symptoms.
- Anxiety disorders are often enduring and can later manifest as a different anxiety or mood disorder or substance abuse problem.
- New or worsening anxiety in a child can be a red flag for violence, trauma, or stress in the home or community and should trigger assessment for environmental conditions or stressors.
- Oftentimes, treatment of anxiety involves not only treating the child, but also treating the whole family and, in particular, recognizing patterns of accommodation and avoidance.
- Children presenting with mild anxiety can sometimes be treated with supportive counseling in the pediatric office setting.

Bibliography

FOR PARENTS

BOOKS

Dacey JS, Fiore LB. *Your Anxious Child: How Parents and Teachers Can Relieve Anxiety in Children.* San Francisco: Jossey-Bass; 2000.

Huebner D. *What to Do When You Worry Too Much: A Kid's Guide to Overcoming Anxiety.* Washington DC: Magination Press; 2008.

Manassis K. *Keys to Parenting Your Anxious Child.* New York: Barron's Educational Series Inc.; 1996.

WEB SITES

National Institute of Mental Health is a federal agency that researches mental and behavioral disorders. www.nimh.nih.gov.

Anxiety Disorders Association of America is a nonprofit organization that provides information regarding anxiety. www.adaa.org.

FOR PROFESSIONALS

Wehry AM, Beesdo-Baum K, Hennelly MM, Connolly SD, Strawn JR. Assessment and treatment of anxiety disorders in children and adolescents. *Curr Psychiatry Rep.* 2015;17(7):52.

Connolly S, Bernstein G, Work group on Quality Issues. Practice parameter for the assessment and treatment of children and adolescents with anxiety disorders. *J Am Acad Child Adolesc Psychiatry.* 2007;46(2):267-283

Weitzman C, Wegner L. Promoting optimal development: screening for behavioral and emotional problems. *Pediatrics.* 2015;135(2):384-395.

Strawn JR, McReynolds DJ. An evidence-based approach to treating pediatric anxiety disorders. *Curr Psychiatry.* 2012;11(9):16-21.

Compton SN, March JS, Brent D, AMt Albano, Weersing R, Curry J. Cognitive-behavioral psychotherapy for anxiety and depressive disorders in children and adolescents: an evidence-based medicine review. *J Am Acad Child Adolesc Psychiatry.* 2004;43(8):930-959.

Wang Z, Whiteside SPH, Sim L, et al. Comparative effectiveness and safety of cognitive behavioral therapy and pharmacotherapy for childhood anxiety disorders. A systematic review and meta-analysis. *JAMA Pediatr.* 2017;171(11):1049-1056.

WEB SITES

AAP Mental Health Screening and Assessment Tools for Primary Care. www.aap.org/en-us/advocacy-and-policy/aap-health-initiatives/Mental-Health/Documents/MH_ScreeningChart.pdf.

AAP Bright Futures Mental Health Toolkit. www.brightfutures.org/mentalhealth/pdf/tools.html.

AAP Anxiety Module. This module provides information on initial management and recognition of children with mild to moderate anxiety in the primary care setting. www.aap.org/en-us/advocacy-and-policy/aap-health-initiatives/Mental-Health/Pages/Module-2-Anxiety.aspx.
http://www.aacap.org/aacap/Families_and_Youth/Resource_Centers/Anxiety_Disorder_Resource_Center/Home.aspx.

Web site listing various pediatric anxiety scales, some with links to downloadable PDF versions. www2.massgeneral.org/schoolpsychiatry/screeningtools_table.asp.

SCARED parent and child scales in PDF versions, multiple translations, and scoring instructions. http://pre.pediatricbipolar.pitt.edu/resources/instruments.

Spence Children's Anxiety Scale parent, child, and preschool versions with scoring instructions. www.scaswebsitecom.

CHAPTER 27

Attention-Deficit/Hyperactivity Disorder

Tanya Froehlich | Jayna B. Schumacher

I. DESCRIPTION OF THE PROBLEM

A. Overview. Overview. Attention-deficit/hyperactivity disorder (ADHD) is not a simple medical diagnosis. Rather, it is a neurodevelopmental disorder, suspected when persistent difficulties with attention regulation, impulse control, and excessive motor activity are consistently observed by parents and other caregivers early in the child's life. In young children, these symptoms cause significant dysfunction in most important aspects of the child's life, leading to challenging relationships with caregivers, teachers, and peers and contributing to behavioral and discipline problems in multiple settings, including home, school, and childcare. In adolescents and adults, ADHD may impair academic achievement, work performance, and relationships and be associated with serious long-term outcomes, such as substance use disorders, criminal activity, and death related to accident and suicide.

1. The *Diagnostic and Statistical Manual of Mental Disorders*, **Fifth Edition (*DSM-5*) diagnostic criteria for ADHD** are found in Table 27-1. The *DSM-5* differentiates three ADHD presentations: predominantly inattentive, predominantly hyperactive-impulsive, and combined presentation. These criteria should be assessed by the pediatric clinician during the diagnostic process.

2. In addition to those symptoms described in the *DSM-5*, difficulties with attention regulation, inhibition, and other executive functions experienced because of having ADHD may be associated with the following:

   - **Decreased responsiveness to environmental reinforcement** (therefore, compared with typical children, children with ADHD require a more explicit and structured presentation of rules and instructions, as well as an amplified system of rewards and consequences, to support appropriate behavior)
   - **Difficulties with delaying gratification** (as a result, children with ADHD tend to live in the "now" and lack the ability to modify or delay behavior in view of future consequences)
   - **Poor social skills and immaturity** (social intrusiveness and poor peer relations, leading to difficulties maintaining friendships)
   - **Low self-esteem** (likely linked to difficulties with relationships with peers, siblings, parents, and teachers, as well as challenges with school and extracurricular endeavors)
   - **Low frustration tolerance and irritability**
   - **Emotional dysregulation or mood lability** (when mood swings are extreme, especially with hyperirritable periods, diagnoses of disruptive mood dysregulation disorder and bipolar disorder may be considered)
   - **Oppositional and/or aggressive behavior** (likely related to emotional dysregulation and impulse control problems; suboptimal parenting practices [e.g., inconsistent discipline, irritable/explosive discipline, inflexible discipline, low supervision] have also been linked to the development and maintenance of oppositional behavior and disordered conduct)
   - **Reduced sense of danger and increased risk-taking** (leading to increased accidents)
   - **Difficulties with timeliness and estimating the amount of time a given task will take to complete**
   - **Cognitive deficits on tests of attention, executive function, or memory** (although these tests have inadequate sensitivity and specificity to serve as diagnostic tools, as not all children with ADHD show deficits on these measures)
   - **Academic underachievement** (likely related to problems with attention, planning, and organization)

Table 27-1 • ADHD: *DSM-5* CRITERIA

A. A persistent pattern of inattention and/or hyperactivity–impulsivity that interferes with functioning as characterized by (1) and/or (2):

1. **Inattention:** Six (or more) of the following symptoms have persisted for at least 6 mo to a degree that is inconsistent with developmental level and that negatively impacts directly on social and academic/occupational activities:
   a. Often fails to give close attention to details or makes careless mistakes in schoolwork, work, or other activities
   b. Often has difficulty sustaining attention in tasks or play activities
   c. Often does not seem to listen when spoken to directly
   d. Often does not follow through on instructions and fails to finish schoolwork, chores, or duties in the workplace
   e. Often has difficulty organizing tasks and activities
   f. Often avoids, dislikes, or is reluctant to engage in tasks that require sustained mental effort (such as homework)
   g. Often loses things necessary for tasks or activities (such as toys, school assignments, pencils, books, or tools)
   h. Is often easily distracted by extraneous stimuli
   i. Is often forgetful in daily activities

2. **Hyperactivity and impulsivity:** Six (or more) of the following symptoms have persisted for at least 6 mo to a degree that is inconsistent with developmental level and that negatively impacts directly on social and academic/occupational activities:
   Note: Symptoms are not solely a manifestation of oppositional behavior, defiance, hostility, or a failure to understand tasks or instructions.
   a. Often fidgets with or taps hands or feet or squirms in seat
   b. Often leaves seat in situations when remaining seated is expected
   c. Often runs about or climbs excessively in situations in which it is inappropriate (in adolescents or adults, may be limited to feeling restless)
   d. Often unable to play or engage in leisure activities quietly
   e. Is often "on the go," acting as if "driven by a motor"
   f. Often talks excessively
   g. Often blurts out answers before questions have been completed
   h. Often has difficulty waiting his or her turn
   i. Often interrupts or intrudes on others (such as butting into conversations or games)

B. Several inattentive or hyperactive–impulsive symptoms were present before age 12 y.[a]

C. Several inattentive or hyperactive–impulsive symptoms are present in two or more settings (such as at home, school, or work).

D. There must be clear evidence that the symptoms interfere with, or reduce the quality of, social, academic, or occupational functioning.[b]

E. The symptoms do not occur exclusively during the course of schizophrenia or another psychotic disorder and are not better explained by another mental disorder (such as a mood, anxiety, dissociative, or personality disorder; substance intoxication or withdrawal).

Reproduced from the American Psychiatric Association, Diagnostic and Statistical Manual of Mental Disorders. 5th ed. Washington, DC: American Psychiatric Association; 2013.
[a]For individuals (especially adolescents and adults) who currently have symptoms that result in impairment but no longer meet full criteria, "in partial remission" should be specified.
[b]Current level of severity (mild, moderate, severe) should be specified to indicate the degree of impairment in social or occupational functioning.

B. Epidemiology

- Prevalence estimates depend on the diagnostic criteria used and means for ascertainment. ADHD rates in US children generally range from 5% to 11%. In worldwide studies, ADHD has been found to occur in most cultures in about 5% of children and about 2.5% of adults.
- Higher rates are seen in boys, with a male to female ratio of 2:1 in the general population. Girls are more likely than boys to manifest primarily inattentive symptoms.
- Higher rates are seen in children with low socioeconomic status. This may be related to the increased exposure to ADHD risk factors in this group (such as lead exposure, pre- and perinatal exposures and complications, and childhood trauma; see Environmental factors below).
- Owing to the natural progression of ADHD symptoms, an individual may change "presentations" during his or her lifetime. ADHD often presents in toddlers as excessive motor activity, but it can be challenging to differentiate this from typical

Table 27-2 • COMORBID DISORDERS

Comorbid Disorders	Prevalence Rate in Children with ADHD
Delays in language, motor, or social development	20%–60%
Specific learning disorder	30%–75%[a]
Oppositional defiant disorder	>45%[b]
Conduct disorder	>15%[b]
Anxiety disorders	25%–35%
Depressive disorder	10%–30%
Bipolar disorder	10%
Chronic tic disorders	20%
Posttraumatic stress disorder	10%

[a]Depending on criteria and means for assessment. Written expression disorders are the most common specific learning disorder comorbid with ADHD.
[b]Higher comorbidity with combined presentation than inattentive presentation.

behavior before the age of 4 years. Hyperactivity often continues as the predominant symptom during the preschool years, with inattentive symptoms becoming more apparent and problematic in elementary school. Over time, hyperactivity may become less obvious and manifest as feelings of restlessness or impatience in adolescence and adulthood. Difficulties with inattention, planning, organization, working memory, and impulsivity are typically ongoing.

C. **Comorbidity.** Comorbidity of other diagnoses and ADHD is quite high, although it is often difficult to discern if the additional diagnosis is the cause of behaviors that mimic ADHD symptoms or if it coexists with ADHD as a discrete disorder. Some estimate that comorbid diagnoses are the rule, not the exception, and can be found in more than two-thirds of all children with ADHD. Table 27-2 lists some principal ADHD comorbidities and rates of these conditions in children with ADHD.

D. **Etiology.** ADHD has no single invariant cause but likely represents the final common pathway for a host of genetic, neurologic, and environmental factors.

1. **Genetic factors.** The concordance rate of ADHD in identical twins is strikingly high (0.6–0.8). In addition, first- and second-degree relatives (parents, siblings, and grandparents) of children with ADHD have a much higher incidence of the disorder (20%–25%). As a result, investigations are ongoing to identify genetic causes of ADHD, which is considered a complex genetic disorder in which many genes of small effect are likely involved. Thus far, ADHD candidate gene studies have found replicated associations of minor effect size across a number of genes, including *SLC6A3* [DAT], *DRD5*, *DRD4*, *SLC6A4*, *LPHN3*, *SNAP-25*, *HTR1B*, *NOS1*, and *GIT1*. Genetic studies using quantitative trait designs also suggest links to Cadherin13 and glucose–fructose oxidoreductase domain 1 genes. In addition, copy number variants (CNVs) in glutamate receptor genes (*GRM1*, *GRM5*, *GRM7*, and *GRM8*) have been implicated in ADHD etiology. Of note, no one genetic variant is considered a necessary or sufficient causal factor, and it is likely that gene–gene and gene–environment interactions are important in the development of ADHD in each individual.

2. **Medical risks.** Children with a history of prematurity, low birth weight, and other perinatal complications have an increased prevalence of ADHD. Rates of ADHD are also higher in children who have experienced traumatic brain injury or early brain infections (e.g., encephalitis).

a. **Differences in the brain.** Animal studies and the effects of psychoactive medications have led to speculations of altered neurotransmitter profiles and brain function in persons with ADHD. Dysregulation of brain dopamine and norepinephrine systems is implicated in the pathophysiology of ADHD. As a group, compared with peers, children with ADHD display increased slow-wave electroencephalograms (EEGs), reduced total brain volume on magnetic resonance imaging, and possibly a delay in posterior to anterior cortical maturation. Positron emission tomography and functional magnetic resonance imaging studies suggest underactivity in parts of the cerebral cortex, especially the prefrontal and cingulate areas of the frontal lobes, perhaps leading to the challenges in executive function and self-regulation described in ADHD. Other areas that have been implicated in studies as having altered function include the cerebellar vermis and basal ganglia. Studies have also suggested multiple functional and structural neural network abnormalities in ADHD, including most prominently the fronto–striatal, but also fronto–parieto–temporal, fronto–cerebellar, and even fronto–limbic networks. Although these ADHD-related brain differences have been demonstrated on the group level, it should be noted that the degree of overlap between individual children with ADHD and their typical peers is such that neuroimaging and EEG studies lack adequate sensitivity and specificity to be used in isolation as diagnostic indicators.

    b. **Environmental factors.** While it is well accepted that ADHD is highly heritable, it is estimated that between 10% and 40% of the variance associated with ADHD is likely to be accounted for by environmental factors. A number of environmental factors have been linked to increased rates of ADHD and ADHD-related symptoms, including neurotoxins (e.g., in utero alcohol and other exposures, lead, polychlorinated biphenyls (PCBs), pesticides, bisphenol A) and psychosocial risk factors (e.g., childhood abuse or neglect, multiple foster care placements), although it is not definitively known if these associations are causal. Of note, children with in utero tobacco exposure have higher rates of ADHD, but at least a portion of this association may be explained by genetic risk factors, as mothers with ADHD are more likely to smoke. Of note, studies have NOT implicated poor parenting as a cause of ADHD, although it may magnify the symptoms of ADHD. On the other hand, harsh and inconsistent parenting practices have been implicated in the development of oppositional and aggressive behaviors.

E. Theories of ADHD. The most popular current theory of ADHD is that it represents a **disorder of executive function**. This theory proposes that ADHD symptoms arise from a primary deficit in *behavioral inhibition*, which leads to difficulties in additional domains such as working memory, self-regulation of affect/motivation/arousal, and goal-directed behavior. An elaboration of this theory posits a **dual pathway**, involving both the executive dysfunction model and a **delay aversion** model. The delay aversion model proposes impaired neural signaling of delayed rewards due to disturbances in motivational processes, such that children prefer immediate small rewards to delayed larger rewards and manifest a negative reaction to imposed delays. An additional ADHD explanatory theory proposes that deficits arise from increased activation in the brain's **default mode network (DMN)**. The DMN is a constellation of brain-related areas that are activated when the brain is at rest (awake and alert, but not actively involved in an attention-demanding task). To engage in a goal-directed activity, the DMN must be deactivated. The DMN theory of ADHD derives from observations that individuals with ADHD, compared with controls, have stronger connections among DMN nodes than those within the response inhibition network.

F. Prognosis
    1. Problems with attention and organization persist in most young adults and adults with ADHD.
    2. Hyperactive symptoms are less prominent and often change in nature (hyperactivity replaced by feelings of restlessness), as individuals age and enter puberty.
    3. Favorable prognostic indicators include higher intelligence, higher socioeconomic status, and fewer peer relationship problems.
    4. Factors linked to a less favorable prognosis include parental psychopathology, conflict and hostility in the parent–child relationship, increased aggression, and disordered conduct.

II. MAKING THE DIAGNOSIS. There is **no sine qua non** for the diagnosis of ADHD. Rather, the pediatric clinician must analyze and integrate the reports of characteristic behaviors by multiple observers, occurring in a variety of different settings, over an extended period. These behaviors are described as occurring with greater intensity and frequency than is typical for other children of the same developmental age and, most importantly, **are causing significant problems in the child's functioning and/or relationships in more than one setting.**
    A. History: key clinical questions
        1. *"Tell me about the behaviors that concern you. What, exactly, does he/she do? Give me a specific example."* It is important to obtain specific examples to see if the behaviors sound truly more severe than other children at the same developmental level, or if the parent has a low tolerance for a typical, albeit temperamentally active and intense, child.

2. *"Who else is concerned about these behaviors?"* Because ADHD symptoms are usually problematic in most or all settings across time and space, if only the parent is concerned but other significant caregivers or teachers are not, one's index of suspicion should be raised for an etiology other than ADHD. However, it is important to keep in mind that ADHD symptoms may be less obvious or even absent when the child is in a novel setting, is engaged in highly interesting or motivating activities, has close supervision or consistent external stimulation (e.g., electronics), or is interacting in one-to-one situations.

3. *"When did you first become concerned about these behaviors?"* Often the symptoms have been present for a long time before coming to your attention and should be present at least to some degree in early childhood. Conversely, the abrupt onset of behavioral problems may suggest a stressful trigger and a different etiology than ADHD.

4. *"Tell me about his/her attention span."* Remember that the ability to watch TV or play video games for an extended period does not necessarily connote a good attention span, as these activities provide consistent external stimulation. Instead, ask about the child's ability to pay attention to less compelling, more boring activities that require sustained attention to be successful. Ask questions such as follows: *"Is he/she a daydreamer? Easily distracted? Does he/she have a hard time completing tasks and following through on instructions? How are his/her listening skills?"*

5. *"Tell me about his/her activity level."* Some children are obviously extremely active. For others, fidgety and nonpurposeful activity may be more prominent than gross motor hyperactivity. Ask: *"Does he/she seem to be in constant motion? Is he/she fidgety, even when quiet? Does he/she talk a lot more than other kids his/her age?"*

6. *"Does he/she often act without thinking? Does he/she interrupt and butt in on others when they are doing something? Does he/she engage in dangerous activities without a sense of fear? Is he/she often remorseful and apologetic after an impulsive act?"*

7. *"Tell me about how he/she expresses his/her emotions. Does he/she seem angry or depressed or anxious or incredibly irritable sometimes?"* The search for another cause (e.g., depression, anxiety, disruptive mood dysregulation disorder, bipolar disorder) or comorbidity begins with the initial history taking.

8. *"How does he/she get along with other kids? Does he/she have many friends?"* Most children with ADHD experience problems with social relationships, which is a significant cause of unhappiness and low self-esteem.

9. *"Tell me about how he/she is doing in school or childcare."* It is important to get a sense of the level of dysfunction these behaviors may be causing in important aspects of his/her world, including day care/preschool/school.

10. *"Given all the problems you describe, how do you think they have affected his/her self-esteem?"* Given the increased issues with anxiety and depression seen in children and adolescents with ADHD, it is helpful to raise the issue early on, especially for parents who have never considered this question before.

11. *"How do you deal with these behaviors? What has worked and what has not?"* Often a child with ADHD has engendered many negative, ineffectual, and punitive responses from parents and teachers. Owing to problems with executive function, self-regulation, and motivation inherent to ADHD, do not be too quick to blame the parents for inadequate limit-setting in a child for whom it requires heroic efforts to set consistent limits. Rather, it is important to connect parents to much-needed behavioral support resources.

12. *"Why do you think these problems are occurring? What do others say is the cause?"* The parents' theories of causation are important to make explicit. Often, they have a direct impact on their response (e.g., stances such as "He's just a bad boy who could behave better if he wanted" can lead to punitive and deprecating interactions). This question can also bring out caregiver disagreements that can affect later treatment ("His father says he's 'just a boy' and there is no problem, but I'm with him all day and I am very concerned.").

B. **Office observations/evaluation**
1. Many children with ADHD can contain themselves during a short clinical visit. They may be on their best behavior, as the physician is considered an authority figure, and the setting is mostly one on one with few distractions. Such "good behavior" in the office should not be used to rule out ADHD, as the diagnosis is dependent on the child's behavior in familiar home, school, and extracurricular settings.

2. On the other hand, if a child has many ADHD behaviors in the office, this may help to confirm the diagnosis when it is otherwise suspected and may represent a level of symptomatology that is more pervasive and intense than a child who can contain himself or herself in the office.

3. **Physical examination** allows a window into the child's behavior and affect during the examination. Furthermore, elements of the physical examination, which are particularly important for ruling out mimicking and/or comorbid medical conditions (such as thyroid and endocrine dysfunctions, sleep apnea and other sleep-related disorders, as well as genetic disorders), include growth parameters (height, weight, and head circumference), vital signs, skin examination, neurologic examination, and evaluation for dysmorphic features. Basic hearing and vision screening are also needed to rule out hearing and visual impairments as mimicking or comorbid conditions. In addition, a complete cardiovascular examination, including blood pressure and heart rate, should be performed, especially if ADHD medication treatment is being considered.

C. **Diagnostic tests.** Aside from an ADHD questionnaire, other testing is rarely indicated *unless suggested by the history and physical examination* (e.g., laboratory tests assessing thyroid function; EEG or neuroimaging when unexpected neurologic findings or symptoms are prominent). Although children with ADHD may exhibit problems on tests of attention, executive function, or memory, computer-based studies of sustained attention (e.g., the "continuous performance task") are neither reliable indicators of the diagnosis nor response to treatment. **Psychological and educational testing** can be illuminating if academic problems are significant and suggest a comorbid learning disability or other learning challenges.

D. **Principles of the diagnostic process once ADHD is suspected**
   1. **Do your homework!** It is rarely sufficient or acceptable to take a history from a parent, observe the child in the office, and make a definitive diagnosis. To meet full diagnostic criteria, ADHD-related symptoms and impairment must occur in more than one setting.
   2. Obtain a description and seek corroboration of the child's behaviors from caretakers in all settings in which he or she spends substantial time.

   Because interviews with these providers can be impractical, use ADHD-specific questionnaires such as the National Institute for Children's Health Quality (NICHQ) Vanderbilt Assessment Scales. Ask the mother, father, and/or other caregivers in the home to complete the questionnaires, as well as all significant outside professionals and caretakers (e.g., babysitters, grandparents, teachers, preschool and Head Start providers, childcare providers).
   3. Review the behavioral descriptions and integrate them with the history and your understanding of the child and family.

   Remember that these descriptions are not diagnostic. *They merely state whether the behavioral descriptions are consistent with (but not necessarily due to) a diagnosis of ADHD.* Clinical judgment must be carefully applied to sort out such information.
   a. Look for consistency of the reported behaviors and whether ADHD is suggested in more than one setting.
   b. Inconsistencies of the reported behaviors in different settings are harder to interpret.
   • For example, extreme behaviors described at home but not at school may imply psychosocial stress and/or problematic relationships at home, rather than true ADHD.
   • Conversely, problematic behaviors seen only in school may imply a learning disability or a poor student–teacher "fit," rather than true ADHD.
   • On the other hand, some parents are quite accepting of their child's inattentive, impulsive behaviors at home, or do not challenge the child to exert sustained attention. Therefore, they may downplay those symptoms in a child with true ADHD.
   c. Remember that a diagnosis of ADHD requires impairment due to the ADHD-related symptoms, not just the presence of the requisite number of symptoms. A child who is functioning reasonably well and not demonstrating impairment does not warrant a diagnosis of ADHD.
   4. Be mindful of potential mimicking conditions and/or comorbidities.

   Because ADHD and related symptoms can be associated with learning disabilities, depression, anxiety, posttraumatic stress disorder, developmental disability, an unrecognized genetic syndrome, language delays, etc. (Table 27-2), a diagnosis of ADHD should never exclude the possibility that other challenges are co-occurring or may even be the cause of the behaviors.
   5. Discuss with caregivers your judgment on the diagnosis.

   It is always helpful to ask caregivers to read about ADHD and state whether they think their child fits the criteria, as diverging clinician and parent views should be made explicit and discussed.

     a. If a caregiver disagrees with your diagnosis, intervention efforts are likely to fail. Hence, clinicians should always employ a shared decision-making model and in such cases allow caregivers time to learn more and observe the child's progress. *"Based on your and the teacher's reports, your child's symptoms and problems at home and school meet criteria for ADHD. But he's your child and you have to make the final decision. Why don't you read some more about it, talk to parents of kids who have ADHD, and let's see if things improve. I think because your child is having such serious problems at school (and at home, with friends, etc.), we really need to try to help him out. If you are not ready to try medications, behavioral treatments for ADHD, which can be put in place at home and at school, can be effective and I can give you more information about them. In any case, we should make an appointment to check in with each other in a month or two to make sure that things are improving, rather than worsening."*

     b. It is helpful to explain ADHD to parents with simple metaphors: *"Your child is like a fast car in which the accelerator is stuck down and the brakes don't work very well. One way or another—through behavioral treatments, medication, or both—we need to get the brakes to be more effective."*

     c. A diagnosis of ADHD is often helpful because it **takes the onus off the child**: *"I know that behaviors of children with ADHD are often exasperating, but believe it or not, it's not all intentional. ADHD is caused by differences in the brain, not because he/she is a 'bad kid' or 'lazy.'"* Without the understanding that *biological* factors lead to the child's behavior, his or her actions are often interpreted as willful and manipulative and may provoke an angry response, which aggravates the child's feelings of being misunderstood and unfairly targeted.

     d. Explain that ADHD is a **chronic condition** and is unlikely to go away on its own.

     e. Encourage the caregivers to learn as much as they can about ADHD to best help their child.

III. MANAGEMENT. Managing ADHD includes behavioral and educational interventions as well as pharmacotherapy. Using a shared decision-making model is recommended, whereby the family is actively involved in determining target behaviors and selecting components of the intervention.

    A. Primary goals. The goals of all treatment for ADHD are to enhance the child's successful functioning in the domains that are impaired and causing distress. This almost always includes his or her academic or preschool functioning, family and peer relationships, and self-esteem.

    B. Information for the family. Explain to the family the nature of ADHD and what is known and recommended regarding its treatment. Specifically, for preschool children, the American Academy of Pediatrics (AAP) ADHD Clinical Practice Guideline recommends that the clinician "prescribe evidence-based parent and/or teacher-administered behavioral therapy as first line treatment...and may prescribe methylphenidate if the behavior interventions do not lead to significant improvement." For school-age children and adolescents, the AAP guideline recommends that the clinician "prescribe FDA-approved medications for ADHD...and/or evidence-based parent and/or teacher-administered behavioral therapy for ADHD, preferably both." Although stimulant medications alone have been shown to produce significant improvements in ADHD-related symptoms, for many important facets of a child's life, such as parent–child relations, academic outcomes, social skills, anxiety symptoms, and oppositional/aggressive symptoms, combined medication and behavioral management achieves the best results. Combining medication and behavioral treatments may also allow for better results at lower medication dosages. In addition, behavioral treatment provides the family with much-needed skills and tools to manage behaviors when medication is not "on board."

    C. Medication treatment

       1. **Fundamental rules of ADHD medication treatment**

         • **All decisions are reversible.** Once a decision has been made either to treat or not to treat with medications, it can be changed as circumstances warrant.

         • **Obtain ongoing feedback regarding efficacy and side effects** from the caregivers and teachers. This can be accomplished by caregivers and teachers completing ADHD rating scales (and returning to the clinician online, via fax, or via mail) upon initiation of treatment, after medication dose changes, and several times during the school year thereafter.

         • **If one medication does not work, try another.** Studies have shown that 70%–75% of children with ADHD respond to any given stimulant medication, and >90% of children are responders if both methylphenidate and amphetamine preparations are tried. The efficacy of the methylphenidate and amphetamine families does not differ *on average*, but some individuals do respond differently. Studies have shown that up to 25% of children with ADHD may respond preferentially to either the methylphenidate group or the amphetamine group, but not both. Nonstimulant ADHD medication options (atomoxetine, extended-release guanfacine, and extended-release clonidine) are also considered if the stimulant medications are ineffective, have intolerable side effects, or are contraindicated.

- Improvement should be gauged in areas such as **academic performance** (classwork and homework efficiency, completion, and accuracy) as well as **classroom behavior, behavior in the home setting, self-esteem, disruptive behaviors, safety-related concerns, and relationships with parents, siblings, teachers, and peers**.

- In general, one is looking for **a clearly beneficial response to the medications**. Reports that maybe there *might* be some subtle or minor changes are not sufficient to view the trial as successful. It should be noted that the lack of beneficial response to ADHD medication does not necessarily mean that the diagnosis is incorrect and response to medication should not be used to rule-in or rule-out ADHD.

- **Parental agreement with a medication trial is essential.** Some parents are understandably reluctant to give their child a psychoactive medication. They may have read or heard of frightening side effects and do not want their child to become "a zombie." The clinician should acknowledge and respect such concerns: *"I understand why you are concerned. The most important thing to remember is that if your child is having side effects that worry you or if the medications don't seem to be helping, we'll stop or change the medicine. Just because we start medications, doesn't mean we have to continue them if you are not satisfied with their effects. Second, these medications have a long safety track record, since methylphenidate was improved by the FDA in 1955, and amphetamine was approved in 1960. If there are any side effects—and these are mild in the majority of children who try stimulant medications—they go away when the medication is discontinued. So, think about it. We are not going to start ADHD medications unless you feel comfortable with this choice. If you decide against it now, we can also reconsider it in the future if things don't improve for your child."*

2. **Pharmacologic agents**
   a. **Psychostimulant medications** remain the first-line medication treatment for ADHD, as they have the highest response rate (>90% of patients will have a positive response to one of the psychostimulants) and effect size (amount of change in symptoms) of any of the ADHD medication classes. The psychostimulant family includes the various preparations of methylphenidate and amphetamines whose primary mechanism of action involves blocking dopamine transporters and thereby increasing dopamine levels in the synaptic space. Table 27-3 contains information concerning their use. Both the methylphenidate and amphetamine families can be effective, but as many as 25% of patients may respond to only one family. It should be noted that, for the preschool age group, there is a stronger body of evidence documenting the efficacy and tolerability of methylphenidate than amphetamine. Therefore, the AAP ADHD Clinical Practice Guideline recommends methylphenidate as the medication treatment of choice for preschoolers with ADHD.
      - **Cardiovascular risk factors and side effects.** Concerns regarding the cardiovascular safety of psychostimulant medications, specifically the risk of sudden cardiac death (SCD), have sparked controversy and received much attention in the academic literature. Although tragic, SCD is fortunately a very rare event in children. Statements by the AAP and the American Academy of Child and Adolescent Psychiatry conclude that there is currently no compelling evidence that the risk of SCD is higher in children receiving medications for ADHD than in the general population.
        - Psychostimulant medications are generally associated with mild increases in blood pressure (2–4 mm Hg systolic and 1–3 mm Hg diastolic) and heart rate (3–5 BPM), which are not clinically significant. However, in a small subset of individuals (5%–15%), more substantial increases can be seen, making monitoring of heart rate and blood pressure essential when prescribing ADHD medications. In addition, there is at least a theoretical risk that children with underlying cardiac disease taking ADHD medications may be at increased risk for SCD. Therefore, all patients should be screened for SCD risk factors

Table 27-3 • DOSING FOR FOOD AND DRUG ADMINISTRATION (FDA)-APPROVED ADHD MEDICATIONS

Pharmacologic Agent	Starting Dose	Maximum Dose (FDA-Approved)	Usual Dosing
First Line			
Short-Acting			
Amphetamine and dextroamphetamine (Adderall, Evekeo)	2.5–5 mg qd (bid)	40 mg	bid—tid (duration 4–6 h)
Dextroamphetamine (Dexedrine, Zenzedi)	2.5–5 mg qd (bid)	40 mg	bid—tid (duration 4–6 h)
Dexmethylphenidate (Focalin)	2.5 mg bid	20 mg	bid (duration 4–6 h)
Methylphenidate (Ritalin or Methylin)	5 mg bid	60 mg	bid—tid (duration 3–4 h)
Long-Acting			
Dextroamphetamine sulfate (Adderall XR)	10 mg qd	30 mg	qd (duration 8–12 h)
Methylphenidate (Concerta)	18 mg qd	72 mg	qAM (duration 12 h)
Methylphenidate (Daytrana patch)	10 mg patch	30 mg	Up to 9-h "wear time" (duration ~12 h)
Dextroamphetamine (Dexedrine Spansule)	5–10 mg qd (bid)	40 mg	qd—bid (duration 6–8 h)
Dexmethylphenidate hydrochloride (Focalin XR)	5 mg qd	30 mg	qd (duration 8–12 h)
Methylphenidate (Metadate CD or Ritalin LA)	10–20 mg qAM	60 mg	qd (duration 8 h)
Methylphenidate (Metadate ER and Methylin ER)	10 mg qd	60 mg	qd (duration 8 h)
Methylphenidate (Aptensio XR)	10 mg qd	60 mg	qd (duration 12 h)
Methylphenidate (Quillivant XR 25 mg/5 mL liquid formulation)	10 mg (2 mL)	60 mg (12 mL)	qd (duration 12 h)
Methylphenidate (QuilliChew ER [chewable tablet])	20 mg	60 mg	qd (duration 12 h)
Amphetamine (Adzenys XR-ODT [orally disintegrating tablet])	6.3 mg	18.8 mg	qd (duration 12 h)
Lisdexamfetamine (Vyvanse)	20 mg qd	70 mg	qd (duration 13 h)
Dexamphetamine (Dyanavel 2.5 mg/1 mL liquid formulation)	2.5 or 5 mg qd	20 mg	qd (duration 13 h)

Table 27-3 • DOSING FOR FOOD AND DRUG ADMINISTRATION (FDA)-APPROVED ADHD MEDICATIONS   (CONTINUED)

Pharmacologic Agent	Starting Dose	Maximum Dose (FDA-Approved)	Usual Dosing
Second Line			
Atomoxetine (Strattera)	<70 kg: 0.5 mg/kg per day × 4–7 d, then increase to 1.2 mg/kg per day >70 kg: 40 mg × 4–7 d then increase to 100 mg/d	Less of 1.4 mg/kg per day or 100 mg	qd–bid (in AM if no drowsiness or HS if there is)
Guanfacine extended release (Intuniv)	1 mg	Less of 0.12 mg/kg per day or 4 mg	qd
Clonidine extended release (Kapvay)	0.1 mg	Less of 0.012 mg/ kg per day or 0.4 mg	qd–bid

Adapted from Practice parameter for the assessment and treatment of children and adolescents with attention-deficit/hyperactivity disorder. *J Am Acad Child Adolesc Psychiatry.* 2007;46(7):894-921.

before the initiation of an ADHD medication trial. In addition to a careful cardiac physical examination, screening should include the following:
- Ask whether the patient has a history of syncope, dizziness, chest pain, palpitations, unexplained change in exercise tolerance or shortness of breath with exercise, high blood pressure, and/or history of cardiac disease.
- Ask whether there is a family history of sudden, unexplained, or cardiac-related death in persons aged <35 years; cardiac arrhythmias; cardiomyopathy; long QT syndrome; or Marfan syndrome.
- Electrocardiograms are generally not recommended for healthy children without identifiable cardiovascular risk factors or cardiac disease.
- When cardiovascular risk factors or known cardiac disease are present, input from a pediatric cardiologist should be obtained before ADHD medication is initiated.

b. **Non-stimulant medications.** Additional Food and Drug Administration (FDA)–approved medication options for ADHD include **atomoxetine, extended-release guanfacine,** and **extended-release clonidine.** These medications are considered second-line medication treatments for ADHD because their response rate and efficacy for core ADHD symptoms lags behind that of psychostimulants. Unlike psychostimulants, atomoxetine is a specific noradrenergic reuptake inhibitor, whereas guanfacine and clonidine are alpha-2 agonists. As such, they have no potential for abuse and are not FDA-regulated controlled substances, thereby enabling clinicians to write for refills.
- Like psychostimulants, atomoxetine, guanfacine, and clonidine generally cause mild changes in heart rate and blood pressure, which are not clinically significant but warrant ongoing monitoring. In the case of atomoxetine, mild *increases* in heart rate and blood pressure can be seen, whereas *decreases* can occur with guanfacine and clonidine.
- As with psychostimulants, there are rare reports of more significant cardiovascular events in patients taking atomoxetine, guanfacine, and clonidine. Therefore, before starting these medications, it is prudent to conduct the same screening for personal and family cardiovascular risk factors, which is recommended for psychostimulant medications (see above) and obtain input from a pediatric cardiologist if there are pertinent positives.
- Owing to the small increased risk of suicidal thinking associated with atomoxetine, the FDA has added a black box warning to its label. Although the risk is small, the pediatric clinician should discuss this risk with the patient and his or her family. Children should be monitored for the onset of suicidal ideation, particularly over the first few months of treatment (see Chapter 23).

- Atomoxetine is associated with a lower rate of sleep initiation difficulties than psychostimulants, and studies have suggested that it may have mild beneficial effects on anxiety disorders. Therefore, atomoxetine is a reasonable alternative for patients experiencing significant anxiety or insomnia with psychostimulant treatment.
- Combination therapy with more than one ADHD medication class may be used if one class does not provide adequate symptom coverage or problematic side effects occur. For example, nonstimulants can be combined with psychostimulant treatment when psychostimulants do not provide adequate evening coverage. In cases of ADHD comorbid with aggression or tics, the addition of guanfacine or clonidine to psychostimulant treatment can be helpful.

c. **Predicting ADHD medication response.** No consistent predictors of ADHD medication response have been identified to date. Owing to the large interindividual variability in ADHD medication response, there is currently great interest in pharmacogenetic tools and even neuroimaging tools, which can help the clinician to predict the best medication and dose for each child. However, at this time, ADHD pharmacogenetic tests and neuroimaging studies are *not* recommended, as the available scientific literature does not provide sufficient evidence to support their clinical utility in predicting ADHD medication response.

d. **Dosage.** In general, a medication is started at the lowest dose and then gradually increased until optimal response is achieved, intolerable side effects occur, or the maximum dosage is reached. Dosages can generally be titrated up every 1–3 weeks. Side effects can usually be minimized by altering the dosage, timing, or form (short- or long-acting) of medication. Table 27-4 lists the common clinical questions, side effects, and side effect management strategies for stimulant medications.

- It is best to **start medications or any changes on the weekend** or any time the parents can be the first to witness the effects. They can then be instructed to call the clinician to relay any benefits or concerns.
- Follow-up monitoring should be scheduled within a month of initiating treatment to review side effects and overall progress.
- Throughout treatment, **height, weight, blood pressure, and heart rate should be monitored**. Some, but not all, studies suggest that children treated with psychostimulants or atomoxetine may experience some mild growth suppression of height. Other studies have demonstrated catch-up growth when treatment is stopped. As the issue of linear growth suppression with ADHD medication treatment has not firmly been settled, close monitoring of growth parameters is warranted.
- Once the appropriate dosage is established, it should be reevaluated and adjusted upward if symptom control wanes or downward if intolerable side effects occur. Follow-up visits should be scheduled several times throughout the year to evaluate medication efficacy, monitor for side effects, and assess for the development of comorbidities.
- The decision to treat with psychostimulants only on weekdays or only during the school year is best made in consultation with the parents. **Improved school performance is always a priority**. When the child's symptoms seem to have a lesser impact on home and peer relationships, weekday use only may be acceptable and will help minimize growth effects. However, when the child's relationships with family and peers are a source of great contention and stress, taking medication every day, including holidays and vacations, may be the best option.
- ADHD nonstimulant medications must be administered every day, without breaks or "medication holidays," to be effective.

e. **Potential for abuse.** Clinicians should be aware of psychostimulant diversion, misuse, and abuse when treating ADHD with medication. Extended-release (especially prodrugs or osmotic controlled-release oral delivery systems) or transdermal stimulant formulations have lower potential for abuse. A nonstimulant such as atomoxetine can also be considered.

f. **Duration of treatment.** In general, ADHD treatment—in the form of medication or home and school behavioral interventions—will need to be continued into and through adolescence (except in the 10%–20% of children with ADHD who may completely "outgrow" the problem). The decision to end pharmacotherapy can be periodically tested via trials off medication during times of low stress.

Table 27-4 • STIMULANT MEDICATION: COMMON CLINICAL QUESTIONS AND SIDE EFFECTS AND MANAGEMENT STRATEGIES

Common Clinical Questions	Management Strategies
Short-acting or long-acting?	In general, long-acting preparations (8–12 h) are preferable, unless the cost is prohibitive, as they produce a slower rise and fall of psycho-stimulant levels in the brain, which decreases potential for abuse and may decrease side effects. Improved adherence has also been shown with long-acting preparations.
Decreased appetite?	Administer medication with or shortly after meals. Offer high-calorie foods when hungry, and encourage eating after school and/or before bedtime. When severe, institute short periods off medication on weekends or breaks from school.
Difficulty falling asleep?	Improve sleep hygiene.
	Decrease dose or try an alternate stimulant class or formulation (such as an 8-h rather than 12-h preparation). On the other hand, if the child is restless and overactive at bedtime, and sleep problems are thought to be due to a rebound effect from waning stimulant medication levels, consider adding a short-acting PM dose.
	Try melatonin for sleep-onset delay.
	Consider discontinuation of stimulant and trial of atomoxetine.
Dazed and/or with-drawn behavior?	Reduce dosage or discontinue medication and try a different class.
Gradual return of hyperactive behaviors?	Determine time of day when hyperactive behaviors return. Increase dosage if resurgence of hyperactive behaviors is evident throughout the day. If resurgence of hyperactivity is only present in the after-noon or evening, consider adding a short-acting PM dose of stimulant medication ½ hour before hyperactive behaviors generally become evident.
Onset of symptoms of depression?	Discontinue medication and try another class. Refer for cognitive behavioral therapy to address depressive symptoms, with the adjunct of pharmacotherapy for depression if symptoms are moderate to severe.
Development of tics that were not pres-ent before starting medication?	Educate families that, although tic exacerbation with psychostimulant treatment may occur in a small minority of patients, there is a lack of evidence, on average, that stimulant medications cause or exacerbate tics.
	Trial discontinuation of stimulant with possible later rechallenge to determine if the temporal course of the tics truly coincides with the stimulant administration, or if the tics are an independent problem. If the stimulant treatment does correlate tightly with onset or worsen-ing of tics, consider dose reduction, switching to an alternative stimu-lant preparation, or switching to a nonstimulant ADHD medication.
	Additional options include adding an intervention to address tics, such as Comprehensive Behavioral Intervention for Tics (CBIT) or a tic-reducing medication (e.g., guanfacine or clonidine).

3. **Multimodal treatments.** In addition to medication, several psychological, social, and school-related treatments should be considered. For preschoolers (4–5 years of age), parent- and/or teacher-administered behavioral therapy is the first-line treat-ment, with medication being used for children for whom behavior interventions do not provide significant improvement.
   • **Behavioral parent training (BPT).** This treatment aims to teach parents how to set limits, provide positive reinforcement for appropriate behaviors, and mini-mize emotionally destructive responses. Training adults (either parents or teach-ers) in behavioral management skills often requires referral to a specialized program for parents of children with ADHD. *Of note, evidence-based ADHD parent training interventions have also shown benefits in improving opposi-tional and defiant as well as ADHD-related behaviors.* For parents, BPT may be

delivered in small groups, which have the advantage of providing psychosocial support as well as training. Importantly, the goal of BPT is improvement in the child's environment to set the stage for the child's success, not to change the child's fundamental nature.

- **Behavioral peer interventions (BPI).** In BPI, behavioral procedures are applied to address peer-related problems experienced by children with ADHD, including skills deficits (lack of knowledge regarding appropriate peer interactions) and inappropriate social behaviors (such as verbal and physical aggression). Skills deficits are typically addressed in weekly group training sessions, whereas behavioral excesses (e.g., teasing or aggression) are addressed in the setting in which they occur through behavioral management plans implemented by teachers, counselors, or other adults who provide supervision in these settings. Of note, the evidence for peer skills training alone, administered in the clinic setting, is not robust. However, BPI interventions involving a behavioral management plan administered in the target setting, such as at school or summer camp, have demonstrated substantial beneficial effects.
- **Organizational skills training (OST).** In OST, older elementary-age children and adolescents are trained to organize their learning materials, track assignments, and formulate plans for work completion. Typically, OST includes consultation to caregivers and/or teachers so that they can provide support to students in these endeavors. Evidence supporting OST is emerging, with studies showing benefits of medium effect size for children receiving OST compared with control groups.
- **Classroom accommodations.** Teacher-implemented strategies such as posted classroom rules, positive reinforcement for appropriate behavior and work completion/accuracy, and appropriate consequences for rule violations help decrease the impact of ADHD on a child's functioning at school. There are also demonstrated benefits of using a teacher-implemented daily report card, which establishes daily goals for the individual child as well as a system of evaluating and providing feedback daily to the child and his or her caregivers. Most children with ADHD need a 504 Plan at school to ensure consistent implementation of these accommodations and some children with ADHD (especially those with a comorbid learning disability or severe behavior problems) may meet criteria for an Individualized Education Program (IEP).
- **Additional therapies** may be needed depending on the circumstances of the family and the child.
  - Cognitive behavioral therapy with exposure sessions is recommended in the case of comorbid anxiety.
  - Cognitive behavioral therapy or interpersonal therapy is recommended in the case of comorbid depression.
  - For children with comorbid oppositional/defiant or aggressive behaviors, evidence-based ADHD-related behavioral interventions such as BPT and BPI have shown comparable, even if not stronger, benefits in addressing these concurrent problems as for ADHD alone. However, adolescents with serious conduct problems may need intensive multisystemic therapy.
  - There is no evidence that individual psychotherapy improves the child's ability to pay attention or reduces impulsiveness. However, as the child gets older and becomes more self-aware, psychotherapy may facilitate an understanding of how his or her own behavior affects others.
  - Family therapy may be useful for families with significant parent–child conflict, impaired communication, or psychosocial discord.
  - At present, there is no sufficient evidence to support a generalized recommendation for cognitive training and/or neurofeedback for children and adolescents with ADHD. Play therapy, vision training, interactive metronome training, and occupational therapy addressing sensory processing issues have also not been shown to improve symptoms and impairment related to ADHD.

IV. CRITERIA FOR REFERRAL. Most primary care clinicians will be involved in these aspects of ADHD treatment: (1) explaining the condition to the child and the family, (2) providing appropriate referrals for behavioral therapy, (3) educating the family about the importance of communication with the school and how to secure needed school accommodations (see above), and (4) prescribing and following medication. The AAP Guideline on Diagnosis and Treatment of ADHD recommends that the diagnosis of children aged 4–18 years is appropriate in the primary care setting. Psychosocial treatments will be administered by others, although the clinician should be familiar with each type of treatment and the goals of each treatment strategy. The clinician should develop resources for behavioral therapy referrals and establish ongoing communication with those resources. Referral to a specialist, such as a developmental and behavioral pediatrician or child psychiatrist, is indicated when the diagnosis is ambiguous or FDA-approved ADHD medications are ineffective or associated with unacceptable side effects.

Bibliography

FOR PARENTS

CHADD (Children and Adults with Attention Deficit Hyperactivity Disorders). CHADD is a national organization with local chapters throughout the country that is dedicated to providing support and advocacy for individuals with ADHD and their families. CHADD provides in-person as well as web-based trainings, including the Parent to Parent training program, which can be remotely accessed for caregivers who lack evidence-based ADHD parent training resources in their communities. CHADD's National Resource Center for ADHD can be accessed through its website and includes additional resources for individuals with ADHD, families/caregivers, and professionals. http://www.chadd.org/.

National Institute of Mental Health. The National Institute of Mental Health provides an overview on ADHD as well as links to additional resources at: https://www.nimh.nih.gov/health/topics/attention-deficit-hyperactivity-disorder-adhd/index.shtml.

ADD Warehouse. The A.D.D. Warehouse is a one-stop shopping site with books, videos, and other products to help children with ADHD and their families to understand and manage ADHD-related problems. Contains an excellent annotated bibliography. http://addwarehouse.com/shopsite_sc/store/html/index.html.

FOR PROFESSIONALS

AMERICAN ACADEMY OF CHILD AND ADOLESCENT PSYCHIATRY ADHD CLINICAL PRACTICE GUIDELINE

Pliszka S, The American Academy of Child and Adolescent Psychiatry Work Group on Quality Issues. Practice parameter for the assessment and treatment of children and adolescents with attention-deficit/hyperactivity disorder. *J Am Acad Child Adolesc Psychiatry*. 2007;46(7):894-921. http://www.jaacap.com/article/S0890-8567(09)62182-1/pdf.

AMERICAN ACADEMY OF PEDIATRICS ADHD CLINICAL PRACTICE GUIDELINE

American Academy of Pediatrics Subcommittee on Attention-Deficit/Hyperactivity Disorder. ADHD: clinical practice guideline for the diagnosis, evaluation, and treatment of attention-deficit/hyperactivity disorder in children and adolescents. *Pediatrics*. 2011;128:1-18. http://pediatrics.aappublications.org/content/pediatrics/early/2011/10/14/peds.2011-2654.full.pdf.

SUPPLEMENT TO THE AMERICAN ACADEMY OF PEDIATRICS ADHD CLINICAL PRACTICE GUIDELINE

Implementing the Key Action Statements: An Algorithm and Explanation for Process of Care for the Evaluation, Diagnosis, Treatment, and Monitoring of ADHD in Children and Adolescents. http://pediatrics.aappublications.org/content/suppl/2011/10/11/peds.2011-2654.DC1/zpe611117822p.pdf.

AMERICAN ACADEMY OF PEDIATRICS POLICY STATEMENT ON CARDIOVASCULAR MONITORING OF CHILDREN ON STIMULANT MEDICATIONS

Perrin JM, Friedman RA, Knilans TK. Cardiovascular monitoring and stimulant drugs for attention deficit/hyperactivity disorder. *Pediatrics*. 2008;122(2):451-453. http://pediatrics.aappublications.org/content/pediatrics/122/2/451.full.pdf.

NATIONAL INSTITUTE FOR CHILDREN'S HEALTH QUALITY ADHD TOOLKIT

Contains very useful, free, downloadable information, handouts for parents, questionnaires, history forms, etc. https://www.nichq.org/resource/caring-children-adhd-resource-toolkit-clinicians.

THE ADHD MEDICATION GUIDE©

Developed by Cohen Children's Medical Center, The ADHD Medication Guide© is a free, downloadable visual aid for professionals caring for individuals with ADHD. It has color pictures of all FDA-approved ADHD medication preparations and their dosage forms, indicates which are available in generic form, and lists ages for which each has an FDA-approved indication for the treatment of ADHD. http://www.adhdmedicationguide.com/.

CHAPTER 28

Autism Spectrum Disorders

Elizabeth B. Caronna | Eileen M. Costello | Marilyn Augustyn

I. DESCRIPTION OF THE PROBLEM. Autism spectrum disorder is a heterogeneous neurodevelopmental disorder. It is defined clinically by characteristic behavioral impairments in:
- Reciprocal social interactions and verbal and nonverbal communication
- Restricted and repetitive behaviors and interests

The *Diagnostic and Statistical Manual of Mental Disorders*, Fifth Edition (*DSM-5*) uses the umbrella term "autism spectrum disorder" (ASD) to include several disorders, which in the *DSM-IV-TR* were separately categorized as autistic disorder, childhood disintegrative disorder, Asperger syndrome, and pervasive developmental disorder–not otherwise specified (PDD-NOS). All these prior diagnoses are now encompassed under ASD. This shift in nomenclature reflects the wider conceptualization of the disorder to include individuals with a broad symptom presentation who share the two core deficits above.

A. Epidemiology. The prevalence of ASD is hotly debated. As recently as the 1980s, prevalence estimates were in the range of 0.5–1/1000. More recent estimates have suggested a prevalence of ASD in the United States as high as 1 in 68 children according to estimates from CDC's Autism and Developmental Disabilities Monitoring (ADDM) Network. ASD is reported to occur in all racial, ethnic, and socioeconomic groups. ASD is about 4.5 times more common among boys (1 in 42) than among girls (1 in 189). Studies in Asia, Europe, and North America have identified individuals with ASD with an average prevalence of between 1% and 2%.

The dramatic increase in rate of diagnosed cases may be attributed to several different factors, including changes in diagnostic criteria and the broader definition of ASD, variation in case-finding methods and diagnostic substitution, increased public and professional awareness of the disorders leading to earlier diagnosis and treatment, and a possible true increase in the prevalence.

B. Etiology/contributing factors. Historically, autism was attributed to cold, distant parenting, widely known as the "refrigerator mother theory." The accumulation of evidence that the disorder had a neurologic basis (associated seizures, obvious genetic links, and pathologic abnormalities in the brain) made psychodynamic theories of etiology untenable. In most cases, the etiology of ASD is idiopathic. There are a small number of cases in which there is an identified underlying metabolic, infectious, or genetic disorder (such as untreated phenylketonuria, congenital cytomegalovirus or rubella, tuberous sclerosis, fragile X syndrome, CHARGE syndrome, or Down syndrome).

ASD is assumed to be a polygenic disorder resulting from gene–environment interactions. Recent studies have focused on genome-wide studies, identifying microduplications and deletions associated with autism on several autosomal chromosomes. Several studies have identified different genes coding for proteins involved in synaptic connectivity. There is a high rate of fragile X syndrome in individuals with ASD and intellectual disability. Notwithstanding rampant speculation in the lay press and on the Internet, possible environmental triggers of the disorder in genetically predisposed individuals have not yet been identified.

II. MAKING THE DIAGNOSIS

A. Signs and symptoms

1. *DSM-5 criteria for autistic disorder.* The criteria for diagnosis of **autism spectrum disorder** according to *DSM-5* are outlined below. The presence of impairment must be judged compared with children of the same developmental level or mental age. The *DSM-5* requires that all criteria of social communication and at least two of the restricted and repetitive behaviors be met.

   a. Persistent deficits in social communication and social interaction across multiple contexts, as manifested by the following, currently or by history:
   - Deficits in social–emotional reciprocity, ranging, for example, from abnormal social approach and failure of normal back-and-forth conversation to reduced sharing of interests, emotions, or affect to failure to initiate or respond to social interactions.

- Deficits in nonverbal communicative behaviors used for social interaction, ranging, for example, from poorly integrated verbal and nonverbal communication to abnormalities in eye contact and body language or deficits in understanding and use of gestures to a total lack of facial expressions and nonverbal communication.
- Deficits in developing, maintaining, and understand relationships, ranging, for example, from difficulties adjusting behavior to suit various social contexts to difficulties in sharing imaginative play or in making friends to absence of interest in peers.

   b. Restricted, repetitive patterns of behavior, interests, or activities, as manifested by at least two of the following, currently or by history (examples are illustrative, not exhaustive):

- Stereotyped or repetitive motor movements, use of objects, or speech (e.g., simple motor stereotypies, lining up toys or flipping objects, echolalia, idiosyncratic phrases).
- Insistence on sameness, inflexible adherence to routines, or ritualized patterns of verbal or nonverbal behavior (e.g., extreme distress at small changes, difficulties with transitions, rigid thinking patterns, greeting rituals, need to take same route or eat same food every day).
- Highly restricted, fixated interests that are abnormal in intensity or focus (e.g., strong attachment to or preoccupation with unusual objects, excessively circumscribed or perseverative interests).
- Hyper- or hyporeactivity to sensory input or unusual interest in sensory aspects of the environment (e.g., apparent indifference to pain/temperature, adverse response to specific sounds or textures, excessive smelling or touching of objects, visual fascination with lights or movement).

   The *DSM-5* specifies that symptoms must be present in the early developmental period but may not become fully manifest until social demands exceed limited capacities or may be masked by learned strategies in later life. The symptoms must cause clinically significant impairment in social, occupational, or other important areas of current functioning, and these disturbances are not better explained by intellectual disability or global developmental delay. Individuals with a well-established *DSM-IV* diagnosis of autistic disorder, Asperger syndrome, or PDD-NOS should be given the diagnosis of ASD without additional testing required. Once the diagnosis of ASD is given, the evaluator specifies whether there is accompanying intellectual impairment and/or language impairment and whether there are associated medical, genetic, psychiatric, or other disorders. Individuals who have marked deficits in social communication, but whose symptoms do not otherwise meet criteria for ASD, should be evaluated for social (pragmatic) communication disorder.

   In addition to meeting the abovementioned criteria, a severity level is assigned for each of the two symptom clusters with the following ranges:

   Level 3: "Requiring Very Substantial Support": very limited initiation of social interactions and minimal response to social overtures from others.

   Level 2: "Requiring Substantial Support": Marked deficits in verbal and nonverbal social communication skills with social impairments apparent even with supports in place.

   Level 1: "Requiring Support": Without supports in place, deficits in social communication cause noticeable impairments.

2. DSM-5: **social (pragmatic) communication disorder.** This is a new diagnosis in *DSM-5*. It focuses on persistent difficulties in the social use of verbal and nonverbal communication, and individuals must meet all the following criteria:

- Deficits in using communication for social purposes
- Impairment of the ability to change communication to match context or the needs of the listener
- Difficulties following rules for conversation and storytelling
- Difficulties understanding what is not explicitly stated and nonliteral or ambiguous meanings of language

   Like ASD, the onset of the symptoms is in the early developmental period, but deficits may not become fully manifest until social communication demands exceed limited capacities.

3. **Clinical features of ASD.** Each child on the autism spectrum has a unique presentation with various levels of impairment in each of the two core symptom areas. The atypical behaviors are notable for lack of flexibility in social communication,

behaviors, and interactions. Common presentations in the often overlapping domains are outlined below.

    a. **Atypical social interactions.** Deficits specific to ASD include lack of joint attention (ability to share interest with another using language, gestures, and eye gaze). Eye contact is usually decreased or not used to modulate social interactions. Children with ASD may range from being very withdrawn and appearing unaware of other people to having variable or odd interactions with others. Despite common misconceptions, they may be quite affectionate with caregivers and have normal attachment. They have difficulty establishing friendships with peers, ranging from being aloof to being overly intrusive. They may lack the ability to feel empathy or "put themselves in another's shoes."

    b. **Atypical communication.** Regression of language skills in the second year of life occurs in up to 30% of cases. Children on the spectrum who have meaningful language may demonstrate immediate and delayed echolalia, scripted speech (language heard on videos or in adult conversation), unusual prosody (monotone or singsong quality to speech), pronoun reversal (I/you) or speaking about themselves in the third person, and preservative speech. Often they do not spontaneously use gestures usually acquired by a child's first birthday, including pointing and waving.

    c. **Restricted activities/play.** Children with ASD show little imaginative play. Often, they engage in repetitive games or routines with toys (lining up, smelling, tapping). They may focus on sensory aspects of objects (spinning fans, flashing lights) or develop fascinations and obsessions with unusual objects (sprinkler systems, picture hooks, manhole covers, women's purses). They often demand sameness in routines, placement of objects, or other rituals and may become very agitated with any change. They may engage in repetitive hand or body movement (hand flapping, spinning, rocking) instead of meaningful play.

    d. **Rote memory, nonverbal skills.** Children with ASD may have advanced "splinter skills," such as being able to decode words at a much higher level than expected (hyperlexia), although they rarely have commensurate reading comprehension. They may learn to count into the thousands, say the alphabet backward, or be able to complete puzzles with the pieces upside down so that no pictures are showing, although they are not able to communicate their wants or needs to their parents.

    e. **Sensory sensitivities.** Many children appear to be hyper- or hyposensitive to sensory experiences. They may, for example, cover their ears to loud noises, become distressed by textures of food or clothing, or be insensitive to painful stimuli.

    f. **Comorbidities.** Many children with ASD have intellectual disability, although as diagnostic categorization of ASD has broadened, the rates are dropping below 50%. Children with intellectual disability are more likely to develop seizure disorders as well (approximately 30%). Many have symptoms of hyperactivity and inattention, anxiety, obsessive–compulsive behaviors, self-injurious behaviors, pica, or aggression. Sleep disorders, gastrointestinal and feeding disorders, and allergies are also common.

B. Differential diagnosis

    1. **Global developmental delay/intellectual disability.** Cognitive abilities may be difficult to assess in the young, nonverbal child. Severe cognitive deficits may be associated with some of the repetitive behavioral manifestations of ASD.

    2. **Developmental language disorder.** In the absence of significantly inhibited temperament or anxiety disorder, the child with developmental language disorder alone should demonstrate normal reciprocal social interactions and appropriate play for age.

    3. **Hearing impairment.** Although not common, it is important to rule out sensory deficits as a cause of language and social delays.

    4. **Landau–Kleffner syndrome.** Also known as acquired epileptic aphasia, this may cause regression of language and other delays and can be diagnosed by sleep-deprived electroencephalography (EEG).

    5. **Rett syndrome.** Rett syndrome is a sporadic X-linked disorder in girls that shares some behavioral features with ASD. It is, however, a distinct disorder with a characteristic course including deceleration of head growth, stereotypic hand movements, and dementia. Many cases of Rett syndrome can be confirmed by genetic testing for the *MECP2* gene.

6. **Severe early deprivation/reactive attachment disorder.** Children who have experienced significant abuse and neglect may exhibit some of the symptoms of ASD.
7. **Anxiety disorders/obsessive–compulsive disorder.** There is overlap between these disorders and ASD, although typically children with primary anxiety disorders have joint attention and reciprocal social relations that children with ASD lack.
C. **History.**
   Screening tools. There is increasing pressure from both parents and professionals for earlier identification of ASD so that treatment can begin before the age of 3 years. In 2006 and 2007, the American Academy of Pediatrics (AAP) outlined algorithms for routine screening and surveillance for developmental disorders including ASD as part of well-child care. The AAP recommended screening for ASD at 18 and 24 months and suggested a list of possible screening tools. One commonly used screening tool is the Modified Checklist for Autism in Toddlers, Revised with Followup (M-CHAT- R/ F™), which is a two-stage parent-report screening tool that is free and easily administered and scored from www.mchatscreen.com. Pediatric clinicians are advised to use a combination of screening tools and ongoing surveillance to identify children at risk for ASD due to limitations of the sensitivity and specificity of the M-CHAT-R/F alone. Additional screening might be needed if a child is at high risk for ASD (e.g., having a sibling with an ASD, receiving early intervention for other delays) or if ASD-related symptoms are present.

   In February 2016, the US Preventive Services Task Force released a recommendation regarding universal screening for ASD among young children and concluded that there is not enough evidence available on the potential benefits and harms of ASD screening in all young children to recommend for or against this screening. Research is ongoing regarding the efficacy and best method of ASD screening.

   Children identified as being at risk for ASD who "fail" routine screening or surveillance with questions below should be referred to a specialist experienced in evaluating children with ASD (developmental and behavioral pediatric clinician, neurologist, psychologist, or psychiatrist).
   1. **Key clinical questions.** When a concern of ASD is raised, the following questions (modified from the MCHAT-R/F) are informative:
      • *"Does your child respond to his/her name?"* Parents often report concerns that their child may be deaf since he/she does not respond to voice, although he/she does turn to other sounds.
      • *"Does your child prefer to play alone than with others?"*
      • *"Does your child ever use his/her index finger to point and to show you something? Does your child ever bring a toy over to show you?"* These questions look at joint attention, which is impaired in ASD.
      • *"Does your child* (older than 18 months) *ever pretend when he/she is playing (e.g., pretend to talk on the phone or feed a doll)?"* Symbolic play is delayed or absent in ASD.
      • **Red flags of development that warrant further evaluation of possible ASD:**
        • No babbling by 9 months
        • No gesturing by 12 months
        • No single words by 16 months
        • No functional, nonecholalic two-word phrases by 24 months
        • **ANY loss of language or social skills at any age**
   2. Family history of ASD and/or parental concern warrant(s) further investigation including history and observation to determine whether the child requires an evaluation by a specialist in the field of ASD.
D. **Physical examination.** Most children with idiopathic ASD have unremarkable physical examinations. Some have isolated macrocephaly. Most have normal neurologic examinations and no motor abnormalities. Because of the association of tuberous sclerosis with ASD, a careful skin examination is required.
E. **Additional evaluations.** The medical workup of ASD should be guided by clues from the history and physical examination.
   1. Formal audiologic evaluation and vision testing should be performed on all children.
   2. Lead level should be tested if pica or social risk is present.
   3. The genetics of ASD are an area of intense study and clinical recommendations are in rapid evolution, and a genetics consultation should be considered. Chromosomal microarray (CMA) (encompassing a variety of array-based genomic copy number

analyses, including comparative genomic hybridization [CGH] and single nucleotide polymorphism [SNP] microarrays) screens for hundreds of microdeletions/duplications and should be performed in all patients. Fragile X should be considered for those with cognitive delays. If results of those tests are normal, or if the child has a complicated presentation (epilepsy, dysmorphic features, microcephaly), further testing should be considered using a tiered approach in consultation with a geneticist.

4. Repeat newborn screen, if not available or not previously performed.
5. Consider EEG if there is clinical concern of seizures or significant regression (to rule out Landau–Kleffner syndrome).
6. Consider magnetic resonance imaging for seizures or focal neurologic examination.
7. Consider metabolic studies if history or physical examination is notable for hypotonia, regression, decompensation with minor illness, or atypical presentation of ASD.

III. **MANAGEMENT.** The foundation of treatment for ASD includes intensive educational and behavioral intervention with individualized instruction aimed at ameliorating the core symptoms of ASD. The evidence base for various treatments is continuously expanding, and it is important that clinicians stay up-to-date. The different types of treatments can generally be broken down into the following categories:
- Behavior and communication approaches: the most widely used approach is Applied Behavior Analysis (ABA) that includes the following:
  - Discrete Trial Training (DTT): uses a series of trials to teach each step of a desired behavior or response.
  - Early Intensive Behavioral Intervention (EIBI): type of ABA for very young children with an ASD
  - Pivotal Response Training (PRT): a naturalistic ABA-based intervention
  - Verbal Behavior Intervention (VBI): ABA that focuses on teaching verbal skills

  Other approaches include Developmental Individual Differences (DIR or Floortime), Early Start Denver Model (ESDM), Treatment and Education of Autistic and related Communication-handicapped Children (TEACCH), and the Picture Exchange Communication System (PECS).
- Dietary approaches. Such changes include removing specific foods from a child's diet (most commonly those containing gluten and casein) and using vitamin, mineral, or other nutritional supplements. Many of these treatments do not have the scientific support needed for widespread recommendation and may be harmful to the developing child and thus require close monitoring.
- Medication: There are no medications that can cure ASD, but some medications can be efficacious to address associated symptoms including inattention, hyperactivity, and self-injurious behavior (see Chapter 23)
- Complementary and alternative medicine. These types of treatments, often referred to by their practitioners as "biomedical," are very controversial. Current research shows that as many as one-third of parents of children with an ASD may have tried complementary or alternative medicine treatments, and up to 10% may be using a potentially dangerous treatment. The National Center for Complementary and Alternative Medicine is a potential resource for families and clinicians.

IV. **CLINICAL PEARLS AND PITFALLS**
- ASD is very common, yet there is often a significant delay between when parents express concerns about their child's development and when the diagnosis of ASD is given. This may result in unnecessary delay of early intervention at the time when it is thought to have greatest impact. Parents' concerns about their child's development should be evaluated seriously, and watchful waiting is rarely appropriate in toddlers with language and social delays.
- In the primary care office, clinicians should be sensitive to the needs of the child with ASD by speaking in a quiet voice and not pushing the child beyond his or her comfort level with eye contact or social interactions.
- Clinicians should be alert to "hidden" medical conditions that can cause behavioral changes in nonverbal children with ASD (dental pain, constipation, etc.).
- Most primary care pediatricians will have a number of children on the autism spectrum in their panels and will see the child with greater frequency than specialists involved in their care. Understanding where along the spectrum a child falls will help the primary care team to anticipate where a child may have difficulty during an encounter. Engaging the parents and child in conversation about the greatest challenges can make the encounter more comfortable for all.

- Informing all team members when a child with ASD will be coming can help foster a better experience for the child and family. Arranging appointments early or late in the day to decrease wait time or to have additional time to address concerns helps to create a welcoming environment.
- Develop a deep understanding of how the child's autism presents itself to both the family and the community, including school. Each child on the spectrum is unique, yet there are overlapping traits that many children share. See further tips in Table 28-1

V. DISCLOSURE. Working with parents to address disclosure of diagnosis to their child is an important role for the primary care provider. As the medical home and continuous presence throughout the developmental course, it is important to continue to discuss with families how they are talking about the child's diagnosis, the words they are using, and what the child understands. Verbal ASD individuals without intellectual disability are often curious and confused about their difficulties and are relieved to understand that it has a name, and that there are others like them, and people devoted to helping them. Other children and young adults with ASD, as well as their families, reject the notion of their diagnosis or feel that the child "does not need to know." Counselors with experience addressing questions around disclosure are often supports to individuals with ASD and their families leading up to and during discussions of disclosure, for those who do and do not accept the diagnosis.

Table 28-1 • SPECIAL CONSIDERATIONS FOR PRIMARY CARE OF A CHILD ON THE AUTISM SPECTRUM

Behaviors/interests	• Language and communication • Behaviors such as sleep, tantrums, rages, rituals, aggression, toileting • Requirement for supervision • Special interests or obsessions • Activity level • Sensory defensiveness
Impact on family and home life	• How are siblings coping? • Are parents on the same page, do they need support? • Financial implications and cost of services not covered by insurance • Can the family attend extended family events such as weddings or other celebrations? • Need to counsel about media usage and Internet safety • Special advice on air travel and ways to prepare the child
School environment	• What type of school and classroom is the child in (ask the number of children and the number of teachers to get an idea)? • Is there an Individualized Education Plan in place? • Is the child making effective progress? • Is the child receiving any Applied Behavioral Analysis services at school? • What other services are in place: occupational, physical, speech and language services? • Does the family require periodic respite care?
Safety concerns	• Does the child run, wander, or "bolt" (consider a monitoring device)? • Is the home secure? • Any self-injury or injury to others? • Are local police aware of child in the home? Do they need to be informed? • Are there concerning behaviors outside the home that could put the child at risk? Unusual special interests can create high-risk situations as the child approaches adolescence or young adulthood
Medical concerns	• Is there a restricted diet? • Food intolerance or allergies? • Gastroesophageal reflux, constipation? • Hyperactivity/ADHD? • Seizures? • Genetic syndromes? • Future family planning and recurrence risks • Can the child communicate pain (ear, teeth, etc)? • Ability to create an "autism friendly" pediatric practice by recognizing safety, communication, and sensory needs specific to individual child

(continued)

Table 28-1 • SPECIAL CONSIDERATIONS FOR PRIMARY CARE OF A CHILD ON THE AUTISM SPECTRUM (CONTINUED)

Mental health	• Anxiety (frequent occurrence in late childhood and adolescence) • Depression may develop as child develops understanding of differences • Obsessions may need evaluation for obsessive compulsive disorder • Increased risk for more serious psychiatric illness
Adolescents and young adults	• Prolonged dependence on parents or other adults is typical • Transition to adult provider versed in ASD care • Risk of bullying or cyberbullying • Sexuality can be confusing for ASD individuals and may result in high risk behaviors • Open communication about appropriate behaviors is critical • Community resources and social groups can provide an outlet for adolescent and young adults • Overreliance on social media/video games for social contact. This should be monitored by a responsible adult

ADHD, attention-deficit/hyperactivity disorder; ASD, autism spectrum disorder.

Bibliography

BOOKS
Grinker R. *Unstrange Minds: Remapping the World of Autism.* New York: Basic Books; 2007 [Written by an anthropologist who is the father of a child with autism, this book offers both a review of many aspects of the science of autism, and interesting descriptions of the experience of autism in a variety of cultural contexts.].
Wiseman N. *Could It Be Autism? A Parent's Guide to First Signs and Next Steps.* New York: Broadway; 2006.

FOR PROFESSIONALS
Developmental Disabilities Monitoring Network Surveillance Year 2010 Principal Investigators, Centers for Disease Control and Prevention (CDC). Prevalence of autism spectrum disorder among children aged 8 years - autism and developmental disabilities monitoring network, 11 sites, United States, 2010. *MMWR Surveill Summ.* 2014;63(2):1-21.
Johnson C, Myers S, The Council on Children with Disabilities. Identification and evaluation of children with autism spectrum disorders. *Pediatrics.* 2007;120:1183-1215 [reaffirmed 2010, 2014].
Robinson EB, Neale BM, Hyman SE. Genetic research in ASD. *Curr Opin Pediatr.* 2015;27(6):685-691.

WEB SITES
Autism Asperger Network: AANE.org [Website with information for parents and providers, including support groups and educational forums as well as great supports around disclosure].
Autism Society of America. www.autism-society.org [Contains resources for parents in English and Spanish].
Autism Speaks. www.autismspeaks.org [Contains resources for parents in English and Spanish].
Centers for Disease and Prevention. https://www.cdc.gov/ncbddd/autism/facts.html.
First Signs. www.firstsigns.org.
https://nccih.nih.gov/health/integrative-health#1.

CHAPTER 29

Bilingualism

Naomi Steiner

I. DESCRIPTION AND DEFINITION

A. **The importance of foreign language mastery is being increasingly recognized** in the global economy.

B. **Bilingualism** is the mastery of two languages and encompasses different levels of proficiency as follows:

1. **Level 1: Ability to understand a second language (passive bilingualism).** Children who are learning a second language often understand the language before they can speak it.
2. **Level 2: Ability to speak a second language fluently.**
3. **Level 3: Ability to read and write in two languages (biliteracy).**

Each level should be considered as **a stepping stone** to the next. In this manner, a child who has level 1 passive understanding can quite rapidly attain level 2 with increased exposure and start speaking the language. For instance, if a child speaks with her parents in English, but understands her parents and grandparents speaking Spanish together, she could rapidly start speaking in Spanish if placed in a Spanish-only-speaking day care.

Parents should expect that a child will have a **dominant language**, which is the stronger and mostly used language, along with a weaker and less used language. **Balanced bilingualism**, which is high proficiency in two languages, is the exception rather than the rule. The dominant language can flip throughout childhood, as quantity of exposure between the languages also shifts. This often happens at preschool or kindergarten entry when English starts to develop more rapidly and becomes the dominant language.

II. EPIDEMIOLOGY

A. **The National U.S. Census 2010** shows that 20% of people living in the United States speak a language other than English at home. After English, Spanish is the most frequently spoken language in the United States with 37 million speakers, followed by Chinese (2.8 million speakers) and then French (1.3 million speakers).

B. **Worldwide** there are more bilinguals than monolinguals. Bilingualism is the norm.

C. **Children from immigrant families** are defined as having at least one foreign-born parent. A one-fourth have one parent born in the United States and four-fifths are US citizens. 25% of immigrants are unauthorized. **22% of immigrant families are linguistically isolated households.** These families have increased medical concerns and are more likely to live in poverty. The parents are less educated, and the head of the household is more likely to be a woman.

III. LEARNING THEORY

A. What affects the proficiency level of language in bilingualism?

In order of importance:

1. **Priority placed by the family to raise a bilingual child**, which may not be related to the parents' own level of proficiency in the second language. As children grow older, it is important for parents to affirm their beliefs and to discuss this with their children.
2. **Consistency and amount of exposure.**
3. **Child's attitude towards language learning and speaking another language**, which includes temperament and is also affected by family dynamics.
4. **Ability toward learning foreign languages.**

B. **Second-language development and the brain**

1. Most scientists agree that **language functions of both languages are more intertwined than previously thought**.
   - As children learn language concepts in one language (such as the concept of plurals), the **theory of transfer** explains that they then do not have to be relearned in the other; rather this knowledge can be transferred directly from one language to another.

147

- The **theory of suppression** describes how a bilingual person is constantly suppressing one language in order to speak the other. Bilinguals are constantly flipping between two languages.
2. **Bilingualism is considered a natural ability.** Children do not need to have above-average intelligence to become bilingual. All typically developing children can become bilingual. Babies are able to learn sounds from all languages and can tell the difference between two languages. The brain is primed to learn more than one language.
3. **Supporting second-language development.**
   - **The earlier the better.** It seems common sense that learning a second language takes years, so it is better to start early. However, from a neurologic perspective, the younger brain is more plastic and better able to adapt to a new language environment and learn a second language. Scientists believe that the younger brain requires less language input to learn the second language. **There is no critical period.** False beliefs around second-language learning relate that after a certain age it is impossible to learn another language. This misconception comes from the fact that after around puberty one should not expect to learn to speak a new language with a native-like accent. However, there is more to language learning than the accent, such as the vocabulary, expression, and understanding of the language. Therefore, it is more exact to say that a child's brain will adapt to his or her environment and that there will be a gradual decline over the span of a lifetime. Adults too can learn a foreign language.
   - **The greater the language input, the faster the acquisition and the greater the language proficiency.**
   - Contrary to the myth, **children do not learn languages** "like a sponge." They require **ongoing quality language input in both languages to become bilingual**. The ultimate proficiency level will depend on the level of the language exposure. Children who receive poor language input in their heritage language and have difficulty learning English at school are at **risk of developing poor language proficiency in both languages**.
   - **Consistency of language input should be the goal.** This leads to increased input and to success. The **"one parent, one language" (OPOL)** approach is when each parent chooses in which language they are going to speak to their children and stick to it. Parents can either both speak the same language to their children or speak in different languages, *but they should always stick to that language*. This method is highly successful toward raising a bilingual child, because it guarantees ongoing consistency and ongoing language input. Additional support comes when grandparents or other extended family members or caretakers also speak with the child a fixed language.
   - **The brain is able to learn from different sources.** For some parents the OPOL approach does not fit their family dynamic. These parents should know that the child's brain can successfully learn languages even if they are exposed in a more scattered way, although the consistency will probably be decreased and therefore the level of proficiency too.
   - **Use it or lose it.** As many adults have experienced, it requires ongoing language input to maintain a language. If the exposure stops, the language fades rapidly. This is what often happens when children from expatriate families return to the United States. Families should be encouraged to make plans to keep up the language even before returning and think about materials that will be needed, such as books. Of course, downloadable apps and movies make access to the language easier. Parents can also remain engaged through social media groups.
   - **Monolingual parents can raise a bilingual child.** Monolingual parents are a new force in the United States interested in raising their children bilingual. Monolingual parents often feel that schools do not prioritize foreign or world language curricula, and that their children will be at a disadvantage in the global world. Monolingual parents might have minimal language proficiency, such as high school remnants, yet they can learn a language along with their children. When children are young, this technique can be very successful. Later, as children progress to higher levels, they will usually need increased outside support, such as Saturday language school or a tutor.
   - **Children will mix both languages as they learn them.** Being raised, bilingual follows a developmental course, where children will use one language, usually the dominant one, to support expressive fluency in the other as they strive to communicate in a language that they might not fully master. This does not mean to say

they are confused; they are not. In fact, children even very young will not speak to someone in a language that they have not heard them use. Facts to keep in mind about mixing of languages are the following:

* **When parents mix, children mix.**
* **Parents mix even if they do not think that they are mixing.**
* **Parents should try their best to speak only one language.** In this manner children have the opportunity to extend their vocabulary and the complexity of their sentence structure in that language.
* **There is no scientific evidence that bilingualism leads to language delay.** However, because speech and language delay is the most prevalent developmental condition in early childhood (incidence 5%–10%), bilingual children will also present with language delay, and language delays will occur in both languages.

IV. RISKS AND ADVANTAGES OF BILINGUALISM

A. Risks

1. **Poor language development in both languages.** Continued input in both languages is necessary for a child to be raised bilingual. Many children who have just arrived in the United States are struggling at school to progress in English as well as academically. Additionally, their home environment might not offer high-level language input in their heritage language. These children are at risk of limited bilingualism, when a child fails to progress and attain native-like proficiency in either language.

   * **The expressive language debate.** Recent research suggests that bilingual children might learn words at a slower pace than monolingual children. When each of the languages of the bilingual child is considered separately, vocabulary in each language will develop slower in bilingual children compared with that in monolingual children. However, total combined vocabulary from both languages in the bilingual child compares similarly with the vocabulary of the monolingual child. Recent studies also suggest that bilinguals might have mildly decreased verbal fluency.

B. Benefits.
Continual shifting between languages is suggested to explain the possible decrease in verbal fluency, but also the numerous advantages of the bilingual brain. Bilingual children are constantly trying to figure out what different words mean, to explain sentences even if they might not fully understand all the words, and to figure out language. Studies in bilingual infants point toward a more flexible brain, primed to learn new information, as compared with monolinguals.

   * **Language benefits.** Compared with monolinguals, bilingual children show increased phonemic awareness. Phonemic awareness is the ability to breakdown words into sounds and is a precursor for reading and writing.
   * **Academic benefits.** Bilinguals show increased ability in math, to understand how language works, and to figure out what words mean.
   * **Other cognitive advantages** include benefits in abstract thinking, grasping rules, processing information, creativity, and cognitive flexibility toward learning new information.
   * **Cultural advantage.** Bilingual children describe themselves as a "bridge between two cultures." They have enhanced cultural awareness, which is important in this global world.

V. MAKING THE DIAGNOSIS OF SPEECH AND LANGUAGE DELAY IN A BILINGUAL CHILD

A. Understand that, in general, bilingualism is both underreferred and misunderstood.
Professionals that the pediatric clinician might typically reach out to for support with a language question, such as speech and language therapists, might not be trained in the area of bilingualism. Teaching staff in schools is also often poorly equipped to guide families and practitioners. Therefore, professionals might give well-meant, however, incorrect advice to parents, and do not take into consideration the long-term bilingual goals of parents.

B.
When faced with a bilingual child who presents with possible language delay, "following the process" will help you take steps toward decision-making.

1. **Take a history** of the child's language milestones and languages spoken at home. Do not assume that a child is being raised bilingual.
2. **Take advantage of the many questionnaires that have been translated into other languages.** The PEDS (Parents' Evaluation of Developmental Status) and the M-CHAT (Modified Checklist for Autism in Toddlers) have both been translated into around 50 languages. Ages and Stages can be found in five languages.

3. **Observe and interact with the child even if he or she is speaking another language.** Do not be intimidated by a child or family speaking another language, attempt to interact with the child, or ask the parent to converse with the child. Use a trained interpreter or ask the parent to translate as well as she can.

C. **Speech and language assessments.** The golden standard for a speech and language assessment in a bilingual child is the assessment by a speech and language pathologist who can assess all languages that the child speaks. However, this could lead to significant delay in the assessment. Therefore, realistically the bilingual child should be referred to a speech and language pathologist with experience in working with bilingual children. Not all speech and language pathologists have training or experience with bilingual children, so it is good for practitioners to have a list at hand.

D. **Speech and language therapy** can be delivered in English because of transfer. Transfer is the ability of the brain to learn a language concept in one language and use it in the other.

VI. **FROM BIRTH TO GRADUATION.** Fostering the heritage or second-language learning in your practice.

A. **Discuss bilingualism, starting at the prenatal visit or at birth.** Although parents want to transmit their language, they might not feel that their language is valued or would make a difference for their child. The pediatric clinician is in a unique position to answer questions at birth or during a prenatal visit. This is a window of opportunity, because starting to speak two languages at birth is the easiest way for parents. Starting to raise a child bilingual can happen at any age; however, the transition requires an increased effort for the parents and should be done in an incremental way.

B. Recognize that the decision to raise a child bilingual often feels overwhelming to parents who might strive toward perfection. **Parents raising a bilingual child usually have questions.** Clinicians can explain that all levels of bilingualism are stepping stones to the next level. This reassures parents and validates their efforts.

C. Because of the risk of limited bilingualism, **language enhancement should be raised at each surveillance visit** of a child being raised bilingual. This translates into proactively speaking to parents about how to boost language, such as through reading out loud, Head Start, library visits, and after-school and summer programs. Parents who *successfully* raise bilingual children usually have a supportive community of friends and/or family and are constantly searching for materials in their language to ensure a language-rich environment at home.

D. Around preschool or kindergarten entry, parents often wonder if they should switch from speaking their heritage language to English. **There is no evidence that dropping the heritage language and switching to English is going to speed up the English language learning.** On the contrary, parents should not speak to their children in broken language, which transmits poor vocabulary and grammar to their children. **Parents should speak in a language in which they are fluent** to their children, in order to assure continued progress in higher language skills. Because of transfer, *strong language skills in the heritage language will support the learning of English.* Additionally, children need strong language skills to develop and discuss ideas and concepts. Strong heritage language skills enable continued higher level thought process in a child who is an English-language learner (ELL).

E. **Children will typically want parents to speak with them in English around kindergarten age.** If parents feel strongly about transmitting their heritage language or a second language, they should follow their convictions. They can enhance their success by explaining to their children why it is so important for them, all in continuing to speak to them in their language and requesting response back in their language.

F. **Consistency of input is key,** so that the OPOL should be seriously considered, if raising a child bilingual is a priority for a family.

G. As children enter school, a third-language option is usually offered at school. Parents should know that not only bilingual children "still have enough space" in the brain for another language but that bilingual children **learn their third language with greater ease than monolingual children learn their second.**

H. **Children with learning disabilities can learn a second language too.** Because of logistics, children with learning disabilities are often scheduled for academic support during foreign/world language classes. Monolingual parents are often concerned about this because of the importance of foreign/world language mastery in the global world. There is no "brain" reason why children with learning disabilities should not learn a second language, although they might require accommodations (which they require for their other subjects too), thus giving them the opportunity to be included in the classroom and progress in this important area of development.

Bibliography

FOR PARENTS

Steiner NJ, Hayes SL. *7 Steps to Raising a Bilingual Child*. New York, NY: Amacom; 2008.

American Speech-Language-Hearing Association. *Learning Two Languages*. www.asha.org/public/speech/development/bilingualchildren/. Accessed June 12, 2018.

FOR TEACHERS AND PROFESSIONALS

Bialystok E. Bilingualism: the good, the bad, and the indifferent. *Biling Lang Cogn*. 2009;12(1):3-11.

Baker C. *Foundations of Bilingual Education and Bilingualism*. 5th ed. Bristol, UK: Multilingual Matters; 2011.

Center for Applied Linguistics, Ellis R. *Principles of Instructed Second Language Acquisition*. 2008. http://www.cal.org/areas-of-impact/english-learners.

ERIC Digest. *A Global Perspective on Bilingualism and Bilingual Education*. 1999. http://www.eric.ed.gov/ERICDocs/data/ericdocs2sql/content_storage_01/0000019b/80/15/eb/59.pdf.

ERIC Digest. Programs that Prepare Teachers to Work Effectively with Students Learning English. 2000.

Marschall M. Parent involvement and educational outcomes for Latino students. *Rev Policy Res*. 2006;23:1053-1076.

CHAPTER 30

Bipolar Disorder in Children

Janet Wozniak | Nicole M. Benson | Joseph Biederman

I. **DESCRIPTION OF THE PROBLEM.** Childhood or pediatric-onset bipolar disorder is increasingly the focus of research studies owing to the high degree of disability associated with the symptoms, the high rate of comorbid conditions, and the increased rate of diagnosis in the last two decades. Up until the mid-1990s, the condition was thought to be so uncommon that it was generally not included in the training of child and adolescent psychiatrists or pediatric clinicians and was not considered in the differential diagnosis of a moody child. More recently, epidemiologic data from meta-analyses suggest that the increase in the diagnosis of pediatric bipolar disorder may represent a more accurate estimate of the true prevalence of the disorder. Because of this increase in diagnoses and the *concomitant increase in medication prescriptions, concerns have arisen that the diagnosis may be over used*, subjecting some children to mood-stabilizing medications inappropriately. In fact, the reported prevalence of bipolar disorder in children may well be an underestimate of real psychiatric illness in youth, and many children who might benefit from psychiatric intervention may never come to clinical attention. Factors such as symptom overlap with attention-deficit/hyperactivity disorder (ADHD) and developmentally different presentation from the classic form of bipolar disorder have likely led to its underdiagnosis in the past.

A. **Epidemiology.** The true epidemiology of childhood bipolar disorder is not known, as no rigorous epidemiologic studies have addressed the question.
- One study of adolescents suggests **that 1% are affected, with up to 15% suffering from a subthreshold (but highly disabling) form of bipolar disorder**.
- Other studies that address the prevalence of bipolar disorder in youth in epidemiologic and international populations show that **1.8%–2.9% of children and adolescents are affected**.
- As in the pediatric age group, evidence in adults assessing the various subtypes of bipolar disorder, especially those with dysphoria, mixed states, and complex cycling, suggests that the **prevalence of bipolar disorder in the adult population may be 4%–5%**, also higher than previously thought.

B. **Etiology/contributing factors.** A complex interplay of environmental influences and genetic factors has been implicated in the development of bipolar disorder in adults as well as in children. **There is no evidence that "bad parenting" or traumatic experience is responsible for the dramatic mood swings present in bipolar children** and adolescents. However, **parenting techniques, which focus on flexibility and decreased rigidity, are gaining acceptance as essential in reducing the frequency and intensity of the rage aspect of bipolar disorder.**
  1. Family studies have elucidated the important role of genetics as critical in the development of bipolar disorder, demonstrating that a **complex, polygenetic etiology** is more likely than a single gene. Neuroimaging studies implicate the **limbic structures of the brain** as the site of the neurobiologic abnormality.

II. **MAKING THE DIAGNOSIS.** There is no definitive test for bipolar disorder.
   Despite advances in neuroimaging and in identifying candidate genes, there are currently no biological markers for this disorder. Like other psychiatric disorders, the diagnosis is made clinically, by asking about the specific symptoms in a developmentally appropriate manner. Research studies often use the Young Mania Rating Scale. Although this scale was designed for use in adult inpatients, addendums with developmentally appropriate cues make it useful in children and adolescents.

A. **Signs and symptoms.** Bipolar disorder is a mood disorder, and therefore the diagnosis is anchored by the presence of abnormal mood states that fluctuate between depression and mania. Please see Chapter 40 on depression for information regarding the symptoms of depression.
  1. Mania is characterized by two types of abnormal mood: **euphoric and irritable**. The abnormal mood must be associated with persistently increased activity or energy. To be diagnosed as having bipolar disorder, it is necessary to have had an **episode of mania that lasts 1 week or longer** (hypomania refers to episodes of

mania lasting less than a week, but at least 4 days). Most individuals who have episodes of mania also have depression.

2. **Depression can cycle in an alternating fashion** with mania (a week or more of mania followed by an episode of depression). Some such individuals will then experience an **intermorbid period of good functioning**, free from abnormal mood states, although this type of alternating mood states and return to good functioning is rare in pediatric cases.

3. Others experience **"mixed" states in which manic episodes have depressive features and depressive episodes have manic/hypomanic features**. In such states, an individual may be euphoric for part of a day, rageful/irritable for another part of the day, and depressed/suicidal for another part of the day. **Children and adolescents tend to present with mood episodes with mixed features and complicated cycling patterns** rather than classic episodes of mania alternating with depression. A return to a high-functioning, euthymic (even/normal) mood appears to be rare in bipolar youth. Many adults also present with mixed features, and most adults with bipolar disorder suffer more from depression than mania.

4. **Euphoric states** are characterized by goofy/giddy behavior and/or a feeling of being high or hyper, being "on top of the world," or being powerful and able to "accomplish anything."

5. The irritable mood of mania is distinctly different from the irritability associated with depression, ADHD, age-appropriate tantrums, or "bad days." The **irritability of mania is extreme, persistent, threatening, attacking, and out of control**. Rage episodes, when they occur, are characterized by long outbursts (20–60 minutes or more) with destructive, out-of-control, and dangerous anger.

6. In addition to abnormal moods and persistently increased activity or energy, the diagnosis of mania requires at least three (or four in the absence of euphoria) additional symptoms from among those referred to by the mnemonic **DIGFAST** (**D**istractibility, **I**ncreased goal-directed activity/energy, **G**randiosity, **F**light of ideas, **A**ctivities with bad outcome, **S**leep decreased, **T**alkativeness).

B. Differential diagnosis
1. **Unipolar depression.** Although irritability can characterize both mania and depression, the irritability of depression is milder, characterized by more complaining/whining/grouchiness and is associated with low self-esteem, self-denigrating and self-destructive feelings, joylessness, and hopelessness. The **irritability of mania is more severe and dramatic, often with aggressive and explosive behavior**.

2. **ADHD.** Mania and ADHD share the symptoms of distractibility, increased energy or hyperactivity, and talkativeness. In addition, while ADHD can be associated with irritability and decreased frustration tolerance, the irritability of ADHD is of lower intensity. Both disorders can be characterized by impulsivity. In general, **the symptoms of mania include extreme mood dysregulation and are much more disabling and of a greater severity than ADHD**. It is important to note that ADHD frequently co-occurs with mania and that both disorders can be present in youth.

3. **Disruptive Mood Dysregulation Disorder.** Mania and disruptive mood dysregulation disorder (DMDD) share the symptoms of recurrent outbursts (verbal or physical) that are inconsistent with developmental level and are out of proportion in intensity or duration to the inciting event. In both, the underlying mood can be irritable or angry. It is important to note that the diagnosis of DMDD is defined by episodes in multiple settings (two of three—home, school, or with peers) and that other symptoms of mania are not present (recall for the diagnosis of mania, **DIGFAST**: **D**istractibility, **I**ncreased goal-directed activity/energy, **G**randiosity, **F**light of ideas, **A**ctivities with bad outcome, **S**leep decreased, **T**alkativeness).

C. History: key clinical questions
1. To **assess overall moodiness.** *"How often is the child moody (How much of each day? How many days out of the week? How many weeks out of the month?) and how severe and impairing are the child's abnormal mood states? Conversely, are age-appropriate moods and responses to stress also present and how often?"*

2. To **assess mania.** *"How frequent and how severe are the angry mood states? How often does grouchy, cranky, whining behavior occur? How common is hitting, kicking, biting, and spitting? How common (many times per day, once per day, a few times per week) are rage episodes or explosions? Do rages last a long time (20–60 minutes or more)? Are the rages threatening, aggressive, attacking, or dangerous? How common and how severe are euphoric or goofy/giddy/silly mood states? While all children can be silly, does your child take jokes too far? Does the child alienate others with immature behavior or excessive laughing fits?"*

3. To assess **depression and cycling**. *"How common are depressed, sad, blue, or hopeless/joyless mood states? Do these moods occur on the same days as the manic mood states noted above? Do depressed moods occur during weeks or months separate from the manic mood states? Is the child self-destructive, self-abusive, or suicidal?"*

4. To assess **DIGFAST symptoms**.
   a. *"Is the child easily distracted from tasks by noise, sights, or internal thoughts?"*
   b. *"Does the child have high-energy states with increased motor activity? Is it difficult to calm or slow down the child? Does the child's energy fluctuate over the course of the day or over the course of weeks or months?"*
   c. *"Is the child grandiose? Does he/she have an inflated sense of self-esteem or does he/she overestimate his/her ability to do things? Does the child act or feel stronger/smarter/more powerful than others? Take on big projects? Does the child demonstrate a flagrant disregard for adult authority, acting like the boss? Is the child a braggart or show-off?"*
   d. *"Does the child jump from idea to idea quickly or go off on tangents that are hard to follow when they talk? Does the child complain of 'racing thoughts' or thoughts that occur so rapidly they are hard to keep track of?"*
   e. *"Does the child show poor judgment in activities? Is the child reckless? Does the child want to buy or spend money excessively? Is the child sexually inappropriate (e.g., excessive bathroom humor, preoccupation with genitals or sexual matters, excessive or public masturbation, touching others' breasts or private parts, exposing self to others)?"*
   f. *"Does the child function with less sleep than most other children of the same age? How many hours less? Has the child ever functioned on little or no sleep or just a few hours?"*
   g. *"Is the child talkative? Does the child have pressured speech? Is the child difficult to stop or interrupt?"*

III. **MANAGEMENT.** Although some children may "grow out" of bipolar disorder symptoms (longitudinal studies are underway), bipolar disorder is generally considered to be a chronic, lifelong condition. Longitudinal studies of children suggest a pattern of partial recovery, with frequent relapse.

   A. **Pharmacotherapy** is the mainstay of treatment of bipolar disorder, and a combined pharmacotherapy approach (using medications in combination) is typically required. **Mood-stabilizing medications** spanning various categories are the first-line treatment. The Food and Drug Administration (FDA)–approved medications for pediatric bipolar disorder are approved down to age 10 years and comprise second-generation medications also known as atypical antipsychotic medications. Mood stabilizers include **atypical antipsychotics** (e.g., risperidone, olanzapine, quetiapine, ziprasidone, aripiprazole), **lithium**, and **certain anticonvulsants** (e.g., valproate, carbamazepine, oxcarbazepine, lamotrigine).
   - Clinical trials and clinical experience have suggested that atypical antipsychotics work the fastest and most effectively in youth to control the disabling symptoms of mania as compared with the more traditional agents (lithium and anticonvulsants), and several of these agents have FDA approval for use in children down to age 10 years.
   - Pediatric bipolar disorder is difficult to treat and often requires combination therapy using more than one mood stabilizer at a time. Mood stabilizers may control mania, but leave depression untreated, requiring the cautious addition of an antidepressant (cautiously using low doses, as antidepressants can cause worsening of mania and some clinicians suggest they should never be used in bipolar patients). Lamotrigine or lurasidone can also be useful for bipolar depression.
   - Because bipolar disorder is highly comorbid with ADHD and anxiety disorders, medications addressing these conditions are often required. Stimulant medications must be used cautiously, as they can exacerbate mania, but frequently improve the functioning of the child who has both mania and ADHD.

   B. **Other therapies including cognitive behavioral therapy, dialectical behavioral therapy, family therapy, group therapy, and individual psychodynamic therapy** can all be helpful for various individuals. An approach combining medication treatment with these other therapies tailored to the needs of the individual is generally recommended for the treatment of bipolar disorder.
   - Helping the bipolar individual develop insight into his or her condition and to recognize the early signs of relapse aids in treatment.
   - Therapy is helpful to ensure medication compliance, which is important in preventing relapse.

C. **Psychiatric hospitalization** is frequently required in the management of bipolar disorder owing to the **dangerous behaviors associated with mania, the suicidal behavior of depression,** or **psychosis** associated with either. Many children improve with the containment and structure of hospitalization or residential treatment programs.

D. **The presence of comorbid conditions** can complicate the management and course of bipolar disorder in youth.
  * In bipolar children younger than 12 years, **comorbid ADHD** is almost always present (90% or more).
  * In adolescents with bipolar disorder, **comorbid ADHD** occurs in 50%–60%.
  * **Conduct disorder or antisocial personality disorder** (criminal behaviors) may occur in as many as 40% of youth with bipolar disorder and may or may not improve when the bipolar disorder is treated.
  * **Anxiety disorders** are present in 50%–60% of youth with bipolar disorder and may be easy to miss, as it may seem counterintuitive to be disinhibited from mania and ADHD but fearful and inhibited from anxiety simultaneously.
  * **Alcohol and drug abuse and addiction** commonly occur in youth with bipolar disorder and age of onset is frequently earlier than peers, with adolescent-onset bipolar disorder carrying the greatest risk. Random drug screening is recommended even in youth professing abstinence.
  * **Autism spectrum disorders** are increasingly recognized in higher functioning and normal IQ children and adolescents and can co-occur with bipolar disorder.

IV. **CLINICAL PEARLS AND PITFALLS**
  * Pediatric bipolar disorder may be a difficult diagnosis to make because it, with a developmental picture, is characterized by (1) more irritability than euphoria; (2) mixed states and complex cycling; (3) chronicity rather than interepisode high functioning; and (4) high levels of comorbidity especially with ADHD. This type of bipolar disorder may also commonly be seen in adults. Pediatric-onset bipolar disorder represents one subtype of bipolar disorder often seen in adults who present for treatment.
  * Parents often feel unfairly blamed by mental health professionals, pediatric clinicians, teachers, and family members for "causing" the disorder by not being strict enough or disciplining "bad behavior" effectively. In fact, children with bipolar disorder are very difficult to parent, and a genetic etiology is most likely.
  * Pediatric bipolar disorder is a neurobiologic disorder affecting thinking, feeling, and behavior in children in a dramatic way. It is characterized by out-of-control mood swings and frequent episodes of rage, irritability, and poor judgment.
  * Some children present with a different array of symptoms in different arenas. At certain stages of the disorder and at certain ages, rage and depression may only be evident to those family members closest to the child and not apparent to teachers, friends, or pediatric clinicians. The reasons for this are unclear but may relate to the progression of the disorder (most evident to parents initially, later spilling over into other arenas). This feature does not mean that parents are "doing something wrong" and should not discourage parents from seeking professional treatment.
  * Although medications used to treat bipolar disorder in children carry many potentially serious side effects, not treating bipolar disorder in children can lead to worsening of the condition and/or the complications of suicidal behavior, substance abuse, or criminal arrest due to disinhibited behaviors in public.
  * Children who initially present with subthreshold symptoms of mania without the full spectrum of bipolar symptoms must be carefully monitored, as this can be disabling and require treatment in itself and/or can develop into full syndrome bipolar disorder over time.

Bibliography

FOR PARENTS

Greene R. *The Explosive Child: A New Approach for Understanding and Parenting Easily Frustrated, "Chronically Inflexible" Children*. New York, NY: Harper Collins; 1998.

McDonnell MA, Wozniak J, Brenneman JF. *Positive Parenting for Bipolar Kids*. New York: Random House; 2008.

Papolos D, Papolos J. *The Bipolar Child and Reassuring Guide to Childhood's Most Misunderstood Disorder*. New York, NY: Broadway Books; 2002.

FOR PROFESSIONALS

Birmaher B, Axelson D, Goldstein B, et al. Four-year longitudinal course of children and adolescents with bipolar spectrum disorders: the Course and Outcome of Bipolar Youth (COBY) study. *Am J Psychiatry*. 2009;166(7):795-804.

Geller B, Tillman R, Bolhofner K, et al. Child bipolar I disorder: prospective continuity with adult bipolar I disorder; characteristics of second and third episodes; predictors of 8-year outcome. *Arch Gen Psychiatry*. 2008;65(10):1125-1133.

Lee T. Pediatric bipolar disorder. *Pediatr Ann*. 2016;45(10):e362-e366.

Merikangas KR, He JP, Burstein M, et al. Lifetime prevalence of mental disorders in U.S. Adolescents: results from the National Comorbidity Survey Replication–Adolescent Supplement (NCS-A). *J Am Acad Child Adolesc Psychiatry*. 2010;49(10):980-989.

Wozniak J, Petty CR, Schreck M, et al. High level of persistence of pediatric bipolar-I disorder from childhood onto adolescent years: a four year prospective longitudinal follow-up study. *J Psychiatry Res*. 2011;45(10):1273-1282.

WEB SITES
arielslegacy.net.
www.DBSA.org.
www.ryanlichtsangbipolarfoundation.org.
www.stepup4kids.com.

CHAPTER 31

Biting Others

Barbara J. Howard

I. DESCRIPTION OF THE PROBLEM

A. Epidemiology

1. Almost all children bite at some time during the first 3 years with a peak in biting at 20–22 months in typically developing children and declining thereafter.
2. 50% of toddlers in childcare are bitten three times every year. Bites constitute 6% of injuries to males and 3% to females in childcare. Biting is reported by parents of 19% of children under 26 months.
3. As with most other aggressive behaviors, boys are more likely than girls to be higher biters, although overall rates are similar by gender.
4. Biting is more persistent in children from families of teen mothers, where parents are depressed or anxious, have lower income or education, where physical punishment is used, or when there is chronic stress.
5. Exposure to violence predisposes to aggressive behaviors, such as biting.

B. Contributing factors

1. **Environmental.** Children are more likely to bite others when they are in social situations beyond their coping abilities. Biting in these situations is usually intended to obtain objects, gain attention, or express frustration. It is also a powerful way of acquiring attention from adults. For example, some parents remove the child from the childcare setting for the day after a biting incident. Such *secondary gain* from the environment may prolong the time to decline in biting.
2. **Developmental.** Biting emerges at predictable developmental stages.
   a. The first peak, at the **time of tooth eruption**, is rarely reported as a problem because caregivers interpret it as normal experimentation. Interestingly, nursing infants generally learn very quickly not to bite the breast, probably because of their mother's shriek, her affective distress, and the prompt removal of the infant from the breast.
   b. The next peak in biting occurs around **8–12** months when infants bite as an expression of excitement. A strong negative emotional response by caregivers accompanied by putting down the infant generally leads to rapid extinction.
   c. The **second year of life** is normally a time when skills develop unevenly, and there is a strong desire to act autonomously. Fledgling or delayed abilities in expressive language and fine motor skills serve to cause frustration and set the child up for aggressive outbursts, peaking at 20–22 months. Biting in toddlers may be used to dominate, to acquire an object, or as an expression of anger or frustration. In addition, children undergoing stressful separation experiences (such as to go to childcare) may get emotional relief from causing distress in others by biting. This phase of biting typically disappears quickly. If it does not abate, the child is likely failing to acquire expected coping skills such as verbal negotiation, primacy of social relationships, or general frustration tolerance. Such children may also have a past or current history of stressful experiences.
   d. Biting in typically developing children **older than 3 years** should occur only in extreme circumstances (e.g., if they are losing a fight, perceive their survival to be threatened, or are very stressed).

II. RECOGNIZING THE ISSUE

A. History: key clinical questions

1. *"When did the biting start? What else was different around that time"*? Look for recent stress (such as new childcare or a new child in the household).
2. *"In what situations does it occur?"* Look for situations in which frustration is common and the child has poor coping skills. This may be a clue to developmental weaknesses such as fine motor delay (e.g., if biting occurs when stacking blocks is attempted). Biting that occurs when there has been a long period between meals may suggest hunger as a cause.
3. *"How have you handled it so far?"* Determine the previous measures used to address the problem and whether there is any secondary gain for the child to continue to

bite (such as increased attention). Parental ambivalence about steps they have taken may need to be acknowledged to implement a better plan, e.g., the parent bit back or washed the child's mouth out with soap.

4. *"What other concerns do you have about your child's behavior or development?"* Other signs of aggressive behavior or specific developmental delays may point to an important contributing cause.

5. *"How is anger expressed in your home?"* Children may model other family members' behaviors around expression of anger and violence. Mothers with a history of conduct problems are more likely to have an aggressive child. Although there is a genetic component to high aggression (>50% concordance), there may also be a familial pattern of poor management or high stress.

6. *"Have you had any concerns about how your child is cared for?"* Abuse, neglect, violence, or poor-quality care by the family or childcare provider may contribute to the problem.

III. MANAGEMENT

A. Information for the family. Adults view biting as a very primitive behavior that elicits strong emotional reactions, especially in childcare settings. Families need to understand that biting by toddlers younger than 3 years is usually a normal developmental phase and does not predict later aggression.

B. Treatment (see Table 31-1)

1. **Determination of cause.** Before formulating a treatment plan, the clinician must determine the reason for the child's biting. Developmental assessment will dictate the need for management of specific delays, especially expressive language and fine motor. Children who are frustrated by their relative weaknesses in skills compared with peers, for example, often do better when placed with younger children or in a less demanding setting. Other children push themselves

---

Table 31-1 • TECHNIQUES TO DIMINISH BITING IN TODDLERS

Directed to the Child

- Provide close supervision.
- Ensure attention to positive behaviors.
- Redirect when anger or frustration appears.
- Verbalize feelings for the child.
- Assess all skill areas and habilitate deficiencies.
- If a bite occurs, shout a loud "NO!" and place child in time-out.
- Be sure that the child receives no interaction in time-out.
- Offer lots of positive attention to the child who was bitten.
- Offer teething ring or cloth to bite.
- If most bites are toward a certain peer, separate the children.
- If biting persists, remove to home or smaller childcare.

Directed to the Caregivers

- Set consistent limits, especially on aggressive acts.
- Avoid physical punishment or exposure to violence including in media.
- Express negative emotions verbally in moderation and stay in control.
- Avoid interfering in the partner's discipline: Whoever starts handling an event should finish.
- Do not bite back. This models the undesirable behavior, elicits fear and anger in the child, and makes the adult feel so guilty that his or her effectiveness in limit setting is diminished.
- Ensure that the child is not the least competent in his or her group.
- Assure adequate sleep and food, as deficiencies may be responsible for poor coping.
- Assess the behavior of other children in the home who may be provoking.
- Ensure that all caregivers are properly responsive and not using physical punishment.

Directed to the Parents If the Child Is About to Be Removed From Childcare

- Meet with childcare staff.
- Determine exactly how incidents are being handled.
- Establish a consistent plan for managing incidents (which does not include taking the child home, if possible).
- Consider a shorter day in the childcare setting if the child is too tired to cope.
- Negotiate a time-limited trial of intervention, documenting incidents to determine improvement.
- If necessary, move the child to home or a smaller, closely supervised, structured setting or one with younger or less aggressive children, or staff who are more open to dealing with biting.

to perform beyond their abilities. Such children may need support by arranging same-age peer play, placement in smaller groups, and avoidance of or support for difficult tasks.

2. **Aversive reinforcement and redirection.** The chronic biter will need to be observed closely for a period so that appropriate social interactions can be praised and biting encounters interrupted quickly with a shout that declares the seriousness of the offense. The child should then be put in time-out, with a short explanation such as "I know you are angry, but people are not for biting." Sympathizing with the victim is helpful and may also serve to avoid secondary gain for the biter. Later, the incident can be reviewed with the child, and alternatives for negotiating conflict and for expressing feelings role played. A teething ring to bite can be offered or attached to the clothing, allowing the child expression of the feelings through an acceptable alternative outlet.

3. **Parental attitudes toward aggression.** Parental attitudes toward aggression need to be discussed. Because corporal punishment is a contributor to persistent biting, it should be eliminated. Parents often need coaching to moderate their own expression of negative affect. Counseling regarding reasonable limits for the child's behavior and nonphysical ways to attain them are the centerpiece of treatment. When parents interfere or criticize the other's discipline, the child experiences the tension and mixed feelings and may become unusually aggressive, including biting.

4. **Childcare setting.** When biting occurs in a childcare setting, a crisis often ensues. Having the parents of the victim meet the equally distraught parents of the biter (or even a meeting of the entire center) can help defuse these situations. The nature of the supervision and activities should be evaluated. Young children need an active curriculum focused on small-group play with responsive adults who are positive in their interactions and able to redirect untoward behaviors. There also should be enough toys to discourage disputes. Larger toys for shared play are associated with fewer struggles. A child in group care who persists in biting often will do better at home or in a family childcare setting with children of a variety of ages. Corporal punishment, mistreatment, or neglect in the childcare should also be considered.

Bibliography

Block RW, Rash FC. *Handbook of Behavioral Pediatrics*. Chicago, IL: Year Book; 1981.

Solomons HC, Elardo R. Biting in day care centers: incidence, prevention and intervention. *J Pediatr Health Care*. 1991;5:191-196.

Nærde A, Ogden T, Janson H, Daae Zachrisson H. Normative development of physical aggression from 8 to 26 months. *Dev Psychol*. 2014;50(60):1710-1720.

CHAPTER 32

Breath Holding

Barry Zuckerman | Micaela A. Jett

I. DESCRIPTION OF THE PROBLEM. Breath-holding spells (BHS) involve the involuntary cessation of breathing in response to a painful, noxious, or frustrating stimulus. If prolonged, they can lead to loss of consciousness, seizures, and/or myoclonic movements. Rare adverse outcomes associated with breath holding have been reported.

A. Epidemiology
- Simple breath holding without loss of consciousness may be seen in up to 25% of children.
- True BHS with transient loss of consciousness has been reported in approximately 4%.
- The peak frequency is between 1–3 years of age, although they may begin in the newborn period.
- BHS after 6 years of age are unusual and warrant further investigation.
- They occur equally in males and females.
- There is a positive family history in approximately 25% of cases.
- 50% resolve by the age of 4 years; 90% by the age of 6 years.

B. Etiology. The etiology of BHS is speculative.
- Pallid spells may be facilitated by an overactive vagus nerve; cyanotic spells may be related to a more central nervous system inhibition of breathing in response to stress.
- Hematologic differences (iron deficiency, transient erythroblastopenia) have been reported.

C. Types
1. **Cyanotic spells (80%).** The most common type of BHS is a cyanotic spell, which is precipitated by anger or frustration. A short burst of crying, usually less than 30 seconds, leads to an involuntary holding of the breath in expiration, resulting in cyanosis that can lead to a loss of consciousness and occasionally a seizure (Table 32-1).
2. **Pallid spells (20%).** The second type is precipitated by fright or minor trauma (e.g., occipital trauma due to a fall). Following the precipitating event, there is an **absence of crying** or a single cry, followed by pallor and limpness. This sequence of events is thought to be due to a hyperresponsive vagal response that results in bradycardia (and even asystole), causing pallor and loss of consciousness. Some of these children (about 15%) go on to faint when they are injured or frightened as adults.

II. MAKING THE DIAGNOSIS
- History is the mainstay of diagnosis; videotape documentation may be possible. The key to diagnosis is to differentiate BHS from seizures (Table 32-2). The presence of a precipitating factor followed by crying and cyanosis before the loss of consciousness and/or seizure is specific to BHS.
- A complete blood count and iron studies should be done to rule out iron deficiency anemia.
- An electroencephalogram (EEG) is rarely necessary unless a clear precipitating event is not apparent or if there is concern for prolonged seizures or status epilepticus after the BHS.
- Consider an electrocardiogram (ECG) if there is a family history of cardiac disease or early sudden death to rule out long QT syndrome.

III. MANAGEMENT
A. Information for parents. BHS need to be explained and demystified for parents and reassurance given. The clinician should explain in simple, concrete terms the sequence of events leading to the loss of consciousness and seizure. The benign nature of these events should be emphasized because parental concerns about epilepsy, brain damage, or death are common.

Table 32-1 • PROGRESSION OF BREATH-HOLDING SPELLS

Cyanotic Spell

Precipitating event (anger or frustration associated with temper tantrums)

Period of crying (frequently less than 20 s)

Holding of breath in expiration

Cyanosis

Progressive loss of consciousness

Occasional twitching, opisthotonos, or clonic movements

Pallid Form

Precipitating event (minor trauma, especially occipital trauma or fright)

Absence of crying or single cry

Bradycardia and often asystole

Simultaneous loss of consciousness and breath holding

Pallor

Occasionally generalized seizure or twitching

Table 32-2 • DISTINGUISHING BREATH-HOLDING SPELLS FROM SEIZURES

	Severe Breath-Holding Spells	Epilepsy
Precipitating factor	Always present	Usually not present
Crying	Present before convulsion	Not usually present
Cyanosis	Occurs before loss of consciousness	When it occurs, it is usually during prolonged seizure
Electroencephalogram	Almost always normal	Usually abnormal but may be normal
Incontinence	Uncommon	Common

B. Management strategies
- **Iron supplementation** may be used in cases with hematological abnormalities. The suggested dose is 5–6 mg/kg per day for 8–16 weeks.
- Other **medications** are generally neither indicated nor helpful unless the patient has severe BHS with either status epilepticus or prolonged bradycardia/asystole. Atropine has been tried in some cases of pallid spells with bradycardia or asystole. For severe refractory cases, cardiac pacemakers have been used.
- For cyanotic spells, an **intense stimulus** (e.g., a cold cloth on the face) may terminate the breath holding if applied before or within the first 15 seconds of apnea. Although the window of opportunity for this intervention is brief, many parents find it comforting to have *something* to try, rather than just feeling helpless.
- If the event progresses for either type of BHS, the **child should be placed on the floor to prevent falling**.
- When the child awakes (usually immediately after the seizure or loss of consciousness), **parents should not fuss over the child** so that inadvertent secondary gain does not occur.

Bibliography

FOR PARENTS

www.childneurologyfoundation.org/disorders/breath-holding-spells.

http://www.webmd.com/parenting/tc/breath-holding-spells-topic-overview.

FOR PROFESSIONALS

Breningstall GN. Breath holding spells. *Pediatr Neurol.* 1996;14(2):91-97.

Evans OB. Breath holding spells. *Pediatr Ann*. 1997;26(7):410-414.

Singh P, Seth A. Breath holding spells - a tale of 50 years. *Indian Pediatr*. 2015;52:695-696.

Zehetner AA, Orr N, Buckmaster A, Williams K, Wheeler DM. Iron supplementation for breath-holding attacks in children. In: *Cochrane Database of Systematic Reviews*. John Wiley & Sons, Ltd.; 2010. doi:10.1002/14651858.CD008132.pub2.

CHAPTER 33

Bullying

Douglas L. Vanderbilt | Robert D. Keder

I. **DESCRIPTION OF THE PROBLEM.** Bullying is a form of violence. The Centers for Disease Control published a definition of bullying as: "any unwanted aggressive behavior(s) by another youth or group of youths who are not siblings or current dating partners that involves an observed or perceived power imbalance and is repeated multiple times or is highly likely to be repeated. Bullying may inflict harm or distress on the targeted youth including physical, psychological, social, or educational harm."

Bullying is on a continuum with teasing on one end and violent assault on the other. Teasing involves mild aggression and humor that can create social embarrassment but does not have the intent to harm. Physical assault and "hate speech" (discriminatory harassment) are intentionally harmful and against the law.

Bullying can come in multiple forms:

- *Physical bullying* is overt physical aggression such as hitting, stealing, and threatening with a weapon.
- *Verbal bullying* is verbal aggression such as name-calling, public humiliation, and intimidation.
- *Relational bullying* is often covert and can involve spreading rumors, social rejection, exclusion from peer groups, and ignoring.
- *Cyberbullying* is verbal aggression that takes place via the use of social media, e-mail, text messaging, blogging, online gaming communities, etc.

A. **Epidemiology**
   1. **Prevalence**
      a. National Survey of Children's Exposure to Violence (2011) found that almost half (48.4%) of the entire sample of school-age children experienced at least one form of bullying (peer victimization) in the past year.
      b. The Youth Risk Behavior Surveillance System (YRBSS; 2015) found that during the past year 20% of high school students reported being bullied on school property and 16% were bullied electronically.
      c. 55% of 8 to 11-year-olds and 68% of 12 to 15-year-olds rated teasing and bullying as big problems.
      d. Types of bullying experienced or committed in a 2-month timeframe: 21% physical bullying, 54% verbal bullying, 51% relational bullying, or 14% cyberbullying.
   2. **Age**
      a. Different types of bullying peak at different ages. Physical intimidation and bullying peaks in primary school. Relational bullying peaks during middle school. Cyberbullying peaks during high school.
      b. Older children are less likely to talk about their victimization with only 50% of all children confiding in anyone.
   3. **Gender**
      a. Boys are more likely to use and be the target of overt physical or verbal bullying.
      b. Girls are more likely to use and be the target of relational bullying and cyberbullying.
      c. The type of cyberbullying tends to differ by gender: Girls are more likely to spread rumors, whereas boys are more likely to post hurtful pictures or videos.
B. **Etiology/contributing factors**
   1. **Settings.** Bullying occurs most frequently at school where there is minimal supervision: breaks, recess, and lunch. Common places are playgrounds, hallways, and to and from school. Cyberbullying, by definition, takes place online through the Internet and social media.
   2. **Social risk factors.** Families may encourage bullying by showing a lack of consistent consequences, using discipline that is negative or physical, and modeling bullying behaviors to their children.

   School climate refers to the overall quality and character of school life; this includes teaching practices, organizational structures, norms and values, and relationships. There is a link between positive school climate and reduction in bullying

behaviors. Schools have more episodes of bullying if they ignore or tolerate such behavior through weak supervision. Peer bystanders can also support bullying through acceptance or encouragement of the behavior.

Community values and media images can promote aggression and violence as normative and appropriate methods of social behavior and conflict resolution.

3. **Characteristics of children who are the targets of bullying.** *Subtypes*: There are two main subtypes of targets:
   • The *passive target* tends to be cautious, sensitive, quiet, and withdrawn. Boys tend to be physically weaker than peers, whereas girls tend to physically mature earlier than their peers. Overall, these children tend to have few friends and find it easier to associate with adults.
   • The *provocative target* tends to behave in ways that cause irritation and attract negative attention. They tend to be reactive and have poor self-control. They can be labeled as "annoying" or "awkward." They can share characteristics with children who bully as they tend to fight back when provoked. They are at risk for becoming targets of bullying who bully others.

   Children who are perceived as "different" are at an increased risk to be the target of bullying. Children with attention-deficit/hyperactivity disorder (ADHD), learning disabilities, autism spectrum disorder, emotional problems (anxiety, depression, etc.), and other special health care needs (i.e., food allergies, wheelchair use, etc.) are notably vulnerable. Children who identify as a relative minority (sexual, gender, racial, ethnic, and/or religious) to their local population or who are overweight or obese are also vulnerable populations. Both types of targets often experience problems with social skills, insecurity, and low self-esteem.

   Developmental trajectory: Long-term consequences include increases in depression, abusive relationships, poor physical health outcomes, and anxiety disorders such as agoraphobia, generalized anxiety, and panic disorder.

4. **Characteristics of children who bully others.** Children who bully may have a range of conduct, behavioral, or emotional problems. They tend to blame others for their problems and often do not accept responsibility for their actions. Some have similar aggressive behaviors modeled at home.

   Developmental trajectory: Those who self-identify have higher rates of depression and psychological distress as compared with those who deny their behavior. They have more drug use and negative attitudes toward school and a fourfold increase in criminal behavior by their mid-20s. They are at higher risk of dropping out of school, carrying weapons, and fighting as well as having increased odds of having antisocial personality disorder.

5. **Characteristics of children who are both targets of bullying and who bully others (bully-victim).** This represents a small percentage of less popular children who are often easily aroused and highly reactive and tend to target others who are clearly weaker than they are. They have experienced victimization to the extent that they now target others.

   Developmental trajectory: These children experience the largest burden of problems and disorders. They are more likely to be both anxious and depressed. They have the most problems with peer relationships and higher rates of loneliness, substance use, and psychosis. Two-thirds of children from intended or conducted school shootings were found to fit this profile. As adults they are at increased odds of having depression and panic disorder; males from this group had 18 times the odds of suicidality and females 27 times the odds of agoraphobia.

6. **Characteristics of children who are bystanders.** *Subtypes*: These children can have different levels of involvement in bullying:
   • *Disengaged onlookers* who have no direct involvement
   • *Supporters* who do not instigate but support children who bully
   • *Upstanders* who provide assistance/intervention on behalf of the target of bullying

   Risk factors: The school climate of fear of bullying distracts children from learning and takes up teachers' time and resources. These groups serve as an intervention point as several studies demonstrate that school programs that promote upstanding result in reduction of school-based bullying.

II. **MAKING THE DIAGNOSIS.** The clinician has four roles to address bullying:
   • Identification
   • Screen for comorbidities and refer for treatment if needed
   • Counsel the families and children
   • Advocate for bullying prevention and appropriate intervention

A. Signs and symptoms

1. **Identifying targets of bullying.** Bullying is often not a presenting complaint. Questions about being a victim should be explored on all visits (Table 33-1). Presenting complaints of a child being bullied include physical complaints such as insomnia, stomachaches, headaches, and new-onset enuresis. Depression, loneliness, anxiety, and suicidal ideation and gestures may occur. Behavioral changes are broad and common such as irritability, poor concentration, school refusal, change in physical activity, changes in eating patterns, substance abuse, academic failure, social problems, and lack of friends. Additional vigilance must be made for those children with chronic medical illnesses, physical deformities, and students in special education who may be potential targets.

2. **Identifying the child who bullies.** Signs of a child being a bully are more difficult to discern because of the bully's desire to obscure the behavior. Children who bully others can present with any of the following: physical or verbal fights, increasingly aggressive behavior, have friends who bully, have frequent disciplinary measures at school, have unexplained extra money/new belongings, blame others, do not accept responsibility for their actions, and/or worry about their reputation/popularity. Children who are aggressive, overly confident, lack empathy, and are having oppositional or conduct problems may need careful screening. These children are at high risk if they come from families who use physical punishment or model violent behavior in conflict resolution.

3. **Identifying the bully-victim.** Signs of a child who is a target of bullying who bullies others can range from subtle to major red flags. They can demonstrate any of the problems of a child who bullies or is the target of bullying. They tend to be loners and often have poor social skills. These children are reactive and usually may have depressed affect/mood or anxiety. Any child who has experienced significant trauma, has a history of low parental involvement, or has notable mood/affect problems should be identified and screened for immediate safety including access to potential self-harm and harm to others.

4. **Differential diagnosis.** Bullying involvement can be viewed as a form of trauma or a symptom. Care must be made not to miss psychological disorders that pose safety issues such as suicidal ideation and plans, substance abuse, and risk-taking behaviors. The physical, behavioral, emotional, and school symptoms of bullying may overlap with other medical, learning or psychological problems. For example, a child with high functioning autism spectrum disorder is both at increased risk to be a target and perpetrator of bullying. They are also at increased risk to misperceive social interactions as bullying. Serious disorders require appropriate behavioral health evaluation and management. Critical states such as active suicidal or homicidal ideation or risk-taking behavior require immediate safety assessment (access to firearms, means, etc.) and referral to emergency behavioral health services.

B. History: key clinical questions (see Table 33-1)

III. **MANAGEMENT.** Management for bullying involves interventions with families/parents, children in all roles of bullying involvement, and school personnel. Interventions should include giving information, supporting families and the individual child, referring as needed, and expecting behavior change from the child who bullies. Management may also include working with the child's school and advocating for appropriate change/intervention within the school environment. Many children are bullied going to or from school. Changing routes, time, or getting school involved even though it is not happening on school grounds should be explored. Children experiencing bullying should be seen for follow-up to monitor the situation.

A. Individual

1. **Targets of bullying.** The clinician should empathetically listen to the parent and child to help empower them. Interest and explicit statements to help are viewed by parents and the child as not being in this alone. Remember that a child may be reluctant to volunteer information, especially regarding cyberbullying. The child and family need reassurance; do not blame the victim or trivialize the child's/parent's concern. For example:

   "No one deserves to be treated this way."

   "You are not alone."

   "Your parents and I will work together to help things get better for you."

   "Let's work together to stop the bullying." What will help you feel safe?

   Clinicians should always assess for immediate safety and screen for comorbid behavioral health problems. Invite families to contact the school with their concerns and to keep a log of what happens, where it happens, and when it happens. Offer to speak to the school. Remind families that schools are not required to notify families of what disciplinary measures are taken against a child who bullies.

Table 33-1 • SAMPLE SCREENING QUESTIONS TO INVESTIGATE IF A CHILD IS BEING BULLIED

Questions for Children

1. Have you ever been teased or bullied at school or going to and from school?
2. Do you know of other children who have been teased?
3. How long has this been going on? Where is it happening?
4. Have you ever told the teacher about the teasing?
5. What kinds of things do children tease you about?
6. Have you ever been teased because of your illness/handicap/disability? ... for not being able to keep up with other children? ... about looking different from them?
7. At recess do you usually play with other children or by yourself?
8. Have you ever changed schools because you had problems with the other students?
9. Who is your "go to" adult at school?
10. What kinds of social media do you use?

Questions for Parents

1. Do you have any concern that your child is having problems with other children at school?
2. Does your child go to the school nurse frequently for physical complaints?
3. Has your child's teacher ever mentioned that your child is often by himself/herself at school?
4. Do you suspect that your child is being harassed or bullied at school for any reason? If so, why?
5. Has your child ever said that other children were bothering him/her?
6. Does your child have access to social media sites? Smartphone? Online gaming community?

Suggestions should include having the child seek support from teachers and friends and avoid situations where the bullying may occur. The phrase *"Walk, Talk, and Squawk"* can help a child to deal with the bully. The child should "Walk" by ignoring the hurtful remarks, "Talk" by making confident yet nonprovocative statements to the bully, and "Squawk" by disclosing the episodes to adults. Role-playing can be helpful in practicing these techniques with the child. Strategies can be used to help to bolster the child's insecurities and increase self-esteem, e.g., extracurricular activities such as drama clubs and sports.

Special considerations:

Children with special needs. Discuss appropriate accommodations for a 504 plan or appropriate interventions for a child receiving special education services with their school. Children with autism spectrum disorder, ADHD, and/or other special needs may benefit from social skills training.

Cyberbullying: Cyberbullying is particularly difficult to manage. Children can be reluctant to disclose because they fear of losing access to related devices and social media accounts. Tell families to never delete texts or online postings before saving. All parents should discuss blocking and privacy settings online with their children. Families should encourage "in real life" positive supports and relationships.

2. **Children who bully.** Once a bully is identified and appropriate screening for risk factors is completed, the clinician should educate the parents and the child about the seriousness of the behavior and its potential consequences. Care must be made to label the behavior and not the child as the problem. The first step in changing the bully's behavior is helping the family and the child to acknowledge the behavior as hurtful. For example:

"How do you feel when other children hurt your feelings?"

"Bullying hurts other children's feelings."

Interventions should include clear accountability of the child's behavior through observations at home by parents and at school by teachers and administrators. Interventions should also deconstruct any blaming and depersonalization of the target of bullying. Clinicians should invite families to work with their school. Parent–teacher conferences and loss of privileges are particularly effective at reducing the reoccurrence of bullying. Clinicians can also discuss venues through which to provide these children alternative opportunities for leadership skills. Consider referral to behavioral health for family counseling and/or cognitive behavioral therapy if the child is demonstrating poor insight into their behavior.

3. **Children who are targets of bullying and who bully others.** In addition to the interventions noted above, clinicians should focus working with families to establish a relationship with a behavioral health provider to assess and treat comorbid psychiatric conditions. These children should be assessed for safety at home and school. Consideration should be given to appropriate referral to emergency behavioral health services or child protective services.

B. **Systemic.** *What works*: Bullying occurs in a permissive and encouraging environment. Evidence-based interventions use a whole-school approach to foster a safe and caring school climate. Programs that promote *upstanding* (empowering the bystander to protect the victim and censor the bully) are proven to be effective.

  What does not work: Zero-tolerance policies, direct conflict resolution and peer mediation between the child who bullies and their target, group treatment for children who bully, use of detention, use of suspension, and parent phone calls (as opposed to live parent–teacher conferences).

  Clinician's role: Clinicians should encourage the use of whole-school programs that foster positive school climate through use of school-wide rules and sanctions, teacher training, classroom curriculum, conflict resolution training, and individual counseling. The clinician must collaborate with appropriate school and community organizations to inform practices and encourage interventions to change social norms regarding violence and access to firearms. Finally, the clinician should be aware of their state's laws surrounding bullying and help refer families to them when needed; the Web site stopbullying.gov has a summary of each state's related laws.

Bibliography

FOR PARENTS

WEB SITES
http://www.bullying.org/.
http://www.pacer.org/bullying/.
https://www.stopbullying.gov/.
http://www.thebullyproject.com/tools_and_resources.

APPS
Be Strong (Apple iOs & Google Android).

BOOKS
Hart L, Caven K. *The Bullying Antidote: Superpower Your Kids for Life*. Hazelden Publishing; 2013.

FOR PROFESSIONALS

WEB SITES
https://www.aap.org/en-us/advocacy-and-policy/aap-health-initiatives/resilience/.
http://pediatrics.aappublications.org/cgi/reprint/peds.2009-0943v1.
https://www.stopbullying.gov/laws/index.html.
https://www.stopbullying.gov/what-you-can-do/community/index.html.

BOOKS
Laminack LL, Wadsworth RM. *Bullying Hurts: Teaching Kindness through Read Alouds and Guided Conversations*. 2012.

FOR CHILDREN & TEENS

WEB SITES
https://pacerkidsagainstbullying.org/.
https://pacerteensagainstbullying.org/.
http://stopbullyingnow.hrsa.gov/kids/.
http://kidshealth.org/teen/school_jobs/bullying/bullies.html.

APPS
Be Strong (Apple iOs & Google Android).

BOOKS
Cook J. *Tease Monster: A Book about Teasing Vs. Bullying*. Boys Town, NE: Boys Town Press; 2013.
Dismondy M. *Spaghetti in a Hot Dog Bun: Having the Courage to Be Who You Are*. Wixom, MI: Cardinal Rule Press; 2008.
Frankel E. *Weird!* Minneapolis, MN: Free Spirit Publishing; 2013.
Romain T. *Bullies Are a Pain in the Brain*. Minneapolis, MN: Free Spirit Publishing; 1997.

CHAPTER 34

Cerebral Palsy

Norah Emara | Laurie Glader

I. DESCRIPTION OF THE PROBLEM.

Cerebral palsy (CP) is a chronic, lifelong disorder of movement and posture resulting in activity limitation caused by a nonprogressive injury or disruption to the developing brain. Although neuromuscular problems are the central feature of CP, the diagnosis can be associated with a spectrum of nonmotor-associated neurodevelopmental disabilities in the cognitive, behavioral, and communication domains, as well as epilepsy and musculoskeletal sequelae. These associated disabilities reflect the fact that motor centers of the brain are rarely affected in isolation. CP, a clinical diagnosis, may be due to a wide range of insults to the developing brain. When the clinical diagnosis of CP is established, it is important to investigate the etiology, which may have implications for management, prognosis, and recurrence risk. Although the brain lesion is, by definition, nonprogressive, its motor and nonmotor manifestations can be expected to change over time. Thorough, ongoing medical and developmental surveillance, ideally via a multidisciplinary approach, is essential to the management of children with CP to promote their optimal functional ability and quality of life.

A. Epidemiology
- CP is the most common motor disability in childhood, affecting 2.1 per 1000 live births.
- In the 85%–90% of cases that are congenital, brain injury occurs before or during birth. Contrary to earlier perception, only 10% of these cases relate to peripartum brain injury, whereas the vast majority of cases result from developmental brain anomalies or prenatal insults. Risk factors include low birthweight, prematurity, multiple gestation, genetic abnormalities (including brain malformations), environmental exposures (medications, substance abuse), maternal/fetal infection (TORCH), and birth complications. The remaining 10%–15% of cases are acquired, associated with postnatal events. Risk factors in these cases include traumatic brain injury, infection, stroke, and severe hypoxic events.

B. Etiology/contributing factors. CP can often be attributed to known risk factors and supported by MRI findings. In many cases, however, a specific cause for CP is not found. Advances in neuroimaging and genomic study are allowing for increasingly sophisticated understanding of the etiologies of CP.

II. CLASSIFICATION.

Clinical classification of CP describes the type of CP an individual has, which in turn allows for anticipation of associated medical issues and the development of individualized treatment plans. There are a number of different classification systems based on severity level, topographical distribution, motor manifestations, and gross motor function. CP has historically been broadly classified as mild, moderate, or severe although that language has been supplanted by more specific functional nomenclature.

Classification by motor manifestations describes the impact of the brain injury on the quality of movement, coordination, and muscle tone (Table 34-1).
- Spastic CP represents 70%–80% of patients with CP. Spasticity is a form of velocity-dependent hypertonia or increased muscle tone. This continuous muscle contraction causes stiffness and can interfere with normal movement, speech, and gait.
- Athetoid, or dyskinetic, CP represents approximately 20% of patients with CP and is characterized by involuntary movements including chorea and dystonia.
- Ataxic CP is characterized by problems with balance and coordination.

Classifications based on topographical distribution describe body parts affected.
- Hemiplegia describes the condition in which one side of the body, involving both the arm and the leg, is more affected than the other.
- Diplegia describes more significant involvement of the bilateral lower extremities as compared with the upper extremities.
- Quadriplegia represents involvement of all extremities.

There are more nuanced combinations as well, such as triplegia to describe hemiplegia superimposed on diplegia. Using this nomenclature, a motor function descriptor is

Table 34-1 • CLASSIFICATION BY MOTOR MANIFESTATIONS

Classification	Description
Spastic	Upper motor neuron signs: velocity-dependent hypertonus (clasp-knife), increased deep tendon reflexes, pathologic reflexes, often associated with weakness, loss of motor control, and dexterity
Dyskinetic	Involuntary movements: chorea, athetosis, dystonia
Mixed	Features of both spastic and dyskinetic CP
Ataxic	Balance, coordination, and postural difficulties

CP, cerebral palsy; DTRs, deep tendon reflexes.

typically combined with a topographical distribution to yield an anatomic diagnosis. For example, "spastic quadriplegia" means a child has spasticity in all four extremities with the lower extremities often more affected than the upper.

Functionality has proven to be one of the single most important descriptors in allowing for comparison between large groups of individuals with CP for research and assessing outcomes and has been revolutionized by the development of the Gross Motor Function Classification System (GMFCS). The GMFCS uses a five-level scale that corresponds to the extent of ability and impairment limitation (Fig. 34-1). A higher number indicates a more significant degree of severity. Each level is determined by an age range and set of activities the child can achieve on his or her own. The goal of this scale is to present an idea of how self-sufficient a child can be at home, at school, and in their community.

Because of challenges associated with consistency across different providers using an anatomic system alone, there has been a movement toward a universal classification system for CP that instead emphasizes broader descriptive information. The elements consist of (1) motor abnormalities, including the presence or absence of spasticity (along with unilateral or bilateral presentation), the presence or absence of dyskinesia, and functionality (GMFCS level); (2) anatomic distribution and radiologic findings; (3) associated findings; and (4) causation (if known).

III. DIAGNOSIS. The diagnosis of CP remains clinical and is typically made by the age of 2 years. However, ongoing studies in Europe indicate that recognition of abnormal spontaneous general movements during the first weeks of life may provide a sensitive tool for much earlier detection. A neurologist, in conjunction with other providers, typically makes the diagnosis. Symptoms warranting further investigation include motoric delay and/or a variety of red flags that suggest abnormal neuromotor function (Table 34-2).

On neuromotor examination, muscle tone may vary from excessive hypotonia to hypertonia (spastic, dystonic, or mixed in character). Hypotonia in an infant may be manifest as head lag on pull to sit, slip through at the shoulders when held under the axilla, or an exaggerated curve in ventral suspension. Early hypotonia may persist, normalize, or evolve into hypertonia. Hypotonia with significant weakness and diminished deep tendon reflexes is uncommon in CP and suggests a neuromuscular disorder. Classic findings that suggest upper motor neuron dysfunction include spasticity, clonus, and preserved primitive reflexes (particularly the Babinski reflex in the lower extremities after age 18 months) and may emerge later in infancy.

The nonprogressive nature of CP is essential to the diagnosis. Serious consideration should be given to other organic etiologies if a progressive pattern is suspected, particularly if the clinical picture includes regression/loss of skills or hypotonia or if examination reveals dysmorphic features, neurocutaneous stigmata, organomegaly, or other atypical findings. In these cases, metabolic, genetic, or neurodegenerative conditions should be suspected. Because many genetic and metabolic diseases may have overlapping symptoms with CP, genetic and metabolic evaluations can be very helpful in diagnosing a child with a potentially reversible or treatable cause for their presentation.

There are a number of associated conditions strongly correlated with CP, such as epilepsy, sensory impairment, and neurodevelopmental delays or differences. Recommended testing for every child with a new diagnosis of CP thus consists of MRI, hearing and vision assessments, and developmental screening. Further testing is guided by clinical suspicion and may include karyotype, chromosomal microarray, metabolic studies (serum lactate and amino acids, urinary organic acids), or evaluation for prior infection, among other studies.

GMFCS for children aged 6–12 years:
Descriptors and illustrations

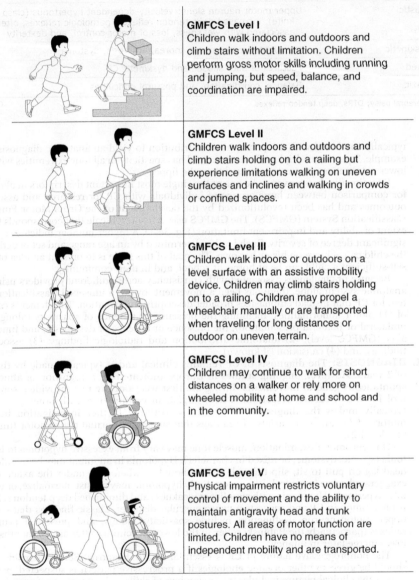

GMFCS Level I
Children walk indoors and outdoors and climb stairs without limitation. Children perform gross motor skills including running and jumping, but speed, balance, and coordination are impaired.

GMFCS Level II
Children walk indoors and outdoors and climb stairs holding on to a railing but experience limitations walking on uneven surfaces and inclines and walking in crowds or confined spaces.

GMFCS Level III
Children walk indoors or outdoors on a level surface with an assistive mobility device. Children may climb stairs holding on to a railing. Children may propel a wheelchair manually or are transported when traveling for long distances or outdoor on uneven terrain.

GMFCS Level IV
Children may continue to walk for short distances on a walker or rely more on wheeled mobility at home and school and in the community.

GMFCS Level V
Physical impairment restricts voluntary control of movement and the ability to maintain antigravity head and trunk postures. All areas of motor function are limited. Children have no means of independent mobility and are transported.

Figure 34-1 Gross motor function classification system (GMFCS).

IV. MANAGEMENT. Because of the complex nature of CP, many medical specialists are usually involved in the care of a child who carries the diagnosis. Multidisciplinary teams often enhance and improve clinical management. They represent a variety of health care workers who interact and coordinate their efforts to diagnose, treat, and plan for children with CP. Care teams often comprise neurologists, orthopedic surgeons, pediatric clinicians with expertise in developmental medicine/complex care, physiatrists, physical and occupational therapists, speech pathologists, and orthotists, among many other disciplines. The activities of the team are often brought together in a group setting to foster collaboration. Even in the absence of a multidisciplinary team that physically meets together, this range of

Table 34-2 • RED FLAGS SUGGESTIVE OF CEREBRAL PALSY

Delay in motor milestones
Abnormal tone
Involuntary movements
Asymmetric movement of extremities
Delay in disappearance of primitive reflexes
Weakness
Abnormal gait (i.e., toe-walking)
Difficulty with fine motor tasks
Difficulty maintaining balance

Table 34-3 • MULTIDISCIPLINARY APPROACH TO MANAGEMENT OF THE CHILD WITH CEREBRAL PALSY

Specialty	Purpose/Indication
Orthopedics	Hip and spine surveillance; surgical management of functional impairment; pain caused by deformity, contracture, or muscular imbalance
Physiatry	Tone management, functional optimization through equipment and therapeutic recommendations
Neurology	Diagnosis, tone management, seizure management
Pediatric clinicians	Anticipatory guidance, developmental surveillance, medical management, team communication, and family support
Physical therapy	Preventative management, functional optimization
Occupational therapy	Preventative management, functional optimization
Nutrition	Nutritional optimization
Audiology	Baseline evaluation, communication enhancement, assistive devices
Speech and language	Communication enhancement, assistive devices, feeding/oromotor evaluation, and management
Behavioral psychology	Behavioral management, integration of plans at school and at home
Social work	Family coping, access to school and community, advocacy, Early Intervention, curriculum modification, IEP services, community agency supports, and affiliation

IEP, individualized Education Plan.

specialists is often involved in the care and management of children with CP and forms a "virtual" team that can be headed by the primary care clinician (Table 34-3).

Goals of care for the child with CP are centered on several fundamental principles:
1. Preventing/minimizing physical deformities and discomfort
2. Improving/enhancing mobility
3. Maximizing capacity for independent functioning at home, at school, and in community
4. Enhancing overall health by managing comorbid conditions with integrated health care plans
5. Optimizing quality of life

A. Spasticity Management. The goals of spasticity management include functional improvement and comfort in addition to the fundamental goal of tone reduction. Objective measurement through functional scales is important when determining the impact of interventions. Treatment typically involves a combination of approaches such as therapies, orthotic devices, adaptive equipment, medications, and, in many cases, surgery. The following represents the variety of treatment modalities commonly seen in CP management and progresses from least to most invasive. In general, the complexity of the child's presentation along with discussion of the goals of care should help determine the direction and aggressiveness of treatment.

Targeted spasticity treatments include the use of orthotics, adaptive equipment, and therapies to support comfort and mobility. Orthotics are braces worn to help provide stability and optimize alignment to promote function, often while maintaining the range of motion across affected joints. There are several types, ranging from shoe inserts and wrist supports to more complex hip-knee-ankle-foot orthotics that provide varying degrees of stability and support designed to correct abnormal mechanics related to the neuromuscular differences seen in CP. Adaptive equipment may also include the use of standers, gait trainers, and wheelchairs, both manual and electric. The use of adaptive equipment and orthotics is often enhanced by services designed to optimize strength, stamina, and function, including physical and occupational therapy, aquatherapy and hippotherapy. Chemodenervation procedures using botulinum toxin and phenol are often used in conjunction with orthotics and physical therapies to tar-. get particular muscle and nerve groups. These injected medications are helpful in balancing forces across joints to decrease contractures associated with spasticity and are typically administered every 6 months.

Systemic treatments targeting spasticity have both enteral and intrathecal formulations. Mainstays of treatment include baclofen (generally administered enterally but for select children with more significant spasticity such as those functioning at a GMFCS level IV or V intrathecal administration via pump may be appropriate), benzodiazepines (e.g., diazepam), and dantrolene. Each has a unique side effect profile (e.g., transaminitis with baclofen) and should be carefully titrated and monitored by a clinician familiar with its usage. Although they are often quite successful in modulating spasticity, systemic treatments are commonly accompanied by the relatively undesirable side effects of unmasking generalized weakness, which can actually diminish function, as well as fatigue. Careful consideration to candidacy for systemic medications should be given before initiation of any systemic therapy. As always, clinicians should listen carefully to parental/caregiver concerns about any changes in their children after medication initiation or dosage change.

Surgical management is not uncommon in children with CP. Some goals of surgical intervention include improving comfort, facilitating positioning and function, correcting limb alignment, and preventing progressive contracture or deformity. For children with more complex CP, orthopedic surgeries go beyond soft tissue releases to address bony issues pertaining to the hip and spine, including procedures such as hip and femoral osteotomies or spinal fusion. Selective dorsal rhizotomy, or SDR, reduces muscle spasticity in the lower extremities by cutting nerve rootlets in the spinal cord that send abnormal signals to the muscle. The best candidates for SDR are typically patients with spastic diplegia affecting the legs more than the arms and children who function at a GMFCS I, II, or III level. Every child's circumstance is unique and his or her treatment will be unique as well.

B. **Effectiveness of interventions.** The CP evidence base has rapidly expanded in recent years, providing clinicians and families with guidance regarding newer, safer, and more effective interventions. Novak et al. developed the traffic light system by which they classified common CP interventions as green, yellow, or red, indicating their effectiveness and overall recommendation based on systematic review of CP interventions. Green light effective interventions are interventions with the most evidence to support their effective utilization. Some of these interventions included anticonvulsants in seizure management, botulinum toxin, diazepam, and SDR for reducing muscle spasticity, bisphosphonates for osteopenia, casting, fitness training, goal-directed training, hip surveillance, home programs, occupational therapy after botulinum toxin, and pressure ulcer care for reducing risk of ulcers. The majority of interventions reviewed were classified as yellow light interventions and had less evidence supporting their effectiveness; red light interventions were interventions that have been shown to be ineffective and are therefore not recommended. Red light interventions include craniosacral therapy, hip bracing, hyperbaric oxygen, neurodevelopmental therapy, and sensory integration. This framework has been helpful in developing evidence-based guidelines in the standardized moving towards more evidence-based management of children with CP.

V. **COEXISTING CONDITIONS.** There are many coexisting impairments and functional limitations associated with CP. These include (1) epilepsy, (2) intellectual disability, (3) hearing impairment, (4) vision impairment, and (5) oromotor impairment causing feeding difficulties, sialorrhea, and communication challenges. The variety of comorbidities demonstrates the importance of a multidisciplinary care team in the management of patients with CP.

With increasing severity of CP, particularly children who function at GMFCS IV–V levels, it can and should be expected that additional comorbidities may arise that are not necessarily directly related to CP but are related to overall medical complexity. Conditions that should be anticipated and screened for include (1) bladder and bowel impairment, (2) osteoporosis, (3) nutritional and vitamin deficiencies, (4) respiratory compromise, and (5) disordered sleep. Guidelines for the evaluation and management of some of these common comorbidities can be found on the American Academy of Cerebral Palsy and Developmental Medicine (AACPDM) Web site.

VI. MORBIDITY AND MORTALITY. Survival prognosis is largely a function of medical fragility. Children with CP who have very low weights have more major medical conditions and are at increased risk of death. Medically fragile children with CP may have increased morbidity and mortality related to infections, respiratory insufficiency, and epilepsy. Survival prognosis for adolescents and adults has been correlated to functional skills and ability to self-feed. Routine evaluations should include screening and management of these conditions to optimize health and decrease morbidity and mortality.

VII. THE ROLE OF THE PEDIATRIC CLINICIAN. Primary care pediatric clinicians are critical in the diagnosis and management of children with CP. Pediatric clinicians are often the first provider a patient comes into contact with during his or her life and, with the appropriate index of suspicion, can often be the first provider to suspect a diagnosis of CP. Primary care clinicians, first and foremost, must continue to provide routine health care maintenance for patients with CP. In addition, screening for known and anticipated complications in children with CP is an important aspect of care. Knowledge of available local intervention programs, their services and ever-changing details of eligibility, access, and payment is an invaluable resource to share with families who have a child with CP. The pediatric clinician is also tasked with the responsibility of coordinating the recommendations of the many subspecialists into an integrated health care plan and providing reinforcement of subspecialist recommendations. Longitudinal relationships, such as those fostered between patients, families, and their primary care provider, lend themselves to identifying patient and family goals and assisting with the psychosocial aspects of living with a chronic disease. Pediatric clinicians can help parents of children with more complex CP in accepting and assuming their roles as primary advocates for their child's needs and often aid in transition of care to adult providers to ensure an efficient, effective, and coordinated transfer of care. For children with milder CP, pediatric clinicians play a critical role in fostering independence so that they can self-advocate as they become independent adults.

Bibliography

Novak I, McIntyre S, Morgan C, et al. A systematic review of interventions for children with cerebral palsy: state of the evidence. *Dev Med Child Neurol.* 2013;55:885-910.

Oskoui M, Coutinho F, Dykeman J, Jetté N, Pringsheim T, An update on the prevalence of cerebral palsy: a systematic review and meta-analysis. *Dev Med Child Neurol.* 2013;55:509-519.

Rosenbloom L. Definition and classification of cerebral palsy. *Dev Med Child Neurol Suppl.* 2007(109):43.

www.cdc.gov/ncbddd/cp/index.html.

ORGANIZATIONS AND WEB SITES

American Academy for Cerebral Palsy and Developmental Medicine, 555 East Wells, Suite 1100 Milwaukee, WI 53202. (414) 918-3014. www.aacpdm.org.

Association of University Centers on Disabilities, 1010 Wayne Avenue, Suite 920, Silver Spring, MD 20910; (301) 588-8252. www.aucd.org/.

Cerebral Palsy Foundation has a number of educational materials for families and providers and can be found at www.yourcpf.org.

Disabled Sports USA, 451 Hungerford Drive, Suite 100, Rockville, MD 20850; (301) 217-0960. www.dsusa.org.

Exceptional Parent Magazine, 555 Kinderkamack Road, Oradell, NJ 07649–1517. Also see www. eparent.com for an extensive online resource for parents of children with disabilities compiled by *Exceptional Parent Magazine*.

The Cerebral Palsy Tool Kit is a useful compilation of information by and for families, particularly those grappling with a new diagnosis, and is now available as an app as well as online. https://cpnowfoundation.org/wp/wp-content/uploads/2015/11/CP-ToolKit.pdf.

The Council for Disability Rights, 205 West Randolph, Suite 1650 I Chicago, IL 60606; (312) 444-9484. www.disabilityrights.org.

United Cerebral Palsy Associations, 1660L Street, NW, Suite 700, Washington, DC 20036; (800) 872-5827. www.ucp.org.

CHAPTER 35

Child Maltreatment: Physical Abuse and Sexual Abuse

Kimberly A. Schwartz | Genevieve Preer

I. **DESCRIPTION OF THE PROBLEM.** Both physical abuse and sexual abuse are common and can have profound and long-lasting impacts on child and adult health. Detection can be complicated by the reality that the presentation of child maltreatment is rarely straightforward. Clinicians must maintain a low threshold to consider physical and sexual abuse as they weigh other diagnostic possibilities.
   A. **Physical abuse** is defined as any inflicted physical injury to a child that may include striking, burning, or biting the child, or any action that results in physical harm to the child.
   B. **Sexual abuse** is defined as the engagement of a child in sexual activities that the child cannot comprehend, for which he or she is developmentally unprepared and cannot give informed consent, and/or that violate laws and/or societal taboos. A spectrum of activities constitutes sexual abuse, from exposure to pornographic materials or sexual situations, to use of a child to produce pornography, to inappropriate touching and penetration. Coercion and threats by the perpetrator are common.

II. **EPIDEMIOLOGY.** In the United States in 2016, Child Protective Services evaluated approximately 3.5 million children and identified 676,000 victims. The majority of children (75%) were found to have been the victims of child neglect. Approximately 18% were victims of physical abuse and 8.5% were victims of sexual abuse, and some were victims of more than one type of maltreatment. It is generally believed that child maltreatment is significantly underreported.
   A. **Contributing factors.** Although both physical abuse and sexual abuse occur in children of all ages, ethnicities, and socioeconomic groups, there are child, parent, and community/society factors that contribute to an increased risk of maltreatment. Child factors that increase vulnerability include emotional/behavioral difficulties, chronic illness, physical/developmental disabilities, preterm birth, and unwanted/unplanned pregnancy. The parent factors that increase risk of child abuse include low self-esteem, substance/alcohol abuse, personal history of child maltreatment, mental illness, lack of understanding or negative perception of normal development/behaviors. Finally, the environmental factors that increase risk of child maltreatment include social isolation, interpersonal violence, poverty, low educational achievement, and the presence of a nonbiologically related male in the home.

III. **MAKING THE DIAGNOSIS: PHYSICAL ABUSE.** Sentinel injuries are seemingly minor injuries to infants and young children, which are common in abused children and rare in those who are not abused. Because some of these injuries are common in ambulatory children, it is important to evaluate an injury in the context of the child's age and level of development.
   A. Consider physical abuse for the following:
   - Any injury (bruise, burn, fracture, or oral injury) in a nonambulatory child
   - Any patterned injury
   - Any injury in an unusual location such as mouth, ears, neck, or torso
   - Significant injuries with no history, insufficient history, illogical, or changing explanations for an injury.
   - Multiple injuries with different stages of healing
   B. Workup for physical abuse:
   1. **History.** A careful injury history should be obtained in a nonjudgmental manner, recognizing the common goal of ensuring the child's safety. **History from parents/ caregivers should be obtained separately from each other and the child.** Open-ended questions should be asked to determine how the injury occurred. Detailed notes of the reported history should be documented including the specific source of each piece of information. Aspects of the history that are generally concerning

include a significantly changing history or blaming the child or siblings for the injury. The caregiver history should include identifying the following:
a. The sequence of events just before and leading up to the injury
b. When the child was last completely normal and move forward from that time
c. Identifying all adults and caregivers who were with the child during the time of the injury episode
d. Identifying any other potential witnesses to the injury including verbal children
e. Medical history, developmental history, family history, a behavioral and physical review of systems, and a thorough social history
f. Risk factors include but are not limited to a history of interpersonal violence, substance use including alcohol, mental health issues, history with child protective services, and prior law enforcement involvement
g. Protective factors include but are not limited to family and community supports, assistance with childcare, the child's consistent participation in school and other activities, the family's strong meaningful connections to community agencies, and parental willingness to seek assistance

C. History from the child: Verbal children can be spoken to about the injuries separately without the adults' presence. A history can be obtained from children for whom this is developmentally appropriate. A child younger than 4 years is unlikely to be able to provide a meaningful history. Understanding any developmental delay or other relevant developmental or behavioral diagnoses is critically important in deciding whether a child should be asked to provide a history.
1. It is important to speak with children at their eye level in a developmentally appropriate way and ask open-ended questions:
   • *"What happened here (while pointing to an injury)?"* <u>NOT</u> "Is this where your father hit you?"
   • If the child discloses, follow up with a statement such as *"Please tell me more about that."*
   • When possible, immediately document what the child exactly says within quotes. Also, write down the question that elicited the disclosure when appropriate. If there is a delay between the disclosure and documentation of the child's statements, frame the disclosure with a phrase such as *"the child said something like..."* or *"in response to open-ended questions, the patient indicated that...."*
2. Obtain only information necessary for the medical diagnosis and treatment of the child. A detailed interview should be done by specially trained professionals in response to a report of the suspicious injuries to the local child welfare agency.
3. Reassure the child that it was okay to tell you, and whatever happened was not his or her fault.

D. Physical examination. The clinician should provide the child with an age-appropriate explanation of what will happen during the examination before performing the examination and should offer to answer any questions that the child has, if age appropriate. If photographs are to be taken, the clinician should explain to the child and parents/caregivers why this is being done. The examination should be completed in a child-friendly examination room with adequate lighting. **All children should be examined in a gown to assist with inspection of the entire skin.** Attention should be paid to respecting the child's privacy during the examination and the clinician should explain what will happen next as he or she proceeds.

A thorough physical examination should be performed with special attention to the head, ears, mouth, and neck. A full skin examination should be performed including the external genital area and buttocks. The location, size, and pattern of an injury should be completed with photographs and/or clearly documented drawings when possible, for example, right ventral upper arm with a "C"-shaped red purple bruise (approximately 2 cm × 3 cm). (See Table 35-1.)

Infants and young children are at the highest risk for abuse because they are nonverbal and have fewer developmental skills; therefore, an occult injury workup is recommended for any young children with suspected physical abuse.

E. Occult injury workup includes the following:
   • Head imaging (CT or MRI) for any infant younger than 4 months
   • Head imaging for any older infant or young child who has injury to the head and/or any symptoms that may be neurologic
   • Skeletal survey for any child younger than 24 months
   • Skeletal survey in older children who are nonmobile and nonverbal
   • ALT/AST for abdominal trauma

Table 35-1 • PARAMETERS OF THE PHYSICAL EXAMINATION IN CASES OF SUSPECTED PHYSICAL ABUSE

Examination	Important Findings
Growth parameters	Obtain and plot growth parameters (head circumference for <36 mo)
General	Altered level of consciousness
	Distress or discomfort
	Behavior during examination
Head, ears, eyes, nose, throat	Facial bruising (check under the chin and on the neck)
	Traction alopecia
	Subgaleal hemorrhages
	Subconjunctival hemorrhages
	Retinal hemorrhages (if intracranial injury identified, may need dilated examination with ophthalmology)
	Bruising on or behind ears
	Hemotympanum
	Nasal or oral bleeding, laceration, or bruising
	Frenulum injuries
	Dental injuries
	Dental impressions on mucosal surface of the upper lip
Chest/back	Any bruising or injury (palpate clavicles)
	Crepitus from rib fractures
Abdomen	Bruises (lack of bruising on the abdomen and torso does not exclude intra-abdominal injury)
	Distension or tenderness (consider pediatric surgery consult)
Genital area/buttocks	Bruising
	Bite marks
Extremities	Soft-tissue swelling
	Tenderness to palpation
	Deformities
	Asymmetry of movement/usage
Skin	Location of injuries (head, torso, ears, neck)
	Recognizable patterns
	Bilateral injuries
	Circumferential injuries
Neuro	Limping

- Abdominal CT for abdominal bruising or ALT/AST > 80
- With an increasing prevalence in substance abuse disorder in the adult population, a urine toxicology screen to identify concerning exposures in young children (marijuana, opiates, opioids, cocaine, and alcohol being the most common)
- Additional labs or imaging depending on the history and physical examination

F. **Differential diagnosis.** A good history and physical examination can often differentiate competing diagnostic possibilities from physical abuse. Some examples of the differential diagnosis can be found in Table 35-2. It is important to remember that some children may have a mimic of physical abuse such as congenital dermal melanosis and ALSO have injuries suspicious for physical abuse.

Table 35-2 • DIAGNOSTIC POSSIBILITIES TO CONSIDER WHEN EVALUATING CHILDREN FOR POSSIBLE PHYSICAL ABUSE

Findings	Diagnostic Possibilities
Bruising	Accidental bruising (in mobile children)
	Bleeding disorders: hemophilia, idiopathic thrombocytopenic purpura, Von Willebrand disease, vitamin K deficiency, leukemia
	Dye or ink
	Birth marks—dermal melanosis, café au lait spots, hemangioma
	Phytophotodermatitis
	Infectious diseases: meningococcemia or viral suppression of the bone marrow
	Folk remedies—coining/dermabrasion, cupping
	Vasculitis: Henoch–Schonlein purpura
	Medication-related bruising (anticoagulation)
	Ehlers–Danlos syndrome
Burns	Accidental burns
	Infections—impetigo, tinea, staphylococcal scaled skin syndrome
	Folk remedies—cupping, moxibustion
	Contact dermatitis
	Phytophotodermatitis
	Fixed drug eruption
Fractures	Birth trauma
	Congenital syphilis
	Accidental trauma
	Osteogenesis imperfecta
	Leukemia
	Infections: osteomyelitis, septic arthritis
	Scurvy
	Rickets
	Menkes syndrome
Intracranial bleeding	Motor vehicle accidents
	Accidental head injury
	Aneurysms
	Glutaric aciduria type I
	Menkes syndrome
	Herpes simplex meningoencephalitis

IV. MAKING THE DIAGNOSIS: SEXUAL ABUSE

A. History from the parent/caregiver (see Table 35-3): if a parent is concerned about possible sexual abuse of a child, it is important to speak with the parent separately without the child's presence. (Children are highly influenced by what they hear their parent say.)
  • Determine whether or not the child made a disclosure and the nature of the disclosure.
  • Determine the last exposure to the person who may have abused the child.
  • Determine any current safety concerns.

Table 35-3 • SEXUALLY TRANSMITTED INFECTIONS FOR THE DIAGNOSIS AND REPORTING OF SEXUAL ABUSE IN PREPUBERTAL CHILDREN

Type of Infection	Likelihood of Abuse	Reporting Guideline
Gonorrhea[a,b]	Certain	Report[c]
Syphilis[a]	Certain	Report[c]
Chlamydia trachomatis[a,b]	Certain	Report[c]
Trichomonas vaginalis[d]	Probable	Report[c]
Condyloma acuminatum[a]	Possible	Evaluate. Report if sexual abuse is suspected based on history and physical examination
Herpes simplex type 1,2[e]	Possible	Evaluate. Report if sexual abuse is suspected based on history and physical examination
Bacterial vaginosis	Uncertain	Evaluate. If no concerns, medical follow-up

[a]If not perinatally acquired.
[b]Before treatment, recommend confirmatory testing with a different section of the nucleic acid sequence on either same or new specimen.
[c]To agency mandated in community to receive reports of suspected sexual abuse.
[d]Differentiate from Trichomonas hominis.
[e]Serotyping of herpes does not help to determine the source or mechanism of transmission.

There is a spectrum of sexual abuse that include nontouching abuse such as exposure to sexual materials including pornography, inappropriate touching, and finally penetration. **Most cases of sexual abuse have normal or nonspecific examinations even when there has been a history of penetration.**

Within 72 hours of a sexual assault, a child should <u>immediately</u> be referred to a local child protection team, child advocacy center, or emergency department for an emergency examination and forensic evidence collection. An urgent evaluation by a child advocacy center or child protection team is recommended for suspected or reported sexual assault that occurred between 3 and 14 days before. If a child has sexualized behaviors, a nonspecific concern for sexual abuse, or has disclosed abuse longer than 2 weeks before, then a nonurgent evaluation can be scheduled at a child advocacy center or with a child protection team if the family/child is interested.

Identify whether there are developmentally normal versus concerning sexualized behaviors. To assess, determine the context of the behavior and the level of development of the child. Questions to consider include whether the behavior seems consistent with age-appropriate exploration and whether the other involved child is a peer. Concerning behaviors include sexual expression that is more adult-like than child-like, behavior that involves coercion, behavior that continues despite requests to stop, a pattern of a child sexualizing nonsexual things, or references to genitals or sexual acts in a child's drawings or play.

B. **History from the child.** In most cases of suspected sexual abuse, there is no need for the clinician to obtain a history directly from the child. If enough information is gathered from the parent/caregiver, the child interview should be deferred to a trained expert interviewer. **As in cases of suspected physical abuse, history should be obtained from a parent or caregiver separately without the child's presence.**

At times, medical clinicians may need to obtain a history relating to possible sexual abuse and should follow these guidelines:

1. Clinician must speak to the child and obtain the history alone.
   a. Children often are uncomfortable speaking about abuse in front of a parent.
   b. A parent/caregiver may try to influence the child's disclosure.
2. Sit at eye level and take time to establish rapport with neutral topics (e.g., ask about pets, school, and favorite activities).
3. Speak to the child at his or her developmental level and use his or her own terms for body parts.
   a. With young children, line drawings can be helpful.
   b. Anatomic drawings and dolls should <u>NOT</u> be used.

4. Introduce the topic of possible sexual abuse in a general way, for example:
   Do you know why you are here today?
   Is there anything bothering you?
   Is there anything that you feel worried or confused about?
   If these opening questions do not result in a spontaneous account, inquire more specifically:
   > *Has anyone touched you or treated you in a way that made you feel uncomfortable?*
   If the child responds "Yes," then say, *Tell me more about that.*
5. Use nonleading follow-up questions such as what, who, where, and when (if developmentally appropriate). Remain patient and avoid any demonstration of emotion, pressure, or correction of the child. Use prompts such as *Then what happened?* or *Tell me more.*
   a. Disclosures sometimes occur during the physical examination as the affected body parts are examined.
   b. When possible, immediately document what the child exactly says within quotes. Also, write down the question that elicited the disclosure when appropriate. If there is a delay between the disclosure and documentation of the child's statements, frame the disclosure with a phrase such as *"the child said something like..."* or *"in response to open ended questions, the patient indicated that..."*
   c. Obtain only information needed to help with the diagnosis and treatment of the child. A detailed interview should be done by specially trained professionals in response to a report of the sexual abuse to the local child welfare agency.
   d. Reassure the child that it was okay to tell you, and whatever happened was not his or her fault.
   e. Do not make promises to the child, such as they will only have to tell you and not tell anyone else.
C. Signs and symptoms in sexual abuse:
   • Genital or rectal pain, bleeding, injury, or infection
   • Sexually transmitted infection (See Table 35-3)
   • NO ABNORMAL FINDINGS AT ALL
D. **Physical examination.** It is important to do a complete physical examination, as this allows for a familiar context for the child. The genital examination is then a part of a fuller examination to check the child's health and to screen for findings that might raise the possibility of physical abuse. Attention should be paid to respecting the child's privacy during the examination and the clinician should explain what will happen next as he or she proceeds. Confirm any concerning findings with a clinician experienced in examining children for sexual abuse.

   Prepare the child with a developmentally appropriate explanation of the examination. This should include why the clinician is examining the genitals. For example, *"I am a clinician and here to check you from head to toe to ensure everything is healthy."* When it comes time for the genital part of the examination, a useful frame is: *"Next I am going to check the private parts of your body and I am only doing it because I am a clinician here to make sure your private parts are healthy."* Because most examinations are normal and occur at a time distant from the abusive episode, if a child is unable to cooperate with the examination despite attempts to distract/redirect the child, the examination should be stopped at that time. Later, in discussion with the parent/caregiver, it can be determined whether an examination should be attempted again in the future and where that examination should take place (primary care office or the office of a child abuse specialist).

   Female genital examination: Careful inspection of the vulva (external only), unless internal trauma is suspected. (In rare circumstances, when an internal exam is needed, prepubertal girls require the pelvic/internal examination under anesthesia.)
   1. Examination is done in supine frog-leg, prone knee-chest, or lithotomy position with both labial separation and labial traction.
   2. Use a good light source with magnification (i.e., otoscope head, handheld or headpiece lens, magnifying florescent light, or a colposcope).
   3. Know genital anatomy and normal developmental variant.
      • All girls are born with a hymen.
      • Newborn hymens are fleshy and redundant due to maternal estrogen effect.
      • Prepubertal hymens have thinner tissue.
      • Pubertal hymens are thickened and redundant from estrogen.
   4. Be aware of normal anatomic variation.
      • Most hymens are one of the five shapes: annular (circumferential), crescentic (posterior rim), fimbriated (redundant), sleeve-like, or septate

- Nontraumatic variations include periurethral and perihymenal bands, small hymenal mounds adjacent to internal vaginal ridges, perineal midline raphe, and hymenal tags.
5. Abnormal findings not due to sexual abuse: urethral prolapse, lichen sclerosis, genital hemangiomas, and straddle injuries.
6. Genital findings that can represent sexual abuse include the following:
   - Acute: lacerations, abrasions, ecchymoses, edema, transection of the posterior hymen
   - Chronic: scarring of hymen or other genital structures, healed transection of the posterior hymen, absent or markedly diminished sections of posterior hymenal tissue
   - Most often, there are no abnormal findings even with clear disclosures of sexual abuse

Male genital examination should include a careful inspection of the penis, urethra meatus, scrotum, and the surrounding skin for evidence of trauma or infection.

Anal examination:
- Know anal anatomy and variations:
  - Smooth areas at the 6- and 12-o'clock position: diastasis ani
  - Midline skin tags
  - Venous congestion
  - Increased pigmentation
  - Erythema
  - Dilation during an examination if there are feces in rectum
- Anal findings that can represent trauma/sexual abuse:
  - Acute: lacerations, abrasions, ecchymoses, fissures that extend past the anal verge
  - Chronic (very rare): scars, persistent dilation without feces in the rectum

Laboratory testing:
1. When indicated by the history or physical findings, test for gonorrhea in the throat, anus, and vagina or urethra, and for chlamydia in the vagina/urethra and anus. If there is a positive result, confirm with another section of the nucleic acid on the same or a new specimen. In most instances, treatment should be deferred pending confirmation of diagnosis.
2. Serologic testing for syphilis, human immunodeficiency virus, hepatitis B (both surface antigen and surface antibody), and hepatitis C should be performed if warranted by the history. Incubation period can be up to 3 months for syphilis and 6 months for HIV; therefore repeat testing is recommended, if initiated before the end of the incubation period.
3. Symptomatic children should be cultured for other genital infections including those caused by *Trichomonas*, *Gardnerella vaginalis*, *Streptococcus pyogenes*, and *Candida*. Testing for herpes simplex can be considered if it would change management, although differentiating HSV-1 from HSV-2 does not assist in determining whether an HSV infection was transmitted through sexual contact. Condyloma acuminata is diagnosed clinically.
4. If having dysuria, consider a urinalysis and urine culture.
5. Perform a pregnancy test on pubertal or peripubertal girls.

V. BEHAVIORAL INDICATORS IN CHILD PHYSICAL AND SEXUAL ABUSE. Behaviors seen in children who have been abused are similar to symptoms due to other stressors and trauma. They are not specifically indicative of abuse.
- Fears/phobias, especially triggered by circumstances that remind the child of the abuse
- Nightmares and other sleep disturbances
- Appetite changes or eating disorders
- Enuresis or encopresis
- Change in behavior, attitude, or school performance
- Depression, withdrawal from social situations, or suicidality
- Excessive anger, aggression, or running away
- Multiple sexual partners at a young age
- Substance abuse

VI. MANAGEMENT. The goals of management are to provide medical treatment if indicated, arrange for psychosocial support for the child and family, and protect the child from further abuse by reporting to child protective services. This is to ensure the safety of the child and other children within the same environment. In all states, clinicians are responsible by law for reporting suspicion for abuse to child welfare agencies. These cases require a multidisciplinary approach from medical personnel, child welfare authorities, and law enforcement officials.

Next steps:
  File a child abuse report with child protective services. When possible, explain your concerns to the parent/caregiver and inform them that you are filing a report.
  Any positive findings warrant a conversation with or referral to a child abuse specialist.
Help guide family toward healing:
* Alert the family to some possible behavioral and emotional reactions that the child may have, especially if the family constellation is disrupted.
* Encourage a sense of physical security for the child after the disclosure, including reassurance of children who were threatened with harm that there is no danger.
* Provide or arrange for crisis intervention counseling, if needed.
* Parents should neither try to make children forget nor pry into details, but rather be open to children's expressions about and reactions to their experience.
* Encourage parents to maintain normal routines, physical affection, and limit setting whenever possible.
* Remind parents/caregivers to attend to the needs or the rest of the family and themselves.

As a child enters each successive developmental stage, new questions and feelings often arise. Be prepared to normalize these feelings for the family/caregivers and the child.

Most children who have been abused should be referred to an experienced mental health clinician (ideally one who has training in trauma-informed therapies) to evaluate the need for ongoing treatment. Even children without overt symptoms can harbor negative or confused feelings that might be revealed only in the context of a full evaluation or an ongoing relationship with a trusted therapist.

Be aware of local resources:
* Parent groups, offender treatment, witness advocates, and children's groups
* Mental health resources who specialize in trauma treatment

VII. CLINICAL PEARLS AND PITFALLS
A. Physical abuse
* Obtain all information in a nonjudgmental manner.
* Nonmobile children with unexplained bruising should have a workup completed for possible child physical abuse.
* Rely on history and physical examination findings to narrow the differential diagnosis.

B. Sexual abuse
* Rely on history to make the diagnosis of sexual abuse, as most abused children have no physical findings. (This is because many forms of abuse do not physically injure the child, or when injuries occur, they heal quickly. Even hymenal tears can heal completely without scarring.)
* A normal examination neither rules out nor confirms the possibility of sexual abuse or prior penetration.
* Take the child's statements and behavior seriously. The incidence of genital complaints is higher than the incidence of genital findings in sexually abused children.
* Children who imitate adult sex acts or touch other children inappropriately should be evaluated for possible sexual abuse. Normal sexual behavior among peers is exploratory and limited (i.e., showing each other private body parts).
* Children who demonstrate overt sexual behaviors may also have been exposed to age-inappropriate media and information.
* Make sure that the parent/caregiver(s) have adequate support. The child's adjustment is related to the family adjustment.
* Sexually abused children need reassurance that their bodies are healthy and fine.

VIII. SUMMARY.
Clinicians should maintain awareness of physical or sexual abuse as diagnostic possibilities when confronted with a concerning injury, behavior, or physical examination finding. The objective facts of a patient's presentation should guide next steps. These next steps include consultation with a child abuse specialist and/or referral to a local emergency department for further evaluation so that the suspected maltreatment can be promptly and appropriately addressed.

Bibliography

FOR CLINICIANS
Adams JA, Harper K, Knudson S, Revilla J. Examination findings in legally confirmed child sexual abuse: it's normal to be normal. *Pediatrics*. 1994;94:310-317.
Christian CW, Committee on Child Abuse and Neglect. The evaluation of suspected child physical abuse. *Pediatrics*. 2015;135:e1337-e1354.

Jenny C, Crawford-Jakubiak JE, Committee on Child Abuse and Neglect, American Academy of Pediatrics. The evaluation of children in the primary care setting when sexual abuse is suspected. *Pediatrics*. 2013;132:e558-e567.

Johnson TC. *Updated and Expanded - Understanding Children's Sexual Behaviors: What's Natural and Healthy*. Family Violence & Sexual Assault Institute; 2015.

Kellogg ND. Clinical report—the evaluation of sexual behaviors in children. *Pediatrics*. 2009;124:992-928.

Sheets LK, Leach ME, Koszewski IJ, Lessmeier AM, Nugent M, Simpson P. Sentinel injuries in infants evaluated for child physical abuse. *Pediatrics*. 2013;131:701-707.

CHAPTER 36

Chronic Conditions

Jodi K. Wenger | Jack S. Maypole

I. DEFINITION AND DEMOGRAPHICS

A. In 1998 the American Academy of Pediatrics (AAP) defined children with special health care needs (CSHCN) as those who have or are at increased risk for a chronic physical, developmental, behavioral, or emotional condition and who also require health and related services of a type or amount beyond that required by children generally. In 2009–2010 the Maternal and Child Health Bureau reported that there were 11 million children or 15% of all children in the United States in the category of children and youth with special health care needs (CYSHCN).

B. Children with medical complexity. In 2011, a subcategory, called children with medical complexity (CMC), was identified and defined as patients with chronic conditions, multiple family-identified service needs, functional limitations requiring medical equipment, and extraordinarily high health care use and cost. This population makes up less than 1% of the pediatric population and 5% of the population of CYSHCN but consumes a disproportionately large portion of all pediatric health care spending costs. CMCs comprise the most complex segment of CYSHCN. Altogether they comprise a heterogenous span of medical, neurodevelopmental, and, very often, associated psychosocial conditions. Over time, individuals may fall into or out of this category as conditions improve or progress.

C. Systems of care. At present, the growing number of CYSHCN has outpaced a consistent national strategy for managing their multifaceted needs. Professional and academic organizations as well as federal and state health agencies have increasingly identified this population as a priority for care innovation and quality improvement by dint of the challenge they present to systems of care.

II. FAMILY AND CLINICIAN PERSPECTIVE OF CARING FOR CYSHCN

A. Social, emotional, and behavioral impact of complex conditions on parents

In addition to the amount of time involved and the extra care required for families who care for CMC, parents consistently convey the burden and stress they face from inadequate and fragmented care coordination, frequent provider visits, financial difficulties, complex and time-consuming bureaucracy, and household and relationship stress, while compensating for missed days at work or caretakers' inability to work. In addition, families face long-term and persistent challenges to find appropriate respite, in home nursing support and appropriate childcare or after-school programs. The caregiving and emotional burden of neurodevelopmental disorders including seizures, autism spectrum disorder, cerebral palsy, and global developmental delay also have important implications for family and marital functioning.

Depression, and/or the so-called medical post-traumatic stress disorder, and other behavioral and emotional disorders have higher prevalence among the adult caretakers of CYSHCN and CMCs, and research suggests that many parents are unsuccessful or unable to seek care for themselves. One study showed that mothers of children born with birth defects died at an earlier age compared with mothers whose newborns did not have such problems. Availabilities of social media, Web sites, chronic condition online forums, and special education Listservs offer newer ways to communicate with providers, peers, and virtual communities to access medical information.

B. Social, emotional, and behavioral impact of complex conditions on children

Children with chronic problems have diminished family functioning, more school absences, and less participation in community activities compared with healthy peers. Parents of CMC experienced more difficulty with childcare, employment, and parenting skills. Financial stress in addition to these social determinants of health are particularly challenging with families from lower socioeconomic or underserved communities, known in the literature as "double jeopardy."

CYSHCN and CMCs have up to four times higher rates of psychiatric comorbidities, such as anxiety and depression, than their healthy, neurotypical peers. Consequently, screening for depression and emotional health concerns remains a priority for care team members in a patient's medical home, with established pathways to connect children and household members of concern with behavioral health supports. Linking children with others via support groups, camps, organizations, and Web sites are helpful ways to ensure they feel connected to others. Cognitive behavioral therapy may be a very helpful approach for most verbal children.

C. **Clinician perspectives**

In general, primary care providers based in community- or hospital-based practices frequently describe their work with CYSHCN and CMCs as intellectually stimulating and professionally rewarding. Relationships with parents and patient can be especially satisfying although not without periodic intense challenges. Providers also identify a number of barriers including inadequate time for patient encounters, metrics for productivity that don't allow for the extra time needed for complex care visits, insufficient reimbursement for the extra administrative time required between visits, and very often, a lack of support services to offer comprehensive care management. Further, for children with less common chronic conditions, additional factors negatively impact care including unfamiliar diagnoses with a dearth of practice guidelines, fragmented care that may involve large numbers of subspecialists and caregivers, dysfunctional communication systems and poor interoperability between electronic health records, polypharmacy, multiorgan system involvement, and family systems that may be stressed and overwhelmed.

Recent practice innovations have sought to address such complex patients to lower cost and improve health outcomes, while building resilience and preventing burnout of care team and family members with remodeled multidisciplinary teams.

D. **Medical education and training programs on complex care**

Increasingly, curricula emphasize understanding of and exposure to care coordination, emerging technology, the interplay of social determinants with overall health of a family, shared decision-making and having more longitudinal experiences.

III. **MANAGING CYSHCN AND CMC IN PRACTICE.** The Triple Aim of the Institute of Healthcare Improvement: finding a balance between patient and parent satisfaction, money saved, and improved health care outcome needs to be the driving priority. Many pediatric tertiary care centers offer either primary care for patients with CYSHCN and CMC or secondary care for patients of community-based providers. Studies of families who obtain their care from this specialized patient-centered tertiary medical home are more likely to encounter expanded care teams, including care coordinators, social work support, and community health workers with experience in complex care and community-based services. In outlying and rural areas, future innovations will continue to leverage the use of telemedicine and other technology to access the concentrated expertise and support at larger centers of care. While payment systems are evolving in this realm, well-respected and growing initiatives such as Project ECHO may eventually decrease the prominence of in-person visits to subspecialists. A related version is the use of secure videoconference technology that may allow medically fragile patients to be managed remotely, at least in part, via direct communication with the patient or family member, or facilitated by a care team member, such as a community health worker or nurse.

IV. **BUILDING IN EFFICIENCY AND INNOVATION FOR COMPLEX VISITS.** Community-based practices may lack the infrastructure and the capacity to deal extensively with large volumes of CYSHCN and CMC. However, given that most programs will have a small number of such patients in each provider's panel, we offer some short- and longer-term strategies that may allow for more efficient workflow and ways to "divide and conquer" the oft encountered "multiple, unmet urgent needs" of these patients and families.

A. **Organize your system**

1. Use the best principles of short-term quality improvement to pilot innovations and changes for your system of care. Identify a workgroup drawing upon the experience of any staff with savvy on the patient-centered medical home. Early on, designate your target population of CYSHCN, how they will be identified, and how they can be tracked and monitored for scheduling and follow-up purposes.

2. **Special scheduling.** Consider the use of alternative iterations of scheduling encounters, using longer appointments (booking slots back to back) or booking early or later in the session. In practices well integrated with specialty programs, multiple appointment bookings on the same day may allow for enhanced communication and problem-solving. The Center for Medicare/Medicaid is developing new codes that capture complex care billing. Document accordingly to optimize the revenue for the effort.

3. **The medical home.** Use best practice aspects of the AAP Patient-Centered Medical Home. When possible, identify a **care coordinator** for high- and rising-risk patients. Consider asking a nurse, social worker, or family navigator to oversee care

plan implementation. Delegate a provider who can assist with associated work such as prescription refills, prior authorization, and ordering durable medical equipment.

B. Organizing your visit

1. Previsit

- Create a rough outline of your agenda in an editable Shared Plan of Care (SPoC) (Fig. 36-1) based on guidelines and medical research on diagnosis. Store in an easy to access, editable page of your electronic medical record (EMR).
- Include a section for your medical goals, parent/guardian and patient goals as well.

Goals of care per 3/2018 encounter

1. Prosthetic replacement
2. MRI in 6/2018
3. Immunology follow-up appointment

Family goals

1. Family wants to learn about epilepsy camps
2. Parents want two appointments on same day when they come to hospital

Barriers to care

1. Will need Arabic translator
2. Children's need for constant supervision and full support with all self-care and ADLs

Team members

1. Immunology/allergy, Dr. Leuko, 555-1212, or message through EMR, patient on penicillin, had Prevnar
2. Neurology—Dr. Theo, 555-1212 or page
3. Physiatrist—Dr. Femur, not in on Mondays, 555-1212
4. Orthotist—Local community orthotist
5. GI and dietician—Dr. Antrum, Wednesday/Fridays

ID: A 5-year-old girl with tuberous sclerosis, epilepsy, developmental delay, s/p leg amputation after septic shock, G-tube

1. **Tuberous sclerosis/epilepsy**

    a. Dr. Theo, Neurology 1/2018, recommended yearly brain MRI, abdominal MRI. Call neuropsychologist about TAND (Tuberous Sclerosis Associated Neuropsychiatric Disorders)

    b. On AEDs well controlled, LTM EEG 10/2017, levels checked 9/2017

2. **Immunology**—Dr. Leuko, Allergy/immunology 9/2017, s/p septic shock and amputation of lower extremity, s/p bacteremia, immunology felt like all cells were ok, but is checking on function of cells, follow-up with immunology 3/2018

3. **Amputation of left leg**—Dr. Femur, Physiatry 12/2017 needs follow-up with physiatrist after orthotist appointment for new prosthetic

    a. Is school encouraging use?

4. **G-tube**—Dr. Antrum 1/2018, G-tube size 3.5 mm, no longer using, good growth, consider removal after winter

5. **Developmental Delay**—IEP at school, gets extended school year, handicapped bus

Routine health care maintenance

1. **Immunizations**—UTD including influenza vaccine 2017/2018
2. **Dental**—Dr. Pulp follow-up two times a year
3. **Hearing screening**—Passed 3/2018
4. **Vision screening**—Ophtho 10/2017, no glasses

Figure 36-1 Shared plan of care for fictional patient, Jill Doe. EMR, electronic medical record; MRI, magnetic resonance imaging; ADL, activities of daily living; s/p, status post; AED, antiepileptic drugs; LTM, long term monitoring; UTD, up to date.

- The SPoC is helpful for subspecialists, covering providers, school nurses, and family. It is also a great way to remind you about medical details and family goals before the next visit.
- Access, review, and update SPoC with interval procedures, subspecialty, and admission notes.
- Determine the best way to communicate or query subspecialists to clarify concerns. Electronic means are often easier than a phone call.
- For the family, consider implementation of a previsit checklist to prompt provider of the current needs and concerns, including symptoms, treatment plan changes, refill and durable medical equipment needs, or communication with other medical, school-based, or community-based team members.

2. **The outpatient visit**
   - Before the visit, consider a rough outline of your agenda for this visit: Consider templated and reusable plain language, discharge instructions of family needs written in checklist fashion that may outline the next steps of care and/or build in transparency and accountability for all concerned (including the patient!). Ideally, offer an SPoC when appropriate, and update it at least every 6 months.
   - Templates: Consider creating or reaching out to others about reusable smart phrase templates for the outpatient visit in the EMR that contain critical information based on diagnosis and can be edited and placed in an easy-to-access part of the EMR. A box format may be easier to navigate than a paragraph.
   - Create or borrow action plans, medical orders for life-sustaining treatment forms, guardianship paperwork, medical authorizations for school medication use, and durable medical equipment prescription information on formulas, diapers, shower chairs, or hospital beds.
   - Anticipatory guidance: Little is published on appropriate anticipatory guidance for children based on their diagnosis. Modify the anticipatory guidance you offer these families to ensure that it is tangible to their circumstance. Become available with resources in your community and have information and Web sites available for families. Learn about local Special Olympics or programs at your local YMCA.
   - Consider safety recommendations: Parking placard for children who may bolt, shoe ID, or MedicAlert applications, police programs that may keep track of high-risk patients, contact with emergency medical service to ensure they understand do not resuscitate, medical needs, home locks for windows and doors. Consider creating an editable safety action plan for seizures, G-tube issues, and shunt issues that can be shared with others.
   - Psychosocial needs: With high rates of mental health issues for both patients and parents, have a plan to offer support, connections to others living with same issues, and mental health services to these families.

3. **Postvisit.** Catalog and use a secure means to track and assign tasks for care management.
   - SPoC/after-visit summary: A plan of care is jointly developed and shared among the primary care provider, the CYSHCN, their family, and the broader health care team. It identifies the strengths and needs of the child and family and is routinely evaluated and updated in partnership with the family (at least) every 6 months; and clearly identifies all entities that participate in a child's care coordination activities and the family's shared goals. In the emerging models of accountable care organizations, increasingly patient engagement and family activation is considered a key measure of performance or as a quality metric of a practice. Electronic health record–based plans of care, with shared access with caregivers and eligible adolescents, may be an area where these aspects can be measured and where accountability for following through on next steps of treatment—collaboratively by providers or by families—may be monitored.

V. TRANSITIONING TO ADULT CARE
- Historically, research shows CYSHCN and CMC encounter fragmentation of their care and potential setbacks or complications as they "graduate" from pediatric-oriented providers.
- A paucity of well-equipped, dedicated providers or the sudden and simultaneous change of medical and behavioral health teams in addition to community-based and school-based services may challenge even the most well-supported young adult. Surveys of family members document the difficulty they encounter with adult systems of care, finding them to be more fragmented and less accommodating to a family-centered approach.

Table 36-1 • DURABLE MEDICAL EQUIPMENT NEEDS

1. **Cardiovascular/respiratory devices**: oxygen and vital sign monitoring, ventilators, nebulizers, blood pressure monitors, tracheostomy supplies, and suction pump and supplies

2. **Feeding and Nutrition Kitchen accessories:** feeding chair or high chair, special bottles, spoons, G-tube, feeding pump, bags, tubing, special formula, blender

3. **Self-care/hygiene:** shower chair, commode, shower mat, diapers and pull-ups, shower hand bars, latex-free gloves, chux, wipes

4. **Bedding/sleep:** hospital bed, bed side rails, video baby monitor

5. **Positioning/mobility**: wheelchair, stroller, walkers or crutches, gait trainers, standers, braces, orthotics, prosthetics, adaptive car seat, recreational, home and vehicle modifications (ramps, integration of special seating or wheelchair)

6. **Adaptive tech**: communication devices, PECs, adaptive computer or tablet attachments, low-vision or low-hearing adaptive equipment

- Studies have shown that adults with intellectual disabilities and/or multiple disabilities experience fewer hours and lower pay for employment, they have lower rates of graduation from university, they have lower rates of marriage, and they are less likely to live independently.
- Over the last two decades, the principle societies of adult and pediatric providers, including the AAP, the American Academy of Family Practice (AAFP), and the American College of Physicians (ACP), have collaborated to establish guidelines for and to bring attention to transitioning CYSHCN and CMC to adult care. Ideally, each patient-centered medical home has an established approach to these children and adolescents that integrates these key concepts:
  - Transition planning begins at age 13 years and may be done using tools or checklists to guide questions and inform tasks at each step.
  - Transition planning should involve the adolescent/young adult as much as possible, specifically informing their preferences when forming shared goals of care.
  - Implementing a system of transition management for complex patients may be an excellent opportunity for quality improvement project for practices and/or may allow designation of responsibilities and roles among patient-centered medical home team members.
  - For providers who may not have a grasp of available programs for primary care to graduate their complex young adult patients, it may be appropriate to reach out to their region or state's medical society or professional society, such as the AAP, AAFP, or ACP.
  - Tools and resources for managing the transition process (including documentation and guardianship planning), may vary per state.

Bibliography

FOR PROFESSIONALS

Forum on Promoting Children's Cognitive, Affective, and Behavioral Health, Board on Children, Youth, and Families, Division of Behavioral and Social Sciences and Education, Health and Medicine Division, National Academies of Sciences, Engineering, and Medicine. *Ensuring Quality and Accessible Care for Children with Disabilities and Complex Health and Educational Needs: Proceedings of a Workshop.* Washington (DC), US: National Academies Press; October 24, 2016.

Packard report. https://www.lpfch.org/publication/achieving-shared-plan-care-children-and-youth-special-health-care-needs.

Packard report. https://www.lpfch.org/publication/standards-systems-care-children-and-youth-special-health-care-needs-version-20.

Project ECHO. https://echo.unm.edu.

Russell CJ, Simon TD. Care of children with medical complexity in the hospital setting. *Pediatr Ann.* 2014;43(7):e157-e162.

Sadof M, Gortakowski M, Stechenberg B, Carlin S. The "HEADS AT" training tool for residents: a roadmap for caring for children with medical complexity. *Clin Pediatr.* 2015;54(12):1210-1214.

CHAPTER 37

Chronic Abdominal Pain

Claudio Morera

I. DESCRIPTION OF THE PROBLEM

A. Definition. Chronic abdominal pain (CAP) is episodic or continuous abdominal pain for at least 2 months. It might or might not interfere with daily functioning. Recurrent abdominal pain (RAP) is a clinical description and not a diagnosis. To avoid confusion from initial descriptions of the problem, it is better called CAP and it can be organic abdominal pain and functional abdominal pain (FAP).

B. Epidemiology

- CAP can be 2%–4% of all pediatric visits.
- Weekly abdominal pain is reported in 13% of middle school and 17% of high school students.
- FAP prevalence in pediatric gastroenterology, using very strict criteria, has been reported in 7.5%.

C. Etiology

1. **Organic abdominal pain.** Although the list of possible etiologies is large, only 10%–25% of children presenting with CAP have an identifiable organic etiology. Table 37-1 shows a list of disorders that can present as CAP that can mimic FAP.

2. **FAP.** FAP is the main cause of CAP in the pediatric age group. It is not an exclusion diagnosis; currently diagnostic criteria have been developed that allows a positive diagnosis. A combined interaction between altered gastrointestinal (GI) motility, visceral sensation, and psychological factors is the main pathophysiologic mechanism. The biopsychosocial model provides the conceptual basis to FAP, including potential etiologies such as genetics, postinfectious, certain foods such as sorbitol and other carbohydrates, psychological stress, school stress, and other anxiety. The concept of health and disease as well as coping skills may also play a role. Parents of patients with FAP have more GI complaints, anxiety, and somatization. Their understanding and acceptance of the biopsychosocial concept is associated with recovery.

II. MAKING THE DIAGNOSIS OF FAP.
The main purpose is to establish the diagnosis of FAP, which was an exclusion diagnosis, but clinical diagnostic criteria have been developed to make a positive diagnosis of FAP with minimal workup (Rome IV criteria, Table 37-2).

A. Signs and symptoms. The abdominal pain is typically periumbilical, lasts 30–60 minutes, and occurs during the day (rarely awakening the child from sleep). It might or might not be associated with alterations in daily functioning. In most cases, the pain pattern cannot differentiate organic from functional, but the presence of red flags (Table 37-3) has a high-positive predictive value for organic disease.

If there is some loss of daily functioning and additional somatic symptoms (headaches, limb pain, or difficulty sleeping), FAP syndrome is present.

B. Differential diagnosis. The initial differentiation is between organic and FAP. Other functional bowel disorders associated with pain should also be considered, that is, irritable bowel syndrome, abdominal migraine, functional dyspepsia, etc.

C. History: key clinical questions

1. *"When did the abdominal pain begin? How often does it occur? Where does it hurt? Has the child located the area by pointing with one finger?"* Establish the origin point in time (at least 2 months), frequency (at least four times per month), and localization.

2. *"Has there been weight loss?"* Investigation of red flags.

3. *"How is the stooling pattern?"* Constipation or diarrhea must be investigated as a potential red flag as well as other functional GI disorder such as irritable bowel syndrome or functional constipation.

4. To both the parent and child: *"What do you think is going on? What do you do when the pain starts or to control it? How does it interfere with daily functioning, school missing, etc.? Are there similar symptoms or other functional disorders in family members?"* It is important to start with open questions and let both parents and patient

Table 37-1 • ORGANIC ABDOMINAL PAIN THAT CAN MIMIC FUNCTIONAL

- Carbohydrate malabsorption
- Parasitic (*Giardia*)
- Inflammatory bowel disease
- Constipation
- Allergic enteropathy
- Celiac disease
- Antibiotic-associated diarrhea
- Peptic ulcer
- Gastroesophageal reflux disease
- Eosinophilic esophagitis
- Crohn disease
- Cholelithiasis
- Pancreatitis

Table 37-2 • DIAGNOSTIC CRITERIA FOR CHILDHOOD FUNCTIONAL ABDOMINAL PAIN

Criteria fulfilled at least four times per month for at least 2 months before diagnosis

Must include all the following:
- Episodic or continuous abdominal pain that does not occur solely during physiologic events (e.g., eating, menses)
- Insufficient criteria for irritable bowel syndrome, functional dyspepsia, or abdominal migraine
- After appropriate evaluation, the abdominal pain cannot be fully explained by another medical condition

Table 37-3 • RED FLAGS

- Involuntary weight loss
- Decreased linear growth
- Pubertal delay
- Significant vomiting
- Gastrointestinal blood loss
- Chronic diarrhea
- Anemia
- Persistent pain in right upper abdomen or right lower abdomen
- Nocturnal pain: pain awakening the child at night
- Dysphagia
- Arthritis
- Perianal disease
- Unexplained fever
- Dysuria
- Inflammation signs (elevated erythrocyte sedimentation rate, elevated C-reactive protein, etc.)
- Family history of inflammatory bowel disease or peptic ulcer disease

elaborate. We need to determine how much the symptoms impair functioning, what is the reward system in the family, what behaviors are reinforced (health or disease), and what are the fears and prior experiences with chronic pain. The objective is to understand the family concept of health and disease, their understanding of the biopsychosocial concept of disease, coping skills, and presence of anxiety, depression, or somatization in the family as well as in the child.

D. Behavioral observations. Observe parent–child interaction (is the patient allowed to answer questions, is he or she treated as if he or she was younger, etc.?) and reaction to pain complaints. Observe developmental state of the patient as well as body posture, dressing, etc.

E. Physical examination. A complete physical examination is essential. Any area not examined at this time should be clearly noted so it can be examined in the future.

F. Laboratory evaluation. If the history and physical examination suggest a specific etiology, appropriate tests should be ordered. Otherwise, the initial laboratory evaluation should be quite limited and is oriented to rule out most organic conditions (Table 37-4).

Table 37-4 • INITIAL WORKUP

Complete physical examination—including rectal examination, examination of spine, and neurologic examination
Initial laboratory examination Urinalysis (culture in females) Complete blood cell count, erythrocyte sedimentation rate, and C-reactive protein Celiac serologies Liver and kidney profiles Stool for ova and parasites Fecal occult blood Fecal lactoferrin or calprotectin (if suggested by history and physical)
Lactose breath test (if suggested by history and physical)
Abdominal ultrasound (if suggested by history and physical)

III. MANAGEMENT

A. **Objectives.** Identify and treat organic diseases producing CAP, decrease pain, and modulate the impact of chronic pain in daily functioning. These are met by a thorough clinical evaluation and the establishment of a clear management and treatment plan with realistic expectations with the patient and the family.

B. **Initial treatment strategies**

1. **Education.** On the initial evaluation, the clinician should explain that most children will not have an identifiable organic etiology for their pain and will fulfill the criteria for FAP. The clinician should explain that the objective of the initial visits is to find organic disease, if present, and to manage the symptoms with available interventions. Explain the interaction between GI motility, enhanced sensation, and psychological factors including anxiety. It is important to explain that FAP is better understood using a biopsychosocial model. Close to 75% of children whose parents understood and accepted the psychological component improved their symptoms.

2. **Medication.** In most patients the initial visit is enough to establish a positive diagnosis of FAP, to order a minimal workup plan, and to design a management plan.

   Histamine-2 receptor blockers: In a double-blind placebo-controlled trial in patients with FAP and dyspeptic symptoms using famotidine at 0.5 mg/kg twice a day, 68% of patients in the treatment group improved versus 12% in the placebo group.

   Migraine medication: (See Chapter 23.) For patients with FAP and diagnosis of abdominal migraine.

   Antidepressants: Have been used extensive with good results in adults with functional abdominal disorders including functional abdominal pain. The evidence of its effectivity in children is not that strong (although a strong placebo effect was also reported), with possible concerning side effects especially with selective serotonin reuptake inhibitors (SSRIs).

   Others: Antispasmodics (mint oil, hyoscyamine, and dicyclomine) have been used with good long-term effect for mint oil and short-term effect for hyoscyamine and dicyclomine.

   Cyproheptadine: Few studies but significant improvement in the treatment group compared with placebo.

   Others include probiotics, antibiotics, and prokinetics.

3. **Diet**

   Fiber: The evidence supporting the use of fiber to treat FAP is weak and inconclusive. On the other hand, it is an inexpensive intervention that might benefit some patients. The Daily Reference Intakes (RDI) for fiber from 2–10 years varies from 15 to 25 g/d. The recommended dose for adults is 30 g/d. It can be provided through diet or by adding extra fiber supplements. It is important to increase fiber intake on a step-up approach, increasing the daily intake weekly to decrease bloating and gassiness that can happen with abrupt increases in fiber intake.

   Lactose: There is inconclusive evidence that a lactose-free diet decreases symptoms in children with FAP. Two studies have compared lactose-free diet with lactose-containing diet. There were no differences in rate of recovery or increased pain in lactose digesters versus lactose nondigesters. Lactose intolerance and FAP seem to be two different entities.

4. **Behavioral interventions.** There have been several trials of cognitive behavioral therapy (CBT) and they provide evidence that it may be useful in improving pain

and disability. Programs include reinforcement of well behavior, distraction, and cognitive coping skills training such as self-efficacy statements, self-induced relaxation, and self-administration of rewards. The training is directed to both patients and parents.

The American Academy of Pediatrics subcommittee on chronic abdominal pain recently concluded that CBT might be useful in "improving pain and disability outcome in the short term."

Adding behavioral intervention to the use of fiber has been shown to offer better results to fiber alone.

Other behavioral interventions include guided imagery, hypnotherapy, and other relaxations techniques. These have also shown to reduce the days with pain and improve functioning.

Overall, CBT appears to be an efficacious treatment for children with chronic abdominal pain. Incorporation of psychological treatments into the management of patients seems to be a reasonable consideration.

    5. **Parents' role.** As stated before, caretakers play a key role in the management of pediatric FAP. Cognitive behavioral interventions are reinforced by the parents, so it is essential that they understand and accept the psychological component of FAP to improve outcome. Also they report the presence of red flag symptoms and should be instructed to recognize and report them to the clinician.

  C. **Backup strategies.** Because the pain of FAP can persist even after initial interventions, it is essential for the clinician to remain vigilant for an etiologic cause and not to be discouraged. Support and reinforcement of the functional nature of the condition is vital. We are aiming for care and control rather than cure, using a similar approach of coping as is used for other chronic conditions. It is also important to understand that failing to find an organic cause or failure of control with initial management does not mean that FAP is not the diagnosis. Do not transmit your uncertainty to the patient by escalating diagnostic tests; rather refer to a specialist *"not because I don't know what you have but to have specialized management."*

IV. CLINICAL PEARLS AND PITFALLS

- There is no substitute for a complete and thorough initial history and physical examination. Unnecessary laboratory and radiologic tests often lead parents to believe that there is an organic etiology for the abdominal pain. Clinical criteria and minimal negative initial workup (Table 37-4) are enough to diagnose FAP.
- Reassure and explain the biopsychosocial concept of FAP.
- Explain to the child that abdominal pain is common in children of their age and that the pain does not mean that there is something wrong. Most patients resolve their symptoms. It is not life-threatening.
- It is important for parents to understand that the pain is a product of a combination of physiological and psychological stressors with no one more important than the other.
- Keep close follow-up. Initially, monthly visits and more frequent phone follow-up calls are advisable. It reinforces the idea that you are not ignoring the pain and also helps coaching the behavioral interventions.
- Do not discourage second opinions or referral to specialist if a family is uncomfortable with your evaluation of their child's abdominal pain. Offer options of specialists, which you consider have a reasonable approach to FAP and discourage "doctor shopping."
- If FAP escalation in treatment is considered, refer the child to a specialist (gastroenterologist or mental health professional) who has an expertise in the management of these conditions.

Bibliography

Brown LK, Beattie RM, Tighe MP. Practical management of functional abdominal pain in children. *Arch Dis Child.* 2016;101:677-683.

Chiou E, Nurko S. Management of functional abdominal pain and irritable bowel syndrome in children and adolescents. *Expert Rev Gastroenterol Hepatol.* 2010;4(3):293-304.

DiLorenzo C, Coletti R, Lehmann H, et al. American Academy of Pediatrics Subcommittee on Chronic Abdominal Pain and NASPGHAN Committee on Abdominal Pain; Clinical Report. Chronic abdominal pain in children: a clinical report of the American Academy of Pediatrics and the North American Society for Pediatric Gastroenterology, Hepatology and Nutrition. *J Pediatr Gastroenterol Nutr.* 2005;40:245-248.

DiLorenzo C, Coletti R, Lehmann H, et al. American Academy of Pediatrics Subcommittee on Chronic Abdominal Pain and NASPGHAN Committee on Abdominal Pain; Technical Report. Chronic abdominal pain in children: a technical report of the American Academy of Pediatrics and the North American Society for Pediatric Gastroenterology, Hepatology and Nutrition. *J Pediatr Gastroenterol Nutr.* 2005;40:249-261.

Huertas-Ceballos AA, Logan S, Bennett C, et al. Pharmacological interventions for recurrent abdominal pain (RAP) and irritable bowel syndrome (IBS) in childhood. *Cochrane Database Syst Rev.* 2008.(1):CD003017. doi: 10.1002/14651858.CD003017.pub2.

Weydert J, Ball T, Davis M. Systematic review of treatments for recurrent abdominal pain. *Pediatrics.* 2003;11:e1-e11.

FOR PARENTS

WEB SITES

International Foundation for Functional gastrointestinal Disorders IFFGD. http://www.iffgd.org/site/gi-disorders/kids-teens.

CHAPTER 38

Excessive Crying and Colic

Larry Gray | Amy Turner | Tracy Magee |
Steven Parker (deceased)

I. **DESCRIPTION OF THE PROBLEM.** All babies cry; however, some cry more than others. Excessive crying can frustrate parents and pediatric caregivers. Parents worry about the reasons for this crying and about their ability to console their crying child. While the amount of early infant crying individually varies, a consistent pattern of early infant crying has been identified. Called the "normal crying curve," the time infants spend crying progressively increases until it peaks at 6–8 weeks of age and then gradually decreases until about 4 months. This pattern includes a clustering of crying in the evening hours, most notably at the peak weeks of crying, and has been demonstrated with different cultural care-giving practices. The mean duration for crying during this peak period is around 2 hours per day. The conventional standard for excessive crying and colic has traditionally been the parent's report of total crying surpassing 3 hours a day for more than 3 days in any 1 week. In Western cultures, the prevalence of parents reporting early crying at this level ranges from 8% to 40% depending largely on the definition used, but 20% seems to be the most consistently reported frequency. A recent meta-analysis of 28 crying studies pooling more than 8500 infants supported these general trends. Excessive crying is not "colic," but both share the core symptom of high levels of crying. Colic, by definition, is excessive crying "plus" additional features despite being "healthy and well fed." The defining behavioral features of colic are (1) inconsolability (despite adequate parenting), (2) crying that begins and ends without warning, (3) a high-pitched quality to the cry, and (4) clenched fists, flexed legs, grimacing, or distended abdomen.

A. **Epidemiology**
   - Estimates range from 7% to 40%, depending on the criteria for diagnosis
   - No differences by gender, breast- versus bottle-fed, full-term versus preterm, or birth order
   - Two times increased risk if maternal smoking during pregnancy
   - Whites > nonwhites
   - Parents older and more educated
   - Industrialized countries > nonindustrialized
   - Occurs the further you live from Equator
   - Increased incidence of physical abuse in colicky infants, especially shaken baby syndrome

B. **Clinical features**
   1. Colic and excessive crying typically begins at 41–42 weeks of gestational age (including preterm infants), which is earlier than the normal expected increase in crying at 6–8 weeks of age.
   2. Behavioral features help the clinician distinguish colic apart from excessive crying:
       a. "Healthy and well fed"
       b. Inconsolability (despite adequate parenting)
       c. Crying that begins and ends without warning
       d. A high-pitched quality to the cry
       e. Clenched fists, flexed legs, grimacing, or distended abdomen
   3. Colic **stops as mysteriously as it starts,** by 3 months in 60% and by 4 months in 80%–90% of infants. Infants with excessive crying past the 4-month period are at higher risk for developmental problems.
   4. There are **no predictable long-term infant outcomes** (behavioral, temperamental, or psychological) that emerge from excessive crying or colic that resolves, although later sleep problems are often seen, and parents and caregivers with excessively crying infants are at higher risk for parental anxiety, family conflict, and conflict among the parenting partners.

C. **Etiology.** No single theory of excessive crying has proven the cause. Theories of what causes colic change with the decade, and the most recent area of research involves the role of gut microbiota and gut inflammation and its effect on the

193

Table 38-1 • THEORIES OF THE ETIOLOGY OF COLIC

Gastrointestinal

Gut inflammation (higher fecal calprotectin—a marker of inflammation released by WBCs)
Gut microbiota (breastfed infants with colic may have more gas-forming coliform species that contribute to abdominal distension)
Cow's milk protein intolerance (considered the most common organic cause of excessive crying)
Gastroesophageal reflux (highly debated role in cause of excessive crying)
Lactose intolerance (higher breath H_2 level in some colicky infants)
Immature gastrointestinal system (ineffective peristalsis, incomplete digestion, gas)
Faulty feeding techniques (e.g., under- or overfeeding, infrequent burping)
Gut hormones causing gastric spasms (motilin and ghrelin stimulate gastric motility and are higher in colic infants)
Decreased cholecystokinin levels ($\rightarrow$gallbladder contractions)

Hormonal

Increased circulating serotonin (hypothetical only, but an attractive hypothesis because serotonin has a circadian rhythm in infancy, which could explain the curious timing of paroxysmal fussing)
Progesterone deficiency (one study in 1963, never repeated)

Neurologic

Imbalance of autonomic nervous system (sympathetic $\gg$ parasympathetic)
Immature neurotransmitters
Circadian rhythm disorder

Temperamental

Difficult temperament (but there is poor correlation of colic and later temperament)
Hypersensitivity (crying at the end of day represents discharge after a long day of shutting out intrusive environmental stimuli, parents may be overstimulating)
Parental behaviors/handling
Most studies do not show a relationship between parental anxiety, psychopathology, and/or emotional difficulties and colic; at most, nonoptimal handling may exacerbate but not cause the symptoms

gut–brain axis. Because no single cause of colic has been identified, excessive crying may simply represent the final common pathway for a number of etiologic factors (Table 38-1).

II. MAKING THE DIAGNOSIS

A. History: key clinical questions

1. *"When does the crying occur?"* The timing of the cry provides useful information. For example, if it occurs directly after a feeding, aerophagia, or gastroesophageal reflux may be considered. If it occurs reliably 1 hour after feedings, a formula intolerance is possible. If the crying occurs only from 5 to 7 PM everyday, it is difficult to posit an organic problem that would cause pain at only one time of the day.

2. *"What do you do when your baby cries?"* It is important to determine how the parents have tried (successfully and unsuccessfully) to console the infant. In some cases, their techniques may have inadvertently worsened the situation (e.g., anxiously overstimulating a hypersensitive infant); in other cases, the technique may be inappropriate (e.g., giving half-strength formula or dangerous/suspect home/folk remedies).

3. *"What does the cry sound like?"* Most parents can distinguish a cry of pain from that of hunger. In addition, the description of the cry provides insight into parental distress, empathy, or anger with the cry. Research suggests that colicky cries have a higher pitch and are described as "urgent" or "piercing."

4. *"Tell me how and what you feed your baby."* Underfeeding, overfeeding, air swallowing, and inadequate burping have all been implicated in colic.

5. *"How does it make you feel when your baby cries?"* "What worries you most about the crying?"* History taking is an opportune time to begin the process of parental support. Opening up the subjects of parental guilt, helplessness, and anxiety sends the message that these topics merit discussion. Some parents are especially worried about their anger toward the screaming child, believing that such anger is the mark of a bad parent. Others seek pediatric attention because they are afraid of actually harming the infant during a crying spell or that the infant has a mysterious illness.

6. *"How has the colic affected your family?"* Colic is a *family* issue. In some cases, it may disturb the parents' relationship with each other, cause distress in a sibling, or serve as a forum for blaming the parents (e.g., by grandparents).

7. *"What is your theory of why the baby cries?"* To support the family, their hypotheses for the crying must be understood. Some may view it as a curse, others as a rebuke to their parenting skills, and others as a sign that something is terribly wrong with the baby.

B. Physical examination. Infants with high levels of crying and "red flags" of additional clinical features such as the following have increased likelihood that their crying is caused by organic pathology:

* High-pitched crying and arching the back
* Regurgitation
* Vomiting
* Diarrhea or blood in the stools

Using these criteria estimates that only 5%–10% of all excessively crying babies have a treatable medical or organic problem. Despite this low percentage, all infants require a thorough history and physical examination to "rule out" any painful cause for the infant's crying. The differential diagnosis list for excessive colic is extensive (bullets below). The majority of causes are identified by a thorough history and physical examination, not laboratory testing. Repeated examinations are often required to increase the sensitivity of the diagnostic process and can provide additional reassurance to parents that an identifiable and hence treatable cause for the crying does or does not exist.

* Infections (otitis media, urinary tract infection, oral herpes)
* Gastrointestinal (diarrhea, constipation, gastroesophageal reflux)
* Genitourinary (posterior urethral valves)
* CNS (intra- or extracranial hemorrhage, hydrocephalus)
* Ophthalmologic (corneal abrasion, glaucoma)
* Cardiac (supraventricular tachycardia)
* Narcotic withdrawal syndrome (especially methadone)
* Fracture, hernia, anal fissures
* Tourniquet (on toe or finger)

A note on GER: Gastroesophageal reflux is a normal, physiologic process in infants, which is self-limited, typically peaking around 4 months of age. Reflux can be managed with nonpharmacologic approaches, including upright positioning, thickening or changing formulas, and small, frequent feeds. Considering reflux as a self-limiting process in this age group that ultimately resolves without intervention, physicians should encourage families to utilize these nonpharmacologic approaches. Many medications exist to address reflux through acid suppression, although current research indicates that infants experience nonacidic reflux. Considering this fact, as well as prior studies showing limited success in reducing reflux symptoms in infants, physicians should avoid initiating medications such as proton pump inhibitors (PPIs), which have risks and side effect profiles physicians should not ignore.

III. MANAGEMENT

A. Family-centered approach. Because excessive crying and colic is a *family* issue, a solely biomedical perspective about treating infant crying and colic is often not helpful. Because the cause of colic is rarely clear and most treatments for colic work in only 30% of infants and none work for all infants, "trying everything" or "a shotgun approach" isn't effective. A family-centered approach embraces the complexity of excessive infant crying and at the same time does not overlook common medical conditions. Central to a family-centered approach is the concept of clinician–parent attunement, defined as an individual's or parent's sense of feeling connected and understood by the clinician. The experience of attunement is especially important to parents of fussy babies who so often report that they have not felt seen or heard by others, even family, friends, or professionals who want to help.

Table 38-2 lists suggestions for parents to help them deal with colic. The history and physical examination may point to one technique as potentially more useful than another. As a general rule, parents first need high levels of empathy when they express feelings around their infant's crying. By asking "how hard has this crying been **for you**," the clinician quickly can gage from the parents response the need for an emphatic response before jumping to solutions. When parents' feelings are contained and have a clear theory for their infant's crying, it is best to collaboratively explore the issue together rather than offer personal suggestions. When families are seeking information or are ready to try new ways, clinician generated suggestions can be heard and received by parents more effectively.

Table 38-2 • SUGGESTIONS FOR PARENTS TO HELP COLIC

Strategy	Comments
Feeding/Nutritional	
Change from milk-based formula to hypoallergenic or elemental formula	Expensive but sometimes effective
If breastfeeding, have mother stop cow's milk, caffeine, etc.	One study showed increased bovine IgG in the breast milk of mothers of colicky babies. Ask the breast feeding mother which foods seem to be associated with increased irritability
Change nipple or bottle; feed in upright position with frequent burping	Try to decrease air swallowing (e.g., by using bottle with a plastic liner)
Probiotics	*Lactobacillus reuteri* has been shown to decrease crying in 4 randomized control trial (breastfed babies > formula babies)

Soothing Techniques		
Common Strategy	**Changing Position and Adding Rhythm**	
	Supplemental daytime carrying	One study found little benefit of supplemental carrying for truly colicky infants (front carrier, e.g., Snugli, allows hand to be free while carrying)
	Ride in the car	Not advisable if the driver is sleepy
	Change of scenery or no scenery	New sights can distract from the distress or the baby may be overstimulated and no scenery may be needed
	Swing	Allows for brief periods of relief, but too much time in swing can delay development
Common Strategy	**White Noise**	
	White noise machine	Noise without rhythm; for babies who don't respond to rocking or swings
	Heartbeat tape	Especially good for babies who are hypersensitive to noise
Common Strategy	**Closeness and Sensation**	
	Swaddling	Especially good for babies who are hypersensitive to body movements or touch
	Belly massage	Use a lubricating lotion
	Warm water bottle on belly	Should be only warm, not hot
	Sleep tight (a device that generates white noise and vibrates the bed)	Some pediatric practices have the device available to loan to patients. (Two controlled studies, however, have shown disappointing benefits)
	Warm bath	
Medications	Herbal tea (e.g., chamomile, spearmint, fennel)	A study of chamomile/verbena/licorice/fennel/mint tea found improvement in 57% of colicky infants, although the amount needed to get effect could affect nutrition
	Simethicone	Probably harmless, dubiously helpful
	Antispasmodics	**Should not be used.** Despite some evidence of efficacy, there have been case reports of respiratory arrests associated with their use in infants

B. Empathy as parental support. Excessive crying and colic is a benign, self-limited problem with negative results only on the early parent–child relationship. Long after the crying resolves, the consequences of an impaired parent–infant relationship may long affect the child's development and the family system. Therefore, the primary role for the clinician in the management of excessive crying and colic is to support the family through a difficult period and attempt to buffer any loss of pleasure in the relationship and emphasizing periods of "relaxed dialogue" or "joy" between the parent and infant.

1. **Collaborate with the family.** Some families will come to the care provider with their own theories or beliefs about why the baby is crying so much. This is when to collaborate with the family using frequent physical examinations to "understand how they see the baby" and assure the family that nothing has been missed and provide reassurance that nothing is physically wrong with the infant. The infant's growth and development may support the parent's theory of the crying too.

   Most parents (especially inexperienced ones) feel that the crying occurs because of something that they are doing wrong. They require reassurance that this is not the case and that excessive crying and colic occurs with even the most attentive, loving, and experienced caregivers. This is the time to explore with parents (especially inexperienced ones) how they are creating moments of pleasure and enjoyment with their baby.

2. **Building the family's capacity.** When a provider or family attempts a new technique to help their baby's crying, parents should call the clinician within 48 hours to report on progress. If no progress is evident, a follow-up visit can be scheduled in short order to continue the discussion and to reassure them that often there is no easy solution even when there is no organic problem. The parents need to be able to count on the clinician's availability during this difficult time and get continued support for what they are trying to do to help their baby.

   Parents need reassurance when the first thing they try does not seem to help and support to stay the course. Some find it reassuring that crying is healthy for the lungs and is not emotionally damaging for the infant; time crying alone may even provide opportunities for the baby to learn how to self-console. Some parents find letting their infant cry unattended to be intolerable. They should be supported in handling the problem in the way that is most comfortable to them.

   Some families find support in knowing it is permissible to take breaks from the baby's crying and put the baby down and let him or her cry for increasingly longer periods of time before attempting another consoling maneuver. Some families find it difficult to take breaks from the baby by letting a friend, family member, or babysitter attend to him or her for a few hours while the parents go out of the house for some personal time. They may find support in knowing a nonparent cannot console their baby either and they are not doing anything wrong.

3. **Be Mindful of feelings/take care of yourself.** Recognize that caring for parents with excessively crying babies may bring up feelings in the provider that dysregulate. Monitor these feelings and find or use personal strategies to protect the encounter and communication with the family from unintended bias due to provider feelings of frustration. Monitoring your own feelings may open the window to addressing parental feelings of resentment and anger engendered by their crying infant. Recognizing one's own feelings and perhaps similar parental feelings about their infant's excessive crying is the first step in addressing crying as a trigger for possible abuse, parental depression, or parent/infant relationship problems.

Bibliography

FOR PARENTS

WEB SITES

http://www.purplecrying.info/.

https://www.webmd.com/parenting/baby/what-is-colic#1.

FOR PROFESSIONALS

Barr RG, Paterson JA, MacMartin LM, Lehtonen L, Young SN. Prolonged and unsoothable crying bouts in infants with and without colic. *J Dev Behav Pediatr*. 2005;26(1):14-23.

Brazelton TB. Crying in infancy. *Pediatrics*. 1962;29:579-588.

Wessel MA, Cobb JC, Jackson EB, Harris GS, Detwiler AC. Paroxysmal fussing in infancy, sometimes called colic. *Pediatrics*. 1954;14(5):421-435.

Wolke D, Bilgin A, Samara M. Systematic review and meta-analysis: fussing and crying durations and prevalence of colic in infants. *J Pediatr*. 2017;185:55-61.e4.

CHAPTER 39

Death During Childhood

David J. Schonfeld

I. DESCRIPTION OF THE PROBLEM. When a child is dying, the child and the family need reassurance, support, and guidance. The primary care provider who has a supportive and ongoing relationship with the child and the family is in a unique position to provide them with that support throughout this difficult period. Some general principles to consider in providing care to dying children and their families are presented in Table 39-1.

II. ISSUES IN HELPING THE DYING CHILD

A. Health care providers must attend to the immediate physical needs of these children.
It is crucial to relieve pain and suffering and to assure the children that adults are always available. Children should be told by both the parents and the health care providers, "*We want you to tell us whenever anything is bothering you. I will always be here (or be able to be reached) anytime you want me. We will all do our best to make sure that you feel as comfortable as possible.*"

B. Children at different developmental stages have different conceptual understandings of the meaning of death.
This will affect their ability to understand and adjust to their impending death. Children with a terminal illness usually do appreciate the seriousness of their illness and may develop a precocious understanding of death and their personal mortality.

C. Many parents and clinicians are uncomfortable when children openly acknowledge an awareness of their impending death.
Children often feel that it is their task to provide emotional support to their parents and to carry on the mutual pretense that they are unaware of their health status. This conspiracy of silence isolates the child from available supports. Most children, in fact, fear the *process* of dying more than death itself.

D. To the extent possible, children should be informed about their health status.
Children often turn to members of the health care team to ask questions, directly or indirectly, about their illness and impending death. Children who are dying may also directly ask family members and staff, "Am I going to die?" Adults should initially clarify the motivation for such questions: Is the child seeking reassurance that all efforts will be made to minimize pain, that parents and family members will remain available, or that every reasonable effort will be made to treat the underlying illness? Is the child merely attempting to determine the seriousness of his/her illness? Once the motivation for the question is identified, the adult family member or health care provider can provide the necessary reassurances or information. Prohibitions on informing children about their condition force parents and professionals to lie, thereby jeopardizing a caregiving relationship built on mutual trust and respect. The principles to consider in informing children about a terminal illness or impending death are summarized in Table 39-2.

E. Facilitating discussion about children's concerns often involves projective techniques such as play or picture drawing. Many children choose not to discuss their impending death directly. It is rarely necessary (or appropriate) to confront children with the reality that they are dying after they have been appropriately informed. Instead, clinicians should remain available and offer indirect outlets for addressing the child's concerns. Children will avail themselves of these opportunities when, and if, they are ready.

F. Clinicians are often anxious that they will not know what to say to a child who is dying.
The goal of counseling children who are dying is not to take away their sadness or to find the "right" answers to all their questions. Rather, it is to listen to their concerns, to accept and empathize with their strong emotions, to offer support, and to assist them in finding their own coping techniques (e.g., "*Some children find it helpful to talk to others about what is worrying them; other children prefer to draw pictures or keep a diary. Whatever you decide to do is fine. I'm always available to talk with you about your feelings, or just to sit and talk about something else.*"). In many cases, the best approach is to talk about a topic of interest to the child or merely to sit quietly and hold the child's hand. Although regressive behavior may be normative and appropriate at times of stress, excessively regressive behavior (e.g., a 6-year-old who begins biting staff)

Table 39-1 • GENERAL PRINCIPLES FOR PRACTITIONERS IN THE CARE OF DYING CHILDREN AND THEIR FAMILIES

Physical Context

Minimize physical discomfort and symptoms
Optimize pain management

Emotional Context

Provide an opportunity for the expression and sharing of personal feelings and concerns for both the children and their families in an accepting atmosphere
Tolerate unpleasant affect (e.g., sadness, anger, despair)

Social Context

Facilitate communication among members of the health care team and the children and their families
Encourage active participation of the children and their families in the treatment decisions and the management of the illness

Personal Context

Treat each child and family member as a unique individual
Form a personal relationship with the child and the family
Acknowledge your own feelings as a health care provider and establish a mechanism(s) to meet your personal needs

Table 39-2 • PRINCIPLES INVOLVED IN INFORMING CHILDREN ABOUT A TERMINAL ILLNESS OR IMPENDING DEATH

Inform the child over time in a series of conversations. During the initial conversation, it is important to convey that the child has a serious illness.
If the child asks directly whether he or she is going to die, initially explore the reason for the question and the child's concerns (e.g., "Are you afraid that you might die?" "What are you worried about?"). Do not provide false reassurances ("No, don't worry, you're going to be okay."), but always try to maintain hope ("Some children with your sickness have died, but we are going to do everything we can to try to help you get better.").
Focus initial discussions on the immediate and near future. Young children have a limited future perspective. Dying "soon" to them may mean minutes, hours, or days and not months or years.
Answer questions directly, but do not overwhelm the child with unnecessary details.
Assess the child's understanding by asking him or her to explain back to you what you have discussed.
Reassure the child of the lack of personal responsibility or guilt. For this reason, avoid using "bad" in the description of the illness (e.g., "You have a bad sickness.").

should be addressed supportively but firmly, often employing a behavioral management approach developed by the treatment team and the family.

   G. Children must be allowed, even encouraged, to continue to have hope and to go on with their lives.

   These children should be regarded less as children who are dying and more as individuals living with a serious and/or life-threatening condition. The goal must be to optimize the quality of their remaining life and not merely to prolong its duration. Important routines should be continued with as little disruption as possible, such as allowing them to attend school or to do schoolwork in the hospital. Consultation should be offered to schools to help them know how best to support children with serious and life-threatening conditions and to assist peers and school staff to deal with the child's serious illness and ultimate death.

   H. Many children and adolescents feel guilty and ashamed about their illness.

   Children who rely on magical thinking and egocentrism to explain the cause of illness may assume that terminal illness and death are the result of some perceived wrongdoing ("immanent justice"). Children need to be reassured periodically that they are not responsible for their illness.

   I. To the extent possible, children should be informed about and participate in the decisions regarding their health care.

Older children and adolescents may possess the intellectual and emotional maturity to allow them to play a significant role regarding critical and difficult decisions (e.g., whether to discontinue aggressive treatment). All children need to be aware of the nature and rationale of planned treatments and should be active participants in the treatment process even if they are able to make only seemingly minor decisions (e.g., whether they should take the pill with juice or with soda).

III. ISSUES IN HELPING THE PARENTS

A. Parents faced with the impending (or actual) death of their child may demonstrate shock, denial, anxiety, depression, or anger.

Almost any reaction can be seen; there is no "correct" way to deal with the death of a child. In addition, parents may alternate among these emotional states without demonstrating any clear pattern of progression. In general, it is important to accept parents' reactions without making judgments about whether or not they are appropriate, unless there are concerns related to personal safety (e.g., drinking and driving, suicidal or homicidal threats).

B. The response of family members to the death may be affected by the duration of the illness.

Anticipatory grieving allows family members to experience graduated feelings of loss while the child is still alive. In the setting of open communication, many families will take advantage of this time to resolve conflicts with the dying child and to express love. Clinicians should appreciate that other families may approach this impending loss with a different coping style and may not choose to engage in this form of leave-taking behavior.

C. Members of the family may proceed with anticipatory grieving at different rates.

Conflicts may result when one family member's course of grieving is not synchronous with that of another member of the family. Primary care clinicians can help families to identify when someone (either a family member or a health care team member) has functionally abandoned the child after having prematurely reached resignation and acceptance of the child's death.

D. As part of anticipatory grieving, family members and health care professionals may wish for the death of a terminally ill child.

This wish may result in excessive guilt and cause the individual to compensate by becoming overly protective or indulgent with the dying child. The health care provider can assist parents with comments such as: *"Many parents of children who have been critically ill for a prolonged period sometimes find themselves wishing their child would just die quickly. This is a common and normal feeling, even for parents who love their children dearly."*

E. Family members should be allowed, even encouraged, to continue to have hope and to go on with their lives.

While the desire for second opinions should be honored, excessive searches for cures that compromise the health of the child or the financial well-being of the family should be discouraged. Parents must be actively assured that they have done everything reasonable to ensure the highest quality of care for their child and that they have no reason to feel guilty.

F. To the extent possible, parents should be informed about and participate actively in decisions regarding their child's care.

The health care providers must provide families with clear professional recommendations and be willing to discuss alternate options when appropriate options exist. When families are faced, for example, with the difficult decision of whether to continue aggressive therapy when little hope of cure remains, the clinician must provide information on the likelihood of success and the anticipated morbidity associated with the treatment process. Palliative and supportive care should always remain available even if children and their families choose a management plan that is not the preferred option of the provider. For terminally ill children maintained on life support at the time of death, the clinician should elicit and attempt to honor the parents' wishes about the timing of termination of life support. Care should be taken so that parents do not infer that they are being asked about whether to allow their child to die.

G. Sudden or unexpected death requires an immediate recognition of the loss.

In this setting, families often initially use denial to cope. Family members should be allowed additional time to hold or be with the child's body in a quiet and private area of the hospital and often need an opportunity to express their shock, disbelief, and anger before further and more detailed explanations of the cause of death can be discussed.

H. Support systems for families of dying children are often hospital-based and frequently withdrawn at the time of the child's death.

Providers should remain available to families after the death has occurred and should help the family establish ties, before the death, with community-based support systems, such as parent or sibling groups, clergy, and counseling services. Hospital support networks should not become an additional loss coincident with the death of the child.

I. At the time of the child's death, parents and other family members should be offered assistance with immediate and pragmatic needs.

Such diverse needs include ensuring safe transportation home for grieving family members at the time of the death, making funeral and burial arrangements, and deciding how to notify family members and friends. Families should be given an appointment for a follow-up meeting (often 2–6 weeks after the death, earlier if necessary) to answer remaining questions about the illness and death (e.g., to review the autopsy report) and to inquire about adjustment of family members. A meeting can also be arranged later on with the siblings either individually or with their parents.

J. Families in grief may feel immobilized and incapable of making even simple decisions.

Complex and emotionally laden decisions such as those regarding autopsy or organ donation may seem especially overwhelming at this time. When death is anticipated, the primary care provider may suggest that family members consider their personal feelings about such decisions before the fact. In sudden and unanticipated deaths, families may need a period of time (1–2 hours) to adjust to the reality of the loss before such questions are asked.

IV. ISSUES IN HELPING THE SIBLINGS

A. The needs of the siblings are often neglected when a child in the family is dying.

Parents have limited reserves of energy, time, and money and strained emotional and psychological resources. Providers must ensure that outreach is provided to siblings to meet their needs.

B. The siblings should be included in receiving information about the child's health status and treatment plan and should participate to some extent in the provision of care for the ill child.

Young children may be given simple tasks such as bringing and opening mail, watering plants in the room, or bringing toys to a child in bed. Parents must be careful not to overburden the siblings, especially the older children and adolescents, with unreasonable chores or responsibilities. Siblings should be encouraged to maintain their peer groups and continue involvement in activities outside the family.

C. Siblings respond to the death with the same diversity of emotional responses seen in adults.

They may be angry at the child who has died or experience guilt over having survived. Primary care clinicians need to monitor how families reorganize after the death of a child so that siblings are not made a scapegoat or the focus of projected defenses. For example, parents who continue to feel guilty about their child's death may overprotect the surviving siblings and interfere with normative attempts to achieve independence.

V. HELPING THE HEALTH CARE PROVIDERS

A. Health care providers must understand their personal feelings about death to be effective in providing support to others.

Often this will involve some introspection about one's own losses and an awareness of the impact of the deaths of their patients on their professional and personal lives.

B. Providers must extend the same quality of care to themselves, as they would offer to patients.

The death of a patient is one of the most stressful personal and professional experiences faced by health care providers. It triggers a similar, albeit less intense, grief response as would a personal loss. Permission and tolerance for professionals to discuss and have their personal needs met regarding bereavement (e.g., for support or reassurance of lack of personal responsibility for a patient death) is necessary. Psychosocial rounds (especially in intensive care settings), retreats, and other support services dealing directly with providers' responses to patient death are important aspects of professional development.

C. All members of the health care team should be involved in important decisions regarding the care provided to a dying child.

Conflicts that arise when one or more members of the team disagree on the appropriateness of care being provided can seriously undermine the clinical care. For example, clinicians who avoid clarifying do-not-resuscitate orders with the family of a dying child may place the nursing staff in the uncomfortable position of having to initiate resuscitation efforts when the death occurs. House staff forced to continue treatment that they feel is not in the best interest of the child or family may be angry if they were not involved in the decision. Often staff differences are best resolved through team meetings.

   D. Primary care providers should avail themselves of the expertise and skills of members of related disciplines, such as the clergy, child life, nursing, psychiatry, psychology, and social work, when responding to the needs of the child and family members, as well as their own personal needs.

Bibliography

FOR PARENTS

ORGANIZATIONS

National Bereavement Resource Guide – a comprehensive listing sponsored by the New York Life Foundation (www.achildingrief.com) and Moyer Foundation (www.moyerfoundation.org) of grief camps, children's bereavement centers, and hospices for children and their families experiencing loss, organized by state. https://moyerfoundation.org/national-bereavement-resource-guide.

PUBLICATIONS
INFORMATION ON HOW TO SUPPORT GRIEVING CHILDREN

Emswiler M, Emswiler J. *Guiding Your Child through Grief*. New York, NY: Bantam Books; 2000.

Schonfeld D, Quackenbush M. *After a Loved One Dies—How Children Grieve and How Parents and Other Adults Can Support Them*. New York, NY: New York Life Foundation; 2009. May be freely downloaded as PDF or hardcopies ordered at no cost in either English or Spanish at www.grievingstudents.org (select "Order Free Materials").

FOR PROFESSIONALS

ORGANIZATIONS

Coalition to Support Grieving Students. A collaboration of over 35 major national organizations representing the full range of school and health professions to empower school communities in the ongoing support of their grieving students – www.GrievingStudents.org is a practitioner-oriented website providing widely-endorsed, practical, free information, handouts and reference materials, including over 20 video training modules.

National Center for School Crisis and Bereavement. Offers free assistance and guidance materials to schools related to the death of a student or staff member or other school crisis. www.school-crisiscenter.org; 877-53-NCSCB (877-536-2722); or info@schoolcrisiscenter.org.

PUBLICATIONS

Glazer J, Schonfeld DJ. Life-threatening illness, palliative care, and bereavement. In: Martin A, Bloch M, Volkmar F, eds. *Lewis' Child and Adolescent Psychiatry: A Comprehensive Textbook*. 5th ed. Philadelphia: Wolters Kluwer; 2017:946-956.

Schonfeld DJ, Demaria T, Committee on Psychosocial Aspects of Child and Family Health, and Disaster Preparedness Advisory Council. Supporting the grieving child and family. *Pediatrics*. 2016;138(3):e20162147. doi:10.1542/peds.2016-2147.

Schonfeld D, Quackenbush M. *The Grieving Student: A Teacher's Guide*. Baltimore, MD: Brookes Publishing; 2010.

Wender E, Committee on Psychosocial Aspects of Child and Family Health. Supporting the family after the death of a child. *Pediatrics*. 2012;130(6):1164-1169.

CHAPTER 40

Depression

Natalija Bogdanovic | Michelle P. Durham

I. **DESCRIPTION OF THE PROBLEM.** Major depressive disorder (MDD) is by definition an episodic, recurring disorder characterized by a significant and pervasive sad or irritable mood and inability to feel joy in everyday activities lasting for at least 2 weeks. It is important to understand that sadness and unhappiness are normal human emotions. Sadness after significant loss, death of a loved one, or end of relationship is a natural reaction to situation that cause emotional upset or pain. People frequently use the term "depressed" to simply describe the way they feel during those times. When sadness becomes intense, persistent, and pervasive and starts affecting the child's functioning, clinicians should become concerned. It is important to appreciate the difference between sadness and MDD, as not doing so can lead to the unnecessary treatment and pathologizing of normal human emotions.

Depression prevalence varies among studies; however, most studies agree that about 1%–2% of prepubertal children and about 5%–6% of adolescents suffer from depression at any one time. Cumulative prevalence is much larger, up to 12% for girls and 7% for boys. In prepubertal children, male to female ratio is 1:1. After puberty, depression becomes about twice as common in females than males.

II. **MAKING THE DIAGNOSIS**

A. **Signs and symptoms.** The *Diagnostic and Statistical Manual of Mental Disorders*, Fifth Edition *(DSM-5)* describes specific criteria for the diagnosis (Table 40-1).

B. **Differential diagnosis.** The most common differential is adjustment disorders, bereavement, medical conditions, medications, or substance use. Bereavement or adjustment disorders can be diagnosed when the onset of symptoms follows a significant life event or loss and do not meet criteria for MDD. It is important to obtain medical and medication history as a variety of medical conditions (e.g., traumatic brain injury, thyroid problems, mononucleosis) or medication (e.g., isotretinoin, corticosteroids, stimulants) can mimic depression. Given the frequency of substance use among adolescents, it is always important to elicit if depressed mood is a result of ingestion or withdrawal from the substances.

C. **Comorbidity.** The most common psychiatric disorders comorbid with depression are anxiety disorders, and the link between depression and anxiety has been well established. Other comorbid disorders include PTSD, ADHD, ODD, and substance abuse.

D. **Course.** Major depressive disorder may be diagnosed in prepubertal children; however, prevalence increases significantly in adolescence.

Prepubertal children with depressive symptoms are more likely to develop nondepressive disorders in adulthood, while depression that starts in adolescence is more likely to have a recurrent course.

There is about 40% probability of recurrence within 2 years and is high even after treatment. Participants in the 5-year follow-up of the Treatment of Adolescent Depression Study (TADS) showed that, although the vast majority (96%) of patients recovered from the primary episode, after 5 years almost half (46%) had a recurrence.

There are several predictors of recurrence including greater severity of illness, having previous episodes, poor response to treatment, history of maltreatment, negative coping styles, family conflict, and having a comorbid illness.

Suicidal thoughts with intent or plan must be taken seriously and should automatically lead to a careful suicide assessment and referral for psychiatric evaluation and follow-up the risk for suicide attempts increases if there is a family history of suicide, past attempts of suicide, presence of comorbid psychiatric disorders (impulsivity, aggression, substance use), adverse life experiences (such as abuse) or access to lethal means (see Chapter 79).

E. **Etiology and risk factors.** Etiology of depression is a multifactorial, largely diathesis-stress model in which stressful experiences trigger depression in those who have vulnerability owing to a combination of biological, psychosocial, and environmental stressors.

Table 40-1 • SIGNS AND SYMPTOMS OF DEPRESSION

Depressed or irritable mood, loss of interests, or pleasure most of the day, nearly every day for at least 2 weeks. The symptoms must cause significant distress or impairment in social, academic, or other important areas of functioning and must be accompanied by changes in *at least four* of the following:	Feeling sad, blue, miserable, hopeless, irritable, "blah," cranky, edgy "Dysphoric mood"—sadness along with irritability; exaggerated sense of frustration over minor things Please note that this can either be subjective feeling or observation made by others (e.g., appears tearful all the time, looks sad all the time, nothing makes him/her happy, "not caring for things anymore") In milder forms of depression, functioning may appear normal but requires markedly increased effort
1. Poor appetite or weight loss/gain	In children, this can be seen as failure to make expected weight gain. Appetite loss or appetite increase nearly every day Changes of more than 5% of weight gain (if not dieting/exercising) is always concerning
2. Change in sleep patterns	Insomnia, frequent awakenings, or hypersomnia nearly every day
3. Change in the level of activity	Psychomotor agitation (pacing, moving a lot, cannot sit still, hand wringing) or retardation (slowed speech, slow body movements) Observable by others; not just subjective feelings
4. Fatigue or loss of energy	Feels tired all the time, even the smallest things perceived as needing great effort
5. Feeling of worthlessness or excessive and inappropriate guilt	Feeling as they cannot do anything right, "a failure," exaggerated sense of responsibility for the negative events, feeling as if they are "shame" for the family
6. Change in concentration or indecisiveness	Less able to focus in class, complete assignments, can present as a drop in school grades, cannot complete tasks that was able to in the past
7. Suicidal ideation	Recurrent thoughts or death and dying, thinking life would be better off without him/her, undeserving of life, unable to cope with the pain of depression

Biological vulnerabilities include genetically based variability in functioning of serotoninergic, neurologic, hormonal, immunologic, and neuroendocrinologic pathways. Genetic studies demonstrate a heritability of depressive disorders. The biologic offspring of depressed adults are up to two to four times more likely to have MDD, which may present earlier and recur more frequently. Family psychiatric history is an important predictor of childhood risk. The incidence of depression in mothers, in general, is approximately 5%; mothers of young children or those facing marital discord are at higher risk.

Psychological vulnerabilities such as negative coping styles (self-blame, rigidity, avoidance, rumination, or disengagement), low self-esteem, or comorbid anxiety disorder causing maladaptive processing of emotional information can make a child more vulnerable to depression. Social and environmental stressors including parental depression or mental health disorder, acute life events such as loss, separation from the caregiver, chronic stress such as physical and sexual abuse, bullying, social isolation and childhood exposure to adversity can also contribute to or trigger depression.

F. History: key clinical questions. Depression falls under "internalizing" disorders, meaning that the person who suffers from depression will often keep the feelings to themselves. Thus, often, parents and teachers tend to underestimate the problem. It is important to get the history from both parent and youth, as one might miss the diagnosis if solely relying on parental report.

   1. To parents: *"How is your child's mood? How does your child feel about himself or herself? For how many days, weeks, months, has this been the case?"*

   To children/adolescents: *"How have you been feeling? How do you feel most of the time? Everyone feels sad at times, how about you? What makes you sad?"*

2. To parents: *"Has there been a recent change in your child's behavior, school performance, or peer relationships?"* A decrease in functioning or significant change in behaviors can be a key indicator of mood-related stress and disability.

To children/adolescents: *"When was the last time you had fun?" "Do you find that recently things that you enjoyed doing no longer make you happy? Is it hard to focus on school? Why?" "Do you want to stay home more often and do not feel the need to be with your friends?"*

3. To parents: *"Does your child have a past history of feeling down, or has he/she ever seen a mental health professional in the past?"*

4. Gathering family psychiatric history: *"Does anyone in the extended family have a history of depression, mania, anxiety, attention deficits, or alcohol or substance use?"*

5. To parents: *"If depressed, has your child ever brought harm to himself/herself, even accidentally? Has the child ever talked or threatened to hurt himself/herself or others?"*

To children/adolescents: *"Have you ever felt so bad that you wanted to die?" "Have you ever thought that world would be better off without you?"*

III. MANAGEMENT. Based on suspicion or following diagnosis, child health clinicians can refer for further evaluation and treatment and participate in care and monitoring or implement treatment themselves. Treatment for depression should start with psychoeducation and counseling to patients and families about depression. Information should be age-appropriate and should cover the nature, course, and treatment of depression. Clinicians should make every effort to engage families in treatment decisions. Most cases of depression can be safely treated in the outpatient setting; however, in treating depression it is important to establish safety first, as suicidal thoughts are frequently a part of depression. About 60% of depressed youth have suicidal thoughts and 30% will make a suicide attempt. Once safety is established, treatment will vary depending on severity of depression and family preferences. Because of the high rates of treatment response to placebo, a stepped approach of treatment and management of depression is advised and is based on severity of depression. The goal of treatment should be remission or marked reduction in symptoms and functional impairment.

Mild depression—few (if any) symptoms in excess of those required to make diagnosis; minor impairment in functioning.

- *Watchful waiting*: if children and adolescents or parents do not want an intervention or, in the opinion of the health care professional, youth may recover without intervention, a further assessment should be arranged within 2 weeks.
- *Guided self-help*: this may include providing the youth and the families with educational material, Web sites, and books about depression and/or dealing with stressful life situation, teaching regarding elimination of stress and situation that produce it, and advising around strengthening of parent–child relationship. Follow-up care should be arranged within 2 weeks, and if youth continues to have symptoms, supportive psychotherapy should be offered.
- *Supportive psychotherapy*: focuses on teaching positive self-talk, effective problem-solving, teaching relaxation techniques, and ways to increase physical activity and start doing more pleasurable activities. It can also include reinforcing and strengthening resilience, maintaining or building up self-esteem, and encouraging youth to share their feelings and thought. This can be done in either individual or group setting.

Antidepressant medication should not be used as the initial treatment for youth with mild depression; however, it may be considered in the youth who did not respond to 4–8 weeks of supportive psychotherapy.

Moderate depression—produces moderate impairment in functioning.

Severe depression—the number of symptoms substantially is in excess of that required to make diagnosis, e.g., all or almost all symptoms present; the intensity of the symptoms is seriously distressing and impairing functioning in all settings.

Treatment for both moderate and severe depression should include manualized psychotherapies, medication management, or both, based on family and patient preference as well as severity of the illness.

- *Cognitive behavioral therapy (CBT)*: therapy with most evidence and modest effect size. CBT is typically delivered in 8–12 weekly visits and focuses on the premise that our thoughts can affect the way we behave and feel. Therapists review and challenge negative thoughts, actions, feelings, and beliefs in a systematic and logical way.
- *Interpersonal psychotherapy:* focuses on enhancing interpersonal problem-solving and social communication. It is an empirically supported treatment that follows a highly structured and time-limited approach and is intended to be completed within 12–16 weeks. Effect size is modest as well.

- *Medication:* The placebo effect is stronger in children and adolescents than adults. Antidepressants that show strong evidence in adults such as tricyclic antidepressants (TCAs) are not effective in children. As a group, selective serotonin reuptake inhibitors (SSRIs) are the safest antidepressants and most well tolerated. Given the strong placebo effect, clinicians should be explicit about effectiveness and telling families it can take up to 6 weeks for full medication response.
  - In the United States, fluoxetine is the only medication that is Food and Drug Administration (FDA)–approved for depression in children above 8 years of age and escitalopram is FDA-approved in adolescents. Children treated with SSRIs experience mild side effects, such as gastrointestinal effects, headaches, and changes in sleep. Some experience more distressing effects, such as restlessness, increase in anxiety, and behavioral activation.
  - FDA issued a **"black box warning"** in 2003 about the possibility of increase in suicidal thoughts and behaviors in some children and adolescents with MDD. The absolute risk for suicidal thoughts is about 3% in the youth treated with antidepressant medication versus 2% in those given placebo. As a result of this risk, the FDA recommends weekly contact for a month, followed by contact every 2 weeks for another month when an antidepressant is started.
  - Approximately 40% of children that do not respond to the first medication trial will respond to a second medication trial, so one should consider a trial with a different antidepressant. Before switching to another antidepressant, one should make sure that the trial was adequate and the dose was maximized.
  - Owing to high recurrence rate, once the child/adolescent responds to medication, treatment should continue 6–12 months after the response.

IV. RATING SCALES/AIDS IN DIAGNOSIS AND TREATMENT. Most commonly used scales are self-report scales that can be freely found on the Internet. They are much more useful in adolescent population and their benefit in children is less known and generally not advised. Although they are used as screening, not diagnostic, tools, they can be helpful in recognizing the problem and tracking progress. Some of the more commonly used scales include Center for Epidemiological Studies Depression Scale for Children (CES-DC), Patient Health Questionnaire-9 (PHQ-9), the Kutcher Adolescent Depression Scale (KADS), Mood and Feelings Questionnaire (MFQ), Patient Health Questionnaire for Adolescents (PHQ-A), Beck Depression Inventory–Primary Care (BDI-PC) version, and the Depression Self-Rating Scale (DSRS).

Bibliography

FOR PARENTS

American Academy of Child and Adolescent Psychiatry Facts for Families. https://www.aacap.org/aacap/families_and_youth/facts_for_families/FFF-Guide/FFF-Guide-Home.aspx.

National Alliance on Mental Illness. https://www.nami.org/.

National Institute of Mental Health. http://www.nimh.nih.gov/health/topics/child-and-adolescent-mental-health/index.shtml.

Parents Medication Guide for Depression from the American Psychiatric Association and AACAP. www.ParentsMedGuide.org.

FOR PROFESSIONALS

Cipriani A, Zhou X, Del Giovane C, et al. Comparative efficacy and tolerability of antidepressants for major depression in children and adolescents: a network meta-analysis. *Lancet.* 2016;388(10047):881-890.

Curry J, Silva S, Rohde P, et al. Recovery and recurrence following treatment for adolescent major depression. *Arch Gen Psychiatry.* 2011;68(3):263-269. doi:10.1001/archgenpsychiatry.2010.150.

IACAPAP Textbook of Child and Adolescent Mental Health: Depression in Children and Adolescents, 2015 Edition. http://iacapap.org/wp-content/uploads/E.1-Depression-2015-update.pdf.

March JS, Silva S, Petrycki S, et al. The Treatment for Adolescents with Depression Study (TADS) long-term effectiveness and safety outcomes. *Arch Gen Psychiatry.* 2007;64(10):1132-1143. doi:10.1001/archpsyc.64.10.1132.

The Reach Institute. Guidelines for Adolescent Depression—Primary Care. Available from: www.glad-pc.org.

CHAPTER 41

Divorce

Margot Kaplan-Sanoff | Melora Wiley | Carol C. Weitzman

I. **DESCRIPTION OF THE PROBLEM.** Divorce is not a single event. Rather, divorce is a process that begins with parental conflict or tension, leads to a physical separation of the parents, and culminates with the legal divorce proceedings. Even before the acute parental separation, oftentimes children have already begun coping with the parental conflict that leads to or is the consequence of an unraveling relationship between their parents. As the divorce process typically spans several years, children may experience the divorce differently based on their age and developmental level, and their reactions may change as they progress through the stages of development.

A. **Incidence**
   - More than 1 million children experience parental separation or divorce per year.
   - Approximately 50% of all marriages end in divorce, usually within the first 8 years of marriage.
   - 85% of parents who divorce remarry, and 40% of these new marriages also end in divorce.

B. **The parent's adjustment to the divorce.** In many divorcing families, each parent is in a different stage of the process. Often one parent is ready to let go of the relationship whereas the other may not. Parents may experience a range of negative emotions such as anger, guilt, humiliation, fear, anxiety, or depression before ultimately moving into the stage of acceptance. During this difficult period, parents are often preoccupied by their own problems and may demonstrate less emotional availability to meet the needs of their children.

C. **The child's adjustment to the divorce.** The goal for a child experiencing parental separation or divorce is that he or she adapts to the changes and copes with the perceived losses with minimal long-term emotional or adjustment problems. The process of successfully adjusting to their new "normal" will look different for each child based on a variety of factors described in the following.
   1. **Understand the divorce.** Children must understand the immediate changes that the divorce brings and differentiate between their fantasies and fears with the reality of the divorce. They may respond to one or both parents or themselves with blame, sadness, anger, guilt, and/or anxiety to the separation and decision to divorce. How children are told about the divorce and the way the family separates, in part, determines the nature of the postdivorce year. Children who blame themselves for the divorce may try to be the "perfect child" in hopes of reuniting the family.
   2. **Strategically withdraw.** Children need to move forward with their own lives and to have permission to remain children by continuing or joining extracurricular activities, such as sports or art programs. Very young children may be unable to avoid the anger and hostility of the divorce, whereas involvement in extracurricular activities can provide older school-aged children and adolescents an escape from tensions or distress in the home.
   3. **Cope with loss.** In a divorce, children often lose daily contact with one of their parents and they lose the family makeup into which they were born. Other losses and changes for children may include a decrease in financial resources and a move to a new neighborhood, school, and/or peer group.
   4. **Deal with anger.** Although divorce is a voluntary action for at least one of the adults in the marriage, it is an event completely out of control of the children who often feel deprived of cohesive family experiences and exposed in front of peers.

II. **FACTORS THAT AFFECT CHILDREN'S ADJUSTMENT TO DIVORCE**
A. **Temperament.** Children with an easygoing and flexible temperament may have an easier time adapting during this period. Children with difficult temperaments, who do not adapt easily or have intense reactions to changes in routine, may elicit more negative attention and become the object that distracts the family from the real issue of conflict—the divorce. Shy, inhibited children may become even more withdrawn and reclusive, but because they do not demand parental attention, their confusion, sadness, and anger may be misinterpreted as adjustment.

Table 41-1 • RESPONSES OF CHILD TO PARENT'S DIVORCE WITHIN THE FIRST YEAR

Developmental Status	Child's Response	Primary Care Clinician's Role
Preschool	Regressive behavior Sleep disturbance Bowel and bladder difficulties Change in sleep and eating patterns Tantrums, aggressive behavior Fears of abandonment, separation anxiety	Encourage stable, predictable daily routines Help parents develop consistent patterns of joining and separating from the child Encourage continued contact with non-custodial parent Provide reassurance Promote parental understanding of child's coping mechanisms
Younger school age	Sadness, anger, fearfulness Loyalty conflicts Attempts to determine responsibility for divorce, self-blame Hopes for family reconciliation Declining school performance	Empathize with child's feelings Provide regular opportunities for the child to talk Support child's continuing relationship with both parents Offer reassurance Encourage open communication with teachers Provide referrals for therapeutic interventions as appropriate for the child's needs
Older school age/ prepubertal	Grief, intense anger Declining school performance Disrupted peer relationships Attempts to clarify responsibility for the divorce Caretaking of a parent	Express interest in and availability to the child Support child's school and peer involvement Provide clear acknowledgment and support for child's working through feelings on the divorce Provide referrals for therapeutic interventions as appropriate for the child's needs
Adolescence	Mood changes including depression and anger Increase in adolescent "acting out" Declining school performance Substance use Suicidal ideation	Empathize with adolescent's feelings Provide opportunities for discussion Encourage parents to support school and peer involvement and appropriate independence in their teens Provide referrals for therapeutic interventions as appropriate for the child's needs

Adapted from Wallerstein JS. Separation, divorce, and remarriage. In: Levine MD, Carey WB, Crocker AC, eds. *Developmental-Behavioral Pediatrics.* 2nd ed. Philadelphia, PA: Saunders; 1992.

B. **Developmental level.** As Table 41-1 shows, the age and developmental level of children at the time of the divorce greatly affects their response to the event.

C. **Predivorce developmental achievements.** Although we cannot predict what developmental progress children might have made had their parents stayed together, their achievements before the divorce continue to affect their abilities postdivorce. Additionally, children with average or above-average cognitive abilities are more likely to pursue additional support from others as a means of coping.

D. **History of previous loss.** For children who may have experienced earlier losses such as the death of a grandparent or a pet or the loss of a beloved childcare provider, the distress caused by parental separation can trigger memories of these difficult periods in the child's life.

E. **Gender.** Effects of gender on a child's adjustment to divorce have been inconsistent.

F. **Extent of parental hostilities before and after the divorce.** The prime determinant of adverse outcomes for children, regardless of age or gender, is ongoing parental hostility. Parents involved in a conflictual relationship are less emotionally available and less effective disciplining their children, and divorces that require a prolonged legal process lead to more negative co-parenting relationships. The outcomes of a high-conflict parental relationship include more externalizing problems, difficulty regulating emotions, and a drop in the child's academic functioning.

G. **Level of economic stress.** For many families, divorce brings a dramatic change in their financial security. Mothers are more likely to experience financial challenges and this has led to a higher percentage of children in divorced families living in poverty. A newly single parent may have to return to school or work, work longer hours, and/or move to a less expensive home and neighborhood, necessitating more changes in the children's lives and less availability of a parent.

H. **Emotional stability of the custodial parent.** Although both parents may experience emotional lability, depression, emotional dependence or disengagement with their children, difficulty maintaining consistent limit setting or discipline, the risk for alcohol or substance abuse, or the excitement of a new active social life, they need to be mindful of the child's need for a stable, familiar environment.

I. **Stability of visitation.** If one parent has sole custody, or if the child resides primarily with one parent, seeing where and how the other parent lives and ideally his or her place in that home can help a child create a new image of family, whereas inconsistent visitation offers children no such relief from their anxiety and fear of abandonment.

J. **Support systems.** Children who can access social supports outside the home, especially a consistent, empathic relationship with another family member, supportive adult, friend, or sibling, are better able to manage their anxieties and anger about the divorce. Many schools offer support groups for children of divorcing parents within the structure of the school day.

III. **MANAGEMENT**

A. **Help families develop a plan.** Helping parents develop a plan for how to tell the children about an impending divorce is invaluable. Children who experienced the most precipitous regressions were those children who had been given no explanation for the separation or for their parent's departure. Children need to be reassured clearly and repeatedly that "divorce is a grown-up problem" and that they were not responsible for the breakup of the marriage. They need to be told explicitly about what will stay the same for them and what will change. Parents may need help to assess the routines in their child's life and problem solve how to try to keep as much of those aspects intact as possible. Trigger questions can be used to ask each parent about discipline problems and changes in the child's sleep and play patterns to generate information about each one's style of parenting and the child's functioning across different households. Although talking to children about a divorce is difficult, providing parents with the following recommendations can help the family initiate and navigate this challenging discussion:

- Do not keep it a secret or wait until the last minute.
- Tell the children together, with both parents participating in the conversation.
- Keep things simple and straightforward.
- Tell children that the divorce is not their fault.
- Acknowledge that this will be a hard and upsetting time for everyone and that it is acceptable to feel sad, angry, or confused.
- Reassure the children that both parents still love them and will always be their parents.
- Do not discuss the other parent's faults or problems with the children or take sides.
- Allow children opportunities to have time to talk privately with a trusted adult, who may or may not be the parent, about their experience of the divorce.
- Do not force children to resolve their complicated feelings prematurely.

B. **Provide anticipatory guidance for the parents throughout the stages of the divorce.** An important opening to begin this discussion might start with "*Has anything changed in your family since we last met?*" If the clinician is aware of the separation/divorce he or she might ask: "*What has it been like for you parenting your child the past few months?*" Meeting with the parents to discuss their child's experience and reactions to the divorce is an important role of the pediatric clinician, especially during the period of parental separation, which is often the most vulnerable time for the child. Other particularly stressful times include birthdays, holidays, and the introduction of a new love interest for either parent or a step-family. Clarifying the pediatric clinician's role early on is critical and may be completed during a parent-only meeting. Reviewing that the pediatric clinician's goal is to meet and advocate for the child's needs also provides an opportunity to set limits with the parents. Maintaining a neutral relationship with each parent should be the goal and will allow for open communication regarding the divorce process, including custody arrangements, each family member's emotional status, and possible beneficial interventions such as therapy. The pediatric clinician should try not to take sides but should listen to each parent when determining what is best for the child. These meetings may need to take place as the child matures, as their understanding of the divorce will shift as they progress developmentally.

C. **Know legal considerations.** Rarely, a pediatric clinician may be subpoenaed by the court as part of the divorce process, often when there are custody disputes, which entails providing testimony and/or the release of documentation relating to the case. In this situation, seeking legal advice would be appropriate to determine which records and what type of information is required from the clinician. The pediatric clinician should also understand whether he or she is being called as a "fact" or an "expert" witness. Whereas the former involves providing facts of the case only, the latter involves a legal procedure qualifying the clinician as an expert on the subject and subsequently allows him or her to offer an opinion on the case. However, maintaining a positive relationship with the entire family is imperative to best meet the needs of the child and every effort should be made to avoid siding with one parent over the other.

D. **Advise parents to inform their child's pediatric clinicians and teachers about the divorce.** Pediatric clinicians should be made aware if one or both parents are able to make medical decisions for the child. If possible, both parents should sign a "consent to treat" form so that medical decisions can be made quickly if necessary. A communication plan between the parents and the pediatric clinician's office should be implemented and this may involve sending copies of medical reports to both parents. Similarly, it is advisable that each parent request in writing to receive school reports and notices so that they can be equally informed about their children's progress.

E. **Emphasize the importance of maintaining structure and organization.** All children have difficulty exerting self-control and organizing their lives when their family arrangement is changing; they need more external control and structure during the stress of a divorce. Regardless of the parents' feelings about each other, continuity of the child's relationships with both parents should be promoted. Parents should discuss and agree upon appropriate rules and limits to be enforced in each household. Consistency with the school environment, extracurricular activities, and peer relationships should also be maintained when possible.

F. **Address children's concerns.** Parents should be informed that when children ask questions about the divorce, they should try to give truthful answers, even if they need to omit certain information. It can be extremely confusing and painful for parents to acknowledge their child's wish for reconciliation. Parents should acknowledge their child's hope for reunion while making it clear that the request will not happen—"You really wish that Daddy and Mommy would live together again in this house. That is not going to happen, but you will see Daddy in his new house every weekend." Reassure parents that it is expected that children will feel sad and that they should give their children permission to grieve and to cry, regardless of their age and gender.

G. **Counsel parents to avoid conflictual interactions around the children.** Watching parents argue without a positive resolution is particularly difficult for children. They bear the guilt of thinking that they are the reason for the conflict. Parents should be encouraged to seek mediation and/or therapy to help them resolve their conflicts without the children needing to witness their anger.

H. **Should parents stay together for the sake of the children?** Although there is never a good time for a family to divorce, growing up in a family in which there is an "emotional divorce" characterized by high levels of tension and low levels of warmth between parents, parents who discredit each other, where one parent aligns with the children to form a coalition against the other parent, or where the child manipulates the parents is also not in the best interests of the child. Staying together for the children places an enormous burden on the children to fill the emotional void between the parents.

I. **When to refer.** Although many children adjust well after their parents' divorce, some children need more than just time and support. Intervention by a therapist or counselor is warranted for children demonstrating significant mood or behavior changes such as depression, regression in self-help skills such as toileting and sleeping, suicidal ideation, aggression, delinquent behavior, substance abuse, or declining school performance. In addition, some children may request to see a therapist to talk about difficult and complex feelings with an impartial, trained person. Parents should not assume that the child has a significant psychiatric problem as a result and should also not feel excessive guilt and shame for having triggered this need. It is more important to address the concerns rather than place blame on either parent or the child.

J. **Long-term consequences.** The majority of children who experience parental divorce or separation adjust well over time, especially those with a strong support system. For children who continue to have difficulty adjusting, therapy has been shown to be effective in helping them cope and work through their emotions. Intense feelings such as sadness, anger, or guilt may be triggered by birthdays, holidays, anniversaries, weddings, or additional losses, even years after the divorce is finalized.

Bibliography

FOR CHILDREN

Blume J. *It's Not The End of the World*. Scarsdale, NY: Bradbury Press; 1972.

Ford A, Blackstone-Ford J. *My Parents Are Divorced Too: A Book for Kids by Kids*. New York, NY: Imagination; 1998. (Ages 9–12).

Holyoke N. *A Smart Girl's Guide to Her Parents' Divorce: How to Land on Your Feet When Your World Turns Upside Down*. Middleton, WI: American Girl Publishing Inc.; 2009. (Ages 8–11).

Masurel C. *Two Homes*. Somerville, MA: Candlewick Press; 2003. (Ages 2–5).

Rogers F. *Let's Talk About It: Divorce*. New York, NY: Putnam; 1996. (Ages 3–7).

Thomas P. *My Family's Changing*. Hauppauge, NY: Barron's Education Series; 1999. (Ages 3–8).

FOR PARENTS

Gardner RA. *The Parents Book About Divorce*. New York, NY: Bantam; 1991.

Jones-Soderman J, Quattrocchi A, Steinberg S. *How to Talk to Your Children About Divorce*. Scottsdale, AZ: Family Mediation Center Publishing Co LLC; 2006.

Lewis J, Sammons W. *Don't Divorce Your Children: Parents and Children Talk About Divorce*. Chicago, IL: Contemporary Books; 1999.

Teyber E. *Helping Children Cope With Divorce*. New York, NY: Lexington Books; 1992.

WEB SITES FOR FAMILIES

Sesame Street: Divorce. https://www.sesamestreet.org/toolkits/divorce.

FOR PROFESSIONALS

PUBLICATIONS

Ang RP, Ooi YP. Impact of gender and parents' marital status on adolescent's suicidal ideation. *Int J Soc Psychiatry*. 2004;50(4):351-360.

Cohen GJ, Weitzman CC; AAP Committee on Psychosocial Aspects of Child and Family Health; AAP Section on Developmental and Behavioral Pediatrics. Helping children and families deal with divorce and separation. *Pediatrics*. 2016;138(6):e20163020.

Kleinsorge C, Covitz LM. Impact of divorce on children: developmental considerations. *Pediatr Rev*. 2012;33(4):147-154.

WEB SITES

American Academy of Child and Adolescent Psychiatry. http://www.aacap.org/publications/facts-fam/divorce.htm.

Divorce Source. http://www.divorcesource.com/info/children/children.shtml.

CHAPTER 42

Down Syndrome

Katherine Myers | Nancy Roizen

I. **DESCRIPTION OF THE PROBLEM.** Down syndrome (DS) is characterized by limitations in cognitive functioning with associated medical problems due to extra, critical portion of chromosome 21 present in all or some of their cells.
   A. **Epidemiology**
   - DS is the most common chromosomal abnormality diagnosed in the United States.
   - DS occurs in 1 in 700 births in the United States.
   - With increased births to older mothers and terminations of pregnancies with prenatal diagnosis, the prevalence varies geographically but has remained steady.
   - With improvements in medical care, the average life span has increased from *12 years to 60 years.* This prolonged life span increases the prevalence of individuals with DS in the general population.
   B. **Genetics**
   - Trisomy of chromosome 21: Accounts for approximately 95% of cases. It is not an inherited mutation, but rather a cell division error during development of the egg, sperm, or embryo. Can be of maternal (90%) or paternal origin.
   - Translocation occurs in approximately 3%–4% of cases. In this situation, the entire long arm of one chromosome 21 is translocated to the long arm of another chromosome.
   - Mosaicism occurs as a result of an error in cell division after fertilization (1%–2%).
   C. **Etiology.** Most children with DS are born to mothers younger than 35 years. However, the risk for conceiving a baby with DS increases when the maternal age at conception is greater than 35 years.
   D. **Making the diagnosis.** DS is diagnosed via chromosome analysis, which can be done prenatally if there are noted risk factors or postnatally if there are concerns for DS based on physical characteristics.
   E. **Prenatal diagnosis.** The American College of Obstetricians and Gynecologists recommends that all women should be offered aneuploidy screening before 20 weeks and should have the option of invasive testing if desired. There are three screening options that are routinely available.
      1. **Combined test or first trimester screening.** The ultrasound evaluation measures nuchal translucency and the blood screen measures pregnancy-associated plasma protein A (PAPP-A) and human chorionic gonadotropin (hCG). Low levels of PAPP-A and high levels of hCG can be associated with DS. In some centers, additional markers are tested including alpha-fetoprotein (AFP), placental growth factor, and dimeric inhibin A. The addition of these three markers can increase the sensitivity of the screen for DS. This screen is completed in the first trimester.
      2. **The Quadruple test or Quad test.** It measures the levels of AFP, estriol, hCG, and inhibin A. Commonly in DS, AFP and estriol levels in blood are lower than expected, whereas those of hCG and inhibin A are elevated. This screen is completed in the second trimester.
      3. **Maternal cell-free DNA testing via blood.** This is a screening test with high sensitivity and specificity to detect DS and lower false-positive rate than other screening options. This testing is controversial due to cost; however, it is typically offered to women who are considered at high risk.
      4. **Diagnostic testing.** If screening results are abnormal, or a woman is considered high risk, the parents are offered diagnostic testing, which can include a chorionic villus sampling (CVS) during the first trimester or amniocentesis in the second trimester to determine if there are any chromosome abnormalities with the fetus.
   F. **Postnatal diagnosis.** When characteristics of DS are noted by providers after birth, a karyotype is diagnostic for DS.
   G. **Signs and symptoms**
   - Common physical findings that occur in more than 75% of newborns with DS include oblique palpebral fissures, wide space between the first and second toes,

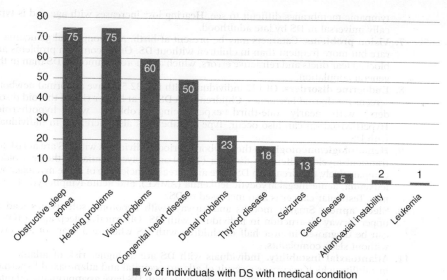

■ % of individuals with DS with medical condition

Figure 42-1 Medical problems common in Down syndrome (DS).

plantar crease between the first and second toes, increased neck tissue, abnormally shaped palate, hypoplastic nose, and brushfield spots. Other common findings are hypotonia, flat nasal bridge, small ears, redundant skin at the nape of the neck, short fifth finger with clinodactyly, and wide spaced fingers.
- Individuals with DS experience a variety of behavioral and medical complications including but not limited to cognitive delays, hearing loss, vision problems, congenital heart defects, gastric malformations, sleep apnea, and leukemia. Fig. 42-1 demonstrates the common medical problems seen in DS.

H. Differential diagnosis. Especially in the newborn period, the phenotypic features of DS may be subtle and can even appear similar to some other genetic conditions. If there is uncertainty, diagnosis of DS can be confirmed via karyotype.

I. Medical concerns with DS
1. **Congenital heart defects (40%–50%).** Most commonly identified congenital heart defects include atrioventricular septal defect, atrial septal defect, and ventricular septal defect. Less common defects include tetralogy of Fallot and aortic coarctation.
2. **Congenital gastrointestinal anomalies.** Duodenal atresia is the most common anomaly noted. Other malformations that may be seen include annular pancreas, imperforate anus, and Hirschsprung disease.
3. **Gastrointestinal problems through the life span.** Children with DS are at risk for celiac disease (3.3%–5%), constipation, and gastrointestinal (GI) reflux. It is important to remember that GI malformations such as Hirschsprung disease and partial obstructions can also be diagnosed after the neonatal period.
4. **Feeding and nutrition.** Feeding difficulties are present in up to 80% of children with DS. This can include chewing and swallowing problems, as well as aspiration of food. Obesity is common and can begin as early as preschool years. Dental problems with malformed teeth as well as too few or too many teeth are common. Dental caries are rare but gingivitis is common.
5. **Neurologic.** Approximately 8% of children with DS will present with seizures in childhood. Of all individuals with DS and seizures, 40% will present before the age of 1 year. West syndrome (infantile spasms) is the most common seizure disorder present in children with DS. Development of Alzheimer disease occurs 10–20 years earlier in individuals with DS.
6. **Hearing loss/recurrent otitis media.** Congenital hearing loss can be found in up to 15% of newborns with DS. Hearing loss can be conductive, sensorineural, or mixed. Most commonly, children with DS experience hearing loss associated with recurrent otitis media and often require treatment with tympanostomy tube placement. Children with DS have smaller and more tortuous ear canals, which makes

tympanic membranes difficult to see. Hearing loss increases with age and is typically universal in DS by late adulthood.

7. **Vision problems.** Cataracts may be present at birth, and congenital glaucoma is rare but more frequent than in children without DS. Other common problems are blocked tear ducts and refractive errors, which are more common in DS than in the general population.

8. **Endocrine disorders.** Of 122 individuals with DS, 32.5% have abnormal newborn screens for thyroid hormones. Children with DS are at higher risk of thyroid disorders, with nearly one-third experiencing problems with hypothyroid. Hyperthyroidism can also occur. Type 1 diabetes is also increased in individuals with DS.

9. **Hematologic/oncologic.** In the newborn period, individuals with DS are at risk for transient myeloproliferative disorder (TMD) and polycythemia. As they get older, comparatively, children with DS have an increased incidence of acute myelogenous leukemia, acute megakaryocytic leukemia (AMKL), and acute lymphocytic leukemia. Testicular cancer is also increased in DS.

10. **Sleep apnea.** Smaller mouths and airways with hypotonic soft tissues lead to upper airway obstruction in individuals with DS. Obstructive sleep apnea (OSA) can be diagnosed in over half of children with DS who are 3 years of age even without sleep complaints.

11. **Atlantoaxial instability.** Individuals with DS are at higher risk of atlantoaxial instability, which occurs as a result of atlanto-occipital and atlantoaxial hypermobility. Approximately 10%–30% of individuals with DS have asymptomatic atlantoaxial instability and about 2% of these experience symptomatic instability.

12. **Orthopedics.** Common orthopedic problems seen in individuals with DS include hypotonia, ligamentous laxity, flat feet, and hyperflexibility. Occasionally, joint subluxation (e.g., patella, shoulder) occurs.

13. **Rheumatologic conditions.** Rheumatologic conditions in DS are eight to nine times more common than in the general population with polyarticular disease in more than half of individuals with DS.

14. **Dermatologic.** In general, children with DS are prone to sensitive skin and have drier skin as they age. They are also more likely to have vitiligo and alopecia including alopecia totalis.

15. **Renal.** Renal and urinary tract anomalies are 4.5 times more common than in the general population.

16. **Development in DS.** Motor development tends to occur at about twice the approximate expected age of a typical child. On average, children with DS sit independently around 11 months and walk around 26 months. On average, first words occur around 19 months of age. Most individuals with DS have mild to moderate intellectual disability. The typical pattern of development includes relative strength in social and fine motor skills and relative weakness in expressive speech and gross motor skills.

17. **Behavioral and mental health concerns.** Children with DS are less likely to have psychopathology than those who have intellectual disability from other etiologies. However, attention-deficit/hyperactivity disorder (ADHD) is as common as in the general population and oppositional defiant behaviors and conduct disorder tend to increase around 10–13 years of age, with noted internalizing problems, such as depression, increasing gradually with age. Autism spectrum disorder is common in DS. Up to 16% of individuals with DS have autism spectrum disorder and the diagnosis is typically later than in children with autism spectrum disorder who do not have DS. If autistic regression takes place, it is at a mean age of 60 months.

II. MANAGEMENT

A. Primary goal. Provide optimal care to achieve the best possible physical and mental health and development as well as psychosocial support for all children with DS.

B. Giving the diagnosis. The DS Diagnosis Study Group created the following evidence-based recommendations for delivering the diagnosis of DS prenatally and postnatally.

1. **Prenatal diagnosis**
   a. When a definitive prenatal diagnosis of DS is made, a health care professional who has specific training on delivering a sensitive diagnosis to parents should discuss it with the family.
   b. This may be an obstetrician, but often he or she will work with an individual who has more experience with DS such as a geneticist, genetic counselor, neonatologist, or developmental–behavioral pediatrician.

c. Be prepared to answer questions about what DS is and what causes the condition. Also, be able to provide realistic expectations of children living with DS today.

d. Offer contact information of support groups that are available for expectant parents.

e. The diagnosis should be given in person whenever possible.

f. Avoid the use of negative language by saying things such as "I'm sorry" during conversations about the diagnosis.

g. Provide up-to-date resources on DS for the family.

h. Make arrangements for follow-up appointments with parents.

2. **Postnatal diagnosis**

a. Obstetricians and pediatric clinicians should meet together with the family to give the diagnosis when possible. When unable to meet together, the clinician team should coordinate to ensure a consistent message to the family.

b. Clinicians should notify the family immediately of their suspicion even if karyotype results are not immediately available. Discretion is advised when determining the exact timing of disclosure in special situations (such as mother is sick after childbirth).

c. Diagnosis should be given in a private location.

d. Parents should be informed together, except in situations when it would significantly delay the conversation.

e. Conversation should begin with positive words (such as congratulating the parents). Avoid apologetic tone during the conversation. Parents will likely remember the first words said during this conversation for years after the discussion is over.

f. Provide the family with accurate information about what DS is and causes for DS. Include lists of up-to-date resources.

g. Limit discussions to medical conditions that the infant has or is suspected of having. Avoid an exhaustive discussion of potential medical conditions.

h. Arrange appropriate follow-up appointments before discharge.

C. **Treatment and medical management**

1. Children with DS are at increased risk for medical disorders affecting arguably every system. There is a risk for *diagnostic overshadowing*, which is to presume that symptoms are simply a consequence of the DS. Because of the diagnostic overshadowing, the diagnosis of an associated disorder such as celiac disease, rheumatoid arthritis, or ADHD may be postponed or missed.

2. Care for children with DS is well described in the 2011 AAP Clinical Report on Health Supervision for Children with DS and is summarized by age in Table 42-1. Organization of care can be divided into several categories.

a. **Evaluation.** *The following recommendations are for ALL children with DS:*

   • **Cardiac**: An echocardiogram read by a pediatric cardiologist is indicated for all newborns with DS *regardless* of whether or not a fetal echocardiogram was performed. If an abnormality is identified, the child should be evaluated by a pediatric cardiologist.

   • **Vision**: It is recommended that babies with DS are evaluated by ophthalmology by 6 months of age or sooner if there are any concerns such as dysconjugate gaze or lack of a red reflex. The recommended schedule for evaluations by an ophthalmologist is annually for 1–5 years of age and then every 2 years for 5- to 13-year-olds and every 3 years for 13- to 21-year-olds. Be vigilant for development of refractive errors, cataracts, and keratoconus.

   • **Hearing**: A newborn hearing screen should be done in the neonatal period. For those who do not pass, a diagnostic evaluation for hearing loss by 3 months of age is recommended. Children with DS who pass their newborn screen can develop conductive, sensorineural, and mixed hearing loss; therefore, audiologic evaluation is recommended every 6 months from 6 months to 5 years of age and then annually.

   • **Sleep apnea**: A sleep study is indicted for symptoms of sleep apnea such as snoring, apnea, restless sleep, daytime sleepiness, frequent night awakenings, and behavior problems. Sleep studies are recommended for all children with DS by the age of 4 years regardless of whether or not they have symptoms due to the high prevalence of OSA in this population. Treatment is usually a tonsillectomy with and without an adenoidectomy, which decreases symptoms in 50% of individuals. Continuous positive airway pressure is sometimes effective, but there are several other interventions being explored to manage OSA.

Table 42-1 • HEALTH MONITORING OF INDIVIDUALS WITH DOWN SYNDROME (DS) BY AGE

Newborn to 1 mo

- Monitor:
  - Echocardiogram (to be read by pediatric cardiologist, even if fetal echo was done) at birth
  - Red reflex check (evaluate for cataracts; require prompt evaluation and treatment if found)
  - Routine newborn hearing screen and follow-up by 3 mo if abnormal
  - Car seat challenge in hospital if child is hypotonic before discharge
  - CBC at birth (newborns are at high risk for transient myeloproliferative disorder [TMD] as well as polycythemia)
  - Obtain thyroid-stimulating hormone (TSH) at birth if state newborn screening measures only free thyroxine (T4)

- Vigilance/management as needed:
  - Referral if noted to have difficulties with feeding or significant hypotonia
  - Pulmonary evaluation for airway assessment if stridor, wheezing, and/or noisy breathing is noted
  - Further GI/surgical evaluation if significant constipation (Hirschsprung) or concerns for duodenal atresia/anorectal atresia

- Things to consider:
  - Support for the family: The family will likely be overwhelmed regardless of the level of medical support the baby requires and know what resources are available to the family locally
  - Developmental services: early intervention services, Down syndrome specialists

1 mo–1 y

- Monitor:
  - Hearing (every 6 mo)
  - Vision (annually)
  - Thyroid (at 6 mo of age, 1 y, and annually)

- Vigilance/management as needed:
  - Growth
  - Heart: If history of CHD, follow up with cardiology as needed based on lesion. If no history of cardiac disease, the child may not need cardiology follow-up
  - Stomach/bowel issues; spitting-up/stooling issues can be a sign that there is a problem
  - Neck instability

- Things to consider:
  - Developmental services: early intervention services, Down syndrome specialists, social supports in community

1–5 y

- Monitor:
  - Hearing (every 6 mo); referral to ENT if hearing loss detected
  - Vision (annually); sooner if noted problems
  - Thyroid (annually)
  - Blood tests for anemia annually
  - Sleep study: All children with DS should have a sleep study by the age of 4 y even if asymptomatic. If symptomatic before or after the age of 4 y prompt referral for sleep study is recommended

- Vigilance/management as needed:
  - Growth: Use DS-specific growth charts
  - Heart: If history of CHD, follow up with cardiology as needed based on lesion. If no history of cardiac disease, the child may not need cardiology follow-up
  - Stomach/bowel issues: Discuss toileting issues at all visits, as constipation and diarrhea are common. May consider celiac testing if signs of disease
  - Neck instability: Discuss safe physical activity and signs of instability
  - Seizures are common in children with DS. Monitor of signs of seizures

- Things to consider:
  - Dental: Patterns of teeth eruption are different in DS. Promote good dental hygiene and care

5–13 y

- Monitor:
  - Hearing every 6 mo until testing can be done in individual ears. When individual ears can be tested, can test annually. Referral to ENT if hearing loss detected
  - Vision (annually), sooner if noted problems
  - Thyroid (annually)
  - Blood tests for anemia (annually)

Table 42-1 • HEALTH MONITORING OF INDIVIDUALS WITH DOWN SYNDROME (DS) BY AGE (CONTINUED)

- Vigilance/management as needed:
  - Growth: Use DS-specific growth charts
  - Heart: If history of CHD, follow up with cardiology as needed based on lesion. If no history of cardiac disease, the child may not need cardiology follow-up
  - Stomach/bowel issues: Discuss toileting issues at all visits as constipation and diarrhea are common. May consider Celiac testing if signs of disease
  - Neck instability: Discuss safe physical activity and signs of instability
  - Seizures: Are common in children with DS. Monitor of signs of seizures
  - Sleep study: If symptomatic, prompt referral for sleep study is recommended

- Things to consider:
  - Sexuality and puberty: As the child becomes older, it is important to begin discussions with the family regarding puberty, managing sexual behaviors (such as masturbation), periods, and teaching children about appropriate touch and correct names for body parts
  - Self-help skills: Developing self-help skills is valuable for the family and the child. Discuss with the families about working toward independence in areas such as bathing, toileting, and other areas of self-care

13–21 y

- Monitor:
  - Hearing (annually); more often if problems are noted
  - Vision (every 3 y); more often if problems are noted
  - Thyroid (annually)
  - Blood tests for anemia (annually)

- Vigilance/management as needed:
  - Growth: Use DS-specific growth charts
  - Heart: If history of CHD, follow up with cardiology as needed based on lesion. If no history of cardiac disease, the child may not need cardiology follow-up
  - Stomach/bowel issues: Discuss toileting issues at all visits, as constipation and diarrhea are common. May consider celiac testing if signs of disease
  - Neck instability: Discuss safe physical activity and signs of instability
  - Seizures: Are common in children with DS. Monitor of signs of seizures
  - Sleep study: If symptomatic prompt referral for sleep study is recommended

- Things to consider:
  - Transitions: Discussions regarding school placement and services. Planning for housing and employment. Guardianship and financial planning
  - Sexuality and puberty: As the child becomes older, it is important to begin discussions with the family regarding puberty, managing sexual behaviors (such as masturbation), periods, and teaching children about appropriate touch and correct names for body parts
  - Self-help skills: Developing self-help skills is valuable for the family and the child. Discuss with the families about working toward independence in areas such as bathing, toileting, and other areas of self-care
  - Aging: Begin to discuss unique adult health issues for individuals with DS (such as early aging and higher risk for Alzheimer disease)

The above information was adapted from the American Academy of Pediatrics Health Care Information for Families of Children with Down Syndrome and the Health Supervision for Children with Down Syndrome.
Bull M and the Committee on Genetics. Health supervision for children with down syndrome. *Pediatrics.* 2011;128:393-406.
Bull M and The Ad Hoc Writing Committee. Health care information for families of children with down syndrome. *American Academy of Pediatrics.* 2013. Available from: http://pediatrics.aappublications.org/content/128/2/393.full.
CHD, congenital heart disease.

b. **Monitoring.** *The following should be monitored for ALL children with DS at varying intervals:*
- **Thyroid:** All states screen for thyroid disease, but in newborns with DS a thyroid-stimulating hormone (TSH) level should be drawn if the newborn screen included only a free thyroxine (T4) level, which may not identify congenital hypothyroidism. An additional TSH level is recommended at 6 and 12 months of age and then annually, as children can develop different types of thyroid disease with age.
- **Hemoglobin:** At birth a complete blood count (CBC) should be done to identify TMD (present in 4%–10% of individuals with DS). TMD generally resolves on its own but can be a serious illness. Also, in those that resolve, by 4 years of

age, approximately 20% of cases develop AMKL. Therefore, those with TMD should be referred for monitoring to pediatric oncology. In addition, monitoring with an annual hemoglobin or ferritin and C-reactive protein if the diet is low in iron is indicated, as children with DS have significantly decreased intake of iron.

- **Growth:** Individuals with DS are often overweight or obese. Weight problems are due in part to a lower resting metabolic rate, which requires fewer calories to maintain weight. Obesity is to be prevented. Monitor weight and height using the 2015 CDC DS-specific growth charts and plot BMI on the standard growth charts for age and gender charts.

c. **Symptomatic management.** When following a child with DS, who is presenting with worrisome symptoms, the following descriptions may help guide management:

- **Atlantoaxial subluxation:** As the first line of defense, parents should be directed to have their child been seen that day by their primary care provider for evaluation if they have signs of spinal cord compromise. Such signs may include gait or motor problems such as limping, having difficulty climbing stairs when they were previously able, new neck pain or a stiff neck, weakness, changes in tone, loss of established bowel or bladder control, or any neurologic changes. The child should undergo plain lateral cervical spine radiography in the neutral position. If there are any abnormalities, the child should be immediately referred for evaluation in a location with a pediatric neurosurgeon or pediatric orthopedic surgeon familiar with atlantoaxial instability. If no abnormalities are noted on, neutral film flexion/extension films can be obtained before immediate referral to a specialist. Routine neck X-rays without symptoms or signs of subluxation are not recommended. In general, children with DS should avoid participation in sports that increase risk of spinal cord injury such as football, soccer, and gymnastics. Trampoline use should be avoided, particularly in those less than 6 years of age.
- **Celiac disease:** If the child has symptoms potentially related to celiac disease such as diarrhea, protracted constipation, slow growth, failure to thrive, anemia, abdominal pain or bloating, and/or worsening behavioral problems, the child should be evaluated further for the disease. Recommended evaluation includes a tissue transglutaminase immunoglobulin A (IgA) level and a quantitative IgA. Refer to a pediatric gastroenterologist for further evaluation if abnormal values or worsening problems are found.
- **OSA:** After passing an initial sleep study, further evaluation is needed if a child develops symptoms of OSA (see Evaluation section for further details).
- **Feeding and swallowing:** A radiographic swallowing assessment should be considered in an infant who has choking with feeds, failure to thrive, recurrent pneumonia, or other recurrent or persistent respiratory symptoms.

d. Vigilance
- **Arthritis, type 1 diabetes, GI malformations, leukemia, renal and urinary tract disorders, and seizures** are all more common in children with DS. They require an awareness of the association with DS and expedited evaluation of symptoms. Sometimes diagnosis has been delayed because of diagnostic overshadowing.
- **Behavioral and mental health concerns:** When there are concerns about behavioral problems, evaluation and intervention with behavioral counseling and medication as needed is indicated. Behavioral problems may be exacerbated or caused by medical problems such as anemia, celiac disease, OSA, thyroid disease, dental pain, or other pain; therefore, proper evaluation and management of medical and behavioral problems is essential to the care of these individuals.

e. Prevention
- **Gingivitis:** Routine dental visit should begin in the second year of life and dental hygiene should be initiated to prevent gingivitis. Braces are frequently needed but not always tolerated.
- **Obesity:** Prevention of obesity is challenging in children with DS because of lower metabolic rates and decreased micronutrient intake. Therefore, food needs to be nutrient rich but calorie poor. Physical activity should be part of a health regimen.

D. Prognosis
- There is no specific treatment or cure for DS; however, medical conditions and behavioral concerns must be monitored and managed closely. The American Academy of Pediatrics (AAP) has designed recommendations for the Health Supervision of Children with Down Syndrome from birth to adolescence. In addition to monitoring and managing the above conditions in DS as needed, the AAP recommends at least annually that pediatric clinicians should discuss with the families the value of support systems within the community and their own family, medical and financial supports that may be available to the family, injury and abuse prevention particularly related to the child's developmental ability, and nutrition and activity as means to prevent obesity.

E. Education and planning for the future
- Discussions about early intervention programs, therapy services (e.g., speech therapy, physical therapy, occupational therapy, and behavioral therapy), and recreational and integrated/inclusive educational programs should be discussed with parents. Educational programs should be developed with consideration of the needs of the individual child and family. Encouraging appropriate therapeutic interventions and educational support can help the children with DS develop self-help skills to live more independently and possibly get and maintain a job in the future. Development of plans for transition to adult medical care and living should begin at 12 years of age and include guardianship, long-term financial planning, adult work, recreation, and places to live.

Bibliography

FOR PARENTS

National Down Syndrome Congress (NDSC): To promote the interests of people with Down syndrome and their families through advocacy, public awareness, and information. Every year this organization holds an annual conference for families. http://www.ndsccenter.org/.

National Down Syndrome Society (NDSS): The NDSS is the leading human rights organization for all individuals with Down syndrome. http://www.ndss.org/.

Health Care Information for Families of Children with Down Syndrome: The American Academy of Pediatrics has information for families on their Web page for children with Down syndrome. The full link can be found here: Health Care Information for Families of Children with Down Syndrome. Available online at: http://pediatrics.aappublications.org/content/128/2/393.full.

Woodbine House: Publishes family-friendly books on topics such as teaching gross motor skills, language skills, reading, math, and others. They have boys' and girls' guides to growing up which discuss puberty as well as a guide to dating for people with disabilities. http://www.woodbinehouse.com/.

FOR PROFESSIONALS

American Academy of Pediatrics Health Supervision Guidelines for Down Syndrome, Bull M, the Committee on Genetics. Health supervision for children with down syndrome. *Pediatrics*. 2011;128:393-406.

Down Syndrome Medical Interest Group (DSMIG-USA): Professionals from a variety of disciplines who provide care to individuals with Down syndrome and/or their families. This organization holds an annual conference for professionals who work with individuals with Down syndrome. https://www.dsmig-usa.org/.

Growth Charts for DS, Zemel BS, Pipan M, Stallings VA, et al. Growth charts for children with down syndrome in the United States. *Pediatrics*. 2015;136:1204-1211.

CHAPTER 43

Eating Disorders in Adolescents

Melissa Beth Freizinger | Sara F. Forman

I. **DESCRIPTION OF THE PROBLEM.** Eating disorders (EDs) are serious psychiatric illnesses with many potential medical complications. In 2013, the American Psychiatric Association added new ED diagnostic categories to the previous group of ED diagnoses. In addition to Anorexia Nervosa (AN), which focuses on restrictive eating behaviors, and Bulimia Nervosa (BN), which includes bingeing and purging behaviors, the DSM-5 now includes ED categories of Binge Eating Disorder (BED) and Avoidant Restrictive Food Intake Disorder (ARFID). The DSM-5 also changed the diagnosis of eating disorder not otherwise specified (EDNOS) to Other Specified Feeding and Eating Disorders (OSFEDs). Each ED diagnosis has unique features although all have shared issues of body weight and shape dissatisfaction and/or difficulty with intake.

Key features of AN include fear of becoming fat and disordered body image in an individual who is malnourished. BN includes purging behaviors in response to bingeing episodes (consuming extremely large amounts of food) while feeling out of control. Individuals with BED have bingeing episodes without compensatory behaviors—these episodes are followed by feelings of distress. The new diagnosis of ARFID includes individuals who are unable to maintain an adequate body weight but who do not have body image concerns. Behaviors that may be seen in individuals with EDs include restrictive intake, binge eating, excessive exercise, self-induced vomiting, and/or laxative/diuretic/diet pill abuse.

- Pre- and postpubertal male and females with AN have a body weight that is significantly below expected body weight for age or growth trajectory. Although patients may deny hunger to rationalize their dieting behavior, they are constantly preoccupied with thoughts about food and weight. Besides restricting calories and exercising excessively, a subset of patients with AN also binge and may vomit or abuse laxatives and diuretics. This purging subgroup tends to have a worse prognosis and is at higher risk of morbidity.
- All patients with BN engage in binge eating (characterized by the ingestion of an amount of food that is distinctly greater than the amount most individuals would consume under similar circumstances over a discrete period of time) followed by purging behaviors: self-induced vomiting, laxatives, diuretics, enemas, and excessive exercise to prevent weight gain. These binge eating episodes that occur minimally once per week over 3 months are accompanied by feelings of lack of control. Additionally, patients with BN have body image disturbances.
- Patients with BED share some features as noted above for BN along with feelings of shame and/or guilt. Binges may occur when patients eat alone because of embarrassment or shame, eat to the point of being uncomfortably full, or eat large amounts of food when not hungry. Patients with BED may be of normal weight, overweight, or obese and are seen in all age groups.
- ARFID patients are most likely underweight and may have had a long-standing history of poor nutritional intake or picky eating because of anxiety related to a traumatic event such as a choking episode, sensory issues with texture or specific foods, or a persistent lack of appetite not specifically due to other medical conditions. There is a persistent inability to meet required energy needs or nutritional requirements and/or the diagnosis interferes with psychosocial functioning. Patients with ARFID may be dependent on nutritional supplements.
- OSFED includes individuals who do not fit into the above categories. The OSFED diagnosis includes Purging Disorder, Atypical AN, and other subthreshold diagnoses. For more detailed information on OSFED, please see the DSM-5.

A. **Epidemiology**
- It is estimated that up to 1% of young females may have AN. Adolescent onset between the ages of 15–19 years is found in 40% of cases.
- Approximately 2%–3% of late adolescent and young adult females may have BN, with age of onset (approximately 18 years) being slightly older than that for AN. A brief period of AN may precede the onset of BN.

- Males account for at least 10% of individuals with EDs, although this is likely to be an underestimate because males often do not seek care as frequently as females.
- ARFID is a relatively new diagnosis and further studies are needed to assess the epidemiology of this diagnosis, although boys seem to have a higher rate of diagnosis compared with AN.
- EDs are seen across all racial, ethnic, and socioeconomic groups.

B. **Etiology.** There is no single cause for an ED. Factors that may precipitate onset or contribute to sustaining an ED include biological, psychological, and environmental causes.

C. **Genetics and biology.** It is now understood that genetics play a significant role in the development of EDs. Heritability estimates obtained in genetic studies are equal to those for other biologically based psychiatric illnesses (bipolar disorder, schizophrenia).

- The concordance rate for AN among monozygotic twins is 55% (vs. 7% for dizygotic pairs), suggesting a genetic basis for this syndrome. First-degree relatives of probands are eight times more likely to develop AN than are first-degree relatives of healthy controls.
- The concordance rate for monozygotic twins with BN (22.9%) is higher than that for dizygotic pairs (8.7%).
- There is less genetic research on BED as it is a more recent diagnostic category.

1. **Psychological factors.** Comorbid psychological illnesses are risk factors for developing an ED. These include affective disorders, anxiety disorders, substance use disorders, and personality disorders. Individuals with AN often have premorbid anxiety disorders (social anxiety/phobia and obsessive–compulsive disorder), which may be exacerbated by malnourishment. Other mood disorders such as depression can be secondary to the weight loss but can also predate the ED. BED is associated with elevated rates of lifetime major depressive disorder.

2. **Sociocultural factors.** Sociocultural influences (i.e., media exposure, perceived pressures for thinness, thin-ideal internalization) are risk factors for disordered eating but only for a subset of females and males who are vulnerable to these influences. Environment factors such as participation in a high-risk sport, a competitive academic or social environment, or a family culture of dieting and exercise can also negatively affect at-risk individuals.

3. **Developmental factors and temperament.** Predisposing traits for the development of an ED include negative emotionality (neuroticism), poor interoceptive awareness, perfectionism, ineffectiveness, drive for thinness, and obsessive–compulsive personality traits. Research has demonstrated that perfectionism and negative emotionality tend to be associated with ED symptoms across the diagnostic spectrum; however, impulsivity is thought to relate specifically to binge eating and purging.

4. **Familial.** There are no data to support the theory that EDs are caused by a certain type of family dynamic or parenting style. As discussed, EDs develop because of a number of complex factors in a multiplicity of family contexts.

5. **Developmental.** The physical transformation that takes place during adolescence is often intertwined with feelings of self-consciousness and low self-esteem. Adapting to a changing body; developing a personal, sexual, and gender identity; and separation from parents are all important developmental tasks. Many adolescents lack the ability to verbally express feelings of depression, low self-esteem, or anxiety. Bullying and teasing, and/or cultural and societal pressures can place them at increased risk for developing disordered eating behaviors.

6. **Physiologic.** Patients with AN and BN have multiple metabolic, hormonal, and neurotransmitter abnormalities due to starvation or purging behaviors.

II. **MAKING THE DIAGNOSIS**

A. **Signs and symptoms.** Making the diagnosis of an ED can be difficult for patients because of the shame and guilt associated with these illnesses. Just as patients with AN may deny hunger as they pursue weight loss, they may minimize various manifestations of their illness. Patients may deny fear of fatness or may be ashamed to discuss their bingeing, vomiting, or abuse of laxatives or diuretics. Clinicians must maintain a high level of awareness and continue to ask questions of the patient and family when symptoms suggest or are consistent with an ED.

The signs and symptoms associated with EDs are highlighted in Table 43-1.

B. **Differential diagnosis.** When developing a differential diagnosis, clinicians should remember that patients with illnesses whose signs and symptoms are similar to AN or BN generally indicate discomfort with these manifestations and do not have a persistent and overriding concern with body shape and weight. Although they may initially

Table 43-1 • SIGNS, SYMPTOMS, AND PHYSICAL EXAMINATION FINDINGS OF EATING DISORDERS

	Associated with Starvation	Associated with Bingeing or Purging
General	Hyperactivity or lethargy Irritability Sleep disturbance Dizziness Syncope Hypothermia Slowed growth	Dizziness Syncope
Skin	Subcutaneous fat loss Dry, brittle hair, or loss of hair Lanugo hair Sallow skin	Callus on back of hand over knuckles (Russell sign) Acanthosis nigricans (with obesity)
Oral		Dental caries Enamel erosion or discoloration of teeth (lingual surface) Parotid gland hypertrophy
Cardiovascular	Hypotension Bradycardia Orthostasis	Arrhythmias
Gastrointestinal	Scaphoid abdomen Constipation Early satiety Decreased bowel sounds	Epigastric tenderness Gastroesophageal reflux Obesity Abdominal distension
Neuromuscular	Muscle weakness/wasting	Muscle weakness
Extremities	Cold, mottled, or cyanotic hands and feet	Edema of feet
Genitourinary/ gynecologic	Thin, pale, dry, atrophic vaginal mucosa Amenorrhea Decreased libido Breast atrophy	Irregular menstruation
Musculoskeletal	Osteopenia Stress fractures	Joint pain if obese

Note: Patients who are malnourished and engaged in purging behaviors will display signs and symptoms from both columns.

be pleased with a limited amount of unexpected weight loss, they may become alarmed as their weight continues to drop. They do not exclusively limit fat and calories, and concerns about weight and body shape do not preoccupy them. In ARFID, individuals may want to gain weight but are unable to do so despite interventions, although they do not have concerns about becoming overweight. Diseases that can mimic EDs are listed in Table 43-2. A thorough history that addresses all aspects of an adolescent's life (HEADSS: Home life, Education/Employment, Activities, Drug use, Sexuality/sexual behaviors, and Suicidal thoughts/mood issues, and Safety), a careful physical examination, and perhaps a few screening laboratory tests (such as a complete blood count, erythrocyte sedimentation rate, electrolytes, urine pregnancy test if amenorrhea is present, thyroid-stimulating hormone, and a celiac panel or stool for occult blood, if indicated) are generally sufficient to exclude these diagnoses.

  C. History: key clinical questions. When indicated by concern, clinicians should ask the following questions.
  1. *How do you feel about your current weight? What would you like to weigh?* These questions begin to elicit information about fear of fatness and body shape dissatisfaction as well as body image distortion (e.g., feeling fat or wanting to lose "just a few more pounds" even when the teenager appears emaciated). Patients with ARFID may express a desire to gain weight.
  2. *What is the most and least you have ever weighed since puberty began and how old were you at each of those times?* (For prepubertal girls: what is the least/most you

Table 43-2 • DIFFERENTIAL DIAGNOSIS OF EATING DISORDERS

CNS	Hypothalamic disorders (e.g., brain tumor)
Endocrine	Adrenal insufficiency Diabetes mellitus Hyperthyroidism, Hypothyroidism, Hypercortisolism
Gastrointestinal	Inflammatory bowel disease Irritable bowel disease *Helicobacter pylori* infection Achalasia Celiac disease
Immunologic	Rheumatologic illness
Gynecologic	Pregnancy
Psychiatric	Depression Anxiety Obsessive–compulsive disorder Thought disorder
Miscellaneous	Malignancy Substance use disorder

CNS, central nervous system.

have weighed in the last few years?). This question establishes baseline measurements and reflects the degree of weight loss. Updating of growth charts is essential.

3. *Tell me what you ate for breakfast, lunch, dinner, and snacks yesterday and was this a typical day for you?* Dietary recall shows caloric intake, meal patterns, and food preferences and helps indicate restriction of food to low-calorie, low-fat choices. Information must be obtained in great detail (e.g., what was on the sandwich? how much of it was eaten?).

4. *Tell me about your exercise routine. How much time do you spend exercising in the average week? Have you increased the amount of exercise you do lately?* Patients with EDs may intensely exercise as a way to increase caloric expenditure and/or to compensate for binge eating episodes. Information about the specific types and duration of exercise should be elicited. Patients often engage in solitary or secretive exercise.

5. *How often do you weigh yourself?* Frequencies greater than once every few days may indicate an over-preoccupation with body weight.

6. *How would you generally describe your mood—happy, sad, worried, etc.? How did you feel last year?* Depression and anxiety are commonly associated with EDs, either as a primary or secondary diagnosis. Screening questions about sleep problems, decreased concentration, fatigue, loss of interest in usual activities, frequent crying, and feelings of self-blame, guilt, or suicidal behavior should be covered.

7. *Have you used any of the following to control your weight: laxatives, water pills (diuretics), diet pills, or dietary supplements?* These represent commonly used compensatory weight control methods. Any positive answers should be followed up with questions about frequency and amount of use.

8. *Do you vomit? If so, how do you induce vomiting? How often do you vomit? How long does each individual episode last?* These questions elicit details of the purging cycle. Some patients with BN have lost their gag reflex and may be able to spontaneously vomit or regurgitate food at will. Patients with severe purging may also experience rumination and gastric reflux.

9. *How often do you binge eat? What did you eat during your last binge?* An objective binge includes consumption of large quantities of food, often several thousand calories. In contrast, some young women mistakenly interpret eating a few cookies or an ice cream sundae as a binge. During a binge episode, food is usually consumed quickly and while alone.

10. *How do you feel before and after you binge? Are there situations or feelings that trigger binge episodes?* Binge eating is typically associated with feelings of lack of control, negative affect, anxiety, shame, or guilt.

11. *How are you coping with situations in your life?* It is important to ask about past or current suicidality. Although EDs have the highest mortality rate of all psychiatric disorders, suicide is the most common cause of nonmedical death among individuals with EDs. Sample questions:
    - *Do you ever feel like just giving up? Or would it be ok if you weren't "here" tomorrow?*
    - *Do you think about dying or suicide?*
    - *Are you thinking about hurting yourself?*
    - *Have you ever engaged in self-injurious behavior i.e. cutting? Do you have any previous suicide attempts?*
    - *Do you have a plan?*
    - *Do you have access to weapons or things that can be used as weapons to harm yourself?*

D. **Behavioral observations.** While eliciting the history, it is important to note the patient's general affect and mood. Patients with EDs may have flat affect—it may be difficult to ascertain whether depressed affect is due to depression or malnourishment. A brief mental health status should be obtained. It is important to note the following:
   - Facial expression
   - General body movement
   - Attitude
   - Thought process and content
   - Mood and appearance
   - Intellectual functioning
   - Memory
   - Insight and judgment
   - Willingness to answer questions

   Patients with EDs often minimize and/or deny their symptoms. Patients may exhibit little concern for a degree of weight loss that others would find alarming. Patients are often ambivalent about entering treatment and recovery. It is also important to note if the patient has engaged in self-injurious behaviors. It may be helpful to first meet with the family and the patient together, and then meet with parents and patient separately. This may help build rapport and trust with the patient who may report behaviors to you that their parents are unaware of. Additionally, family members may offer other information and certain aspects of the family or patient history without the patient being present.

E. **Physical examination.** Key aspects of the physical examination should include accurate measurements of height and weight and orthostatic vital signs, including heart rate and blood pressure. Other physical examination findings are noted in Table 43-1. Severely underweight patients will display more of these features, especially if they also binge and purge. Patients must be undressed completely (except for a gown) to accurately assess their physical condition. Examination of the breasts and external genitalia (pubic hair development, testicular size) to assess sexual maturity rating in adolescents should also be performed. Review of the growth chart with accurately obtained height and weight is essential.

F. **Tests.** Table 43-3 includes the most commonly noted abnormalities that can help to confirm or eliminate the diagnosis, or identify potentially life-threatening conditions. However, in the presence of the classic syndrome of AN marked by fear of fatness and dieting behavior, or BN with binge/purge behaviors and overemphasis on weight and shape concerns, an exhaustive diagnostic workup may not be indicated but should be made on an individual case basis.

III. MANAGEMENT

A. **Primary goals.** Restoration of weight is the primary goal in the treatment of patients with AN and ARFID. Until this goal is achieved, patients with AN may not benefit from other therapeutic modalities as a result of the intense preoccupation with food and weight and psychiatric symptoms sustained by malnourishment. For individuals with ARFID, nutritional rehabilitation is essential for growth and further development. For patients with bingeing and/or purging behaviors, cessation of eating disordered behaviors and normalization of eating is of primary importance.

   Other goals for patients with EDs include the following:
   - Medical stability
   - Monitoring for medical complications
   - Normalization of eating patterns
   - Absence of purging behaviors
   - Healthy coping mechanisms
   - Improved mental health

Table 43-3 • LABORATORY VALUES IN EATING DISORDERS

Hematologic	Anemia (mild) Leukopenia Thrombocytopenia
Endocrine	Follicle-stimulating hormone/luteinizing hormone: low/low normal Thyroxine/thyroid-stimulating hormone: low/low normal or sick euthyroid levels Elevated cortisol (in starvation)
GI	AST/ALT normal or elevated Salivary amylase increased (in vomiting)
Renal	BUN normal or elevated Urine pH >7 Urine specific gravity normal or elevated (may also be very low in patients who drink excessive water)
Metabolic	Hypokalemic, hypochloremic, metabolic alkalosis Hyponatremia Hypocalcaemia Hypophosphatemia, hypomagnesemia Elevated bicarbonate
ECG	Low voltage Bradycardia Depressed T waves Prolonged QTc interval

GI, gastrointestinal tract; AST, aspartate aminotransferase; ALT, alanine aminotransferase; BUN, blood urea nitrogen; ECG, electrocardiogram.

- Improved personal, social, and family functioning
- Treatment of comorbid psychiatric conditions (e.g., depression, anxiety disorders, drug and alcohol abuse)
- Normalization of exercise

B. Treatment. Evidence-based treatment provided by health professionals with expertise in the care of patients with an ED is necessary.

Family-based treatment (FBT) has been shown to be effective for adolescents with restrictive EDs and BN. FBT is a highly structured 20-session outpatient program designed to put parents in control of their child's nutrition and refeeding (sessions 1–10) and then gradually return control of eating back to the adolescent (sessions 11–20).

Patients who fail to gain weight after 1–2 months of outpatient therapy or those with a long-standing ED may require a higher level of care. This may involve an admission to a specialty inpatient treatment program, residential treatment, and/or a partial hospital day program. Immediate hospitalization may be necessary if any of the conditions in Table 43-4 are present.

Cognitive behavioral therapy (CBT) is another useful mode of treatment for patients with BN or BED.

The primary care clinician is ideally suited to serve as coordinator of the treatment process along with the ED specialist. Often, he or she has a long-standing relationship with the patient and his or her family and can explain the nature and severity of the illness. The clinician can also assume the role of monitoring weight gain and the potential medical complications of the illness (such as amenorrhea or hypokalemia).

1. **Weight gain.** Initially, patients should be weighed weekly dressed in a gown only. They should urinate before being weighed because water loading may be used by patients to artificially raise their weight and can be detected by checking urine specific gravity. The goal should be a steady gain of 1–2 pounds per week. The target goal weight for adolescents should be the return to the prior weight or BMI trajectory percentile that was established before the development of the ED. For adolescents who were obese before developing an ED, restoration to the 50%–75% percentile may be an appropriate first weight goal; however, further weight gain may be needed over the course of treatment.

2. **Activity.** Restrictions on activities are necessary for underweight patients, both as a means of assuring the child's safety and because patients are unlikely to gain weight if permitted to exercise. In many cases, no significant exercise should be permitted until the patient is either close to or at their goal weight.

Table 43-4 • INDICATIONS FOR MEDICAL OR PSYCHIATRIC HOSPITALIZATION

Weight less than 75% of median BMI for age, or severe malnutrition per SAHM guideline paper
Failure to respond to outpatient treatment
Cardiovascular compromise
  Cardiac arrhythmias
  Bradycardia (<50 BPM daytime, <45 BPM nighttime)
  QTc prolongation
  Postural hypotension with presyncopal symptoms or systolic blood pressure less than
  90 mm Hg
Hypothermia (<96°F)
Significant dehydration
Electrolyte disturbances
Severe psychiatric symptoms, e.g., comorbid depression or anxiety or substance abuse
Suicidal ideation or recurrent self-injurious behavior
Acute food refusal

BMI, body mass index; SAHM, Society for Adolescent Health and Medicine.

3. **Restoration of health.** Much of the ongoing treatment will revolve around addressing the patient's concern about body changes and weight gain. The clinician may discuss the negative consequences of EDs and the importance of returning to his or her growth curve. The clinician can review the importance of bone health, brain health, and reproductive functions. Finally, it may help to remind patients that body image improves last and often lags behind normalization of eating behavior by 3–6 months, but that body image may improve as the patient maintains his or her goal weight.

4. **Nutrition.** Many adolescents (and their parents) have inaccurate information about the caloric content of various foods and the appropriate food intake for a maturing adolescent. It is important to stress, for example, that a low-calcium diet, coupled with a hypoestrogenic state, can lead to osteopenia that may be irreversible and that this complication occurs early, often within 6 months of the onset of amenorrhea. Many of the symptoms the patient experiences and finds distressful are due to physiologic alterations secondary to weight loss; clarifying this relationship will lend credence to the team's insistence on weight gain. Dietary fat should be consumed with each meal (in a society that emphasizes no-fat foods, teenagers may not be aware of the importance of dietary fat to the body's normal functioning) and no "diet" or "fat-free" products should be eaten.

5. **Purging.** Teenagers may not be aware that self-induced vomiting or regular use of diuretics or laxatives primarily results in water weight loss rather than true weight loss yet can induce dehydration or a variety of life-threatening complications. The clinician should routinely ask if patients have used or are using any of these products or to what extent they are purging. Hypokalemia (serum $K^+ < 3.0$ mEq/dL) suggests a patient is vomiting and is potentially life-threatening. Deaths in EDs may arise from cardiac arrhythmias because of electrolyte imbalances.

6. **Family support.** Treatment goals and expectations among team members and the family must be clear so that the patient, family, and members of the treatment team are united in their approach. The clinician has a critical role in coordinating these treatment efforts and assuring that everyone is in agreement with the treatment plan.

7. **Medications,** such as the serotonergic reuptake inhibitors (SSRIs), have been found to be helpful in decreasing episodes of bingeing and purging in BN; however, no medication has been found to be useful in achieving weight gain among patients with AN. SSRIs may be helpful in patients with comorbid anxiety and depressive disorders but usually will not be effective unless the starved state is reversed. Appetite-enhancing medications such as cyproheptadine may be tried for patients with ARFID with low appetite levels. Oral contraceptive hormonal treatment to induce or regulate menses has not been demonstrated to be effective in preventing osteopenia; furthermore, it eliminates an important marker for gauging the adequacy of weight gain and may falsely reassure a young woman that "everything is okay."

Bibliography

NATIONAL ORGANIZATIONS

Academy for Eating Disorders (AED). http://www.aedweb.org/ An international multidisciplinary professional organization that focuses on advocacy, research, and treatment of eating disorders.

Academy of Nutrition and Dietetics. http://www.eatright.org/ Formerly the American Dietetic Association, the site offers information about eating disorders, including an extensive nutrition reading list and a professional directory that allows visitors to search for registered dietitians specializing in eating disorders.

National Association of Anorexia Nervosa and Associated Eating Disorders (ANAD). http://www.anad.org/ ANAD is a nonprofit (501 c 3) organization working in the areas of support, awareness, advocacy, referral, education, and prevention of eating disorders.

Binge Eating Disorder Association (BEDA). https://bedaonline.com/ The Binge Eating Disorder Association (BEDA) is the national organization focusing on increased prevention, diagnosis, and treatment for binge eating disorder.

F.E.A.S.T. http://www.feast-ed.org/ F.E.A.S.T. is an organization of and for parents and caregivers to help loved ones recover from eating disorders by providing information and mutual support, promoting evidence-based treatment, and advocating for research and education to reduce the suffering associated with eating disorders.

Maudsley Parents. http://www.maudsleyparents.org/ A site for parents of eating disordered children focused on supporting families using family-based treatment.

National Eating Disorders Association (NEDA). https://www.nationaleatingdisorders.org/. NEDA is a nonprofit organization devoted to preventing eating disorders, providing treatment referrals, and increasing the education and understanding of eating disorders, weight, and body image.

The National Association for Males with Eating Disorders, Inc. (N.A.M.E.D.). http://namedinc.org/ N.A.M.E.D. is dedicated to offering support to and public awareness about males with eating disorders.

The National Institute of Mental Health. Eating disorders. http://www.nimh.nih.gov/health/publications/eating-disorders/index.shtml

FOR PARENTS AND PATIENTS

Brown, H. *Brave Girl Eating: A Family's Struggle with Anorexia.* Harpercollins; 2011.

Gürze Books, LLC is a trade book publishing company that has specialized in eating disorders. http://gurzebooks.com/.

Herrin M, Matsumoto N. *Parent's Guide to Eating Disorders, Supporting Self-esteem, Healthy Eating, & Positive Body Image at Home.* Gurze Books; 2007.

Kerrigan C. *Telling Ed No! And Other Practical Tools to Conquer Your Eating Disorder and Find Freedom.* Gurze Books; 2011.

Lock J, Le Grange D. *Help Your Teenager Beat an Eating Disorder.* 2nd ed. New York: The Guilford Press; 2004.

Schaefer J. *Life Without Ed: How One Woman Declared Independence from Her Eating Disorder and How You Can Too.* New York: McGraw-Hill Education; 2003.

Siegel M, Brisman J, Weinshel M. *Surviving an Eating Disorder: Strategies for Family and Friends.* New York: Harper; 2009.

FOR PROFESSIONALS

American Psychiatric Association (APA). *Practice Guideline for the Treatment of Patients with Eating Disorders.* 3rd ed. Washington, DC: American Psychiatric Association; 2006. http://psychiatryonline.org/pb/assets/raw/sitewide/practice_guidelines/guidelines/eatingdisorders.pdf

Calero-Elvira A, Krug I, Davis K, et al. Meta-analysis on drugs in people with eating disorders. *Eur Eat Disord Rev.* 2009;17:243-259.

Claudino AM, Hay P, Lima MS, et al. Antidepressants for anorexia nervosa. *Cochrane Database Syst Rev.* 2006;1:CD004365.

Culbert KM, Racine SE, Klump KL. Research review: what we have learned about the causes of eating disorders—a synthesis of sociocultural, psychological, and biological research. *J Child Psychol Psychiatry.* 2015;56(11):1141-1164.

Eating disorders: Core interventions in the treatment and management of anorexia nervosa, bulimia nervosa and related eating disorders. National Institute for Clinical Excellence; 2004. www.nice.org.uk/CG009NICEguidelines.

Golden NH, Katzman DK, Sawyer SM, et al. Position paper of the society for adolescent health and medicine: medical management of restrictive eating disorders in adolescents and young adults. *J Adolesc Health.* 2015;56:121-125. http://www.jahonline.org/article/S1054-139X%2814%2900686-7/fulltext.

Peebles R, Campbell K. Eating disorders in children and adolescents: state of the art review. *Pediatrics*. 2014;134(3):582-592.

Rosen DS; American Academy of Pediatrics Committee on Adolescence. Identification and management of eating disorders in children and adolescents. *Pediatrics*. 2010;126:1240-1253.

Swanson SA, Crow SJ, Le Grange D, Swendsen J, Merikangas KR. Prevalence and correlates of eating disorders in adolescents: results from the national comorbidity survey replication adolescent supplement. *Arch Gen Psychiatry*. 2011;68(7):714-723.

CHAPTER 44

Encopresis

Laura Weissman | Leonard A. Rappaport

I. **DESCRIPTION OF THE PROBLEM.** Encopresis is defined as repeated passage of stool into inappropriate places in a child older than 4 years, chronologically and developmentally, and the behavior is not due exclusively to the direct physiological effects of a substance (e.g., laxatives) or a general medical condition, except through a mechanism involving constipation.

Retentive fecal incontinence involves functional constipation, whereas nonretentive fecal incontinence does not.

A. **Epidemiology**
   - Encopresis reportedly affects 2.8% of 4-year-olds, 1.9% of 6-year-olds, and 1.6% of 10- to 11-year-olds.
   - Encopresis usually presents in children younger than 7 years although it can present at any age.
   - Encopresis can be more common among children with developmental disabilities including ADHD, autism spectrum disorder, and other disabilities.

B. **Etiology/contributing factors**
   - More than 80% of encopresis is due to functional constipation where retained stool distends the rectum, resulting in soft stool leaking around a stool mass. Distention of the rectum results in abnormal feedback to the stretch receptors in the bowel resulting in leakage. As a result, the child often does not receive a signal to defecate until soiling is nearly complete.
   - Encopresis is not generally caused by underlying psychopathology but can be associated with emotional distress. In addition, encopresis itself can result in considerable embarrassment, humiliation, punishment, and bullying.
   - Rare cases of encopresis are due to damaged corticospinal pathways, bowel inflammation, or anorectal dysfunction such as that seen after pull through or other bowel surgery. Encopresis can also be seen in the case of undiagnosed Hirschsprung disease (although this is rare) or after surgical correction of this disorder.
   - A very small subset of children with encopresis may impulsively pass stool due to anxiety or other emotional stressors, without underlying constipation.
   - There are an even smaller number of children who soil on purpose, but they are rare, and it is best to assume a physiological reason and treatment as an initial approach.

II. **MAKING THE DIAGNOSIS**
A. **History: key clinical questions**
   1. *"Was there a time when the child's bowel movements seemed typical?"* History starts at birth with specifics surrounding bowel function and any treatments used. Medical and surgical history may identify systemic diseases or medical causes of constipation that indicate treatments other than laxatives and maintenance of stool regularity.
   2. *"Did your child have a period of stooling into the toilet? How old was he/she? Did he/she feel the stool coming and get to the bathroom by herself/himself regularly?"* Distinguishing delayed toilet training, where the child never consolidated the ability to stool independently into the toilet and is essentially afraid to use the toilet to stool, from encopresis is essential. Treatment will vary, depending on whether or not constipation underlies the stooling accidents, rather than toilet refusal (although toilet refusal is often associated with constipation as well).
   3. *"How often does your child stool and urinate into the toilet now? How often into underwear? Are the stools large? Hard? Liquid? Do they hurt?"* Review details of present urinary and bowel patterns, such as frequency of stool evacuation into the toilet, stool accidents, stool consistency, and the urge to defecate. More severe, prolonged constipation generally will require more aggressive treatment. Any history of abuse or other trauma should be sought as well. Children who have been abused may become incontinent in times of stress or as part of regressive behavior and are less suitable candidates for rectal suppositories or enemas. They may also soil their underwear to keep someone away from them.

4. *"Often stool problems coexist with wetting accidents. Has he/she had any urinary tract infections? Does she/he have urine accidents in the day or at night?"* Urinary patterns, daytime wetting and nocturnal enuresis, and symptoms of urinary tract infection must be elicited. Approximately one-third of individuals with encopresis have urination issues. Constipation and especially encopresis may be associated with urinary tract infections, especially in females, due to poor hygiene. Even without infection, enuresis can be caused by a dilated rectum pushing on and irritating the bladder, thus causing bladder irritability and spasms.

5. *"I see a lot of kids who have poop sneak out and they don't like it. If you can help me figure out what is going on, I think I can help so things get better."* History taking provides an essential opportunity to communicate with the child. The child must be an active participant for the treatment to be effective, and often children with encopresis are overwhelmed and embarrassed when encopresis is discussed. The child often appears to not even be listening to the discussion, but he or she certainly is. When treatment is successful, the clinician often observes a drastic increase in positive affect in the child. Developing a sense of the child's perspective can create a connection between the caregiver and the child and should include questions about present school and family functioning.

B. Signs and symptoms. A child with functional constipation and consequent encopresis (retentive fecal incontinence) may report uncomfortable and infrequent stooling into the toilet and intermittent large and small bowel movements with uncontrolled stool accidents into underwear or pull-ups. There also may be a history of voluntary holding of stool.

Physical examination of the child with any type of encopresis includes the following:

- Growth parameters.
- Attention to signs of systemic disease.
- Thorough neurologic assessment including a close look for skin abnormalities overlying the spine and the presence of Achilles reflexes.
- Abdominal examination to evaluate for masses and constipation.
- Examine the anal opening. Anal fissures will cause ongoing pain with defecation; tags may reflect inflammatory bowel disease, and an absent anal wink may indicate neurologic abnormality.
- Rectal examination can be useful in assessing for Hirschsprung disease and may provide an indication of the degree of rectal impaction to guide treatment.

C. Differential diagnosis. Any disorder that can cause constipation can cause encopresis. A detailed history and physical examination is required to rule out systemic or organic causes of constipation or incontinence, such as spinal cord dysplasia or tethering, hypothyroidism, and a history of abnormal stools such as a meconium ileus seen in the case of cystic fibrosis.

D. Diagnostic assessment. For most children, no further diagnostic assessment is necessary beyond thorough history and physical examination. Laboratory investigation is indicated only as history or physical examination suggests a specific diagnosis. Laboratories may include thyroid function tests, electrolytes, celiac serology, calcium, lead, and magnesium. An abdominal radiograph may be useful to confirm constipation when the history is vague or the child is unable to comply with the abdominal or rectal examination and also can be used as a tool to educate families. Lumbosacral spine films or magnetic resonance imaging are indicated when lower extremity neurologic examination is abnormal or sacral abnormalities are visualized. Anorectal manometry may serve a purpose in patients who do not respond to treatment but is not typically necessary.

III. MANAGEMENT. Treatment requires a multimodal plan including education, laxatives, and behavioral interventions. First, it is important to educate families regarding the pathophysiology and clinical course of encopresis. Next, a full bowel clean-out is necessary to remove the stool burden so as to start the process of bowel recovery. A maintenance treatment plan along with behavioral interventions is required to ensure ongoing evacuation of stool followed by a reduction of laxatives as appropriate.

A. Psychoeducation

1. **Education.** Demystify the shame and blame around stool accidents. Use the patient's abdominal radiograph or an illustrated explanation (or both) to review the process of retained stool that leads to a distended colon and especially rectum, allowing stool to "sneak out without warning." Discuss that retained stool has to be cleaned out with medication and that there will likely be a lot of stool to clean out. Empathize with the stress and frustration that everyone has experienced, and

Table 44-1 • SAMPLE CLEAN-OUT REGIMENS

Regimen	Comment
Day 1: bisacodyl pill Day 2: bisacodyl suppository Day 3: sodium phosphate enema	Repeat four times for a total of 12 d and then return to clinic
Polyethylene glycol (PEG) without electrolytes	1–1.5 g/kg per day with or without a stimulant laxative (such as senna) for up to 6 d
PEG with electrolytes	25 mL/kg per hour to a maximum of 1000 mL/h
Mineral oil	15–30 mL per year of age, up to 240 mL

emphasize the need to break the cycle of failure that may have developed. Clarify that now the child truly cannot control the stool leaking out and should not be blamed. On the other hand, to cure encopresis, the child needs to commit to following your suggestions for treatment.

  2. **Clean-out.** The first part of treatment includes a clean-out of the retained stool that is dilating the rectum and affecting stool continence. There are many different choices for clean-out regimens, and the clinician's choice often depends on the needs of the child and the family. Although high-dose oral laxative can provide more control for the child, rectal and oral combinations can be quite effective (see Table 44-1). Children aged 7 years and older without a history of trauma may opt for a fast and direct choice using a combination of oral and rectal medications. There are multiple options but one includes a 3-day cycle, which is repeated over four times for a total of 12 days: Day 1—sodium phosphate enema, Day 2—bisacodyl pills, Day 3—bisacodyl suppository. To gain compliance, it is helpful to explain to children that the enemas and suppositories are necessary because the muscle has been stretched by the stool and is not strong enough to get the stool out easily from oral medicine. Starting with the enema makes sense because the pill is likely to give the child a stomachache if the bowel is full. Oral laxative alone can also be very effective and may be preferable in some patients including younger children or those who cannot tolerate suppositories or enemas. Options for oral medications can include high-dose polyethylene glycol without electrolytes, alone or along with a stimulant medication such as senna or bisacodyl, high-dose polyethylene glycol with electrolytes, or high-dose mineral oil given over a 2- to 6-day interval Impaction that is present for many months may require higher dosing. During the initial clean-out, the child and the family should expect a large amount of stool output and are reminded of the radiograph full of stool. The frequency of accidents may increase initially during the clean-out but then should subside. The child should return at the end of the clean-out and at that time, there should really be no accidents. If there are still accidents, either there is stool remaining in the rectum or the child is being given too much laxative resulting in accidents that are iatrogenic.

B. Regular bowel patterns must be established

  1. Once clean-out is achieved, it is important for the patient to be placed on a maintenance laxative medication along with a behavior plan to discourage reaccumulation of stool. It makes sense to meet with the child and family after the clean-out is complete to ensure complete clean-out and to plan the next stage of treatment. A full range of maintenance medications is included in Table 44-2, but options for maintenance medications include polyethylene glycol without electrolytes, magnesium hydroxide, lactulose, and mineral oil. Dosing is adjusted to maintain soft regular stools. As the child may not develop the urge to defecate for 6–9 months after constipation is treated, regular toilet sitting time is necessary. This should occur two to three times a day and compliance should be reinforced using a reward incentive plan. This can include stickers or other tokens as rewards for sitting on the toilet or taking care of his or her bodily needs. Older children may benefit from having games or activities that can only be used in the bathroom as well.

It is helpful to schedule that sitting time about 20–30 minutes after a meal to take advantage of the gastrocolic reflex.

The goal is to stool before the sensation of needing to stool develops because the objective is to keep the rectum as empty as possible so that it can return to its

Table 44-2 • MAINTENANCE MEDICATION DOSING

Medication	Dose
Polyethylene glycol without electrolytes	½ cap to 1 cap (17 g) once or twice per day
Milk of magnesia	1–2 mL/kg per dose one to two times daily
Mineral oil	2–6 tbsp per day
Lactulose	0.5–1.0 mL/kg per dose, qd or bid
Senna	Children 6–12 y: 15 mg sennosides one to two times daily Children 12 y and older: 30 mg sennosides one to two times a day
Bisacodyl	In children 3 y or older to 10 y/o: 5 mg daily Children >10 y: 5–10 mg daily

normal size. The family must work to eliminate any negative associations around toileting that may have developed. Limiting conversation about toileting can be helpful.

IV. CLINICAL PEARLS AND PITFALLS

- Most families of a child with encopresis have never met anyone with the same problem. Reassuring them that encopresis is not so unusual and can be treated successfully is a vital first step.
- Parent and child education around the mechanism of encopresis to increase understanding and decrease blame is essential for successful treatment.
- Constipation and encopresis are often long-term issues, recurring intermittently after great initial improvement with treatment. Children may require medications such as polyethylene glycol without electrolytes, for extended periods (months to years).
- Reviewing signs of stool backup (e.g., hard stools, skipping days between bowel movements, stomachaches, and/or smears) and developing a rescue plan (e.g., increased polyethylene glycol without electrolytes, the addition of a stimulant such as senna, increased sitting, and/or increased fiber) empower the child and family to anticipate, tolerate, and treat recurrences. If you do not warn them, they may be embarrassed to come back and tell you on account of the perceived shame around encopresis.

Bibliography

FOR PARENTS

WEB SITES

Children's Medical Center, University of Virginia. http://www.people.virginia.edu/~smb4v/tutorials/constipation/encotreat.htm.

FOR PROFESSIONALS

Brazzelli M, Griffiths P. Behavioural and cognitive interventions with or without other treatments for defaecation disorders in children. *Cochrane Database Syst Rev*. 2001;(4):CD002240.

Loening-Baucke V. Encopresis. *Curr Opin Pediatr*. 2002;14(5):570-575.

Tabbers MM, DiLorenso C, Bergerr MY, et al. Evaluation and treatment of functional constipation in infants and children: evidence-based recommendations from ESPGHAN AND NASPGHAN. *J Pediatr Gastroenterol Nutr*. 2014;58:258.

CHAPTER 45

Enuresis and Urinary Incontinence

Laura Weissman | Leonard A. Rappaport

I. DESCRIPTION OF THE PROBLEM. Incontinence is defined as uncontrollable leakage of urine:
- Beyond age 4 years for daytime continence
- Beyond age 5–7 years for nocturnal continence
- The loss of continence after at least 6 months of dryness

A. Definitions. The International Children's Continence Society classifies urinary incontinence into two categories **enuresis or nighttime incontinence** also known as nocturnal enuresis defined as nighttime wetting in a child 5 years of age or greater and **daytime urinary incontinence** (previously called diurnal enuresis), which includes daytime wetting at least once every 2 weeks.

Another classification distinguishes between enuresis (intermittent nocturnal incontinence) with and without bladder symptoms, as individuals in these categories differ clinically. **Monosymptomatic enuresis** is wetting without lower urinary tract symptoms or daytime symptoms, whereas **nonmonosymptomatic enuresis** is wetting with lower urinary symptoms such as severe frequency, urgency, or daytime symptoms. Nonmonosymptomatic wetting is associated with a greater degree of organic pathology.

Enuresis can also be divided into **primary enuresis** (incontinence in a child who has never obtained continence) and **secondary enuresis** (when a child has been continent for at least 6 months and becomes incontinent).

There is clearly more than one classification system so it is sensible to be aware of them all.

B. Epidemiology. Although the development of urinary continence varies by culture, gender, race, and country, the prevalence of daytime urinary incontinence in 5- to 6-year-old children is approximately 10% and in 6- to 12-year-olds, 5%. For nighttime incontinence or enuresis the prevalence is 10%–15% in 7-year-olds.

C. Etiology. In the vast majority of cases, the etiology of monosymptomatic enuresis is unknown. There are, however, causes and contributing factors that should be considered. For nonmonosymptomatic enuresis and daytime incontinence, the etiology can be more complex.

   1. Nocturnal incontinence or enuresis
   a. Contributing factors to primary monosymptomatic enuresis
      (1) **Maturational delay** is a commonly accepted cause of nocturnal incontinence. This refers to the enuretic child's inability to send, perceive, or respond to information about a filled bladder during the night. Support for this theory comes from the spontaneous 15% cure rate and relationship between enuresis, maturation of motor systems, and neurophysiologic data.
      (2) **Sleep and arousal factors.** Originally, it was thought that enuresis was a nonrapid eye movement (non-REM) dyssomnia (such as sleepwalking and night terrors). Although wetting is more common in non-REM sleep, it can occur in *all* stages of sleep. Data on the sleep patterns of youth with enuresis are inconclusive. Obstructive sleep apnea (OSA) can be associated with nocturnal enuresis. In some cases, interventions for OSA including a tonsillectomy and adenoidectomy can result in resolution of enuresis symptoms.
      (3) **Central nervous system factors.** Continuing research has focused on the possible role of antidiuretic hormone secretion in children with nocturnal enuresis, leading to an increase in urinary output, and suggests that this may be a contributing feature in enuresis. Although desmopressin is a recognized and approved treatment for enuresis, considerable data have accumulated that make this etiology less likely as a singular etiology.
      (4) **Psychopathology/stress.** There are no data to support enuresis as a neurotic disorder. Similarly, although stress may exacerbate or contribute to enuresis, it is not a primary etiologic factor. However, certain conditions, such as attention-deficit/hyperactivity disorder (ADHD) are related to an increase in

enuresis. However, the ADHD itself may not be causal but representative of a neurochemical marker.

(5) **Genetics.** There is a genetic predisposition to enuresis. If one parent had enuresis, close to 50% of his or her children will have enuresis. If both parents had enuresis, approximately 75% of their children will have enuresis. Identical twins have the highest concordance rate (68%). Several genetic loci have been located by intensive family studies.

(6) **Bladder capacity.** Functional bladder capacity tends to be decreased in children with enuresis compared with their siblings without enuresis. This reflects differences in functional, rather than absolute, bladder capacity, with contractions occurring earlier in filling.

The following may also be contributory to enuresis and nonmonosymptomatic enuresis:

(1) **Increased bladder irritability.** A common cause of secondary enuresis is increased bladder irritability, usually due to a urinary tract infection. In addition, any mass impinging on the bladder (e.g., severe constipation) can increase bladder irritability.

(2) **Increased urinary output.** Any process that increases urinary output can cause enuresis (e.g., diabetes mellitus, diabetes insipidus, and sickle cell disease).

2. Daytime incontinence
  a. Known causes
  (1) **Overactive bladder.** This can be related to increased bladder irritability as described above. It can also include unstable detrusor contractions early in bladder filling. Children with this finding often exhibit holding maneuvers such as squatting (Vincent curtsy) or sitting asymmetrically on one heel in an effort to prevent a detrusor contraction. Symptoms resolve with time, usually by 10–12 years.

  (2) **Micturition deferral.** A common cause of daytime wetting in preschool children is holding of the urine and ignoring the urge to void, usually during play. Incontinence results when detrusor contraction cannot be suppressed. Children with short attention spans often fail to respond to body signals until it is too late. This type of wetting can be more common in children with behavioral issues.

  (3) **Abnormal sphincter control.** This includes dysfunctional voiding (poor coordination of the urinary sphincter and bladder contraction) and abnormalities with the opening of the bladder neck. Dysfunctional voiding can occur in patients with and without neurologic cause. Neurologic causes include spinal cord abnormalities.

  (4) **Structural abnormalities.** Girls with ectopic ureters, which empty into the vagina, have constant wetting with no recognized episodes of incontinence. Partial labial fusion may develop after inflammation, allowing urine to collect in a pocket behind the fused labia minora and subsequently leak. Other structural abnormalities exist but are less common.

  (5) **Vaginal reflux.** Overweight girls or girls who sit with their legs together when urinating can reflux urine into the vagina. The urine will then leak out over the next several hours without the urge to void. This causes almost constant daytime wetting without nighttime episodes.

  b. Contributing factors
  (1) **Giggle incontinence.** Emptying the bladder entirely while laughing may be familial. It is common in school-aged girls and generally resolves with maturity.

  (2) **Stress incontinence.** With increased abdominal pressure, such as during coughing, some children's bladders empty.

  (3) **Postvoid dribble syndrome.** Children may sense wetness after a void but without actual incontinence.

II. MAKING THE DIAGNOSIS
A. History: key clinical questions. A complete history should be obtained with a particular focus on a family history of enuresis, the child's pattern of wetting, and the previous interventions.
  1. *"Has the child ever been dry at night?"* It is important to differentiate primary from secondary enuresis.
  2. *"Does the child have accidents during the day, as well as at night?"* Treat the daytime wetting first if it coexists with nocturnal incontinence.

3. *"Has the child been constipated? How many days does he/she typically go between bowel movements? Are bowel movements hard, particularly large, or painful to produce?"* Treat constipation before more invasive investigation, unless history or physical examination suggests otherwise.

4. *"Was anyone else in the family late in achieving dryness at night or day?"* A positive family history may make the family more sympathetic to the child's feelings. It may be helpful to elicit the parents' own experience with enuresis and how it affects their response to their child.

5. *"What methods have you tried to address the problem?"* Evaluate the positive and negative interventions. Determine if they were appropriately implemented and their secondary effects (e.g., on the child's self-esteem).

6. [To the child] *"How much of a problem is this to you?"* The child must be motivated to be cured if treatment is to be successful.

7. *"Are there other symptoms your child is describing such as pain or needing to use the bathroom frequently?"* Symptoms such as urgency, frequency, urine leaking, abnormalities of urine stream, or daytime and nighttime symptoms should result in further investigation of organic pathology.

B. **Physical examination.** A complete physical examination should be performed, with emphasis placed on the spinal, neurologic, and genital examinations as well as examination for constipation. Constipation is frequently associated with wetting.

C. **Social history.** A social history should focus on history of stress and abuse.

D. **Tests.** The laboratory evaluation should be very limited. A urinalysis is recommended in all children, and a urine culture should be obtained based on the results of the urinalysis. Further workup should be directed by findings in the history and physical examination. There is no indication for the use of imaging techniques or urodynamic studies unless suggested by the history or physical examination or in cases where patients don't respond to initial treatment.

III. **MANAGEMENT**

A. **Primary goals.** The primary goals in the treatment of incontinence are to alleviate the problem and to limit its impact on the child's self-esteem and interpersonal relationships. Although a cure is possible for most children, a small percentage may have to learn to live with this problem. Initial interventions should be directed both at helping the child cope with the problem and working on a solution.

B. **Information for the family.** The family should be told how common enuresis is and made to understand that it is usually a developmental problem over which the child has little to no control. Punishments only lower the child's self-esteem without improving the symptoms. Finally, parents should understand that effective treatments are available and that most treatments require cooperation between them, the child, and the primary care clinician.

C. **Treatment strategies**

1. **Nocturnal enuresis.** The spontaneous remission rate for nocturnal enuresis is 15% per year.

   a. **Constipation.** If constipation is suspected, this should be treated to increase efficacy of any treatment.

   b. **Behavioral modification.** Initial treatments include rewards/incentive, decreasing nighttime fluid, and pre-bedtime voids. This can be effective in up to a quarter of children aged 5–7 years who are already showing signs of multiple dry nights a week.

   c. **Alarms.** Alarms have become the preferred treatment for nocturnal wetting or enuresis because of their high efficacy, low cost, ease of use, and low regression rate. However, their use requires a considerable commitment from the parents (at least for the first week or two) when the child may not awaken to the alarm. Children must be motivated and are generally older than 7 years with the exception of younger, mature, highly motivated patients. The parents and child should be instructed in its use.

   • Use the alarm every night for at least 2–3 months and sometimes as long as 4 months.

   • Both parents and child need to be involved.

   • The child should be instructed to visualize the steps necessary before going to sleep at night, such as waking when the alarm sounds, going to the bathroom, changing into dry clothes, replacing the alarm, and pulling off wet sheets. The child should then act out these steps before going to sleep.

   • When the alarm goes off, the child should wake up and void in the toilet. If the child does not wake up, parents should wake up the child when the alarm rings

and take the child to the bathroom (even if an accident has already occurred). After a week or two, the child usually will awaken independently when the alarm sounds.
- Restart the alarm after the underwear is changed.
- Use a reward/incentive chart for dry nights (sticker or stars).
- Over two-thirds who respond to alarms do so within 2 weeks. The cure rate continues to be above spontaneous remission until 4 months. Fifty percent of those who achieved dryness with alarm therapy remained accident-free after the therapy was discontinued.

d. **Medications**
(1) **Desmopressin** is a synthetic analogue of 8-arginine vasopressin and has shown to be effective in the treatment of nighttime enuresis by decreasing urine production at night.
- Studies have shown that children who use desmopressin have an average of around 1.3 drier nights per week, but there is a very high relapse rate when discontinued.
- There are concerns about hyponatremia from water intoxication while taking desmopressin, so excessive nighttime fluid intake should be avoided.
- There is currently a black box warning for the intranasal form on account of hyponatremic seizures given the long half-life, so it is no longer recommended and the oral formulation is preferred.
- This can be used in children older than 5 years who do not respond or are not candidates for alarm therapy.
- If it works in a trial, it can be used for sleepovers or overnight camps until an alarm can be initiated.
(2) **Imipramine,** a tricyclic antidepressant, has been shown to be successful in the treatment of nocturnal enuresis with reported decrease in one wet night per week, although the mechanism for this improvement remains uncertain. There are two problems with imipramine in the treatment of enuresis: the high relapse rate when stopped and the very high toxic index if taken in overdosage. As a result, this is not recommended as a first-line therapy.
(3) Anticholinergic medications such as oxybutynin are not recommended as individual therapy for nocturnal enuresis but can be used for patients with daytime wetting and nighttime wetting along with desmopressin. This may work by increasing bladder capacity and decreasing overactivity. Side effects of anticholinergics include constipation, flushing, dizziness, increased temperature, and urine retention after voiding. Given the side effects of the combination (constipation and residual urine volume), it should only be used with close monitoring.
(4) **Bladder exercises.** The research is currently inconclusive regarding the use of other bladder exercises for incontinence, but some studies suggest a potential benefit as does clinical experience.
- **Bladder stretching exercises** are not found to be a successful form of treatment.
- **Bladder relaxation exercises** are found to be a successful form of treatment. This includes behavioral techniques, which teach the child to be more aware and relax muscles related to urination.

2. **Daytime incontinence.** When a child has both enuresis and daytime incontinence, the daytime component should be addressed first. It is recommended to treat the underlying pathology. If no organic cause is identified, the following is recommended. In most children, the daytime incontinence will resolve over several months.

a. Treatment of constipation
- Implementation of a regimen to ensure the treatment of underlying constipation is essential. This includes dietary interventions, laxatives if needed, and behavioral interventions to encourage stool evacuation.
- Encourage physical activity.
b. **Behavioral interventions** can be extremely useful. These include the following:
- **Timed voiding.** Encourage voiding every 2 hours and allow for easy access to restrooms. Use a reward/incentive for remaining dry during intervals and complying with the voiding schedule.

   c. **Use of appropriate voiding methods**
   * Encourage liberal fluids during the day, but discourage fluids before bedtime.
   * Discourage the child from holding urine.
   * Encourage a good voiding technique, which allows for relaxation of the pelvic floor.
   d. **Medications** for diurnal enuresis are rarely indicated. Potential agents include anticholinergics (oxybutynin and tolterodine tartrate), which work to decrease bladder spasms, and alpha blockers (doxazosin and tamsulosin), which work by relaxing the bladder sphincter and decreasing the resistance. However, these medications have many side effects commonly including constipation from the anticholinergics, which can exacerbate enuresis.
D. Improving self-esteem/family function. Self-esteem is best preserved by a nonpunitive response to the incontinence. The child and family should be made aware that wetting is common and that it is usually not a sign of emotional, psychological, or medical dysfunction. The child can be empowered to take responsibility for dryness at night following an accident via the "double bubble" technique.
   * Place a plastic sheet over the mattress, followed by the usual sheets and blankets.
   * Place another plastic sheet over those sheets, again followed by another set of sheets and blankets.
   * Keep a dry set of pajamas by the bedside.
   * During the day, rehearse with the child how to take the wet set of sheets off the bed, uncovering the dry second set, and how to change pajamas.
   * This technique can defuse family tensions by allowing the child to handle his or her own needs at night and not awaken the parents. It is not for punishment but to help the child take responsibility for his or her own bodily functions.
E. Criteria for referral. The child should be referred to a urologist when genitourinary pathology is suspected. Psychological counseling should be sought when the child's social function appears to have been impaired by the enuresis or when the family's response appears to be unduly punitive.

IV. CLINICAL PEARLS AND PITFALLS
   * *Always* obtain a complete history and physical examination when beginning the treatment of a child with enuresis, even if they are your primary care patient and you think you know them well.
   * Parents may have not shared with the clinician all the information pertaining to incontinence unless they are asked directly. Parents need to be asked about previous interventions and, in particular, how these interventions were instituted. Frequently, parents will have tried an intervention inappropriately (e.g., Alarm for one night).
   * Involvement of the child is essential. No intervention will be successful without the motivation and commitment of the child.
   * Always pay attention to the evolution of the child's self-esteem. Punitive techniques should be avoided at all costs.
   * Do not forget to ask. Many families are ashamed to tell their pediatric clinicians that their child has enuresis. Sadly, sometimes the more a family likes a pediatric clinician, the less likely they are to share a shameful subject.

Bibliography

FOR PARENTS
Mack A. *Dry All Night*. Boston, MA: Little, Brown; 1989.

FOR CHILDREN
Boelts M. *Dry Days, Wet Nights*. Morton Grove, IL: Albert Whitman & Company; 1994.

FOR PROFESSIONALS
Graham KM, Levey JB. Enuresis. *Pediatr Rev*. 2009;30:165-173.
Neveus T, Von Gontard A, Hoebeke P, et al. The standardization of terminology of lower urinary tract function in children and adolescents: report from the Standardization Committee of the International Children's Continence Society. *J Urol*. 2006;176:314-324.
Robson WL, Leung AK. Daytime wetting. *J Pediatr*. 2001;139(4):609-610.
Robson WLM. Evaluation and management of enuresis. *N Engl J Med*. 2009;360(14):1429-1435.
von Gontard A, Schaumburg H, Hollmann E, et al. The genetics of enuresis: a review. *J Urol*. 2001;166(6):2438-2443.

WEB SITES
American Academy of Family Physicians. http://familydoctor.org/366.xml.
American Academy of Family Physicians. http://www.aafp.org/afp/20030401/1499.html.

SELECTED ENURESIS ALARMS

Nite Train'r Alarm Koregon Enterprises, 9735 Southwest Sunshine Court, Beaverton, OR 97005, 1-800-544-4240.

Nytone Medical Products, 2424 South 900 West, Salt Lake City, UT 84119, 801-973-4090.

Wet Stop Alarm, Palco Laboratories, 8030 Soquel Avenue, Santa Cruz, CA 95062, 1-800-346-4488.

CHAPTER 46

Executive Function: Its Importance and Promotion

Irene M. Loe | Casey Krueger

I. WHAT IS EXECUTIVE FUNCTION? Executive function (EF) refers to multiple, inter-related cognitive skills needed for purposeful, goal-directed behavior. EF skills develop from birth but are more reliably measured after age 3–4 years compared with infancy and toddlerhood. Rapid development occurs through childhood and adolescence into young adulthood, followed by decline with aging. The brain basis for EF skills is often attributed to the frontal lobes, specifically prefrontal cortex, and other brain regions with connections among regions. There is debate about the EF construct and subcomponents; however, EF is often operationalized as three main skills:

- **Working memory** is the ability to hold or manipulate information in your mind despite the presence of competing or distracting information. An example is the ability to hold a new phone number in mind despite having a continuing conversation about another topic.
- **Inhibition** is the ability to stop an automatic or reflexive behavior. An example is the ability to stop oneself from either blurting out an answer or saying the first thing that comes to mind. Impulse control and self-regulation are related constructs used to control and manage these behavioral responses. It is often seen earliest in games such as Simon Says or Musical Chairs.
- **Cognitive flexibility** is the ability to shift or switch between different tasks or rules in response to feedback. At a more advanced level, it refers to the ability to revise plans, problem-solve dynamically, or generate solutions in the face of obstacles, setbacks, new information or situations, or mistakes. An example for a young child is the ability to adjust to a change in plans or routine without major distress; for an older child or teen, she/he can find an alternative solution to a problem when the first one no longer works.

There are other high-level cognitive skills that are also considered EF skills:

- **Planning and organization**, or ability to think ahead, plan, and sequence events or actions
- **Initiation** of activity and idea generation
- **Selection of efficient problem-solving strategies**
- **Monitoring** of performance, behavior, and emotional regulation

Constructs that are core cognitive abilities related to EF include the following:

- **Attention** is a multifaceted construct that includes the ability to concentrate and focus to acquire new skills. Different types of attention include selective (i.e., ability to focus on relevant stimuli despite distracters), sustained (i.e., ability to maintain an alert, focused state for an extended period), and divided (i.e., ability to focus on multiple competing stimuli at the same time).
- **Processing speed**, often measured as reaction time or decision time, refers to the time required to encode, interpret, and respond to incoming stimuli or information.

II. WHY IS EF IMPORTANT?

- EF is associated with important functional outcomes, such as academic achievement, social competence, overall function, and adaptive skills.
- EF impairments are common in behavioral and neurodevelopmental disorders, including attention-deficit/hyperactivity disorder, learning disability, anxiety, depression, and autism spectrum disorder. EF impairments often occur in association with several medical conditions or risk factors, such as preterm birth, fetal alcohol and in utero substance exposure, congenital heart disease, brain injury, seizures, and genetic disorders, among others.
- EF may be a target for intervention to improve function.

III. HOW IS EF ASSESSED?

- **Parent and teacher report of EF skills on standardized rating scales.** Broadband behavior rating scales, such as the Behavior Assessment Scale for Children, Third Edition, and Conners, Third Edition, include EF subscales. Standardized EF-specific rating scales, such as the Behavior Rating Inventory of Executive Function, Second

Edition (BRIEF-2) or BRIEF-Preschool version, provide more detailed information on EF and its components than broadband rating scales do.

- **Direct assessment of EF** can be performed through psychological, neuropsychological, or educational testing with standardized EF batteries (e.g., A Developmental Neuropsychological Assessment, Second Edition [NEPSY-II]; Delis–Kaplan Executive Function System [D-KEFS]; Minnesota Executive Function Scale [MEFS], among others). General cognitive tests of intelligence often include subtests that focus on components of EF, such as working memory, or related skills, such as processing speed.

IV. TAKING THE HISTORY

- Working memory—*"Does your child have trouble remembering where she/he put an object or what homework the teacher assigned earlier? Does she/he often lose or forget things? Does your child have trouble completing chores or tasks that have more than one step (remembers only the first or last step)?"*
- Inhibition—*"Does she/he speak or act without thinking or say things that might be hurtful because she/he doesn't think about it first?"*
- Cognitive flexibility—*"What does your child do if she/he is unable to solve a new problem with the same steps she/he used to solve a similar problem?"*
- Inhibition and organization—*"What is your morning routine like? Is it hard to get out the door?"* or *"Does your child have trouble getting through the morning/after-school/bedtime routine?"*
- Planning—*"Does your child have trouble completing and turning in assignments? How does she/he do when she/he needs to plan for longer-term assignments such as projects or book reports that have multiple steps and need more time to complete?"*
- Initiation—*"Does your child have trouble getting started on homework or chores?"*
- Self-regulation—*"Does your child become tearful easily or overreact to small problems?"*

V. SUPPORTING THE CHILD WITH EF IMPAIRMENTS

- Review risk factors and refer for evaluation typically from the school system or a private neuropsychologist or developmental and behavioral pediatrician.
- EF "coaching" in which a coach or tutor provides customized and comprehensive support to teach skills to compensate for EF impairments or strengthen EF skills is available in some communities, but it may be expensive and the evidence base for such an approach is lacking.

VI. PROMOTING EF? Young children:

- Inhibition. Games such as "Simon Says" or Musical Chairs help children engage actively in a fun game that involves practicing EF skills including when to follow an instruction and when to inhibit a response. Other inhibition games include playing "Freeze" or "Statue" during active dancing/singing play. A visual aid during book reading can remind the child of his/her turn—"When you have the ear, it's your turn to listen" or "When you have the mouth, it's your turn to talk."
- Working memory. Parents can hide bath toys under bubbles during bath time and ask the child to name or find the hidden toys. Ask children to turn over playing cards from a large array two at a time to find the pairs. While walking or driving, take turns reciting the letters and numbers on a license plate and then saying them backward, too.
- Cognitive flexibility. Pretend play using a block to represent a plane or car or reverse roles when playing house (i.e., the child is the mommy and the parent is the baby) also encourages memory of staying in role and inhibition of the tendency to revert to typical roles.
- Planning. Draw a visual schedule to organize, plan, and prepare children for a play activity, morning or bedtime routine, or other activities.

School-age children and adolescents—including organization and planning abilities:

- Attention, freedom from distractibility. Try preferential seating so the teacher can monitor the child's attention and focus. Provide children with an organized work/study area free of distractions, especially to complete homework and to take tests.
- Organization. Books, folders, and materials can be organized by subject with color coding. Other visual aids may help with processing information and maintain engagement with learning.
- Planning. Use calendars to map out steps to complete a project or assignment. Provide checklists for assignments to be shared with the child, teacher, and parents with due dates. Breaking down tasks or daily routines into checklists can help with day-to-day activities such as getting out the door to school or settling down for bedtime. A reminder and reward system can also help.
- Memory. Break down instructions into fewer, concise commands.
- Cognitive flexibility. Encourage "metacognition" or thinking about thinking. For example, "homework wrappers": At the start of a homework session, ask the youth to name

the three things they think the lesson will cover. At the end of the assignment, ask them to name the three things they learned and see how well they matched.
- Planning and organization. Review the long-term goal, steps to be completed, and the time it takes to complete.
  - Completing a recipe (i.e., finding the recipe, reading all of the ingredients, buying/ gathering the ingredients, following the steps, understanding what needs to be prepared first, attending to the timing of the recipe, planning for when it should be compete) is one multistep activity that meets this goal. Other activities include planning the wardrobe for a week or doing laundry. Longer-term school projects such as book reports or team projects take similar long-term planning.
  - Planning a trip (even a pretend trip) is a fun activity. Kids can pick a destination, review maps, determine which mode of travel is realistic, plan how long it will take to travel, explore alternative routes, outline what things will be required for a trip, understand any costs associated (gas, fees for the park/museum/attraction), and understand their goal for this destination (spend time with my family, learn about a specific site, get good pictures of a famous spot).
- Prioritization, planning, and organization. Learning to prioritize is an important skill. Before each week begins, a fun activity is for each family member to identify a priority for the week, even if it is small. Reviewing all the tasks and activities that need to be done and then being able to think through why certain tasks should take priority helps identify goals, learn how to make thoughtful decisions, and prioritize.

Bibliography

RESOURCES FOR PARENTS AND CLINICIANS

https://www.parentbooks.ca/Executive_Function.html.
http://developingchild.harvard.edu/resources/tools_and_guides/enhancing_and_ practicing_executive_function_skills_with_children/.
https://children.wi.gov/Documents/Harvard%20Parenting%20Resource.pdf.
http://www.joinvroom.org/tools-and-activities.

RESOURCES FOR CLINICIANS

Diamond A. Executive functions. *Annu Rev Psychol.* 2013;64:135-168.
Miyake A, Friedman NP, Emerson MJ, Witzki AH, Howerter A. The unity and diversity of executive functions and their contributions to complex "frontal lobe" tasks: a latent variable analysis. *Cogn Psychol.* 2000;41(1):49-100.
Zelazo PD, Blair CB, Willoughby MT. *Executive Function: Implications for Education (NCER 2017-2000).* Washington, DC: National Center for Education Research, Institute of Education Sciences, U.S. Department of Education; 2016. This report is available on the Institute website at http://files.eric.ed.gov/fulltext/ED570880.pdf.

CHAPTER 47

Fetal Alcohol Spectrum Disorders

Yasmin Suzanne N. Senturias | Carol C. Weitzman |
Rachel Amgott

I. **DESCRIPTION OF THE PROBLEM.** Fetal alcohol spectrum disorder (FASD) is an umbrella term that describes the range of effects that can occur in an individual whose mother drank alcohol during pregnancy. These effects may include physical, mental, behavioral, and/or learning disabilities with lifelong implications. The term "FASDs" is *not* meant for use as a clinical diagnosis.

- Fetal alcohol syndrome (FAS)
- Partial FAS (PFAS)
- Alcohol-related neurodevelopmental disorders (ARNDs)
- Alcohol-related birth defects (ARBDs)
- Neurobehavioral disorder with prenatal alcohol exposure (ND-PAE)

The absence of cardinal facial features does not guarantee that the central nervous system (CNS) abnormalities are of less severity, and there is a significant continuum of impairment along the FASD spectrum. In 2016 Hoyme et al. updated the Clinical Guidelines for Diagnosing Fetal Alcohol Spectrum Disorders to reflect neurobehavioral impairments as the principal source of disability for an individual with an FASD.

A. **Epidemiology**
- The Centers for Disease Control and Prevention (CDC) reports FAS prevalence to be from 0.2 to 1.5 cases per 1000 live births, but the broader profile of FASDs are reported to occur in up to 9–10 per 1000 live births, which translates to about 40,000 alcohol-affected births per year in the United States. Studies using in-person assessment of school-aged children in several US communities report higher estimates of FAS: 6–9 out of 1000 children. The newest FASD estimates, based on community studies utilizing physical examinations, experts estimate that FASDs are now even as high as 2 to 5 per 100 school children (or 2% to 5% of the population).
- Alcohol consumption is a global public health issue, and countries with high rates of alcohol consumption also have high rates of FAS. The global prevalence of FASDs among children and youth in the general population was estimated to be 7.7 per 1000 population in a recent study.

B. **Etiology/contributing factors**
1. **Dose.** The more a pregnant woman drinks, the greater the risk of FASDs. However, as reflected in the US Surgeon General's advisory, there is no known safe amount of alcohol during pregnancy. Prenatal alcohol exposure to one or more drinks per day is associated with reduced birth weight and intrauterine growth retardation, spontaneous abortion, preterm delivery, and stillbirth.
2. **Pattern.** Drinking patterns that create high-peak blood alcohol level pose the greatest risk. Binge drinking is felt to be particularly risky. A binge is defined as the consumption of four alcoholic drinks per drinking occasion. One drink is defined as 12 oz of beer or wine cooler, 5 oz of wine, or 1.5 oz of liquor.
3. **Timing.** First trimester exposure poses risks to major structures; second trimester exposure poses risk of spontaneous abortion; and third trimester exposure has the greatest impact on height, weight, and brain growth. However, no period of pregnancy appears to be safe for drinking because damage can occur at any point after conception. The brain can be affected by alcohol in all the three trimesters.
4. **Genetic sensitivity or effects of metabolism.** There may be genetic differences in a woman's ability to metabolize alcohol and in how a fetus is affected. The fetus is limited in its ability to metabolize alcohol, and alcohol levels in the fetus are thought to be higher and present for a more prolonged period when compared with maternal levels.
5. **Maternal nutrition.** Alcohol intake can have direct or indirect effects on the nutritional status of the fetus either because alcohol abusers often have a poor diet or because alcohol can interfere with the absorption or processing of nutrients such as thiamine, magnesium, zinc, and folate.

6. **Maternal age.** Children of mothers who are older than 30 years have a higher risk of negative outcomes following prenatal alcohol exposure.

7. **Parity.** Studies suggest that the risk of having a child with FAS increases with each successive pregnancy. The rate increases from 0.2–1.5/1000 to 771/1000 live births for the younger sibling of a child with FAS.

II. **MAKING THE DIAGNOSIS.** Assignment of an FASD diagnosis is a complex medical diagnostic process best accomplished through a structured multidisciplinary approach by a clinical multidisciplinary team. Nonetheless, pediatric clinicians should be screening mothers for prenatal alcohol use, considering an FASD when they see children with complex neurodevelopmental disorders and implementing intervention even in the absence of diagnosis. Below are the highlights of the criteria for each subtype of clinical knowledge.

A. **Criteria for Institute of Medicine subtypes**

1. **FAS** (with or without a known history of prenatal alcohol exposure) requires all four of the following:

   a. Documentation of two or more minor facial abnormalities; smooth philtrum (rank 4 or 5 on racially normed lip philtrum guide), thin vermillion border (rank 4 or 5 on racially normed lip philtrum guide), and short palpebral fissures (measured as <10% tile according to age and racial norms).

   b. Prenatal and/or postal documentation of growth deficiency (weight and/or length, at or below the 10th percentile). The CDC guidelines state that the weight or height growth deficit can occur at anytime beginning in the prenatal period (adjusted for age, sex, gestational age, and race/ethnicity).

   c. Documentation of CNS abnormality (structural, neurologic, or functional) including more than one of the following: head circumference (HC) <10%tile, structural brain abnormalities, and recurrent nonfebrile seizures (other causes of seizures ruled out).

   d. Neurobehavioral impairments:
   * For children younger than 3 years there needs to be evidence of developmental delay.
   * For children older than 3 years with a cognitive impairment there must be either general conceptual ability >1.5 SD below the mean or cognitive deficient in at least one domain:
     * Executive functioning
     * Specific learning disability
     * Memory impairment
     * Visual spatial impairment
   * For children older than 3 years with behavioral impairment without cognitive impairment: evidence of behavioral deficit in at least one aspect of self-regulation:
     * Mood or behavioral regulation
     * Attention deficit
     * Impulse control

2. **PFAS.** See diagnostic criteria in references below. Used for children who display some but not all of the physical/neurodevelopmental characteristics of FAS.

3. **ARND.** This diagnosis cannot be made definitively in children younger than 3 years and is used for children who demonstrate cognitive or behavior impairment without the characteristic physical features. A confirmed history of prenatal alcohol exposure is needed to make this diagnosis.

4. **ARBD.** This diagnosis is used for children with a physical malformation linked to maternal drinking without the requirement of characteristic facial features or growth anomalies.

B. **DSM-5 subtype**

1. **ND-PAE** was added to the *Diagnostic and Statistical Manual of Mental Disorders, Fifth Edition* (*DSM-5*) as a diagnostic code to describe more fully the range of neurobehavioral and neurodevelopmental effects of prenatal alcohol exposure and is coated under Other Specified Neurodevelopmental Disorder 315.8 (F88). The *DMS-5* requires impairments in at least one neurocognitive domain (IQ, executive function, learning, memory, or visual-spatial impairment) and self-regulatory domain (mood/behavior regulation, attention, or impulse control), plus impairments in at least two domains of adaptive functioning (communication, social communication and interaction, daily living skills, or motor skills) in the presence of prenatal alcohol exposure. Under the adaptive domain, there should be impairment in either communication or social interaction. This diagnosis is highly overlapping with ARND but can be diagnosed in the presence or absence of characteristic dysmorphic facial features.

C. **Documentation of alcohol exposure.** Although it is important to document alcohol exposure, this is often difficult to obtain. Birth mothers may be hesitant to provide the information, and when the child is adopted, exposure to prenatal alcohol may be unknown. When the FAS diagnostic criteria are met on the basis of the characteristic facial growth and CNS abnormalities, confirmation of maternal alcohol exposure is helpful but not essential for the diagnosis. There are clinical criteria to identify the other FASDs, but for the individuals who do not meet full facial growth and CNS criteria for FAS, there must always be confirmed prenatal alcohol exposure. A consensus definition of significant prenatal alcohol exposure is a component of the new criteria. A positive confirmation of alcohol exposure must be available for the diagnosis of ARND or ARBD to be assigned.

D. **Differential diagnosis.** A careful history that includes maternal alcohol use is needed to differentiate the effects of alcohol from those of other teratogens. There could also be growth retardation, facial dysmorphology, and/or CNS disturbance in other disorders such as fetal valproate syndrome, fetal hydantoin syndrome, maternal phenylketonuria (PKU), William syndrome, and velocardiofacial syndrome. It may be helpful to consult with a geneticist if questions about alternative or comorbid diagnoses arise. It is also important to rule out other problems that can contribute to the CNS dysfunction, such as early negative child experiences and comorbid mental illness.

E. **History: key clinical questions**
   1. **Pregnancy history.** *"During this pregnancy, how many times a week did you drink beer, wine, or liquor? How many cans, glasses, or drinks each time?"* (Or in the case of a foster or adopted child, *"Do you know how much alcohol was consumed during this pregnancy?"*) Remember to ask about alcohol consumption before knowledge of the pregnancy with the following question: *In the 3 months before you knew you were pregnant, how many times did you have four or more drinks in a day?*
      More than 50% of pregnancies in the United States are unplanned, and some women may not have had knowledge until several weeks to months into the pregnancy (e.g., certain women with irregular periods or who become pregnant while on a contraceptive). Excessive alcohol consumption in the 3 months before pregnancy is often considered predictive of alcohol use in pregnancy. Binge drinking (consuming four or more standard drinks on a single occasion) is considered particularly harmful and so is chronic drinking throughout the pregnancy.
   2. **Medical history.** Ask about the child's general health and then about specific medical problems seen in FAS/FASD. Inquire about the child's vision (e.g., refractive problems due to small globes) and hearing (i.e., sensorineural/conductive hearing loss). Also ask about a history of heart murmurs (e.g., atrial/ventricular septal defects), kidney problems (e.g., horseshoe kidneys), or spinal abnormalities (e.g., scoliosis), which can occur in children with an FASD.
   3. **Developmental history/educational function.** *"Does your child show unusual sensitivity to touch (overreaction to injury, tags in the back of clothes, hugs), light, or sound (says things are too bright or too loud)? Does the child have difficulty behaving at large, noisy gatherings or at recess or lunch?"* Sensory hypersensitivity is a frequent but poorly recognized feature of FAS, causing children to become easily overstimulated.
      "Does your child understand cause and effect, abstract thinking? Can he/she generalize information learned in one context to another? Does your child seem to 'learn' and 'forget' the same piece of information over and over?" Children with FASDs may have trouble with academics (specifically mathematics or subjects requiring abstract reasoning), problem-solving, processing speed, memory, and even language comprehension. Verbal skills are often a strength, and most children test in the low average cognitive range.
   4. **Social skills.** *"How does your child relate to peers?"* Individuals with FASDs may be indiscriminately friendly or unheedingly fearless and exhibit poor judgment and impulse control. They may be more susceptible to being used or manipulated (even into wrongdoing) by other individuals.
   5. **Adaptive skills.** Inquire about self-care skills. Many children with FAS/FASD's have executive dysfunction, which could affect their ability to develop adaptive skills.
   6. **Maladaptive behavior.** Inquire about problem behaviors. Children may have behavioral problems owing to poor comprehension, limited ability to generalize learning from one situation to another, and cause-and-effect reasoning, with subsequent frustration and externalizing behaviors. Some children are hyperactive and impulsive and have significant mood dysregulation, which can readily contribute to these problem behaviors. They may also act out more in noisy places (e.g., cafeteria or gymnasium).

F. **Physical examination.** A complete physical and neurologic examination is necessary and should evaluate growth, facial dysmorphology, and neurologic function, not only as it pertains to FAS but also to rule out comorbid or alternative diagnoses.

Children exposed to valproate may have some similar features to children with FAS including wide-spaced eyes, short palpebral fissures, long philtrum, and thin vermillion border. Children with velocardiofacial syndrome may have short palpebral fissures and a thin vermillion border. Maternal PKU effects and toluene embryopathy have all three facial characteristics that characterize children with FAS but could be ruled out by obtaining a good history (maternal diagnosis of PKU, maternal toluene abuse). Physical examination and/or subsequent diagnostic tests may be able to identify potential ARBDs such as cardiac (e.g., septal defects or aortic anomalies), renal (e.g., horseshoe kidneys), ocular (e.g., optic nerve hypoplasia), otologic (e.g., sensorineural hearing loss), skeletal/spinal (e.g., clinodactyly, spina bifida), or oral (e.g., cleft palate). Facial features become less easily distinguished as children become adolescents.

G. **Tests.** The diagnosis of an FASD relies on fulfillment of the diagnostic criteria. Developmental, neurologic, psychological, and speech–language evaluation can assist in establishing the presence of CNS dysfunction, identifying alternative/comorbid conditions and planning appropriate services. Genetic evaluation may help establish the diagnosis, rule out comorbid syndromes, or recommend alternative diagnoses.

III. MANAGEMENT

A. **Information for the family**

1. Symptoms are not the result of "poor parenting" or a "bad personality." The child is often "unable" not "unwilling."

2. Individuals with FASDs have a CNS abnormality that is permanent but not degenerative. The CNS abnormality often presents as neurobehavioral or neurocognitive dysfunction with associated difficulty in learning, self-care, behavior, and self-regulation. Persons with FASDs and their families, as well as educators and care providers, can help by providing accommodations that take into consideration the individual's strengths and weaknesses.

3. There is a spectrum of effects related to prenatal alcohol exposure—from subclinical effects to mainly neurobehavioral effects to full FAS. Having an FASD is often characterized as a hidden disability because the physical abnormalities may not be as obvious yet brain-based challenges can be profound.

   Early diagnosis and developmental intervention as well as a nurturing environment can improve outcomes and can be protective against secondary disabilities. Children who are diagnosed with an FASD early have a better prognosis, and not diagnosing children often leads to significant disability including substance abuse, school dropout or underperformance, incarceration, physical and mental health issues, and early death.

B. **Treatment**

1. **Early intervention.** Some children with FASDs may have obvious developmental disabilities as early as infancy or toddlerhood. Early intervention services can be provided to children 0–36 months with significant developmental delay in one or more areas (e.g., language, motor skills, and social skills).

2. **Educational intervention.** Some individuals with FASDs may have subtler neurodevelopmental weaknesses that can be easily overlooked until school-age years, when they are expected to learn by integrating from a wide knowledge base and to generalize from one learning situation to another. School-based services are important for many individuals with FASDs because they may have specific learning disabilities or brain-based difficulties (attention-deficit/hyperactivity disorder, executive functioning deficits, etc.). Currently, FASD is not one of the categories in the Individuals with Disabilities Education Act (IDEA) for which one can obtain special education services (http://www.nichcy.org). Because FAS is a medical diagnosis that can negatively affect educational functioning, some school districts may also categorize it under "Other Health Impairment." School systems may benefit from educational sessions geared toward understanding students with FASDs. Occupational therapy can be very helpful in teaching self-regulation.

3. **Social skills training.** As many children with FASDs have difficulty reading and accurately interpreting social cues, it is important that social skills are taught, practiced, and reinforced. Learning to curtail indiscriminate social approach can be challenging for many of these children and may place them in vulnerable positions if not addressed.

4. **Parenting strategies.** Parenting a child with an FASD can be challenging owing to the outlined neurobehavioral deficits. Children with FASDs benefit from a structured environment where there are reasonable rules, routines, and

supervision. They benefit from instructions that are concrete, consistent, simple, and specific and visual aids may help. They may need several repetitions for them to master concepts. Children with FASDs need help with transitions and may require multiple cues.

5. **Medication management.** Stimulants (methylphenidate, dextroamphetamine) and alpha-adrenergic agonists (clonidine or guanfacine) can be helpful for hyperactivity, impulsivity, and inattention. Selective serotonin reuptake inhibitors (e.g., fluoxetine, fluvoxamine, sertraline); anticonvulsants (e.g., carbamazepine, valproic acid); and antipsychotics (e.g., risperidone, quetiapine [Seroquel]) may help address depression, anxiety, or other mood disorders. It may be helpful to address medication questions with a developmental pediatrician or child psychiatrist with expertise in these issues. Children with FASDs are often treated with higher doses and more psychotropic medications, and some of this may be due to limited responses or more adverse events to treatment.

6. **Advocacy issues.** Individuals with FASDs will benefit from support, apprenticeship, and advocacy in the home, school, and workplace in order that they receive adequate preparation for adult life. Individuals will need help in the transition between the school and the workplace. There may also be need for an advocate to navigate the legal system, as the brain-based cognitive challenges experienced by individuals with FASDs may make them more prone to victimization, poor judgment, and poor cause-and-effect reasoning.

7. **Identification of risk and protective factors.** There are several protective factors that have been shown to improve functioning for individuals with prenatal alcohol exposure. These include a stable and nurturing environment; early diagnosis; absence of violence; stable home placements; and eligibility for social, developmental, and educational services (i.e., developmental intervention or special education). Conversely, risk factors for poor outcomes also have been identified, including multiple caregiving placements, early or continued exposure to violence, and failure to qualify for disability services.

IV. CLINICAL PEARLS AND PITFALLS

- Primary care clinicians are often the first to encounter a child with a possible FASD and will remain the medical home and caretaker for children, thus are critically important in their ongoing care.
- Pediatric clinicians should screen women for prenatal alcohol exposure, which is key to diagnosing children and possibly preventing future pregnancies where there is prenatal alcohol exposure.
- Diagnosis at any point, but especially before the age of 6 years, is a predictor for better outcomes. Diagnosis is not the end point but helps start the process of identifying the individual's inherent strengths and neurobehavioral challenges and the provision of appropriate intervention.
- Diagnosis is often a complex process and is best made by a multidisciplinary team (developmental and behavioral clinician, neurology clinician, geneticist, psychologist/neuropsychologist, parent navigator, social worker).
- Not all children with FASDs will have facial or growth abnormalities. Even in children with FAS, facial features can be subtle.
- Only 20%–25% of children with FAS have intellectual disability, and a normal or average IQ does not mean that a child does not have an FASD. IQs range from 20 to 120 in FAS and 49 to 142 for the other FASDs.
- Learning difficulties that are not remediated or for which there are no accommodations/interventions can lead to longstanding frustration and either internalizing or externalizing symptoms. It is important to address the primary disabilities (learning/language problems, etc.), as this is the best way to prevent secondary disabilities (substance abuse, school failure, mental illness, criminal involvement, etc.).
- Many children with FAS have troubles with low self-esteem owing to the neurobehavioral challenges they encounter on a day-to-day basis. It may be helpful to refer to a therapist with knowledge on FASDs who can support the child and who can guide parents and teachers on appropriate strategies.
- Adolescence is a challenging time for many individuals, but for individuals with FASDs, especially for those who are identified late, there may be more significant behavioral problems such as inappropriate sexual behavior, aggression, lying, and criminal activity.
- The clinician can help the biologic mother to understand that the diagnosis of FASDs does not mean that she drank during pregnancy out of the intent to hurt her child and that both she and the child are victims of the disease of alcoholism. If the parent is

suffering from continued addiction, the clinician should refer a parent for substance abuse evaluation and treatment.
* Prevention is key—frequent screening of teens/young adults, all women of childbearing age, all pregnant women, and nursing mothers for alcohol use.

Bibliography

FOR FAMILIES

BOOKS

Kleinfield J, Wescott S, eds. *Fantastic Antone Succeeds: Experiences in Educating Children With Fetal Alcohol Syndrome.* Fairbanks: University of Alaska Press; 1993.
Kleinfeld JS, Morse BA, Wescott S, eds. *Fantastic Antone Grows Up: Assisting Alcohol Affected Adolescents and Adults.* Fairbanks: University of Alaska Press; 1998.
Malbin D. *Fetal Alcohol Spectrum Disorders: Trying Differently Rather Than Harder.* 2nd ed. Portland, OR: FASCETS; 2002.
Streissguth AP. *Fetal Alcohol Syndrome: A Guide for Families and Communities.* Baltimore, MD: Paul H. Brookes Publishing; 1997.

WEB SITES

Centers for Disease Control and Prevention (CDC). www.cdc.gov/ncbddd/fas.
FASD Center for Excellence. http://fasdcenter.samhsa.gov.
FAS Community Resource Center. www.come-over.to/FASCRC/.
Fetal Alcohol Syndrome Consultation, Education and Training Services. www.fascets.org.
Fetal Alcohol Syndrome: Support, Training, Advocacy, and Resources. www.fasstar.com.
National Institute on Alcohol Abuse and Alcoholism. www.niaaa.nih.gov.
National Organization on Fetal Alcohol Syndrome. www.nofas.org.
The Arc of the United States. http://www.thearc.org.

FOR PROFESSIONALS

American Academy of Pediatrics FASD TOOLKIT. https://www.aap.org/en-us/advocacy-and-policy/aap-health-initiatives/fetal-alcohol-spectrum-disorders-toolkit/Pages/Management.aspx.
FAS Diagnostic and Prevention Network: FASD Diagnostic Tools. https://www.depts.washington.edu/fasdpn/htmls/diagnostic-tools.htm.
Hagan JF, Balachova T, Bertrand J, et al. on behalf of Neurobehavioral Disorder Associated With Prenatal Alcohol Exposure Workgroup; American Academy of Pediatrics. Neurobehavioral disorder associated with prenatal alcohol exposure. *Pediatrics.* 2016;138(4):e20151553. doi:10.1542/peds.2015-1553.
Hoymes HE, Kalberg WO, Elliott AJ, et al. Updated clinical guidelines for diagnosing fetal alcohol spectrum disorder. *Pediatrics.* 2016;138(2):1-18.
Lange S, Probst C, Gmel G, Rehm J, Burd L, Popova S. Global prevalence of fetal alcohol spectrum disorder among children and youth: a systematic review and meta-analysis. *JAMA Pediatr.* 2017;171(10):948-956.
May PA, Baete A, Russo J, et al. Prevalence and characteristics of fetal alcohol spectrum disorders. *Pediatrics.* 2014;134:855-866.
May PA, Gossage JP, Kalberg WO, et al. Prevalence and epidemiologic characteristics of FASD from various research methods with an emphasis on recent in-school studies. *Dev Disabil Res Rev.* 2009;15:176-192.
Rangmar J, Hjern A, Vinnerljung B, Strömland K, Aronson M, Fahlke C. Psychosocial outcomes of fetal alcohol syndrome in adulthood. *Pediatrics.* 2015;135(1):e52-e58.
SAMSHA. https://www.samhsa.gov/fetal-alcohol-spectrum-disorders-fasd-center.
Senturias Y. FASD Fetal alcohol spectrum disorders: An overview for pediatric and adolescent care providers. *Curr Probl Pediatr Adolesc Health Care.* 2014;44(4):74-81.
Senturias Y, Asamoah A. Fetal alcohol spectrum disorders: Guidance for recognition, diagnosis, differential diagnosis and referral. *Curr Probl Pediatr Adolesc Health Care.* 2014;44(4):88-95.
Senturias Y, Asamoah A, Allard A, et al. Fetal alcohol spectrum disorders (FASD): what medical professionals need to know. *J Ky Med Assoc.* 2009;107(5):177-180.
Senturias Y, Burns B. Managing Children and adolescents with fetal alcohol spectrum disorders in the medical home. *Curr Probl Pediatr Adolesc Health Care.* 2014;44(4):96-101.

CHAPTER 48

Fears

Marilyn Augustyn

I. DESCRIPTION OF THE PROBLEM. Fear is an unpleasant emotion with cognitive, behavioral, and physiologic components. It occurs in response to a consciously recognized source of danger, either real or imaginary. From an evolutionary perspective, fear is a key to survival.

A **phobia** is a persistent and compulsive dread of and preoccupation with the feared object or event. Phobias may interfere with the child's functioning in a way that fears do not.

All children have fears at some point in their lives. Most childhood fears are normal, temporary, and eventually outgrown. Some fears, however, may be symptoms of an anxiety disorder. Fears and anxiety are on a continuum, with phobias at the more severe end of the spectrum where symptoms are accompanied by functional impairment. Children with this presentation warrant additional evaluation for specific phobia or other anxiety disorders.

A. Epidemiology

- Fears are present at various times in the lives of *all* children.
- Between 2 and 6 years, most children experience more than four fears.
- Between 6 and 12 years, they experience an average of seven different fears.
- Fears often peak at the age of 11 years and then decrease with age.
- Studies of identical twins suggest a genetic predisposition to fearfulness in some children.
- Females report fears more often than males do.
- Mothers often underreport (by up to 40%) the fears of their children.
- Unconfronted fears are more likely to persist.
- Phobias are seen in 7% of adults (disabling phobias in 2%); the prevalence in children is unknown.

B. Familial trends

1. **Fearful, anxious parents tend to have fearful, anxious children**, probably through a combination of genetic predisposition and social learning.
2. **Simple phobias appear to run in families**, although individuals rarely share the same specific phobic stimulus.

C. Etiology/contributing factors

1. **Environmental**
   a. Although fears in childhood reflect a universal developmental tendency, the **onset often relates to a triggering event**. For example, a child may become fearful of dogs following a startling experience with an unleashed large dog. The (perhaps) innate human fear of large animals is intensified by a developmental level that does not allow a nonthreatening explanation of the event.
   b. New **stimuli from the media** join the roster of later childhood fears (e.g., school violence, sexual abuse, environmental toxins, terrorist attacks) even as old ones have dissipated (e.g., the communists). Sensationalistic news flashes can often heighten children's fear of exposure.
   c. Significant fears may reflect an **accurate assessment of a truly harmful situation** or represent a **displacement of feeling** from another environmental stressor (e.g., physical or sexual abuse).

2. **Developmental.** Fears change and evolve as cognitive development becomes more sophisticated. Fear of falling and loud noises are the only fears children have at birth. The emergence of other common fears reflects a child's increasing awareness of the world around him. Fantasy–reality differentiation is a developmental process that occurs in the first decade and sometimes longer, which can impact children's development of fear. Early childhood fears center on the environment. Exposure to real-world dangers intensifies and expands fear. Table 48-1 provides the timing of selected fears throughout early development.

3. **Temperamental tendencies.** This is the tendency to react with distress and withdrawal when confronted with unfamiliar people or situations.

Table 48-1 • COMMON FEARS IN CHILDHOOD AND ADOLESCENCE

Fear	Age (Years)							
	1	2	3	5	7	9	12	14
Separation	X	X			X			
Noises		X			X			
Falling	X				X	X		
Animals/insects	X		X	X				
Toilet training	X	X						
Bath	X	X						
Bedtime		X	X		X			
Monsters/ghosts			X	X				
Divorce					X			
Getting lost			X	X				
Loss of parent				X				
Social rejection						X	X	X
War						X		
New situations						X		
Adoption						X		X
Burglars							X	X
Injections	X	X	X	X	X	X	X	X
Sexual relations								X

II. **MAKING THE DIAGNOSIS.** The most useful way to differentiate a fear from a phobia is **the degree to which the fear interferes with the child's daily activities** (Table 48-2). If the child is developing normally in all other aspects, most often the behavior is a simple fear. If the fear impinges on important activities, it may have progressed to a phobia and requires specialized attention.

    A. **History: key clinical questions.** The primary care clinician must determine if the symptoms represent a simple fear, a response to significant environmental pathology, or a displacement of other stresses in the child's life.

        1. *"Does your child's fear interrupt his or her daily schedule more than three times per day?"*

        2. *"Can anyone recall a specific trigger to the fear?"*

        3. *"How do you* [the parents] *usually respond to the child's fear?"*

        Useful screening tools include the Fear Survey Schedule for Infants–Preschoolers (FSSIP) and the Preschool Anxiety Scale–Revised (PAS-R).

III. **MANAGEMENT.** Management will depend on whether the problem is a simple fear, a mild phobia, a debilitating phobia, or a response to environmental pathology. In most cases, simple parental support and empathy will suffice. Fears are ubiquitous throughout childhood. The goal is not to *banish* all of them but to help the child learn positive ways of coping with and transcending them. In the words of Selma Fraiberg, "The future mental health of the child does not depend upon the presence or absence of ogres in his fantasy life.... It depends upon the child's solution to the ogre problem."

    A. **Information for parents.** Parents should understand that simple fears are normal and do not necessarily represent a problem in the child or in the environment. The complexity and overwhelming nature of the world, coupled with a child's limited cognitive resources, conspire to create fears in *all* children, even those in the most secure and loving homes.

    B. **Supportive strategies.** Parents can exacerbate children's fears by using them as a threat (e.g., The doctor is going to give you a shot if you are not good), by humiliating the child (e.g., Only babies are afraid of bugs), by indifference to the child's distress, by unrealistic expectations to master the fear, and by overprotectiveness (thereby confirming the child's hypothesis that the stimulus is to be feared). They should follow these guidelines:

Table 48-2 • DIFFERENTIATION OF FEARS AND PHOBIAS

	Fears	Phobias
Response to reassurance	Yes	No
Plausible event as cause	Yes	No
Distractible	Yes	No
Impinges on play/development	No	Yes

1. Parents should **respect the child's inclination to withdraw from that which is feared**.
2. **The parents and the clinician should not exaggerate the fear or belittle it. They should also not overreact.**
3. **Support should be provided to the child as he or she develops an increased mastery of the fearful object. Do not cater to a fear.** This may involve initial avoidance of the fearful stimulus, planned discussions about the fear with attempts to correct cognitive misconceptions, and a gradual introduction to the feared stimulus with much family support, "bibliotherapy," that is, reading a book together about the feared stimulus can be useful. Watching reassuring videos together (such as *Monsters, Inc.*) can also lessen anxiety.
4. In young children, some fears cannot be reasoned away. **Parents may have to resort to comprehensible and concrete actions**, such as "monster proofing" the bedroom.
5. **Unconfronted fears can last.** Although many fears will disappear as quickly as they came, some persist and may become ingrained.
6. **Coping with a fear often involves breaking fear into its parts**: physical aspects, cognitive aspects, and behavioral aspects. Different techniques may help in fear mastery for each, but useful techniques for overcoming fear include imagination, information, observation, and exposure.
7. An additional approach is "bibliotherapy" or the use of reading aloud to children to address fears.

C. **Criteria for referral.** The child/family should be referred to a mental health professional for a phobic condition when fears begin to generalize from the situation of origin or the fears significantly hamper the child's activities of daily living or if the fears are felt to represent a realistic response to a truly threatening environment. Mental health professionals may use techniques such as behavioral modification with systematic desensitization or psychopharmacology to treat severe phobias.

Bibliography

FOR PARENTS

BOOKS
American Academy of Pediatrics. Fears and phobias. In: Schor EL, ed. *Caring for Your School-Age Child Ages 5 to 12. The Complete and Authoritative Guide.* Elk Grove Vill, IL: American Academy of Pediatrics; 1995:263.

WEB SITES
http://kidshealth.org/en/parents/anxiety.html.

FOR CHILDREN
Spinelli E. *When Mama Comes Home Tonight.* New York, NY: Simon & Schuster; 1998.
Viorst J. *Alexander and the Terrible, Horrible, No Good, Very Bad Day.* New York, NY: Simon & Schuster Children's Books; 1972.
Waddel M. *Owl Babies.* Cambridge, MA: Candlewick Press; 1996.

FOR PROFESSIONALS
Dunne G, Askew C. Vicarious learning and unlearning of fear in childhood via mother and stranger models. *Emotion.* 2013;13:974.
Jovanovic T, Nylocks KM, Gamwell KL, et al. Development of fear acquisition and extinction in children: effects of age and anxiety. *Neurobiol Learn Mem.* 2014;113:135-142.
Muris P, Ollendick TH, Roelofs J, Austin K. The short form of the fear survey schedule for children-revised (FSSC-R-SF): an efficient, reliable and valid scale for measuring fear and in children and adolescents. *J Anxiety Disord.* 2014;28(8):957-965.

CHAPTER 49

Foster Care

Moira Szilagyi | Linda D. Sagor

I. **DESCRIPTION OF THE PROBLEM.** Foster care **is government subsidized and reg-**
ulated temporary care for children who have been removed from their families for
reasons of abuse and neglect. The goals of foster care are safety, and well-being for
children through reunification with their family or adoption. The main types of care are
nonrelative family foster care, relative foster care (kinship care), and residential group care
(congregate care). For brevity, the term *foster care* will be used for all three types of care.
With the increased emphasis on keeping families together over the last 15 years, the numbers of children in foster care declined, until 2012 when they began increasing again. The
decline was due to child welfare allowing as more children to remain at home with services
or informally with relatives.

A. **Epidemiology.** As of 2012, the total daily census had declined to less than 400,000
children and youth but has increased every year since. The overall reduction in numbers was the result of increased reliance on preventive services, the emphasis on returning children to parents/extended family sooner, and earlier termination of parental
rights to facilitate adoption when reunification was not feasible. However, the numbers
subsequently increased largely related to a surge in parental substance abuse: 61% of
infants and 41% of older children in foster care come from families with active alcohol
or drug abuse.

In 2016, 44% of children entering care were younger than 5 years while the percentage of adolescents 13 years and older was 22%. Shifts in the demographics have
occurred with respect to race and ethnicity as well, with a relatively greater decline in
the African American population (21% in 2016), even though they are still overrepresented in foster care. This shift is attributed to the efforts around disparities reduction
in investigation, removal and placement undertaken by child welfare in the last
15 years. Mean time in care is now 20.1 months with 28% of children in care for greater
than 2 years.

Other characteristics typically include the following:

Types of care
75% in regular (including kinship) care
4% in preadoptive home
14% in group or residential care
7% in other arrangements

Age of foster children
7% infants
32% 1–5 years of age
31% 6–12 years of age
26% adolescents, 13–17 years of age
4% young adults, 18–20 years of age

Race; ethnicity of foster children
43% white, non-Hispanic
24% African American, non-Hispanic
21% Latino
12% others

B. **Contributory factors.** Although parental substance abuse has always been a significant risk factor for many children who enter foster care, the recent prevalence of opioid
use in the United States has led to a significant increase in this population. The opioid
crisis follows the crack cocaine epidemic and a methamphetamine resurgence, all of
which have affected vulnerable families over the past several decades.

In 2016 the Department of Health and Human Services noted that substance abuse
was a factor in 34% of the cases in which a child was removed from the home, up from
32% the previous year. Approximately 15% of newborn infants are affected **prenatally**
with alcohol or drug exposure. These substance-exposed newborns may face many

physical and developmental challenges, especially when the parents' substance use disorder and possible co-occurring mental illness are not adequately treated. They are also more likely to be placed in out-of-home care and more likely to stay in care longer than other children.

Children entering foster care have typically endured multiple and chronic adverse life experiences, including abuse and neglect, inconsistent and chaotic parenting from multiple caregivers, severe emotional deprivation, and limited access to appropriate services. In addition, their families often live in poverty and experience housing, employment, and food insecurity. Removal from their families and all that is familiar is a traumatizing event for most children, and the uncertainty inherent in the foster care system may further erode a child's sense of well-being. The impact of foster care on individual children depends on their personal strengths and coping skills, prior life experiences, developmental abilities, and the availability of protective environmental factors, the most important of which is the ongoing presence of a safe, stable, nurturing caregiver.

II. IDENTIFYING PROBLEMS

A. General issues. Children in foster care are defined as children with special health care needs by the American Academy of Pediatrics (AAP) because of their high prevalence of medical, mental health, developmental, educational, and psychosocial problems. One-third of children in foster care have a chronic condition (obesity, asthma, and dental caries top the list), 60% have developmental delay, especially speech delay, and, not surprisingly, 80% have a significant mental health need. Thus, providers may wish to consider the following:

1. The periodicity schedule of the AAP for child health supervision may need to be adjusted to reflect the more intensive support and monitoring necessary because of the many junctures in foster care that may adversely affect a child's health and well-being. A checklist that includes the crucial aspects of the health assessment and health care for children in foster care is available through the AAP (www.aap.org/advocacy/HFCA).

2. Intensive health care management to guarantee access to an appropriate array of developmental, mental health, medical, and dental services is essential to good health outcomes for children in foster care.

3. The single greatest health need of children in foster care is for mental health care services and support.

B. Specific issues. The AAP has several specific recommendations for health care of this population with special health care needs.

1. **Primary pediatric care.** Children in foster care should have a "medical home." The AAP recommends visits:
   - Monthly until 6 months of age, particularly if born prematurely or with medical complexity
   - Every 3 months from 6 to 24 months of age with close monitoring of development
   - Every 6 months from 24 months to 21 years

   Primary care clinicians may wish to particularly address the adjustment of the child to the foster care placement, child emotional and behavioral issues, school functioning, and the capacities of all the child's families to meet the child's needs. As thorough a history should be taken as possible to include information about the child's reason for placement, legal status, and the names and roles of child welfare professionals responsible for the child (e.g., foster parents, caseworker, law guardian). On physical examination, it is important to monitor growth parameters and nutrition and assess for skin findings and vision, hearing, dental, musculoskeletal, and neurologic health. Clear communication and collaboration with the other professionals involved in the child's care is essential. Frequent follow-up visits and a high index of suspicion for emotional and psychological problems are fundamental to providing appropriate health care for this population.

   Mental health is the most significant health concern for children and adolescents in foster care. In addition to prior childhood trauma, children in foster care may experience acute traumatic grief related to separation and loss and may feel unloved or abandoned by their parents or experience anger, anxiety, and depression. The careful use of language is important. For example, describing parents as *unable* to care for them is preferred to other terms, such as unwilling. Because of prior trauma, children may display extreme behaviors and distrust of caregivers and others, both of which may have been adaptive in their prior environment. Clinicians can play a valuable role by supporting and educating foster parents, reframing behaviors in terms of child traumatic stress, focusing on the child's strengths and modeling attentive listening and a consistent and caring manner toward the child during visits.

The increased use of psychotropic medication for children in foster care as compared with the general population (13%–52% vs. 4%) has led to increased scrutiny and promotion of monitoring policies and protocols. The US General Accounting Office report of 2015 indicated that recognition of this discrepancy has led to some reduction in psychotropic medication prescribing. The report acknowledges that reducing medication may not be the best course for every child and the overarching goal would be to ensure that all children receive appropriate treatment, including psychosocial services and family support.

2. **Transitions in foster care.** Placement changes, sibling separation or reunion, changes in visitation patterns, and the termination of parental rights are but a few of the traumatizing experiences that occur in foster care and during which children need special support. The primary care clinician can advocate for appropriate preparation of the child to facilitate these transitions and provide anticipatory guidance to the foster parent and caseworker about ways to support the child. The clinician should emphasize the need for abundant patience, affection, consistency, and nurturance during these difficult junctures.

3. **Screening questions for foster parents to assess how the transition is progressing include the following:**
   - *"How do you think your child is doing?"*
   - *"How has this child adjusted to your family and your family to this child?"*
   - *"Are there some behaviors you are worried about?"*
   - *"What has it been like for others in your home since this child moved in?"*
   - *"How are you coping?"*
   - *"Have there been any other significant changes in your family?"*

4. **The child's view of being in care.** Depending on a child's maturity and expressive abilities, it may be possible to ascertain directly how he or she perceives foster care, the foster home, and visitation. Useful questions, without the caregiver present, include the following:
   - *"What is it like for you living in this home?"*
   - *"What do you like best? Least?"*
   - *"How do you get along with the people in your new home?"*
   - *"What would you like to change?"*
   - *"Do you feel loved and cared for where you are living?"*
   - *"Tell me how your visits with your parent(s) are going?"*

5. **Visitation with parents.** Visits with birth parents can evoke strong, ambivalent emotions and difficult behaviors in children. Practitioners should encourage foster parents to maintain a positive view of the birth parents, at least, in front of the child. For example, foster families should help the child prepare for visits, send a beloved transitional object and healthy food/formula/water with younger children, and help them rehearse their response to potentially difficult situations. Occasionally, the clinician may need to recommend a change in visitation that is clearly stressful to a child; for example, the clinician might recommend that the child go for a visit only if the parent calls ahead if there has been frequent noncompliance with visits by the parent. The clinician must be careful to avoid simplistic explanations for children's responses to visits (e.g., interpreting aggressive behavior after a visit as reflecting a child's negative feelings toward his or her parents when, in fact, it is due to the anxiety of separating from them or anger that they did not show).

6. **Discipline in substitute care.** Foster caregivers are rightfully forbidden to use corporal punishment for children placed in their care. Disciplinary techniques should be grounded in positive parenting approaches. Caregivers should focus on using positive words and instructions, distraction techniques, teachable moments, reassurance, and rewarding positive behaviors. Health care professionals can help foster parents by educating them about childhood trauma and how it might lead to dysregulation because of its impact on the developing brain. Common presentations include dysregulated sleep, eating, and elimination patterns as well as poor emotional self-regulation. Shifting the conversation from "what is wrong with this child?" to "what happened to this child?" can help foster parents to respond more calmly and reassuringly to the child. Consistency and emotional support in the foster home environment can help children with the initial adjustment to the placement and with the subsequent challenges that may arise, such as inconsistent visitation with family. Understanding a foster caregiver's parenting skills and abilities is fundamental to offering them parenting advice (e.g., *"How do you cope when your child is acting this way?"*). Some foster parents may benefit from trauma education and/or an evidence-based parenting education course.

7. **Abuse and neglect in substitute care.** Abuse and neglect appear to be infrequent in substitute care. However, primary care clinicians need to remain alert to the physical and behavioral markers of maltreatment and assess whether these resulted from abuse or neglect before or during placement. Weight loss or poor weight gain in a young child is often the first sign of a neglectful foster care placement. Prolonged dysregulated behaviors may reflect either prior trauma or concerning behaviors by caregivers in the current placement. Children with behavioral dysregulation, developmental disabilities, and/or medically complex conditions may be more vulnerable to abuse and neglect in out-of-home placements.

8. **Discontinuous health care.** Children in foster have usually experienced inadequate preventive health care or frequent changes in health care providers. Health information is often sparse or unavailable, and the primary care clinician should be mindful of gathering and maintaining medical documentation that will be useful to future clinicians. Communication with child welfare professionals about health information is crucial to appropriate permanency planning for children in foster care. State immunization registries have improved access of providers to this information and often enable identification of prior providers from whom to obtain health records.

9. **Support for substitute caregivers.** Healing from trauma occurs in the context of a secure attachment relationship and so attachment to the substitute caregiver is to be encouraged. Many children in foster care have serious emotional and behavioral problems rooted in childhood trauma that their foster parents and caseworkers may find difficult to handle. Primary care clinicians can help by providing more frequent visits for education, emotional support, and counseling. They should treat foster parents as members of the team supporting the child. And, while acknowledging this commitment, clinicians can be helpful in advocating for respite for foster parents when needed. Many foster parent groups have newsletters for which some clinicians write a column on health issues. Timely referral to appropriate mental health care, developmental, and home health services may stabilize a foster care placement for a child. The clinician can offer foster parents support and respect by reminding caregivers that child behaviors are usually the result of what has happened to them, discussing trauma reminders that may trigger some behaviors, focusing on child and caregiver strengths, expressing admiration for the stability and consistency caregivers are providing children in their care and their parenting skills, when indicated. Finally, clinicians may explicitly state to foster parents when it seems appropriate *"you are making a big difference in this child's life; thank you."*

10. **Involvement with birth parents.** Birth parents retain legal custody of their children unless they have been freed for adoption. Consent and confidentiality issues are complex in foster care, and the clinician should clarify who has the capacity to consent for a given child with the foster care agency. Involvement of the birth parents in the health care of their child is encouraged when deemed appropriate by the agency.

11. **Support for caseworkers.** Casework staff are often overwhelmed by large caseloads and undertrained and underpaid for the complex work they are required by law and regulation to do. Caseworkers are assigned to the family as a unit, not to the child or children. As a result, they are mandated to work with the birth family toward reunification while simultaneously identifying alternative permanency options for children in the interests of their safety, well-being, and permanency. Clinicians can help casework staff by maintaining clear and open lines of communication, providing useful clinical information, and acknowledging their efforts (e.g., *"You're really making a big difference in his life by finding all the services he needs"*). In some states, primary care clinicians have advocated for dedicated personnel in child welfare agencies to provide care coordination for medical, developmental, psychiatric, and dental issues of children in foster care. These medical social workers function as champions for the health care needs of these children and facilitate collaboration and communication among the agency staff, foster families, and the medical community. In addition, clinicians may be interested in playing a role in their local, county, or state child welfare agency as a consultant or medical director.

12. **Children preparing for independence.** In almost every state, children in foster care are expected to begin preparation for independent living at age 14 years and assume increased responsibility and independence as they reach 18 years of age. Almost every state now enables young adults to remain in care until age 21 years if they are working, in job training or in school. Intellectually impaired young people transition to the state's adult care system between 18 and 21 years. It is important

to be mindful that trauma experiences may have impacted those areas of the brain involved in emotional self-regulation and executive function, so that many adolescents age into adulthood undereducated and underprepared to function adaptively without support. This raises complex ethical and practical issues in terms of preparing young people for their futures and how long the child welfare or some other system should remain involved. The transition to adult health and mental health services may lead to disconnection from needed services. The clinician can suggest measures to prepare the adolescent for independent living. (Materials to assist caregivers and youth in this task are available from the National Foster Care Resource Center.) Ideally, the pediatric clinician will continue caring for the young adult or make a referral to another health care provider.

Bibliography

FOR PARENTS

ORGANIZATIONS
American Professional Society on the Abuse of Children. www.apsac.org.
Child Welfare League of America. www.cwla.org.
National Foster Parent Association. http://nfpainc.org.
National Child Traumatic Stress Network. http://www.nctsn.org/resources/audiences/parents-caregivers.

FOR TRANSITION AGE YOUTH
Foster Care Alumni Association of America. https://fostercarealumni.org/resources/.
iFoster: https://www.ifoster.org.
Guardian Scholars Program: http://www.fosteryouthhelp.ca.gov/pdfs/GuardianScholars.pdf.

FOR PROFESSIONALS

PUBLICATIONS
American Academy of Pediatrics, Committee on Early Childhood, Adoption and Dependent Care. Developmental issues for young children in foster care. *Pediatrics*. 2000;106:1145-1150.
American Academy of Pediatrics Council on Foster Care, Adoption and Kinship Care, Committee on Adolescence, and Council on Early Childhood. Policy statement: health care issues for children and adolescents in foster care and kinship care. *Pediatrics*. 2015:e1131-e1140.
Jee SH, Szilagyi M, Ovenshire C, et al. Improved detection of developmental delays among young children in foster care. *Pediatrics*. 2010;125:282-289.
McMillen JC, Raghavan R. Pediatric to adult mental health service use of young people leaving the foster care system. *J Adolesc Health*. 2009;44:7-13.
Pilowsky DJ, Wu LT. Psychiatric symptoms and substance use disorders in a nationally representative sample of American adolescents involved with foster care. *J Adolesc Health*. 2006;38:351.
Simms M, Dubowitz H, Szilagyi M. Health care needs of children in the foster care system. *Pediatrics*. 2000;106:909-918.
Stein RE, Hurlburt MS, Heneghan AM, et al. Health status and type of out-of-home placement: informal kinship care in an investigated sample. *Acad Pediatr*. 2014;14:559-564.
van der Kolk BA. Developmental trauma disorder. *Psychiatr Ann*. 2005;35:401-408.

WEB SITE
The Future of Children. http://www.futureofchildren.org/pubs-info2825/pubs-info.htm?doc_id=209538.

CHAPTER 50

Failure to Thrive

Caroline J. Kistin | Deborah A. Frank

I. **DESCRIPTION OF THE PROBLEM.** Failure to thrive (FTT) in childhood refers to children whose growth persistently and significantly deviates from the norms for their age and sex on appropriate growth charts.

   A. **Epidemiology.** Nutritional growth failure is seen in 8%–12% of children of low-income families. However, the prevalence of FTT in the general population has not been well described.

   B. **Family transmission/genetics.** Familial short stature may be considered when the child's weight is appropriate to height and when linear growth velocity parallels the normal curve on the growth chart. It is, however, perilous to assume that poor growth, particularly low weight for height, in children is secondary to familial predisposition for several reasons:
   - Parental height may be a poor guide of the child's growth potential if parents themselves were nutritionally deprived as children and therefore did not attain their optimal growth (as is often the case with immigrant and impoverished families).
   - The parents may have an eating disorder, be excessively concerned with obesity, or may be otherwise unwisely overrestricting children's diets.
   - The child may share an underlying medical growth-retarding problem with the parents (e.g., celiac disease).

   C. **Etiology**
   1. **"Organic" versus "nonorganic".** Historically, the etiology of FTT was considered either organic (medical) or nonorganic (social/environmental). However, this dichotomy is of limited use because children with so-called nonorganic FTT are suffering from malnutrition, a serious medical insult, whereas children with major medical diagnoses may, in part, have growth failure attributable to social and nutritional factors. Diagnostically and therapeutically, it is useful to assess each child and family along four parameters: (1) medical, (2) nutritional, (3) developmental, and (4) social. Problems in any or all of these areas may interact to produce growth failure. For example, a temperamentally passive child with iron deficiency may fail to receive frequent enough feedings from an exhausted mother who has other more demanding children.
   2. **Psychosocial causes**
      a. Child may fail to thrive in families of any social class **when parents' emotional and material resources are diverted or not available from for the care of the child**. This can occur because of poverty, parental depression, maladaptive parenting practices, family discord, substance abuse, domestic violence, acute reaction to a recent loss or trauma (such as death of grandparent or unemployment), or depletion of a caregiver's energy by another chronically ill family member of any age, including other children with special health care needs.
      b. **FTT does not necessarily imply parental neglect or pathology.** Feeding disorders that lead to suboptimal weight gain can reflect numerous medical stressors (see below) or can develop in physically well children when not eating serves other purposes (e.g., to express anger, to exert autonomy from overly intrusive caretakers, to gain the attention of otherwise abstracted caretakers, or to divert adults from conflict with each other).
      c. Children with **preexisting minor developmental deficits** (e.g., subtle oral motor difficulties, hypersensitivity to stimulation) may develop feeding problems that lead to nutritional FTT. Apathy and irritability associated with malnutrition may exacerbate parent–child interactional dysfunction and lead to further feeding difficulties.
      d. Children **living in poverty** are often at nutritional risk because of inadequate food supplies in the home ("food insecurity"), homelessness, overcrowding, and the inability of federal feeding programs (e.g., SNAP [Supplemental Nutrition Assistance Program, formerly food stamps] supplemental food program for women, infants, and children [WIC], child care, or school meals) to reach many

Table 50-1 • OFTEN UNAPPARENT MEDICAL CAUSES OF FAILURE TO THRIVE (FTT)

Infectious

Giardiasis (other parasites, e.g., nematodes)
Chronic urinary tract infection
Chronic sinusitis
HIV

Mechanical

Adenoid and/or tonsillar hypertrophy
Dental lesions
Vascular slings
Gastroesophageal reflux

Neurologic

Oral motor dysfunction (gagging, tactile hypersensitivity, decreased or increased oral tone)

Toxic/metabolic

Lead toxicity
Iron deficiency
Zinc deficiency
Rickets
Inborn errors of metabolism

Gastrointestinal

Celiac disease
Malabsorption (various causes including cystic fibrosis)
Chronic constipation

Allergic

Food allergies (often present as FTT with atopic dermatitis)

of the eligible families. In other cases, the benefit levels of such safety net programs are insufficient to meet the nutritional needs of at-risk children.

3. **Medical causes**
   a. The **medical causes** of FTT encompass a whole textbook of pediatrics. Most contributing conditions are suggested by a careful history and physical examination, but some are occult (Table 50-1). Inborn errors of metabolism are rare but catastrophic causes of FTT, often with an associated history of seizures, recurrent dehydration, or developmental regression.
   b. **Perinatal risk factors** include prematurity and intrauterine growth retardation (IUGR). IUGR with dysmorphic features suggests a growth-retarding syndrome (genetic, congenital, or related to teratogen exposure).

D. **Long-term outcomes.** FTT is a major risk factor for later developmental and behavioral difficulties, usually reflecting both the nutritional deprivation of the developing nervous system and the environmental experiences of the child.

II. MAKING THE DIAGNOSIS

A. **Signs and symptoms.** Although there are no universally accepted anthropometric criteria, the following are frequently used:
   1. **Attained weight less than fifth or third percentile.**
   2. **Failure to maintain previously established growth trajectory, particularly after 18 months of age,** with parameters crossing two major percentiles (e.g., 75th to below 25th).
   3. **Decreased rate of daily weight gain for age** (Table 50-2).
   4. **Depressed weight for height,** which always reflects inadequate nutritional intake for the child's metabolic requirements. (Short stature with a weight that is proportionate to height may reflect chronic malnutrition, a normal familial pattern, or may be genetic/syndromal or endocrinologic in origin.)

   Using a combination of criteria—such as depressed weight for height *and* faltering growth trajectory—increases the accuracy of the FTT diagnosis. In general, the World Health Organization (WHO) growth standards are used for children younger than 2 years and the Centers for Disease Control and Prevention/National Center for

Table 50-2 • AVERAGE DAILY WEIGHT GAIN FOR AGE

Age	Median Daily Weight Gain (g)
0–3 mo	26–31
3–6 mo	17–18
6–9 mo	12–13
9–12 mo	9
1–3 y	7–9
4–6 y	6

Health Statistics (CDC/NCHS) growth charts are used for children older than 2 years. However, young children who have low weight for age or low weight for height on the CDC/NCHS charts but not on the WHO charts may suffer increased risks to health and development compared with children who are in the normal range on the CDC/NCHS charts and may still benefit from interventions.

B. **History: key clinical questions.** It is important first to evaluate the growth chart to ascertain the pattern and timing of onset of growth failure.

1. *"What were the changes in your family's or child's life around the time the child's growth slowed?"* Perhaps a parent returned to work and the child was placed in suboptimal childcare at the time; perhaps there was a family loss.

2. *"What, when (how often), where, why, and by whom is your child fed?"* It is useful to ascertain a 24-hour dietary recall. In addition, the child's behaviors and affect at mealtime should be elicited.

3. *"How much low-calorie liquid (e.g., juice, soda, iced tea, coffee, soup, Kool-Aid, water) does your child drink each day?"*

4. *"Does your child choke on food, have trouble chewing or swallowing, vomit or spit up, or take a few bites and then stop eating?"* Oral motor problems, gastroesophageal reflux, sometimes with associated food allergies, and painful teeth usually present with one or more of these symptoms.

5. *"What are your child's bowel movements like?"* Frequency and nature of stools may be a clue for occult gastrointestinal disease. Both constipation and diarrhea should prompt further evaluation and intervention.

6. *"Do you ever run out of food?"* If the clinician does not ask, the parents may never tell.

7. *"Does your child snore, even when they are not sick?"* Tonsillar and/or adenoidal hypertrophy is a frequently missed cause of poor oral intake.

8. *"Are there any foods to which your child is allergic or which he/she is not allowed to eat for religious or other reasons (e.g., vegetarian)?"* Allergies may manifest as anaphylaxis, but may also include symptoms of eczema, isolated urticaria, and stool changes, among others.

9. *"Do you and the child's other caretakers see eye to eye about the growing and eating problem?"*

10. *"Are there any significant stresses in the house?"*

C. **Behavioral observations**

1. The clinician can **observe the child while eating or being fed** in his or her office (or ideally during a home visit by trained observer):
   • Is the child adaptively positioned to eat?
   • Are the child's cues clear, and does the caretaker respond appropriately?
   • Are there oral motor difficulties?
   • Does the caretaker permit age-appropriate autonomy and messiness?
   • What is the affective tone at the feeding interaction for both the feeder and the child?
   • Is the child easily distracted during the feeding?
   • Is the child fed in front of television?

2. The clinician should also observe the **quality of the** caretaker–child *nonfeeding* **interactions:**
   • Is the caretaker irritable, punitive, depressed, disengaged, or intrusive?
   • Is the child apathetic, irritable, noncompliant, or provocative?

D. **Physical examination.** A careful history and physical examination should be performed to identify medical factors contributing to the FTT. In addition, all children with FTT should have formal developmental testing, with particular attention to cognition, language, and subtle fine motor difficulties.

E. Tests

1. Testing should be performed on the basis of the history and physical examination. **Basic screening laboratory tests** to consider include complete blood cell count with differential (as a screen for eosinophilia or anemia, which may result from malnutrition), lead (as lead may be absorbed more readily in the presence of malnutrition), urinalysis and urine culture (to evaluate for chronic urinary tract infection, renal tubular acidosis, or protein or carbohydrate loss), and serum electrolytes, including blood urea nitrogen and creatinine (to evaluate kidney function). Clinicians should have a low threshold for obtaining liver function tests, HIV screening, sweat tests (to evaluate for cystic fibrosis), and screening tests for occult celiac disease, depending on the findings from the history and physical examination. Thyroid studies should be considered if there are symptoms concerning for hyper- or hypothyroidism.

2. If the child is a new immigrant or recent traveler, lives in a homeless shelter, has been camping, or is in childcare and has a history of diarrhea or abdominal pain, **evaluation for enteric pathogens** (e.g., *Giardia lamblia*, *Helicobacter pylori*) should be considered as well as screening for hepatitis. A purified protein derivative (PPD) skin test or QuantiFERON gold test for tuberculosis should be considered for children with immigration or travel history, homelessness, or an experience of visiting incarcerated adults.

3. If the child is short but has an appropriate weight for height, a **bone age** may be useful to distinguish the constitutionally short child (with a bone age equivalent to chronological age) from a child with endocrine or nutritional derangement (with a delayed bone age). Evidence of rickets on wrist films or physical examination mandates evaluation of calcium, phosphorous, alkaline phosphatase, and vitamin D parameters.

III. MANAGEMENT

A. Primary goals. The primary goal is for the child to attain catch-up growth at a rate faster than average for age to repair the growth deficit. This typically requires a calorically dense diet that provides 1.5–2 times the recommended daily allowance of calories and protein. In addition, other identified medical and socioemotional difficulties must be specifically addressed.

B. Treatment strategies

1. **Instruct the parents in high-calorie/high-protein diet** (Figs. 50-1 and 50-2). This may require reassurance for the parents, as a higher fat diet than usual may be necessary to provide adequate calories in small volume. Children older than 1 year

---

Try to keep mealtimes and snack times about the same each day. Children work well with schedules.

Children need to eat often, not constantly. Offer something every 2–3 hours, to allow three meals and two to three snacks per day.

Make sure your child can reach the food. Use a high chair, telephone book, or a small table.

Allow your child to feed himself or herself. Try very small amounts at first. Offer seconds later. *Expect messiness.*

No force feeding, bribing, or cajoling! This will backfire.

Variety is not important. Total *calories* and *protein* are.

Offer solids before liquids.

Limit juice, water, and carbonated drinks. Offer milk or formula instead.

Offer foods that are easy for your child to handle: "finger foods" such as Cheerios®, french fries, slices of banana, cut-up burger, hot dogs, or peas.

Add margarine, mayonnaise, gravies, and grated cheese. For snacks, use peanut butter, cheese, pudding, bananas, or dried fruit.

Junk foods (soda, doughnuts, candy, etc.) have little protein and fewer calories than some other food choices. Junk foods will not help growth; they only take up valuable space in the stomach.

Eat with your child when possible, or allow your child to eat with others, so meals and snacks can be fun.

Figure 50-1 Effective feeding checklist for parents.

24-calorie per ounce formula
    1 can (13 oz) formula concentrate
    8 oz water

Note: Don't make the formula more concentrated than this: overconcentrating can be harmful to a child's kidneys.

Super fruit
    1 jar (4 oz) strained fruit
    1 scoop formula powder

Super milk (use instead of whole milk; 28 calories per ounce)
    1 cup dry milk powder
    4 cups whole milk

Super pudding
    2 cups whole milk
    ½ cup dry milk powder
    1 pkg. instant pudding mix
Mix whole and dry milk together. Then follow package directions for making pudding. Yield: 4 servings (116 calories per serving)

Super shake
    1 cup whole milk
    1 pkg. Carnation® Instant Breakfast
    1 cup ice cream
Mix together in blender. (430 calories)

Note: If making any of these changes causes your child to have diarrhea, stop and call your pediatrician.

Figure 50-2 Recipes for children.

who are able to drink cow's milk should have a goal intake of 20–24 ounces of whole milk per day in divided servings. Low-calorie drinks such as water and juice should be eliminated or at least decreased to no more than 4 ounces total per day. Sugar-sweetened and caffeinated beverages should be eliminated all together.

2. **Feed the child three meals and three snacks** on a consistent schedule. Milk should be given after food.
3. Give a **multivitamin** with iron and zinc (and therapeutic dosages of iron if indicated).
4. **Meet with all caretakers** involved in feeding the child to reduce conflict, to prevent the child from playing one caretaker against another, and to ensure consistency in the feeding regimen.
5. **Discuss adaptive feeding interactions** (e.g., allowing the child to self-feed even if messy, decreasing power struggles at meals, and fewer distractions in the environment). Encourage turning off the television and eliminating other screen time at mealtimes, eating with other family members, and pleasant conversation not related to food. Discourage grazing and constant sipping on low-calorie liquids that decrease appetite.
6. **Ensure access to resources** (e.g., WIC, SNAP [food stamps], food pantries).
7. **Give all immunizations** (including influenza vaccine); aggressively **treat intercurrent infections and chronic conditions such as asthma, atopic dermatitis, or gastroesophageal reflux.**
8. **Follow growth weekly to monthly,** depending on age and severity of malnutrition. Success is manifested as faster than normal rate of weight gain for age.

9. Depending on the needs of the family, **mobilize community services,** including mental health, substance abuse treatment, housing advocacy, and job training resources.

10. **Ensure that the child receives appropriate developmental intervention** through Head Start, early intervention, or public school programs.

C. **Criteria for referral**

1. Children whose **growth rate fails to respond in 2–3 months** should be referred to a multidisciplinary team in an appropriate center.

2. Children with **severe malnutrition, risk of abuse, serious intercurrent illness, or extreme parental impairment or anxiety** should be hospitalized.

IV. CLINICAL PEARLS AND PITFALLS

- Failure to correct for prematurity in plotting growth may lead to a factitious diagnosis of FTT. The chronologic age should be corrected for prematurity until 18 months for head circumference, until 24 months for weight, and until 40 months for height. Even after correcting for prematurity, very low-birth-weight children may remain short for corrected age, but weight for height should be proportionate.

- Children with symmetrical IUGR whether from unknown causes or prenatal exposure to alcohol may remain short but should not be underweight for height. After most intra-uterine exposures, except alcohol, children in adequate caregiving environments usually show postnatal catch up in both height and weight.

- Depressed height for age may be genetic/syndromic, endocrine, or nutritional, but depressed weight for height always reflects primary or secondary malnutrition.

Bibliography

FOR PARENTS

Framingham State University, article on high calorie diet. https://www.framingham.edu/Assets/uploads/academics/colleges/science-technology-engineering-and-mathematics/food-and-nutrition/_documents/high-cal-foods-for-toddlers.pdf.

FOR PROFESSIONALS

Addressing Food Insecurity: A Toolkit for Pediatricians. http://www.frac.org/aaptoolkit.

Blenner S, Wilbur MA, Frank DA. Food insecurity and failure to thrive. In: Wolraich ML, Drotar DD, Dworkin PH, et al, eds. *Developmental-Behavioral Pediatrics: Evidence and Practice.* Philadelphia, PA: Mosby Elsevier; 2008:768-779.

Ficicioglu C, An Haack K. Failure to thrive: when to suspect inborn errors of metabolism. *Pediatrics.* 2009;124:972-979.

Gahagan S. Infant feeding processes and disorders. In: Wolraich ML, Drotar DD, Dworkin PH, et al, eds. *Developmental-Behavioral Pediatrics: Evidence and Practice.* Philadelphia, PA: Mosby Elsevier; 2008:757-767.

Hernandez W, Frank DA, Morton S, Palacios C, Augustyn M. Growth-and documentation-deficits: where to start in helping families. *J Dev Behav Pediatr.* 2017;38(suppl 1):S82-S83.

Kistin CJ, Sandel M, Frank D. Failure to thrive: a reconceptualization. In: Chadwick DL, Alexander R, Giardino AP, Esernio-Jenssen D, Thackeray JD, eds. *Child Maltreatment: Physical Abuse and Neglect: Encyclopedic Volume 1 of 3.* 4th ed. Saint Louis, MO: STM Learning, Inc.; 2014.

Meyers AF, Joyce K, Coleman SM, et al. Health of children classified as underweight by CDC reference but normal by WHO standard. *Pediatrics.* 2013;131(6):e1780-e1787.

CHAPTER **51**

Fragile X Syndrome

Randi Jenssen Hagerman

I. DESCRIPTION OF THE PROBLEM. Fragile X syndrome (FXS) is the most common inherited form of intellectual disability and the most common single gene cause of autism spectrum disorder (ASD). It causes a spectrum of developmental problems, ranging from learning disabilities and emotional problems (in those with a normal IQ) through all levels of intellectual disability. The fragile X premutation can also be associated with developmental problems including attention-deficit/hyperactivity disorder (ADHD) and social deficits in addition to problems with tremor and balance difficulties in aging.

A. Epidemiology
- Causes intellectual disability in approximately 1 in 2500–4000 in the general population.
- Responsible for approximately 20%–30% of all cases of X-linked intellectual disability.
- Approximately 1 in 130–259 females and 1 in 250–810 males in the general population carry the premutation (55–200 CGG repeats).
- No known racial or ethnic differences; identified in all racial groups tested.
- Both males and females can be unaffected carriers although ADHD, anxiety, and social deficits including ASD can occur in premutation carriers. Approximately 40% of older male carriers and 16% of older female carriers can develop the fragile X-associated tremor ataxia syndrome (FXTAS). Fragile X-associated primary ovarian insufficiency (FXPOI) occurs before 40 years of age in about 20% of female carriers.

B. Genetics. FXS is caused by a mutation in the fragile X mental retardation-1 gene (*FMR1*), which is located on the bottom end of the X chromosome. The mutation causes a fragile site or break in the chromosome at that location. The *FMR1* gene was identified and sequenced in 1991. An unusual expansion of a cytosine, guanine, guanine (CGG) nucleotide repetitive sequence was found to be the mutation. Within the *FMR1* gene, normal individuals have a nucleotide CGG sequence that repeats up to 45 times, **carriers with a premutation have an expansion of the CGG sequence between 55 and 200 repeats**, and **individuals affected with FXS have a CGG repeat number greater than 200 (termed a full mutation).** When this occurs, the gene usually becomes methylated or turned off so that little or no *FMR1* protein (FMRP) is made, and the full FXS occurs. Point mutations or deletions can also occur in *FMR1* leading to FXS.

   A carrier male will pass only X chromosome to all his daughters, who will be his obligate carriers and these women will pass the mutation to 50% of their offspring. A significant expansion of the mutation will often occur in their children so that males and females with intellectual disability are common. A detailed family tree must be drawn to sort out possible carriers and other extended family members who may be affected by FXS or by premutation involvement including FXTAS and FXPOI.

II. MAKING THE DIAGNOSIS. Both behavioral and physical features are included in the fragile X checklist (Fig. 51-1), which serves as a reminder for clinicians of the signs and symptoms of FXS.

A. Signs and symptoms in males
   1. Early signs and symptoms
   - Infants with FXS may appear to be normal, although behavior and feeding difficulties have been described including recurrent vomiting.
   - **Recurrent otitis media** begins in the first year of life for the majority of males affected by this syndrome.
   - **Hypotonia** is also notable in young boys, with subsequent mild delays in motor milestones.
   - Most boys with FXS and significantly affected girls with fragile X **are delayed in the onset of language.** Phrases or short sentences are usually delayed until the age of 3 years or older. The language delays in addition to hyperactivity or tantrums are the typical initial concerns leading to medical consultation.

SCORE:	0	1	2

		Borderline or present	
	Not present	In the past	Definitely present
Mental retardation			
Hyperactivity			
Short attention span			
Tactilely defensive			
Hand flapping			
Hand biting			
Poor eye contact			
Perseverative speech			
Hyperextensible finger joints			
Large or prominent ears			
Large testicles			
Simian crease or Sydney line			
Family history of mental retardation or autism			

TOTAL SCORE _____

A score > 15 has a 45% chance of FXS

Figure 51-1 Fragile X checklist. FXS, Fragile X syndrome. Modified from Hagerman RJ, Amiri K, Cronister A. Fragile X checklist. *Am J Med Genet*. 1991;38:283-287.

- **Prominent ears** with occasional ear cupping, **hyperextensible finger joints, double-jointed thumbs, flat feet,** and soft skin are seen in the majority of boys with fragile X in early childhood. These physical findings are considered to be part of a connective tissue dysplasia that is related to the absence of FMRP.
- Young boys with FXS may also have a broad or prominent forehead and a large head circumference.
2. **Later signs and symptoms**
   - **Macroorchidism** becomes prominent in males with FXS during the early stages of puberty. Usually the testicular volume is at least twice the normal size, with an adult range in FXS of 40–100 cc. Although the spermatic tubules are tortuous by histological studies, fertility has been reported in several males with FXS.
   - In addition, a long **face and prominent jaw** are often noted after puberty.
   - Other diagnoses such as Soto syndrome, Tourette syndrome, Pierre–Robin sequence, and other congenital defects such as cleft palate or hip dislocation may be associated with FXS because of the connective tissue problems and behavioral difficulties that occur in this disorder.
B. **Behavioral problems in males.** Behavioral problems are a common presenting complaint in young boys with FXS. These include hyperactivity; impulsivity; an extremely short attention span; perseveration in speech and actions; hand flapping with excitement; hand biting with anger or frustration; oversensitivity to touch, noises, and textures of food or clothing; shyness; poor eye contact; self-talk; and tantrums. These behaviors are often described as "autistic-like," and 60% of boys with FXS have ASD.

Table 51-1 • ASSOCIATED MEDICAL PROBLEMS IN FRAGILE X SYNDROME IN MALES

Medical Problem	Frequency in Males
Flat feet	80%
Scoliosis	<20%
Mitral valve prolapse	50%–80% in adulthood
Recurrent otitis	60%
Strabismus	8%–30%
Nystagmus	Occasional
Refractive errors	20%
Seizures	20%
Macroorchidism	80% at puberty

C. **Signs and symptoms in girls.** Approximately 70% of females who carry the full mutation will have a borderline or intellectually impaired IQ (IQ < 70). The other 30% will have a normal IQ but may have significant learning disabilities, including attentional problems (with or without hyperactivity), math deficits, and language delays. **Significant shyness** is very common, often accompanied by poor eye contact. Females with FXS may be given a psychiatric diagnosis of avoidant disorder or ASD because of their social deficits. Schizotypal features (i.e., oddness in social interactional skills and appearance), depression, mood lability, anxiety, impulsive behavior, ADHD, or emotional problems have also been reported in women affected by FXS.

D. **Tests.** All children with intellectual impairment or ASD of unknown etiology should have **fragile X DNA testing.** If a learning disabled or carrier individual is suspected, fragile X (*FMR1*) DNA testing should be carried out. Once a proband is diagnosed with FXS, other family members should be assessed with *FMR1* DNA testing, including all siblings of the proband and of the carrier parent and grandparent. Premutation carriers older than 50 years, especially males, are at risk for FXTAS and should be referred to a neurologist if symptoms of tremor, neuropathy, cognitive decline, or gait instability occur. Women with the premutation should be counseled regarding FXPOI.

III. **MANAGEMENT**

A. **Goals and initial treatment strategies.** The goals of the primary care clinician are to provide appropriate medical therapy and to coordinate a team of professionals who will provide optimal treatment for the child with FXS. Speech and language therapy and occupational therapy are essential for all young children affected by FXS. A developmental preschool setting can usually provide these therapies, in addition to special education. Whenever possible, mainstreaming or full inclusion with typical peers is preferable because children with FXS usually model their behavior after their peers.

B. **Follow-up.** Medical follow-up includes recognition and treatment of connective tissue problems and associated complications of FXS (Table 51-1). **Because ophthalmological problems** are common, referral to an ophthalmologist before the age of 5 years will facilitate early treatment. Orthopedic referral is appropriate if scoliosis or joint dislocations occur. Mitral valve prolapse is usually noted in the older child or adult, so referral to a cardiologist for evaluation and echocardiogram is necessary if a murmur or click is heard in auscultation. Vigorous treatment of recurrent otitis media in early childhood is indicated and usually includes the use of pressure equalizing tubes, so that a fluctuating hearing loss does not interfere with optimal language development.

C. **Psychopharmacology.** The most common behavioral problem is hyperactivity, which is seen in approximately 80% of affected boys and 30% of affected girls. Therefore treatment of ADHD symptoms in these children is a main focus of intervention. A common concern of families of adolescent children with FXS is treatment of outbursts or aggression, a significant problem in approximately 30% of male adults and adolescents with FXS. Episodic dyscontrol usually occurs during or after significant environmental overstimulation (such as shopping in a busy store), or it may be precipitated by anger or frustration. A variety of medications have been used with some success (including clonidine, selective serotonin reuptake inhibitors [SSRIs], risperidone, aripiprazole, and anticonvulsants), but controlled studies have not yet been performed. SSRIs such as fluoxetine, sertraline, and citalopram can improve anxiety, obsessive–compulsive behavior and irritability, although 20% may have significant behavioral activation. Low-dose sertraline (2.5–5 mg) has been shown to be helpful for development including language in young children with FXS between the ages of 2–6 years in a randomized controlled trial. SSRIs are also helpful for premutation carriers who experience anxiety or depression. Aripiprazole in low dose is usually helpful for anxiety, attention, mood lability, and aggression. Recent studies of metformin have demonstrated efficacy in both animal models and in patients with FXS because it downregulates the insulin receptor and lowers the activity of the mTOR pathway, which is too high in FXS. Additional targeted treatments that reverse the neurochemical abnormalities in FXS are being studied including minocycline, gamma aminobutyric acid agonists, metabotropic glutamate receptor 5 antagonists, cannabidiol, trofinetide, bumetanide, and lovastatin.

D. Other therapies. Sensory integration therapy by an occupational therapist with a specific focus on calming techniques may be helpful. Significant behavioral problems may also respond to a behavioral modification program organized by a psychologist who can also provide support and guidance for the parents. If ASD is diagnosed, behavior intervention treatment for ASD should be carried out.

E. Criteria for referral. All families with FXS should be referred to a geneticist or genetics counselor for a detailed discussion regarding the inheritance of this mutation throughout the family tree. A clinical and genetic assessment of other family members who may be affected by the fragile X-associated disorders including FXTAS, FXS, and FXPOI is indicated.

Bibliography

FOR PARENTS

Braden ML. *Fragile, Handle with Care: More About Fragile X Syndrome, Adolescents and Adults*. Dillon, CO: Spectra Publishing Co.; 2000.

FRAXA Research Foundation. Has a network of support groups and funds research. P.O. Box 935, West Newbury, MA 01985-0935 978-462-1866. www.fraxa.org.

National Fragile X Foundation. Has produced many educational pamphlets, books, and videotapes regarding FXS; has resource centers associated with parent support groups in the United States and internationally; supports research and organizes conferences for parents and professionals. www.FragileX.org.

FOR PROFESSIONALS

Dy AB, Tassone F, Eldeeb M, et al. Metformin as a targeted treatment in Fragile X syndrome. *Clin Genet*. 2017;93(2):216-222. doi:10.1111/cge.13039.

Greiss Hess L, Fitzpatrick SE, Nguyen DV, et al. A randomized double-blind, placebo controlled trial of low dose sertraline in young children with fragile X syndrome. *J Dev Behav Pediatr*. 2016;37(8):619-628.

Hagerman R, Berry-Kravis E, Kaufmann WE, et al. Advances in the treatment of fragile X syndrome. *Pediatrics*. 2009;123:378-390.

National Fragile X Foundation. Identifies laboratories that carry out DNA testing. 1-800-688-8765 or 925-938-9300.

WEB SITES

http://dante.med.utoronto.ca/Fragile-X/linksto.htm.

FRAXA Research Foundation. http://www.fraxa.org.

National Fragile X Foundation. http://www.fragileX.org.

CHAPTER 52

Lesbian, Gay, Bisexual, Transgender, and Queer Youth

Carly E. Guss | Katharine Thomson | Sabra L. Katz-Wise

I. **SEXUAL ORIENTATION AND GENDER IDENTITY.** Pediatric clinicians are well positioned to help patients navigate sexual orientation and gender identity. Both gender identity and sexual orientation may develop before adolescence, although even young children may question their gender or romantic feelings. Table 52-1 lists key definitions for terms related to caring for LGBTQ+ (lesbian, gay, bisexual, transgender, queer, and others) youth. Terminology is frequently in flux, so it is important to stay updated with the most recent terminology and mirror the patient's identified labels and terms. It is worthwhile to highlight that sexual orientation refers to one's romantic or sexual attraction to other individuals. Sexual orientation also includes emotional and romantic attractions, sexual behavior, self-identification, and sexual fantasies.

Gender identity is distinct from sexual orientation and refers to one's intrinsic sense of being male, female, both, or neither. Transgender is an umbrella term for individuals whose gender identity does not match their sex assigned at birth. Children develop a gender identity at a very young age. Some transgender youth identify as a different gender than their sex assigned at birth at a very young age. For others, the onset of puberty and secondary sex characteristics may lead to significant distress, which may prompt an individual to ultimately identify with a different gender. Other individuals may not realize they are transgender until adulthood. Each patient has their own gender narrative.

II. **SOCIAL AND HEALTH INEQUITIES FOR LGBTQ+ YOUTH.** Many LGBTQ+ youth flourish from childhood through adolescence to adulthood, but societal stigma and discrimination can contribute to risk factors for some individuals (see Table 52-2). In 2003, Ilan Meyer proposed the minority stress model, building on the theory that harassment, discrimination, and victimization related to being a minority, as well as the internalization of stigma, can cause "minority stress," resulting in health inequities for LGB individuals. This model has since been expanded to transgender and gender nonbinary individuals. The minority stress model also proposes that coping mechanisms as well as protective factors, such as social support, may lead to resilience in LGBTQ+ individuals.

A. **Issues at school.** As a result of heterosexism, homophobia, and pervasive stigma related to gender identity and sexual orientation, LGBTQ+ youth may underperform in school and may eventually resort to truancy and dropping out. Additionally, school may be an unsafe environment for LGBTQ+ youth. Data from LGB students who participated in the 2015 Youth Risk Behavior Survey (YRBS) found that 10% were threatened or injured with a weapon at school and 35% were bullied at school. Transgender youth may face even more bullying at school than their cisgender (nontransgender, see Table 52-1) LGB peers.

B. **Family conflict.** Family conflicts and possible rejection based on a teen's sexual orientation and/or gender identity exacerbate risks for LGBTQ+ youth, leading to shame, guilt, and low self-esteem. LGBTQ+ teens who disclose their sexual orientation or gender identity to their parents may be met with support in some families, but in other families, teens may experience rejection and may even be told to leave the home.

C. **Homelessness and prostitution.** LGBTQ+ youth are at risk of being ejected from their homes because of their sexual orientation or gender identity. In 2012, the Williams Institute reported that 40% of homeless youth identify themselves as LGBTQ+. As homeless youth, they are exposed to multiple medical and psychosocial risks, including drugs, sexual abuse, and prostitution or "survival sex" (engaging in sex for money, food, or shelter), which in turn places them at high risk for human immunodeficiency virus (HIV) infection, sexually transmitted infections (STIs), suicide, and trauma.

D. **Trauma and discrimination.** LGBTQ+ youth are at increased risk for suffering verbal, physical, and sexual violence compared with their cisgender heterosexual peers, starting in early adolescence. The experience of trauma can further isolate youth and

Table 52-1 • KEY TERMS

Binding	A method to bind flattening breast tissue to create a male-appearing chest. This can be employed to decrease dysphoria related to the chest.
Bisexual	Romantic or sexual attraction to more than one sex or gender.
Blockers	Also known as "puberty blockers," this refers to the use of a gonadotropin-releasing hormone agonist (GnRH agonist) to prevent pubertal progression.
Cisgender	An umbrella term for individuals whose gender identity matches with their sex assigned at birth.
Cisnormative/cisnormativity	A view that promotes being cisgender as "more normal" or the preferred gender identity.
Gay or lesbian	Romantic or sexual attraction to the same sex or gender.
Gender-affirming hormones	Previously referred to as "cross-sex hormones," when a transgender individual receives hormone treatment that matches their gender identity. For transgender men this would include testosterone. For transgender women, this would include estrogen and/or antiandrogens.
Gender binary	The idea that there are only two genders: female/woman and male/man.
Gender dysphoria	Clinically significant distress due to an individual's experience with the biological sex and/or with the gender role assigned to it. This term replaced "gender identity disorder" in the *Diagnostic and Statistical Manual of Mental Disorders* in the 5th Edition. Not all transgender individuals experience clinically significant gender dysphoria.
Gender expression	External manifestations of gender, such as clothing, hair, behavior, voice, or other characteristics.
Gender identity	One's inner sense of gender—that is whether one identifies as a man/boy, woman/girl, both, neither, or another gender. Gender identity is independent of sex assigned at birth.
Gender minority	A group of individuals whose gender identity differs from the majority of the surrounding society. Typically this refers to transgender and/or gender nonbinary individuals.
Gender nonconforming	Someone who does not follow society's expectations or stereotypes of how they should look or act based on their sex assigned at birth.
Heteronormative/heteronormativity	A view that promotes heterosexuality as "more normal" or the preferred sexual orientation.
Heterosexism	A discriminatory attitude or belief against gay individuals. This may also include the belief that everyone is heterosexual.
Homophobia	Dislike or phobia of gay individuals.
Nonbinary	Someone who identifies as something other than exclusively man/boy or exclusively woman/girl.
Queer	An umbrella term that can refer to any nonheterosexual sexual orientation or transgender identity.
Sexual minority	A group of individuals whose sexual orientation differs from the majority of the surrounding society. Typically this refers to LGB people.
Sexual orientation	One's romantic or sexual attraction to other individuals, often based on gender. Components include emotional and romantic attractions, sexual behavior, self-identification, and sexual fantasies.
Transgender	An umbrella term for individuals whose gender identity is different from their sex assigned at birth.

(continued)

Table 52-1 • KEY TERMS   (CONTINUED)

Transphobia	Fear of, discrimination against, or hatred of transgender people.
Tucking	A modality to put one's penis between the legs to make the underwear area look smoother. This can be employed to decrease dysphoria related to the genitals.
Pansexual	Someone whose sexual preference is not limited to assigned sex, gender, or gender identity.

LGB, lesbian, gay, bisexual.

Table 52-2 • SPECIAL RISKS FACED BY LGBTQ+ (LESBIAN, GAY, BISEXUAL, TRANSGENDER, QUEER, AND OTHERS) YOUTHS

Medical	Psychosocial
• Gastrointestinal conditions, hepatitis • Anogenital conditions, urethritis • STIs, including HIV/AIDS • Unplanned pregnancy • Traumatic injury • Chronic pain • Overweight/obesity (female youth only)	• Depression, anxiety, suicidality, self-harm • Substance use • Eating disorders, unhealthy weight control behaviors • Homelessness • Prostitution, survival sex • Bullying • Violence (as perpetrator and as victim) • Family rejection

STIs, sexually transmitted infections.

increase their feelings of vulnerability and isolation, as well as increase rates of anxiety, depression, suicidality, and posttraumatic stress disorder (PTSD).

E. HIV and sexually transmitted infections. In the Centers for Disease Control and Prevention (CDC)'s 2015 estimates of HIV prevalence in the United States, youth aged 13–24 years accounted for 22% of all new HIV diagnoses, with the majority of new diagnoses among gay and bisexual males. In both males and females, racial and ethnic minorities are at substantially higher risk of HIV. Syphilis also is disproportionally prevalent among males who have sex with males. Female adolescents with female partners may also transmit viral STIs such as herpes simplex virus (HSV) or human papillomavirus (HPV).

F. Pregnancy. Sexual experimentation is common among youth of all sexual orientations and gender identities. Many LGBTQ+ youth have had intercourse with someone of a different sex or gender. In a 2016 study using data from the Growing Up Today Study, a national prospective cohort of youth in the United States, 99% of sexual minority (LGB) females reported having sexual contact with a male in their lifetime, and 84% of sexual minority males reported having sexual contact with a female in their lifetime. Health care providers should not assume that all pregnant teenagers are heterosexual, or that lesbian adolescents do not need counseling about contraception. In fact, surveillance studies have found that adolescent lesbian and bisexual females are at higher risk of pregnancy than heterosexual adolescents.

G. Weight and eating disorders. LGB adolescents show a different pattern for weight than heterosexual adolescents. On average, sexual minority females have a higher body mass index (BMI) and sexual minority males have a lower BMI than their same-gender heterosexual peers, with sexual orientation differences in males increasing across adolescence. There is also an increased risk of eating disorders and unhealthy weight control behaviors (e.g., bingeing and purging) in both female and male LGB adolescents compared with heterosexuals. These behaviors may be used to cope with sexual minority stressors, such as victimization and bullying. Research suggests that transgender individuals are also at elevated risks of disordered eating and weight management behaviors such as fasting for over 24 hours and using diet pills or laxatives. This may be related to attempts to suppress secondary sex characteristics associated with their assigned sex (such as menses) to better match their gender identity.

H. Chronic pain. LGB youth are more likely than heterosexual youth to report experiencing chronic pain. A 2015 study using data from the US National Longitudinal Study of Adolescent to Adult Health found that sexual minority females and males were more likely than same-gender heterosexual peers to report headaches. Sexual minority females were also more likely to report muscle/joint pain, compared with heterosexual females. This study found that inequities in chronic pain were partially explained by greater internalizing symptoms (e.g., depression, suicidality) among sexual minorities, which may be related to experiencing minority stress.

I. Substance use. Substance use may represent an attempt to escape from the stigmatization, shame, and discrimination that LGBTQ+ youth face. LGBTQ+ adolescents have almost two times the likelihood of using marijuana, cocaine, and alcohol and are more likely than their heterosexual peers to initiate tobacco use at a younger age and to report ongoing tobacco use. Transgender adolescents also have higher risk of substance abuse than their cisgender peers, including cocaine and prescription drug misuse. Increased substance use in transgender adolescents has been linked to experiencing bullying and victimization in schools.

J. Mental health. LGBTQ+ youth may experience mental health concerns, related to feeling isolated, which may be intensified by being in an openly hostile or unsupportive environment. Deciding when to first disclose sexual orientation and/or gender identity to friends and family can heighten anxiety and may be the time of greatest risk for suicidality and self-injurious behavior. Data from the CDC indicated that nearly one-third of LGB youth have attempted suicide. The risk factors that predict suicide attempts in heterosexual youth (e.g., depression, hopelessness, loss of support, abuse, prior suicide attempt, and substance use) also predict suicidality among LGBTQ+ youth. Transgender youth have a two to three times higher risk of depression, anxiety, suicidal ideation, suicide attempt, and self-injury than their cisgender peers.

III. RESILIENCE AMONG LGBTQ+ YOUTH. Over the past decade, the increasing social recognition and acceptance of diversity in sexual orientation and gender identity, and numerous societal and school-based efforts have increased the availability of resources for LGBTQ+ teens. While it presents some risks, the Internet has also created many safe and anonymous opportunities for youth to explore their emerging sexuality or gender identity. Support from teachers, counselors, and other students have been helpful in reducing consequences from medical and social stressors. LGBTQ+ youth from accepting families have lower rates of depression and suicidal ideation than LGBTQ+ youth from nonaccepting families. In fact, family acceptance leads to higher self-esteem and social support among LGBTQ+ youth. Participation in Gay Straight Alliances (GSAs, also sometimes called Queer Straight Alliances/QSAs) in a supportive school environment can also support LGBTQ+ youth. Table 52-3 summarizes some of the other protective factors that assist in creating resilience among this population.

IV. CLINICIAN'S ROLE

A. Office environment. Many LGBTQ+ youth fear discrimination from health care clinicians, which can delay disclosure and seeking of medical care. This fear is not unfounded; there are still many clinicians with homophobic or transphobic attitudes. In the 2015 US Trans Survey, transgender adults reported alarming levels of health care provider discrimination. A 2010 report of LGBT adults by Lambda Legal found that more than half of LGB people had experienced some kind of discrimination in health care, including being refused essential care or had a health care provider be physically rough or abusive.

Table 52-3 • PREDICTORS OF RESILIENCE

Parental acceptance and support
Sibling support
Extended family support
Peer support (either in person or online)
Community youth groups
School-based "Gay Straight Alliances" or "Queer Straight Alliances" and school safety
Religious or spiritual communities

Pediatric clinicians must be proactive in counteracting these fears and attitudes to best serve LGBTQ+ youth. Pediatric clinicians should foster a safe environment by making it clear to patients and their families that the office supports LGBTQ+ youth. Moreover, all staff, especially frontline staff, should be competent in providing affirming care to LGBTQ+ patients. This may include incorporating Safe Zone training into medical practices, which can provide staff and clinicians with information about sexual and gender diversity and how to provide affirming care for LGBTQ+ patients. For example, staff and clinicians should be counseled to never assume a patient or caregiver's pronouns and apologize for mistakes in a professional manner. Waiting rooms can also be made into welcoming spaces by displaying rainbow imagery (such as posters on the wall, stickers on identification badges, or using rainbow lanyards). Additionally, confidentiality policies should be prominently posted in office waiting areas and examination rooms.

B. Intake form. For medical practices that use intake forms, asking about preferred or affirmed name and pronouns is an effective way to show patients that the office is welcoming. These questionnaires in paper or electronic format may also be a way for youth to indicate a subject they would like to discuss in a format that may be less intimidating. Once an indication is made that the teen has questions or concerns about sexuality or gender identity, it is the responsibility of the pediatric clinician to initiate further conversation with the youth during the confidential portion of the visit. All forms and questionnaires should be reviewed for assumed heterosexuality and cisnormativity and rewritten using gender-neutral language. For practices geared toward adolescents and young adults, asking directly about gender identity on a confidential intake form can facilitate conversation. Updating clinical forms is also beneficial to diverse or nonheteronormative families (e.g., families headed by two women).

C. Documentation. If possible, clinicians should document portions of the visit related to sensitive information, including sexual orientation and gender identity, in a confidential manner. This is particularly important when working with adolescent patients because they may not have disclosed this information to their parent or guardian and discussing this information with guardians present may put youth at risk for negative reactions from guardians or even rejection. Additionally, with patient's consent, clinicians should use affirmed name and pronouns in the patient's chart, even if parents or guardians do not. This is an essential sign of support to the youth and provides modeling for the family and other providers that the youth may encounter. In general, providers should use the same language that the youth uses to describe themselves (e.g., some youth may use different terms to describe their body parts) in their conversations with youth, as well as in medical documentation.

D. Information-gathering
  1. Patient observations. Health care providers should avoid making assumptions of sexual orientation or gender identity on the basis of observation of a patient's gender expression or behavior. A patient's sexual orientation and gender identity cannot *be determined based on appearance, behavior, clothing, or romantic and sexual partners.*
  2. History: key clinical questions. With all adolescent visits, establishing confidentiality at the outset is essential. Patients should be told that questions about sexuality and gender identity are asked of all adolescents. They should also be informed that they do not need to answer all questions, that the clinician is always available for questions or discussions, and that providing honest answers allows the clinician to deliver the best care. Clinicians should ask all questions nonjudgmentally. Using the same approach for all patients increases clinician comfort and performance, which in turn increases youth comfort. Clinicians should not feel that their goal is to have patients "come out" to them as LGBTQ+, but rather to provide a safe, affirming environment if and when the patient is ready to do so.

Care should be taken that questions about sexuality do not assume heterosexuality. Asking only about different-sex relationships may suggest that the clinician is not open to a discussion about same-sex relationships. Some examples of nonjudgmental gender-neutral questions about sexual behavior are provided in Table 52-4 and some examples of how to ask about gender identity are provided in Table 52-5.

Practitioners should attempt to understand the level of support that the youth has for their sexual orientation and gender identity both inside and outside of the family, as less support is associated with more risks to health and emotional well-being. Risk for suicidality, self-harm, depression, substance use, and abuse should be assessed in a confidential manner with all adolescent patients.

Table 52-4 • GENDER-NEUTRAL QUESTIONS ABOUT SEXUALITY

Are you dating anyone or in a relationship?
Who are you attracted to?
There are many ways of being sexual with another person: touching, kissing, hugging, as well as having sexual intercourse. Have you had any kinds of sexual experiences?
Do you have any questions about your sexual feelings or the sexual things you have been doing?
Do you consider yourself gay, lesbian, bisexual, heterosexual (straight) or do you use another label to describe yourself?

Table 52-5 • ASKING ABOUT GENDER IDENTITY

What is your gender identity?
Do you think of yourself as a boy, a girl, or someone else?
What are your pronouns?
What name would you like me to call you?
Do others at home/school use your affirmed pronouns and name?

In addition, it is important to understand the extent of the adolescent's sexual activity because medical management should be guided by the adolescent's sexual *behaviors*, not *orientation*. For example, clinicians can ask: *"How do you protect yourself and your partner against sexually transmitted infections?"* It is especially important to ensure that *all* adolescents have a thorough understanding of HIV/STIs and their prevention. As with all adolescent patients, counseling should emphasize education regarding transmission and prevention of HIV/STIs and stress, limiting the number of sexual partners, avoiding the exchange of bodily fluids, and the regular use of condoms or dental dams during all forms of sexual activity. It is important to remember that even youth who identify as gay or lesbian may engage in sexual activity with an individual of a different sex or gender. It is also key to note that sexual behavior does not necessarily reflect sexual orientation. For example, youth who engage in sexual activity with persons of the same gender may not identify their sexual orientation as LGB.

For patients who are questioning their gender identity or who identify as transgender, it may be appropriate to ask for additional information regarding their transition goals. Not all youth who identify as transgender will want to pursue hormones or surgery.

If the patient has disclosed the sexual orientation or gender identity, the provider should ask questions to assess support. For example, clinicians may ask: *"Have you come out to your parents/guardians or any other adult? How did they respond?"* Providers can offer assistance and guidance to youth and their family around the disclosure process. It should also be determined if there are any safety concerns regarding the youth's disclosure of the gender identity to the family or guardian.

V. PHYSICAL EXAMINATION. Clinicians should assess for history of abuse or trauma before the physical examination and be cognizant of portions of the examination that may be particularly sensitive to LGBTQ+ patients, such as a chest or pelvic examination. Allowing patients to listen to music on their phone or play a game can be a relaxing distraction. Transgender patients may be particularly dysphoric around certain parts of their body. Ask them if they have any preferred names for body parts (such as "chest" instead of "breasts") and use those terms when explaining the examination. Transgender patients may also engage in binding (wearing a compression top to hide breasts) or tucking (placement of the penis and testicles so that they are not visible in the groin area). Patients who bind or tuck may need more time to change for an examination and may appreciate advanced notice regarding when an examination will occur. Binding or tucking with tape can be harmful or limit an individual's ability to use the restroom. Clinicians should counsel patients on how to bind and tuck safely.

For transgender patients, it is important to remember that all screening should be done based on their current anatomy. For example, a transgender male adolescent who has a cervix still requires pap smears per guidelines for cisgender female adolescents.

VI. TREATMENT AND MEDICAL MANAGEMENT

A. Testing for STIs. According to recommendations by numerous professional organizations, including the CDC and the American Academy of Pediatrics (AAP), all adolescents should be tested at least once for HIV, regardless of sexual activity. The CDC additionally recommends annual chlamydia and gonorrhea screening for all sexually active females younger than 25 years. It is also recommended that sexually active gay and bisexual males be screened annually for syphilis, chlamydia, and gonorrhea. Patients engaging in survival sex should be routinely screened for HIV, and clinicians should also consider screening these patients for syphilis and hepatitis C. Patients should receive extragenital screening of the pharynx and anus based on their reported sexual activity. Lesbian and bisexual females may also acquire STIs and HIV depending on their sexual behaviors. Females who have sex with females may transmit HSV or HPV. Oral transmission of syphilis with females who have female partners has also been reported. Although bacterial vaginosis is prevalent among females who have sex with females, routine screening is not recommended. There is a particularly high prevalence of HIV among transgender women, especially transgender women of color.

All sexually active youth should be immunized against hepatitis B. Ideally, patients will be vaccinated for HPV before onset of sexual activity, but if an adolescent male or female patient presents who has not yet had the vaccine, it should be given. Males who have sex with other males should also be offered the hepatitis A vaccine. The CDC continues to update testing and treatment guidelines for STIs; current guidelines can be found at CDC.gov.

B. Preexposure prophylaxis. In 2012, the US Food and Drug Administration approved a chemoprophylaxis for HIV consisting of a single pill with the combination of tenofovir disoproxil fumarate (TDF) and emtricitabine (FTC). The CDC currently recommends that Preexposure prophylaxis (PrEP) should be offered to adults at substantial risk of HIV infection. PrEP candidates include men who have sex with men who have unprotected anal intercourse, people in a sexual relationship with a HIV positive partner, individuals who engage in survival sex, and injection drug users.

Placebo-controlled trials for PrEP have not included participants younger than 18 years. There are several potential barriers to minors using PrEP, including adherence, side effects, and legal concerns. However, expert opinion states that PrEP should be considered for adolescents younger than 18 years at high risk for HIV.

VII. COUNSELING.
Health care providers are a unique source of information and support for LGBTQ+ youth. Besides providing medical information and dispelling myths, clinicians can offer advice to youth who have not yet disclosed their sexual orientation or gender identity to parents or other family members. Because youth are disclosing their sexual orientation and gender identity to their parents at increasingly younger ages, when they are still financially and emotionally dependent on their parents, they may be at increased risk for conflict and even rejection. For some youth who may be at greater risk for rejection, it may be prudent to wait to disclose their identity until they are less financially dependent on their parents. Health care providers may be able to offer assistance and support resources for both LGBTQ+ youth and their guardians.

Referral. Health care providers should refer LGBTQ+ youth to mental health colleagues, as they would do for all youth who present with the following:

1. Suicidality, self-harm, depression, anxiety, substance abuse, or other severe psychiatric symptoms
2. Serious social situations, including abuse, homelessness, school dropout, and prostitution
3. Difficulties with interpersonal adjustment that do not respond to education and social support

It is important to refer patients who are transgender or exploring their gender identity and who are interested in therapy to a mental health clinician who has experience with gender identity. Therapy can be helpful for exploring gender identity as well as for helping youth articulate their goals if they have a desire to transition. However, parents and providers should confirm that the therapist perceives his or her role as one of supporting the youth's development into the youth's self-affirmed gender identity. A therapist who aims to alter the youth's self-affirmed gender identity will likely cause more psychological and emotional harm than good.

It is essential that pediatric clinicians are aware that "conversion therapy" or "reparative therapy," which aims to change sexual orientation and gender identity and/or encourages an individual to become comfortable identifying as heterosexual or with their assigned sex at birth, is not appropriate and is harmful. Numerous organizations have positions or statements against conversion therapy, including the AAP, the American Academy of Child and Adolescent Psychiatry (AACAP), the American Medical Association (AMA), the American Psychological Association (APA), and the World Professional Association on Transgender Health (WPATH). Attempts to change sexual orientation or gender identity are contraindicated, ethically inappropriate, and can lead to further stigmatization and marginalization.

VIII. **TRANSGENDER YOUTH.** Many transgender and nonbinary youth begin with a social transition, which is separate from medical intervention. A social transition typically consists of using their affirmed name and gender expression in one or more settings (such as home, school, or work). The clinician should discuss how they can be helpful to the patient and family. This may include advocacy in school settings.

It is additionally important to note that not all individuals may identify with the binary (that is, male or female) concept of gender. Some may identify as nonbinary, a term often used to describe genders other than male or female. Nonbinary individuals may identify as transgender, though not necessarily. Some individuals may feel that they do not have a gender and are agender. They may use pronouns that are not gender specific, such as they/them or ze/zir. Nonbinary individuals are less commonly included in research, so unfortunately much less is known about their specific health care needs. However, it is likely that they face many of the same risk factors related to minority stress as other LGBTQ+ individuals, perhaps with added stress based on having a nonbinary identity in a society that is organized around two genders.

A. **Medical transition.** Transgender youth who seek medical transition are often medically managed by a multidisciplinary team consisting of endocrinology and/or adolescent medicine, and mental health. Community-based medical teams may also facilitate medical transition. It is important to note that medical transition goals will be specific to the individual, and not all transgender youth have similar transition desires.

A goal of early medical intervention for transgender patients is to allow the patient to complete exploration of their gender without developing permanent secondary sex characteristics associated with their sex assigned at birth. Ideally, this is accomplished by suppressing puberty via GnRH (gonadotropin-releasing hormone) analogue at Tanner 2 genital development. For youth assigned male at birth, this is when testicles increase in size to 4–8 cm without phallic lengthening. For youth assigned female at birth, this is at Tanner 2 breast budding.

This approach includes the following benefits for those assigned female at birth:
- Prevention of menarche and menses, which can be psychologically traumatic
- Prevention of development of breast tissue
- Allowing a longer period of growth via delayed epiphyseal closure

This approach includes the following benefits for those assigned male at birth:
- Prevention of skeletal changes, especially facial bones that accentuate the brow, zygoma, and mandible, and to prevent an Adam's apple
- Prevention of unwanted phallic growth and potentially upsetting spontaneous erections
- Prevention of permanent voice deepening and virilized hair pattern, including temporal balding

Another benefit of GnRH-induced pubertal suppression is that it is completely reversible; if it were to be stopped, puberty consistent with the assigned sex would continue. GnRH agonist therapy has been used for other medical conditions, although long-term effects in transgender youth are not yet known. It is important to note that if a child chooses to go from pubertal suppression at Tanner 2 to gender-affirming hormones (previously referred to as cross-sex hormones) that align with their gender identity, there will not be ovulatory or sperm production. Therefore, it is important to discuss with the patient and the parents/guardian the implications for future fertility and potentially refer them to a fertility expert who has experience caring for transgender youth.

For transgender patients who present at a young age but have already completed puberty, discussion with them surrounding particular aspects of their body and pubertal changes associated with their assigned sex that are troublesome for them provides an opportunity for intervention. For example, a patient who was assigned female at birth and has a male gender identity may find menstrual bleeding upsetting. Medical management can alleviate menses and provide substantial improvement in the patient's quality of life. Transgender male patients often prefer treatment that does not involve estrogen (such as oral contraceptive pills). Therefore, the minipill (norethindrone), norethindrone acetate, or depot medroxyprogesterone may be tried. Intrauterine devices that provide levonorgestrel may also be likely to stop menses but may not be the first choice for these patients because they require a pelvic examination. Addressing menstrual concerns is an opportunity for a primary care provider to provide a transgender patient with relief before an appointment with a specialist.

Currently, professional guidelines recommend starting gender-affirming hormones at age 16 years. However, depending on the patient, many providers will offer gender-affirming hormones at a younger age. Gender-affirming hormones allow the patient to develop secondary sex characteristics of the affirmed gender, rather than the assigned sex. For transgender female patients, the sex steroid is typically estrogen (potentially with an antiandrogen). For transgender male patients, the sex steroid is testosterone. Patients should continue to work with a mental health clinician to address any comorbid psychiatric conditions, if present, as well as emotional or mood changes that may occur with gender-affirming hormones. Primary care physicians are well situated to encourage and refer patients for mental health support.

It is anticipated that gender-affirming hormones should be taken across the life span and desired effects may take months to years. Transgender individuals may choose to transition later in life for many reasons, such as having an unsupportive family environment. Additionally, given that longitudinal research in this area is in its infancy, long-term knowledge about the effects of these medications is limited. Patients and their parents/guardians are typically counseled that hormones permanently affect fertility, although case studies of successful pregnancies after hormone transition have been documented. Thus, it is important to provide counseling regarding contraception for transgender youth who are sexually active. It is essential to note that research demonstrates improved psychological outcomes for youth who transition.

B. Surgical transition. Surgery may also be a goal for some transgender patients, although not all transgender patients are interested in surgery. Mastectomy for transgender male patients who progressed through their assigned puberty may be desired and is increasingly done before age 18 years by surgeons with letters of support by mental health and medical clinicians. Genitoplasty (including neovagina and phalloplasty) are also options. Bilateral oophorectomy and hysterectomy or orchiectomy is typically not done prior to the age of 18 years. It is essential to note that transgender patients who have not had surgery still require screening that is the based on their current anatomy, regardless of gender identity.

Providers should have some general knowledge about medical and surgical options for transgender youth; however, they should also know when to refer patients to a gender affirmative specialist for further information and management.

IX. SUPPORTING THE FAMILY

A. Parents' experience. For many parents, the disclosure of their child's sexual orientation or gender identity only confirms their own wondering; for others finding out that their child is LGBTQ+ may be shocking, discomforting, and difficult. Most parents' initial reactions include fear for their child's health and safety, grief at the loss of the adult child they had anticipated, and guilt about their own imagined role in the formation of their child's sexual orientation. They may initially be reluctant to share information with their other children, grandparents, other family members, or close friends. It is also common for two parents to have different reactions (e.g., one being accepting and the other ambivalent or rejecting), leading to parental or familial conflict.

B. Support and advice. Health care providers should be available to answer questions and dispel myths for parents, just as they are available for LGBTQ+ youth. Many parents equate sexual orientation with gender identity. Clinicians should help educate parents about the difference between sexual orientation and gender identity, as well as the possibility that some individuals may experience changes in their sexual orientation and gender identity across the life span. To address parental fears about their child's future, it is helpful to provide examples of successful LGBTQ+ role models. Parents should be encouraged to focus on loving their child for who they are and the qualities the child possesses. Clinicians should be available to help parents advocate for their children in schools and other settings; letters of support by medical and mental health providers often hold significant weight in these advocacy efforts. For transgender patients, the primary care provider can help the family and child determine if/when a social and/or a physical transition should occur and help them prepare for all aspects of such a transition (e.g., school issues, and reactions of extended family members, friends, neighbors, religious community). This can also be done with coordination with the child's therapist.

C. **Referral/resources.** Encouraging parents to learn as much as they can about LGBTQ+ issues is an important first step in helping them cope and eventually advocate for their child. Clinicians should build a list of referral sources, including local resources and parenting groups for LGBTQ+ youth, as well as reliable Web sites, organizations, and books that are affirming for both LGB and transgender and nonbinary youth.

X. **COMMUNITY ADVOCACY.** Clinicians of LGBTQ+ youth serve an important role in raising awareness and acceptance of diversity in gender and sexuality within their communities. Encouraging families and communities to form GSAs or QSAs in schools, for example, can provide important social support. Pediatric clinicians may serve as advisors to schools, making sure that tolerance policies and curricular materials at every age convey an appreciation of diversity and foster a safe environment. School and community libraries should contain books that describe the full range of sexual orientation and gender identities as well as the variety of family constellations for children of all ages. Clinicians provide an effective presence in local and national politics, as well as a valuable voice within professional associations and medical education programs. A clinician's commitment to learning more about LGBTQ+ youth via continuing medical education is an important element of providing high-quality care.

Bibliography

RESOURCES

American Medical Association LGBT Advisory Committee. http://www.ama-assn.org/ama/pub/about-ama/our-people/member-groups-sections/glbt-advisory-committee.page?.

American Psychological Association—APA LGBT Resources and Publications.http://www.apa.org/pi/lgbt/resources/index.aspx.

Gay-Straight Alliance (GAS) Network. www.gsanetwork.org.

GLBT Health Access Project. www.glbthealth.org.

Human Rights Campaign. www.hrc.org.

Lesbian, Gay, Bisexual, and Transgender National Hotline 1-888-THE-GLNH (1–888-843-4564). Nonprofit organization providing nationwide toll-free and confidential peer-counseling, information, and referrals.

WPATH—World Professional Association for Transgender Health. http://www.wpath.org/.

FOR PROFESSIONALS

Levine DA; Committee On Adolescence. Office-based care for lesbian, gay, bisexual, transgender, and questioning youth. *Pediatrics*. 2013;132(1):e297-e313.

Society for Adolescent Health and Medicine. Recommendations for promoting the health and well-being of lesbian, gay, bisexual, and transgender adolescents: a position paper of the Society for Adolescent Health and Medicine. *J Adolesc Health*. 2013;52(4):506-510.

Grief, Resiliency, and Coping in Children and Families Facing Stressful Circumstances

Maureen A. Patterson-Fede | Angela M. Feraco | Richard D. Goldstein

I. **STRESS.** For both children and adults, stress is an inevitable part of life. "Stress" can refer to a difficult event, the consequences arising from such an event, or the accompanying mental, emotional, or physical states provoked when adapting to the "stressor." Despite its ubiquity, the term itself is often used to connote a negative influence. However, stress can also be a growth-promoting, resiliency-building catalyst. This chapter will provide an overview of the concept of stress and its potential impact on children and families (Table 53-1). A discussion of the factors influencing resiliency will be provided as well as an overview of the role of the pediatric clinician in supporting children and families in times of significant distress.

   A. **Defining stress.** Stress, whether an experience, event, or condition, disrupts physiological homeostasis by eliciting a sympathetic, "fight or flight" response that is experienced as tension. Stress can be experienced by individuals, groups, or systems. Its impact is influenced by a variety of factors including its intensity, duration, and frequency as well as the context. When stress affects individuals, perceptions, expectations, and social context play a role in its effects. For example, a child living in an unstable home may respond differently to a parent's angry outburst than a child living in a more secure and predictable environment. Child temperament and interpersonal factors make the experience of stress more complicated than simply stimulus and response.

   B. **The stress continuum.** Stress exists along a continuum; at one pole is "positive stress," at the other is negative stress, and at the extreme, "toxic stress." Positive stresses are normal and essential stresses of human experience. These positive stresses are accompanied by a brief activation of the stress response system, which provides a boost in focus and ability. Examples include the stress felt during novel experiences, when newly developed skills are tested, or doing common challenges such as athletic competition or tests in school. Positive stress allows an individual to perform better before returning to a baseline state, and success provides an opportunity to build personal competency and confidence, gain mastery, and boost self-esteem. Through positive stress experiences, individuals build their overall competency and capacity to respond to future stress, potentially mitigating against disruptive effects.

   Negative stress refers to major, frequent, and/or recurrent conditions of deprivation and adversity. Negative stress can be acute (e.g., being involved in a serious motor vehicle accident) or chronic (e.g., exposure to neglect in early childhood). When the stress is significant (e.g., witnessing extreme violence or murder or ongoing physical or sexual abuse), it becomes "toxic," leading to persistent activation of the stress response system with permanent or long-term physiological, neurologic, emotional, and physical health implications (e.g., posttraumatic stress disorder, stress-related diseases). Depending on the impact and individual differences, an individual may be able to return to baseline functioning. The negative circumstances typically attributed to negative stress do not uniformly damage a child. A resiliency framework provides a way of understanding the multidimensional, interactive response to stress.

II. **RESILIENCY.** Resiliency describes the quality in stress-resistant individuals that protects them from vulnerability in the face of environmental risk, including the capacity to successfully and meaningfully adapt to stress. Although sometimes presented as an individual trait, a closer look finds three domains of factors that contribute to resistance to stress: (1) positive personality dispositions, (2) a supportive and nurturing family milieu, and (3) advantages coming from a thriving social support system. As such, resiliency is a dynamic process. Although individual differences will affect resiliency, this concept is interactive and relational; an individual's resiliency emerges from the synergistic interaction between person and

Table 53-1 • IMPACT OF STRESS ON CHILDREN ACROSS AGE RANGES

Age Range	Cognitive Symptoms	Affective Symptoms	Behavioral Symptoms	Physiological Symptoms
Very young children (0–3 y)	Demonstrate poor verbal skills Exhibit memory problems Demonstrate developmental delays	Exhibit sadness Act withdrawn Exhibit anxiety/fearfulness; develop new fears or anxieties Increased crying; inconsolable crying Flat or blunted affect Intense/prolonged separation distress	Irritability Engage in attention-seeking Exhibit regressive behaviors Elevated startle response Exhibit aggressive behaviors Head banging	Change in appetite; poor feeding Low weight gain Digestive problems Sleep disturbances Develop rashes; skin irritability
Preschool-age children (3–6 y)	Difficulty focusing; inattention Exhibit memory problems Compromised social skills	Feelings of guilt or shame Exhibit sadness Act withdrawn Exhibit anxiety Lack self-confidence Exhibit separation distress	Irritability Engage in attention-seeking Exhibit regressive behaviors Elevated startle response Exhibit aggressive behaviors Increased temper tantrums Hyperactivity	Change in appetite Somatic complaints (e.g., stomachaches, headaches) Sleep disturbances Nightmares Enuresis/encopresis (after acquisition of skill)
School-age children (6–12 y)	Difficulty focusing; inattention Exhibit memory problems Compromised social skills Decreased school performance	Feelings of guilt or shame Exhibit sadness Act withdrawn Exhibit anxiety Lack self-confidence Feelings of anger Emotional avoidance; flat affect	Irritability; moodiness Elevated startle response Exhibit aggressive behaviors Hyperactivity School avoidance Increased oppositional behaviors; noncompliance	Change in appetite Somatic complaints (e.g., stomachaches, headaches) Sleep disturbance Nightmares
Adolescents (13 y and up)	Difficulty focusing; inattention Exhibit memory problems Decreased school performance	Feelings of guilt or shame Exhibit sadness Act withdrawn Exhibit anxiety Feelings of anger Emotional avoidance; flat affect Exhibit depression Feelings of embarrassment	Irritability; moodiness School avoidance/failure Suicidal ideation Sexual acting out Increased oppositional behavior; noncompliance Engage in high-risk behaviors (e.g., truancy, substance use) Antisocial behaviors Relational difficulties	Change in appetite Somatic complaints (e.g., stomachaches, headaches) Sleep disturbance Nightmares

environment, particularly regarding stress. In this transactional conceptualization, stress provides the opportunity to activate the personal and environmental elements that may allow for mastery of the stress and its self-affirming value. This mastery also predicts greater ability to face future challenges in those children able to locate and utilize their strengths in the face of adversity.

The resiliency literature recognizes two pathways through which exposure to stress can increase or decrease future vulnerability:

- The Strengthening or "Steeling" Pathway: Stressful circumstances result in a response that increases one's capacity to manage stress. Strengthening, therefore, increases resistance to later stress.
- The Sensitization Pathway: Stressful circumstances lead to a response that feels inadequate, overwhelming, and undersupported; individuals may become increasingly sensitized to stress. Sensitization, therefore, increases susceptibility to later stress.

Understanding the factors that promote resiliency can help pediatric clinicians as they support children and families facing stressful circumstances. The domains mentioned above comprise several factors.

A. **Positive personality dispositions.** Each child carries intrinsic characteristics and qualities that define his or her uniqueness.
   - **Temperament**: Temperamental characteristics associated with easily adaptable children tend to predispose them to cope with difficulties more easily compared with children who are slowly adaptable. A child and family's perception of an experience also determines whether it will be interpreted as stressful. Furthermore, some children are innately better able to draw in the support of caregiving adults or peers.
   - **Capacity to plan:** Developing executive functioning skills (Chapter 46), such as advanced thinking and planning ahead, are linked to possessing a growth orientation. Planning ahead not only helps children think about and address challenges but also implies assumptions about predictability. Successful planning can help children feel a greater capability to handle stress.
   - **Sense of purpose:** A sense of efficacy, hopefulness, and purpose are important qualities associated with a child's developing self-regulation and self-concept. Insecurities often cause inflexibility, self-doubt, and a lack of vision, reducing resiliency and enhancing vulnerabilities.
   - **Capacity for self-reflection:** The ability to think reflectively is associated with better outcomes for children and adults. In times of distress, reflective thinking can help individuals assess what is and what is not working, which can lead to more adaptive responses. It also helps them understand themselves especially their unique triggers or vulnerabilities.
   - **Problem-solving:** Children who possess problem-solving skills can respond flexibly and adaptively to stressors. A problem-solving mentality can perceive stress or failure as a challenge instead of an obstacle, thus enhancing an individual's sense of control.
   - **Emotional regulation:** The capacity for emotional regulation allows children to find constructive ways to cope with and process their feelings and contain their influence. The ability to regulate and manage feelings increases a child's sense of self-efficacy and leads to better social relationships.
   - **Self-esteem:** Self-esteem is a dynamic concept that intertwines a child's belief in his or her self-worth with their sense of self-efficacy. Positive, successful interactions in the world can bolster a child's self-esteem and, therefore, his or her ability to feel effective in addressing challenges. Children who have specific vulnerabilities (e.g., a learning disability) should be introduced to other activities (e.g., athletics, music) where they can be successful, thus promoting their self-esteem. These esteem-boosting activities are often referred to as "islands or competence."

B. **Supportive and nurturing family milieu.** Interconnectedness is essential to resiliency. Resiliency can be realized and actualized within a family system that identifies, supports, and develops a child's strengths and skills.
   - **Attachment to primary caregivers:** Attachment is the basic building block for all life's relationships. Children who experience consistent, available, and nurturing caregivers are more likely to feel safe and secure in the world. This type of healthy attachment offers children protection and guidance during times of negative stress and greater sense of agency during times of positive stress.
   - **Familial environment:** The baseline status of a family system has implications for responding to stress. Cohesive systems create a different environment than ones marked by discord. A supportive, responsive caregiving environment is more likely to build on the strengths of the child and encourage the use of the child's skills to respond to a stressor.

C. Thriving social support system. Beyond the family, children are embedded within a series of other systems from their neighborhood to their school to their cultural identity. Each of these systems can offer relationships that encourage and optimize resilience.

- **Schools:** Schools provide countless experiences for children to gain mastery, build relationships, and develop responsibility. As such, schools can play a vital role in fostering resiliency.
- **Sociocultural community:** Socioeconomic, ethnic, religious, and cultural factors matter when conceptualizing the resiliency of children and families. These factors can deeply influence a child's sense of belonging and affect his or her developing sense of identity.
- **Access to resources:** When considering a child's larger environment, it is important to think about the child's access to supportive services. This includes services intended to directly mitigate the impact of stress such as support groups and counseling as well as services intended to expand a child's sense of self including participation in sports leagues, extracurricular activities, and community groups.

   Resiliency develops through interactions between a child, his or her family system, and the sociocultural context. When these three domains combine positively, a child can feel capable, supported, in control, and secure. Resiliency mitigates the potentially deleterious effects of stress by the following:

- Seeing risk and risk exposure as a challenge to master and learn
- Reducing the negative sequelae of adverse experiences
- Promoting a sense of self-efficacy by mastering challenges

   It should be noted, however, that resiliency does not require the presence of every factor for the process to yield a promising response. Instead, the above factors are meant to enumerate the many possible avenues through which resilience can manifest. For example, a child who lacks a consistent, stable home environment may have internal qualities that allow for resilience and success. Despite ever-present challenges in his or her home, such a child may be able to identify strengths, build skills, and develop successful strategies, even in the face of chronic stress. However, children who live in multistressed communities may not have access to as many growth-promoting resources. Providers can play an essential role by acting as buffering, consistent supports and increasing the family's access to resources that can promote adaptive coping.

III. THE PEDIATRIC CLINICIAN'S ROLE IN TIMES OF SIGNIFICANT DISTRESS.
There are times when acute or chronic stress may overwhelm a family's capacity to respond in an affirmative manner. In these circumstances, primary care physicians are well positioned to assist in providing children and families with the support needed to navigate these difficult experiences.

- **Safety first.** No matter how considerable the capacities of a child or family may be, the first responsibility of the clinician is to assure the child's safety and to remove him or her from dangerous threats.
- **Model and encourage open, honest communication.** Children benefit from clear, concrete, and honest explanations during stressful circumstances. Pediatric clinicians can model this type of communication during clinical visits and also provide guidance and coaching to caregivers. For example, following the death of a family member, *"I will try to answer your questions and would like to know what you think or feel when someone dies."*
- **Coach caregivers in providing age-appropriate explanations.** When stress overwhelms families, caregivers may feel at a loss about how to have conversations with their children. Adults may want to use euphemistic language to "protect" children or minimize the impact of difficult news. However, children need clear, concrete, direct explanations. Pediatric clinicians can serve an important function by coaching caregivers on age-appropriate, compassionate, and direct language. For example a 6-year-old questioning "When will Grandma come home?" it is important to encourage a direct and honest response such as "Grandma died. That means her body stopped working. She will not be coming home. We all feel very sad."
- **Be honest without overwhelming.** For most children, a brief explanation works best. Clinicians can remind caregivers to provide a short, simple description that avoids unnecessary details.
- **Allow children's questions to lead discussions.** Clinicians can remind caregivers that listening to their children's questions is the most important element of critical communications with their child during turbulent times. Children often let adults know exactly what information is important to them through their questions. Pediatric clinicians can model this behavior directly during clinical appointments by making room for children's questions.

- **Convey "togetherness."** Worries and stress are made worse by isolation. It is important to remind caregivers to provide their children with support and reassurance during stressful times. Caregivers can boost their children's confidence in facing what is ahead through messages of capability and togetherness. For example, *"Your mother and father will always be there to help you and if they need help, I am always here as well."* or *"We will get through this together."*
- **Provide anticipatory guidance.** Psychoeducation can prepare families to manage a stressor and improve understanding between children and caregivers. By providing normalization, encouraging responsive caregiving techniques, and helping families realize their strengths and resiliency, pediatric clinicians can offer safety and stability during stressful times.
- **Caregivers need to deal with issues first.** No matter what the stressor, caregivers need to face it first. A caregiver's capacity to face the stressor and demonstrate equipoise has a significant impact on the outcome of the child's adjustment. Crisis theory reminds us that reestablishing equilibrium after the onset of a stressor is primarily dependent on how well the adult models appropriate coping skills.
- **Maintain routines.** The predictability of routines such as mealtimes and bedtimes creates a safety net for children during stressful times. Finding a time to read to a young child is a nice routine in general but can be introduced during a stressful time because it involves joint attention, shared affect, physical closeness, and usually an unhurried parent. Caregivers should be advised to avoid any unnecessary changes to the family's normal routine. Families should preserve children's connections to familiar and safe people, places, and things (e.g., visits with a supportive grandparent, going to school, and using a transitional object), as possible.
- **Expect behavioral changes.** Under stress, it is normal for children's behavior to change. This can manifest in a variety of ways including sleeping or eating disturbances, irritability, regressive behaviors (e.g., bed-wetting, "baby talk"), acting out, somatic complaints, or "parentified" behaviors. Pediatric clinicians can provide caregivers with a gentle reminder that these behavioral variations are a child's normal response to an abnormal amount of stress.
- **Encourage emotional expression.** Adults can feel quite helpless when children express feelings such as sadness, anger, confusion, and betrayal. Remind caregivers that it is most important to acknowledge their children's feelings rather than fix them. Caregivers can truly support their children by helping them label their feelings and develop coping strategies. For example, *"How are you feeling about this?"* or *"It is normal for someone to feel sad or angry after a big loss."*
- **Predict anniversary reactions and loss reminders.** After a major change, anniversary reactions and loss reminders are common. Pediatric clinicians can help families feel better prepared by predicting and normalizing that emotional and behavioral variations can occur during holidays, developmental milestones (e.g., the first day of school, graduations), and other important events. Not all triggers are predictable and different children will exhibit different reactions. Caregivers may need reminding that it takes time to move forward after a stressor.
- **Connect with community resources.** The deterioration of communication and connection is often a hallmark of distress. Clinicians can play a powerful role in helping families initiate, maintain, and deepen connections to sustaining community resources.
- **Consult with collaterals.** Pediatric teams can lead communication with collateral agencies working with the family to make a stressful time feel more manageable.
- **Connect to needed resources.** Pediatric clinicians can make referrals to needed resources and programming that can offer a sense of safety and stability during stressful circumstances.
- **Refer to mental health providers.** For some children and families, a referral to a mental health provider may provide additional support during stressful times. Clinicians may encourage both children and caregivers to seek out mental health support if they are persistently distressed or overwhelmed.

A. **Guidance for specific stressors.** It would be an impossible expectation for a clinician to be fully prepared to respond to every type of stress a family may experience. The information below provides guidelines for specific stressors that may affect families.

1. **Supporting families facing homelessness.** Children without a home are more likely to suffer from accompanying conditions of food insecurity, malnutrition, and chronic disease. For these children, consistent access to health care is often

interrupted, which can further contribute to poor health outcomes. Pediatric clinicians can take several steps to support children facing homelessness:

- **Understand the issue.** To best address the health concerns of children and families facing homelessness, a pediatric clinician must first understand the underlying causes of homelessness. It is often necessary to address related conditions such as intimate partner violence, substance use, or unemployment to meaningfully support families. Clinicians can gather this information through thoughtful, routine screening.
- **Understand the population.** Clinicians should familiarize themselves with the health conditions associated with homelessness (e.g., infectious diseases, malnutrition) and the best practices for addressing them. This often involves communication with available supportive resources.
- **Optimize care visits.** Clinicians can take a flexible approach to resolve health concerns in fewer visits rather than scheduling additional appointments. Examples include coordinated appointments in multidisciplinary settings and utilizing a visit to update immunizations rather than scheduling an additional appointment.
- **Develop care plans that address obstacles of homelessness.** By including families in developing care plans, clinicians can work to address obstacles to consistent care. This may include referrals to visiting or mobile care services, transportation assistance, or thoughtful discussion on how to maintain communication with family (if access to consistent mailing address or telephone is limited). Providing a "medical passport" with immunization records and other medical data may be useful.
- **Build a pediatric resource base.** Clinicians should familiarize themselves with the local, state, and federal programs that address economic challenges faced by homeless families and make referrals to resources that can help families comprehensively address these issues.

2. **Family member diagnosed with life-threatening illness.** Parents often seek advice about what to say and how to talk with their children about serious illness and death. Clinicians can serve as both a model to children and families during pediatric visits and a support to caregivers. The following guidelines provide suggestions of how to best prepare children when they are encountering this difficult experience. Based on the age and cognitive development of the child, the focus and depth of explanation will change.

- **Encourage clear, simple description of illness.** It is helpful for adults to clarify the difference between a terminal illness and times when children "get sick." This helps to reduce the anxiety around "catching" the illness or the fear of becoming very ill: *"Kids may worry that they may 'catch cancer' when they visit someone. But cancer isn't a disease that you can 'catch' from someone."*
- **Prepare children for visits.** Children should be prepared for what they can expect: changes in appearance, medical equipment, and the presence of doctors, nurses, and support staff. Clinicians can remind caregivers that accommodating these changes may be difficult for children, so having advanced notice and preparation is helpful: "When we go to visit Grandpa at the hospital, he is going to look different. There is a machine that is helping him breathe that will look like a mask over his face. That mask doesn't hurt him at all; it helps him. Grandpa won't be able to talk and play like he used to. He will be lying down in his hospital bed. But he will be able to hear you when you talk to him."
- **Avoid false statements that are offered to console.** In motivation to protect the child from emotional pain and distress, it can be alluring to use statements such as "Everything will be all right" or "He will get better." Such statements are ill-advised. The best way to prepare and support children is to provide them with age-appropriate, honest information.
- **Encourage caregivers to model emotional expression and coping.** Caregivers lead by example. Showing children their authentic emotional reactions and the ways they cope with the difficult circumstances provides children with a model to emulate. Clinicians can remind caregivers to explain their thoughts, feelings, and reactions to their children. This models effective and open communication within the family system. It can also be important to discuss with caregivers how their style of emotional expression may affect the child. Overcontrolled expression or lack of expression creates a message of intolerance of emotion, whereas large expressions of emotion in a caregiver may cause fear. Sometimes it is helpful to plan for someone less emotionally engaged in the difficulties to be available for the child during the visit.
- **Attune to children's cues.** When children are facing a distressing event, such as the impending loss of a family member, clinicians and caregivers should be observant to the child's cues. These include changes in attentional levels, academic setbacks,

withdrawing, or acting out. These signs may indicate a child who needs further support. Clinicians can be mindful in assessing for changes across appointments. Sitting and listening to a child is frequently more important than answering questions that a caregiver thinks the child has.

3. **Death of a relative, friend, or other close acquaintance.** The impact of a death on a child is dependent on many factors including the child's relationship with the deceased, the child's history of other losses, and the nature of the death. A child's developmental age also plays an essential role in how the child will understand and grieve the loss.

- **Infants and toddlers (0–2 years):** Very young children do not have the cognitive capacity to understand death. They experience death as the loss of an attachment figure and, therefore, may exhibit symptoms of grieving such as changes in sleeping or eating, increased irritability, or heightened distress during transitions or separations. Very young children benefit from consistent, responsive caregiving during these difficult times.

- **Young children (3–5 years):** Young children do not yet understand the finality or universality of death; therefore, they view death as a changed state. As such, they may need sympathetic reminders that the deceased is not coming back. Because children of this age demonstrate egocentrism, they may believe that the death is their fault (e.g., "Mommy died 'cause I told her 'Go away!'"). Young children may need support and reassurance from adults that the death is not their fault.

- **Latency-age children (6–11 years):** In latency, children come to understand the finality and universality of death. With this more sophisticated understanding, latency-age children may seek more detailed information about the deceased, the cause of death, and the impact of the death on the family. Children of this age may appear emotionally unaffected; however, this can be an attempt to maintain a sense of predictability and control. Adults can support children by being responsive to their questions and checking in with them, even if they appear "fine" on the surface.

- **Adolescents (12+ years):** Adolescents demonstrate an adult-like, nuanced understanding of death. They are capable of wrestling with the abstract and philosophical aspects. Most adolescents prefer to process their grief with peers rather than with adults. However, adolescents continue to benefit from the emotional and psychological availability of caring, supportive adults.

  It is important to remember that a death affects the entire family system. As discussed throughout this chapter, clinicians are uniquely positioned to provide essential support to parents and caregivers. Clinicians can provide helpful anticipatory guidance and a responsive environment for caregivers to acknowledge their feelings related to this loss. These interventions can provide needed support to caregivers and significantly mediate the child's adjustment. Caregivers may seek their pediatric clinician's advice on whether their child should participate in rituals and services after a relative's death. Following are guidelines to support families in making this important decision.

- **Provide a clear explanation of the services.** Children should be given a clear, developmentally appropriate explanation of the services including what events will take place, who will be there, and what to expect about the behaviors of others (e.g., "There will be a special mass at our church." "There may be a lot of people there who want to talk to our family and tell us about how they knew Auntie." "Many people may look sad and be crying."). Clear explanations help to prevent unrealistic fears or fantasies about these services.

- **Provide choice, as possible.** When possible, caregivers should give children a choice to participate. If not given a choice, children may feel resentful when excluded or overwhelmed if compelled to participate. Providing choice gives children a sense of control during chaotic times.

- **Find appropriate alternatives.** If children do not want to attend services, caregivers should explore their reasoning and see if alternative ways to participate exist. For example, a child may want to visit the gravesite instead of attending the funeral.

- **Ensure access to a compassionate adult.** If a child chooses to partake or constraints limit a child's choice around participation, the child should be accompanied by a known and empathetic adult. Primary caregivers may be deeply grieving and unable to attend to the child throughout an event. Having another supportive adult available helps to ensure that the child's needs are being met.

- **Find ways to involve children.** Children benefit from having a sense of purpose and responsibility. Providing children with developmentally suitable roles (e.g., picking photos for a display, handing out commemorative cards) can support their resiliency.

Bibliography

FOR PROFESSIONALS

Briggs MA; American Academy of Pediatrics Council on Community Pediatrics. Providing care for children and adolescents facing homelessness and housing insecurity. *Pediatrics*. 2013;131(6):1206-1210. Reaffirmed October 2016.

Center on the Developing Child at Harvard University. Supportive Relationships and Active Skill-Building Strengthen the Foundations of Resilience. Working Paper No. 13. 2015:1-12. https://46y5eh11fhgw3ve3ytpwxt9r-wpengine.netdna-ssl.com/wp-content/uploads/2015/05/The-Science-of-Resilience2.pdf. Accessed January 3, 2017.

Garner AS, Shonkoff JP, Siegel BS; American Academy of Pediatrics Committee on Psychosocial Aspects of Child and Family Health; Committee on Early Childhood, Adoption, and Dependent Care; Section on Developmental and Behavioral Pediatrics. Early childhood adversity, toxic stress, and the role of the pediatrician: translating developmental science into lifelong health. *Pediatrics*. 2012;129(1):e224-e231. http://pediatrics.aappublications.org/content/pediatrics/129/1/e224.full.pdf. Accessed August 10, 2017.

Goldstein RD. Resilience in the care of children with palliative care needs. In: DeMichelis C, Ferrari M, eds. *Child and Adolescent Resilience Within Medical Contexts*. Cham: Springer; 2016:121-130.

Rutter M. Annual research review: resilience—clinical implications. *J Child Psychol Psychiatry*. 2013;54(4):474-487.

Wolraich ML, Aceves J, Feldman HM, et al. American Academy of Pediatrics Committee on Psychosocial Aspect of Child and Family Health. The pediatrician and childhood bereavement. *Pediatrics*. 2000;105(2):445–447. Reaffirmed March 2013.

FOR FAMILIES

A collection of stories from athletes, musicians, and celebrities "who have experienced a major loss at an early age and have gone on to live healthy, happy, and successful lives." www.sharedgrief.org.

National Alliance for Grieving Children's "Find Support" map. Contains resources for grieving children and families. www.childrengrieve.org/find-support.

Cooperative Children's Book Center of the University of Wisconsin-Madison created a collection of books to support families through various life transitions, including the arrival of a new sibling, moving, separation from primary caregivers, dealing with death, and starting school. https://ccbc.education.wisc.edu/books/detailListBooks.asp?idBookLists=175.

The Barr Harris Children's Grief Center has compiled a list of recommended books about death and grieving for children of various ages. The list contains suggestions for children across different age ranges. http://barrharris.org/for-your-child/books-about-death-for-children/.

The New York Life Foundation's comprehensive resource database for bereaved families. Contains guides for caregivers, links to bereavement support programs and camps, and multimedia coping tools. www.achildingrief.com.

Trozzi M, Massimini K. *Talking With Children About Loss*. New York: Putnam-Penguin; 1999.

CHAPTER 54

Headaches

Mandeep Rana | Martin T. Stein

I. DESCRIPTION OF THE PROBLEM

A. Epidemiology

- Headaches represent the most common recurrent pain pattern in childhood and adolescence.
- 40% of children and 70% of adolescents have experienced a headache at some time.
- Chronic recurrent headaches occur in 15% of children and adolescents. Chronic daily headache occurs in 2% of middle school–aged girls and 0.8% of middle school–aged boys; in high school, it occurs in 4% and 2%, respectively.
- Before puberty, boys are affected more than girls, but after puberty, headaches occur more frequently in girls.

B. Etiology.
Children experience headaches from many causes, but only a few pathologic mechanisms induce head pain:

- Inflammation, traction, and direct pressure on intracranial structures.
- Vasodilation of cerebral vessels.
- Sustained contractions, trauma, or inflammation of scalp and neck muscles.
- Sinus, dental, and orbital pathologic processes.
- The brain parenchyma, most of the dura and meningeal surfaces, and the ependymal lining of the ventricles are insensitive to pain. Central nervous system causes of headache result from stretching or inflammation of a limited number of pain-sensitive intracranial structures.

II. MAKING THE DIAGNOSIS.
Most headaches are brief and do not significantly alter a child's life. Recurrent headaches may be accompanied by fears and anxieties about brain tumors and other life-threatening diseases. The diagnostic challenge for the primary care clinician is multifaceted:

- To differentiate benign, self-limited headaches from those that suggest a serious organic disease
- To explore the potential relationship between headaches and a child's home, school, and social environment
- To recognize patients with headaches secondary to internal stressors (depression, anxiety, phobias) and those with environmental causes
- To develop a therapeutic plan consistent with the cause, severity, and significance of the headaches for the child and family

A. Differential diagnosis.
A useful clinical model to differentiate the large variety of headaches in children and adolescents focuses on identifying primary headache syndromes from secondary headache disorders (Table 54-1). Common primary headaches include the following:

- Tension-type headaches
- Migraine headaches
- Trigeminal autonomic cephalgias (short-lived headaches)

Tension-type headaches and migraine headaches occur most frequently. An alternative model of headaches in children deemphasizes the migraine–tension dichotomy and places greater emphasis on a headache continuum. Migraine with associated anatomic nervous system symptoms is at one end of the continuum and muscular tension headache at the other end. Symptoms and signs of both tension and migraine headaches in children are often nonspecific compared with the less common causes. Headaches in younger children, especially infants and toddlers, are more likely to have a specific organic cause. A focused clinical interview, coupled with age-appropriate behavioral observations and a comprehensive physical examination, will result in the probable diagnosis at the initial office visit for most patients (Table 54-1).

B. History: key clinical questions.
Whenever possible, questions should be directed to the patient, inquiring of the parent only after the child or adolescent has had an opportunity to describe the headache to the clinician. Most recurrent forms of pediatric headaches are associated with a behavioral diagnosis (in the presence or absence of migraine). The clinical interview should develop in a manner that raises questions

simultaneously about both organic and behavioral causes. An open-ended question (*"Tell me about your headaches."*) will allow the child and parent to explore what seems important to them and may lead to further exploration in the direction of either organic or behavioral etiologies. Focused questions that may suggest common (sinusitis, migraine) or uncommon (increased intracranial pressure, chronic infection) organic etiologies should be directed to the patient or parent.

The history should begin with a description of the headache pattern. In infants and toddlers, nonspecific symptoms may reflect a headache (e.g., irritability, inconsolability, sleep disturbances, poor appetite, head banging, or repetitive placing of a hand to the head or face). In older children and adolescents, an open-ended question may yield important information about the location, quality, onset, duration, and frequency of the headache.

Table 54-1 • CLASSIFICATION OF HEADACHES

Headache	Mechanism	Features/Etiology
Tension-type headaches (muscle contraction headaches)	Contraction of scalp and neck muscles	Sensation of tightness or pressure over frontal, temporal, occipital regions, or generalized Life-event change/stress: home, school, social relations, activity overload, depression Normal physical examination (occasional tightness or tenderness of posterior cervical muscles)
Migraine headaches	Cortical spreading depression (CSD)—wave of depolarization across cerebral cortex. This triggers trigeminovascular reflex, leading to cerebral vascular dilatation (secondary phenomena) and plasma protein extravasation (sterile neurogenic inflammation)	Family history (70%–80%) Paroxysmal attacks Gender: in childhood, boys and girls equally (4%–5%); in adolescence, girls more than boys **Migraine without aura:** • Unilateral or generalized • Throbbing or aching • Nausea/vomiting **Migraine with aura:** • With typical aura (visual, sensory, or speech symptoms) • Migraine with brainstem aura (vertigo, ataxia, tinnitus) • Hemiplegic migraine • Retinal migraine (monocular scotomata, blindness) Episodic syndrome associated with migraine—cyclical vomiting syndrome, abdominal migraine, benign paroxysmal vertigo, benign paroxysmal torticollis
Trigeminal autonomic cephalgias	Facilitation of trigeminal autonomic reflex	unilateral head pain with prominent ipsilateral autonomic features—lacrimation, conjunctival injection, or nasal symptoms. Include cluster headache, paroxysmal hemicranias, and short-lasting unilateral headache attacks with conjunctival injection and tearing (SUNCT). In migraine, autonomic symptoms often bilateral Pituitary pathology may accompany
Extracranial sources	Inflammation or trauma of structures or sustained contracture of scalp and neck muscles	Typically regional pain in area of pathology but often generalized in young children Otitis media and mastoiditis Sinusitis (chronic purulent rhinorrhea and/or nocturnal cough) Dental infection Tonsillopharyngitis (streptococcal) Refractive errors and strabismus Cervical spine osteomyelitis or discitis Systemic infection with fever Temporomandibular joint syndrome Severe malocclusion

(continued)

Table 54-1 • CLASSIFICATION OF HEADACHES   (CONTINUED)

Headache	Mechanism	Features/Etiology
Intracranial sources	Inflammation	Meningitis, encephalitis, cerebral vasculitis, subarachnoid hemorrhage
	Traction	Central nervous system tumor Cerebral edema Abscess Hematoma Post–lumbar puncture Idiopathic intracranial hypertension
	Toxic substances	Lead-alcohol Carbon monoxide Hypoxia Foods and food additives (nitrates, nitrites, monosodium glutamate, phenylethylamine) Paint, glue (including model glue) Oral contraceptives Renal disease
	Direct pressure	Hydrocephalus Trauma
	Vascular (nonmigraine)	Hypertension Arteriovenous malformation Fever
	Miscellaneous	Noise Sensory overload

An aura, unilateral location, and throbbing pain will be present in some children with migraine. Those with migraine without aura may have a generalized aching headache with nausea or vomiting but without an aura. Recent onset of severe headache or morning headache; awakening with vomiting; worsening of pain with coughing, sneezing, and straining; double vision; and progression of pain in severity and frequency should suggest an intracranial source.

The clinical interview begins the therapeutic process. Detailed, focused, and empathic questions give the child and family a sense of security that the symptoms are being evaluated by a concerned, knowledgeable clinician. It also gives the child and parents the opportunity to explore the interpersonal, educational, and family aspects of their lives that may provide insight into the headache formation.

1. *"Tell me about your headaches. What do they feel like?"* The child who has difficulty describing the headache can be asked to *"draw a picture of what the headache feels like."* The drawing may be concrete (a person or family) or abstract with designs or color. The child's description of the drawing, as well as the parents' and clinician's emotional responses, may provide useful information about the nature of the pain.
2. *"What seems to bring on a headache?"* or *"What are you doing when the headache starts?"* The emotional or physical environment in which the headache occurs may provide a clue to etiology.
3. *"What do you do to stop the headache?"* Migraine without aura typically resolves with sleep. Tension headaches resolve gradually during the awake state.
4. *"Do others in your family experience headaches?"* A history of episodic throbbing headaches in adults will suggest familial migraine headaches. Positive or negative reinforcement of headaches within the family may give an important clue to the etiology of recurrent headaches.
5. *"What is a headache?"* [To the preschool child] *Where do headaches come from?* [School-aged child] *What causes your headache?* [Adolescent] *Why do you think you get headaches?* These developmentally appropriate questions give a clue to the child's explanatory model of headache formation. Responses provide clinical insight into a patient's development, a clue to cognitive adaptation to the headache, and a source for improved communication between the clinician and the child through empathic connections.

6. *"Why do you think that your headaches are more frequent or more severe?"* For most children who experience headaches, it is helpful to explore the child's developmental understanding of headaches. A perceived cause of a headache will be linked to the child's cognitive and developmental stage. For example, an elementary-aged child in concrete operations stage of development may reply his or her headaches are caused by "thinking too hard in school." The child is given an opportunity to reflect on the symptoms. The response may provide a clue to self-esteem, ego integration, superego formation, and interpersonal relationships.

7. *"How are things going at school, ..., at home, ..., with your friends?"* The structure of the family (and a family medical history), friendships, and the school environment are critical to understanding the etiology of and response to the headache and potential therapeutic interventions. It is important to determine the impact of the condition on school and extracurricular activities, including the number of school days missed in a given period.

   a. **Family stress.** Is the child living with someone who experiences headaches? The family constellation should be explored for recent changes in parental relationships, a new sibling, emotional illness in family members, economic stress (lost job, homelessness, and child support), and family violence.

   b. **Social stress.** When factors such as inherent shyness, bullies, class and racial differences, and physical or mental dysfunction affect social relationships, psychophysiological reactions are common. Recurrent frontal, generalized, or temporal headaches (both with and without associated symptoms of pallor, malaise, nausea, and vomiting) are seen in these situations. Importantly, migraine headaches as well as tension headaches may be associated with social or familial stress.

   c. **School stress.** Stress that originates in the classroom may be associated with headache formation. The school may act as an environmental stressor by placing demands on both cognitive achievement and social behavior. Children's adaptive potential to a variety of school pressures varies significantly. The clinical interview should explore the nature of the classroom (number of students, where the child sits), the relationship between the child and the teacher, the quality and quantity of academic work, the child's response to homework, and the parents' attitudes about learning. Parents can be asked when they last spoke to the child's teacher, the content of the conference, whether the child is learning, and if the child is happy at school.

8. *"What do you think we can do together to help the headaches go away?"* This question engages the child in a therapeutic alliance and opens the possibility of managing the problem together. A thorough review of lifestyle practices, including caffeine intake, regularity of meals, sleep habits and exercise, is important in identifying possible sources of modification.

C. **Physical examination and further testing.** Narrating normal physical findings to the child during a comprehensive physical examination is reassuring and helps to demystify the medical evaluation. Organic causes for a child's headaches are usually apparent after a complete history and physical examination. Routine diagnostic studies are not indicated when the clinical history has no associated risk factors (recent onset of severe headache, absence of family history of migraine) and the physical/neurologic examination is normal (absence of abnormal neurologic finding, gait abnormality, seizures). When the signs and symptoms of organic causes of headache are vague or subtle and a specific diagnosis remains elusive, a specialty consultation may be useful.

III. **MANAGEMENT**

A. **Primary goals.** The clinician's goals for management should be to provide a developmentally appropriate understanding of the cause of headaches for both parent and child. The working assumption is that through a greater understanding of the physical and behavioral causes and triggers for headaches, both the child and the parent will be able to cope with and adapt to the pain as well as collaborate in recommended therapies.

B. **Treatment strategies**

   1. **Information.** When migraine or tension headaches are present, the anatomic mechanisms of pain should be illustrated by means of a descriptive narrative and schematic drawings. Visual images of the abnormal anatomic structures may help some children to gain control over the symptoms. Simple drawings of a blood vessel contracting and dilating with an explanation of pain-sensitive nerve endings within the blood vessel illustrates the physical nature of migraine headache and the associated symptoms.

2. **Relaxation exercises.** For tension headaches, children may respond to a progressive relaxation exercise that teaches them to relax specified areas of the body. The exercise may be followed by teaching the child to focus on a pleasant image of his or her choosing. Other children respond to an explanation directed at "tight muscles around the head" that cause pain at times of stress and tension ("worry," "nerves," and "daily hassles"). The clinician can demonstrate this phenomenon by tensing her or his biceps and asking the child to mimic that maneuver. This should be followed by an explanation that the biceps muscle is similar to the thin muscles around the head, which tighten at the point where the headache occurs. The child can learn to image—through visual imagination—the tense, painful cranial muscles' relaxing gradually and voluntarily as the pain diminishes.

These forms of voluntary relaxation follow the principles of self-regulation that have been successful in the elimination of migraine and tension headaches in school-aged children and adolescents. Controlled studies of children with headaches have shown that relaxation therapy and imaging (with or without biofeedback) significantly decreases headache frequency with lasting effects. It is a safe and simple intervention that can be practiced by the primary care clinician (see Chapter 20).

3. **Headache diary.** A headache diary may be a useful adjunct intervention. The older child or parent is asked to chart the headaches (time of day, intensity on a 1–10 scale, associated symptoms, hours of sleep night before headache, food/meal eaten before headache [caffeine, diet soda, chocolate, artificial sweeteners, processed foods], activity before headache, intervention, and duration) and record any stressful events that occur in the life of the child or family around the time of the headache. This exercise may encourage parents and children to talk about environmental triggers for headaches specifically and improve parent–child communication in general. Following an initial treatment period, it may be useful to shift the emphasis of the diary to headache-free days, which can shift family focus to successes rather than failures.

4. **Medication.** A pharmacologic approach to acute, chronic, and recurrent headaches may be beneficial for pain relief and prevention. Most children and adolescents with occasional migraine and tension-related headaches respond to **acetaminophen and ibuprofen** when the pain is of mild to moderate severity. Parenteral medication is available for the very severe migraine. More severe recurrent headaches respond to prophylactic suppression therapy, although there are few controlled drug studies in children. The primary care clinician will rarely need to resort to suppression therapy because episodic, severe headaches are uncommon in children and adolescents.

C. **Follow-up.** In general, a child with recurrent headaches should always be followed up within 2–4 weeks after the initial office evaluation. Support for behavioral interventions, monitoring of headache frequency and functional severity, and reviewing the parent–child understanding of the symptoms are the goals for the follow-up visit. New information or clinical observations may either alter the initial diagnosis or provide a new direction for management.

Bibliography

Denmark JO, Bes A, Kunkel R, et al. The international classification of headache disorders, 3rd edition (beta version). *Cephalalgia*. 2013;33(9):629-808. https://www.ichd-3.org/.

Lewis D, Ashwal S, Hershey A, et al. Practice parameter: pharmacological treatment of migraine headache in children and adolescents. *Neurology*. 2004;63:2215-2224.

Quality Standards Subcommittee of the American Academy of Neurology and the Practice Committee of the Child Neurology Society. Practice parameter: evaluation of children and adolescents with recurrent headaches. *Neurology*. 2002;58:1589-1596.

Slover R, Kent S. Pediatric headaches. *Adv Pediatr*. 2015;62(1):283-293.

FOR PARENTS

American Migraine Foundation. www.achenet.org.

The National Headache Foundation. www.headaches.org.

CHAPTER 55

Hearing Loss and Deafness

Laurel M. Wills | Karen E. Wills

I. DESCRIPTION OF THE CONDITION. A broad understanding of childhood deafness or hearing loss goes beyond traditional medical or audiologic definitions to include developmental, linguistic, and sociocultural implications as well. Advances in communication therapies, progressive special education policy, and "high-tech" devices, such as cochlear implants, digital hearing aids, and frequency modulation (FM) listening systems, have dramatically changed the developmental outlook for children with hearing loss. Individualized, family-centered care management decisions must account for the following characteristics:

A. Degree or severity of hearing loss
- "Normal" hearing is defined as the ability to detect a full range of environmental and speech sounds at a whispering volume of less than 15 decibels (dB), whereas conversational speech typically registers at 50–60 dB range.
- Slight (15–25 dB), mild (26–40 dB), moderate (41–55 dB), moderately severe (56–70 dB), severe (71–90 dB), and profound (91 dB or higher) degrees of deafness are associated with diminishing capability to detect and discriminate speech and environmental sounds.
- The configuration or profile of hearing loss, depicted as an *audiogram* (Fig. 55-1), varies for each child, with better hearing in certain frequencies than in others, and with separate profiles displayed for the right and left ears.
- The audiogram may or may not accurately reflect the *functional* listening level. For example, a child with moderate hearing loss might be able to comprehend what he or she hears better than a second child with only mild hearing loss. Deafness is not simply turning down the volume on normal hearing; it may also involve distortion of speech sounds. Listening skills are influenced by multiple factors including the child's biomedical status, cognitive and social-communicative skills, and past experiences (family support, schooling, hearing aid use, speech-language therapy, etc., as described further below).

B. Types of hearing loss
- Conductive hearing loss results from conditions that interfere with the form and/or functioning of the eardrum or ossicles, such as middle ear infections, effusions, or cholesteatoma. The hearing *nerve* is typically still intact. Conductive hearing loss is generally in the mild to moderate range and is often reversible, depending on the cause.
- Sensorineural hearing loss is defined as a dysfunction, absence, or loss of the cochlear hair cells in the inner ear or of the 8th cranial (auditory) nerve, preventing neural transmission of sound signals to the brain.
- Auditory neuropathy or dyssynchrony refers to dysfunction at one or more points along the central auditory pathway (8th nerve, auditory brainstem nuclei, auditory cortex), with or without an otherwise normally functioning cochlea.
- Mixed hearing losses involve both *peripheral* (outer and middle ear) and *central* (inner ear and neural) components of the auditory pathway.
- Children with mild or unilateral hearing loss may have age-typical speech skills. They may go undiagnosed until well into their elementary school years. They may present with symptoms of inattention, distractibility, language or learning deficits, or irritable mood. Therefore, a basic hearing screen should be a standard part of developmental–behavioral pediatric assessments.
- Children with fluctuating hearing loss in early childhood (associated with chronic severe otitis media, or severe bilateral cerumen impaction) may show distorted or delayed speech and language development, and behavioral dysregulation, which sometimes can persist into later childhood.

C. Age of onset of hearing loss
- Children who are born deaf or who lose their hearing before acquiring spoken language ("prelingual deafness"), relative to those who lose their hearing later on ("postlingual deafness"), are usually at a communicative disadvantage with regard to developing and/or preserving spoken language skills.

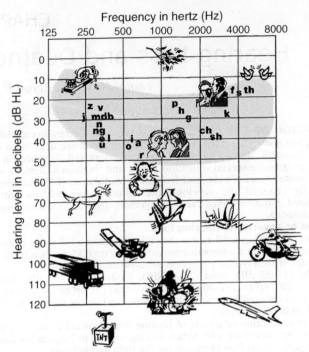

Figure 55-1 Audiogram showing a comparison of the frequency and intensity of various environmental and speech sounds. (Figure 1—4 from "Hearing and Hearing Loss in Children" in Hearing in Children, Sixth Edition (p. 13) by Jerry L. Northern and Marion P. Downs. Copyright © 2014 Plural Publishing, Inc. All rights reserved. Used with permission.)

- Older children or adolescents who are *late-deafened* (e.g., from meningitis or progressive hearing loss), but still fluent in their native spoken language, are usually optimal candidates for restoration (rehabilitation) of oral–aural communication skills.
- Hearing loss that is *progressive* may be detected and treated later than *stable* hearing losses. Often, older children or adolescents attempt to minimize or deny the increasing severity of a progressive hearing loss, just as older adults often do, to avoid the psychosocial stigma of wearing hearing aids or acknowledging a disability.

D. Identification and intervention: the 1-3-6 rule
- Universal newborn hearing screening has dramatically improved the rate of early detection of childhood hearing loss, and tracking systems are in place at the state or regional level in many areas. The current standard of care recommends:
  - hearing screening at birth or by *1 month* of age,
  - referral when indicated for formal audiologic assessment by *3 months* of age,
  - audiologic, medical, and early intervention services initiated by *6 months* of age.
- Prelingual or congenital deafness confers risk for loss of stimulation to the auditory pathways during sensitive early neurodevelopmental periods. Earlier intervention enables access to oral–aural (spoken) and/or manual–visual (signed) communication, which improves developmental prognosis. This is equally important in cases of acquired or postlingual deafness.
- When parents report concern about a child's hearing because of symptoms such as "not responding to sounds at home," "not listening," or "not talking" at the expected age, formal referral to a pediatric audiologist is indicated. Informal office methods of testing hearing (such as clapping or ringing a bell and then watching for response) are considered unreliable because the baby may react to a visual cue, vibration, or movement and the decibel level of the noise presented is uncontrolled; this may inadvertently result in delayed diagnosis. See section "IV. Making the diagnosis" for details on formal assessment methods.

E. Coexisting disabilities related to cause of hearing loss
- Approximately one-third of children with hearing loss have additional medical or neurologic diagnoses. The other two-thirds of children tend to be healthy, otherwise typically developing youngsters with isolated hearing loss, usually genetic in origin.
- For all deaf and hard of hearing children, it is critically important to protect and optimize vision for purposes of speech-reading and/or signing. Formal periodic evaluation with a pediatric ophthalmologist is strongly recommended. Dual sensory loss (deaf-blindness) occurs in several conditions, such as CHARGE or Usher syndrome.
- Children born in developing countries (including many internationally adopted and new immigrant children), as well as foster, low-income, and rural children with less access to health care, are more likely to have late-identified hearing loss or coexisting disabilities.

F. Psychosocial experience and home environment
- Positive adjustment and social–emotional well-being among deaf children is closely linked to the quality and quantity of parent–child communication (spoken and/or signed), as well as to warm, responsive nurturing, and developmentally appropriate behavioral expectations (see "For parents and clinicians" in Bibliography).
- Chronic frustration, conflict, and chaos in the home are linked to behavioral and emotional problems in deaf children. The diagnosis of deafness can be a crisis that tries the family's coping resources, demanding support systems within their extended family and community, as well as support from health care and special education professionals. Ongoing monitoring, as the child grows and develops, can help to optimize family adjustment and functioning.
- Only 10% of deaf babies are born to deaf parents, whereas ~90% of deaf babies are born to hearing parents. Deaf-of-Deaf children are more likely to grow up as native signers, because of the rare natural circumstance of having exposure, from birth, to one or more fluent sign language models. In the Deaf Community, deaf, with a lowercase "d," refers to audiologic status, whereas Deaf, with a capital "D," refers to cultural affiliation and self-identity. In contrast to the reaction of most hearing parents, parents who identify as culturally Deaf may be pleased or relieved to learn that their child is also Deaf, like themselves.

II. EPIDEMIOLOGY
- 20 million Americans of all ages have a hearing loss. Roughly 1 million children and adolescents have a "communicatively significant" hearing loss.
- 1–2 per 1000 live births will have severe or profound deafness.
- 6–10 per 1000 will have milder degrees of hearing loss.
- Males and females are equally affected.
- Preventative measures, such as vaccines against rubella, *Haemophilus influenza* B, and meningococcal and pneumococcal diseases, as well as appropriate treatment of otitis media and neonatal hyperbilirubinemia, have all markedly reduced the incidence of childhood hearing loss.
- Although developmental and occupational outcomes are rapidly improving, academic underachievement, functional illiteracy, and underemployment remain significant concerns for many adults with severe to profound hearing loss.

III. ETIOLOGY
A. Genetic causes account for roughly 50%–60% of all children with hearing loss, and of these genetic causes, about one-third are "deafness-related syndromes" and two-thirds are "nonsyndromic." Laboratory testing and DNA molecular analysis is now available for some of the more common gene mutations, such as Connexin 26 (*GJB2*). Malformations of the cochlea or other inner ear structures can result in hearing loss and, in some children, problems with balance or equilibrium. Other examples include Usher syndrome (sensorineural deafness associated with progressive vision loss from retinitis pigmentosa), Treacher–Collins syndrome (conductive or mixed hearing loss, associated with dysmorphic facies), and Waardenburg syndrome (sensorineural deafness and pigmentary changes of the hair and irises). These syndromes are usually associated with normal intelligence.

B. Nongenetic or "acquired" **hearing loss** can be separated into etiologies occurring in the prenatal, perinatal, and postnatal periods:
- **Prenatal:** Maternal infections, including CMV (cytomegalovirus), toxoplasmosis, rubella, and zika should be considered in the setting of a newborn with microcephaly, intrauterine growth retardation, seizures, or unusual eye findings. Newborns with these infections may be asymptomatic. Deafness from congenital infection may be present at birth or may emerge and progress later in childhood (in which case,

the newborn hearing screen is passed). New laboratory techniques may enable retrospective analysis for CMV on blood-spot specimens collected at birth in the nursery and kept in storage.

- **Perinatal:** Severe hyperbilirubinemia can result in damage (kernicterus) to the auditory nuclei and other central, "retrocochlear" neurologic regions. Neonatal sepsis or severe neonatal cardiorespiratory compromise often requires treatment with ototoxic antibiotic or diuretic medications, or extracorporeal membrane oxygenation. Thus, newborn intensive care unit graduates and premature babies have a much higher incidence of hearing loss than full-term healthy neonates.
- **Postnatal:** Chronic suppurative otitis media or other types of middle ear pathology can result in a transient or permanent conductive or mixed hearing loss. Bacterial meningitis, though much less common in this vaccine era, remains a common cause of acquired hearing loss. Ototoxic medications include certain antibiotics and cancer chemotherapeutic agents. Noise trauma (think teens with ear buds!) or physical trauma can result in conductive or mixed hearing loss. Acoustic neuroma, rare in childhood, can also cause deafness, usually unilateral.
- **Unknown etiology:** 20% or more of children have a hearing loss of undetermined etiology, despite thorough evaluation.

IV. MAKING THE DIAGNOSIS

- **History and physical examination.** A thorough prenatal and birth history, medical, developmental, and family (genetic) history may identify the cause of deafness and coexisting conditions. On physical examination, particular attention should be given to growth curves, facial features and other potentially syndromic markers (e.g., skin and hair pigment changes), appearance of the external and middle ear, eye examination and vision screen, and a complete neurologic examination, including muscle tone, coordination, gait, and balance.
- **Developmental screening tools** that are standardized and validated and used during routine health care maintenance to primary care practices query parents about speech and language milestones. Parental observations and concerns should be taken seriously to make an early diagnosis of hearing loss.
- **Subspecialty evaluation** and input regarding treatment options is usually indicated, including otolaryngology, clinical genetics, child neurology and child psychology, infectious disease, and ophthalmology, among others.
- **Hearing and speech evaluations.** It is important to realize that hearing acuity can be formally tested in the newborn period—no infant is too young! Consistent follow-up with a pediatric audiologist can help to detect and document any change or progression in the child's hearing loss. These clinicians can also assess for fit and proper functioning of hearing aids, cochlear implants, or other assistive listening devices, for example, those used at school.
- **Physiologic measures (requiring no cooperation):** Universal newborn hearing screening relies on noninvasive physiologic methods such as otoacoustic emissions (OAE) and/or brainstem auditory evoked response (BAER or ABR). OAE testing is performed by presenting a click stimulus via a soft-tipped probe in the external ear canal. The computer receiver then detects the "acoustic emissions" or echo-like sounds produced by the hair cells of the cochlea. False-positive OAE tests can result from middle ear fluid or vernix in the external ear canal at birth. If these emissions are not detected, the baby or young child is referred for BAER testing, the current "gold standard" physiologic measure of hearing acuity. BAER testing involves placement of scalp electrodes to measure electrical waveforms produced along the auditory pathway in response to a sound stimulus presented by an earphone. Older children who are unable to cooperate with behavioral tests, such as some with developmental or autism spectrum disabilities, can also be evaluated with these types of "passive" hearing tests. Handheld hearing screening devices, using OAE technology, have become available for use in primary care settings.
- **Behavioral testing (requires cooperation or active participation):**
  - *Visual reinforcement audiometry* is performed by having the toddler sit facing outward on a parent's lap in a sound-treated room. The audiologist presents a series of tones at specific frequencies and volumes from a speaker at one or the other side of the room, watching for the child's reaction. Visual reinforcement is offered (e.g., with a dancing toy in one or the other corner of the room) when the baby clearly localizes and looks toward the sound source.
  - *Conditioned play audiometry* is performed in a sound-treated room in which the preschooler is taught or "conditioned" to respond with a play activity (e.g., put a block in a box) in response to hearing a specific tone. When the child is too young

or unable to tolerate headphones, hearing acuity can only be determined for "the better ear in a sound field" as opposed to more precise measures of hearing, in each ear, made possible by using headphones in older children and adolescents.

- *Routine behavioral audiometry* involves the older child simply raising a hand when a tone is heard through the right or left side of the headphones. School- and clinic-based hearing screens are useful tools but can miss milder degrees of hearing loss. Referral to an audiology clinic is recommended whenever hearing status is questioned, even for a child who has passed routine screening.
- The audiologist will be able to measure and compare air conduction of sound waves, as well as bone conduction of vibratory sound, to help distinguish between conductive and/or sensorineural hearing loss. With conductive hearing losses, air conduction is diminished, while bone conduction may be relatively preserved, whereas in a sensorineural loss, both air and bone conduction may be compromised.
- Tympanometry and pneumatic otoscopy are measures of eardrum mobility and middle ear disease, which may be abnormal in the setting of conductive hearing impairment. These are performed by many primary care offices, as well as audiologists. It is not uncommon for parents to mistake an office-based tympanogram for a "hearing test." For example, a child with profound sensorineural deafness may have normal tympanograms.
- The audiologist will also perform measures of speech detection and discrimination, in addition to "pure tone" audiometry, at the initial hearing assessment and later, when testing hearing aid function. It is important to make a distinction among speech detection (knowing when one is being spoken to), speech discrimination (being able to recognize certain speech sounds or words), and comprehension of connected speech (being able to listen and understand the meaning of spoken phrases and sentences in conversation).
- In addition to audiology testing, children with hearing loss require assessment of communicative competence, that is, a thorough evaluation of spoken, signed, and gestural communication abilities by an experienced speech-language clinician and/or special educator. Interdisciplinary team clinics, with the required expertise, are available at some pediatric medical centers or schools for deaf and hard of hearing children.

V. MANAGEMENT
- **Hearing aid technology** continues to advance with programmable digital devices that are tailored to the individual child's audiogram. Behind-the-ear aids are most common for children with sensorineural losses. A bone-anchored hearing aid may be indicated for children with a conductive loss.
- **Cochlear implants:** A cochlear implant is a surgically implanted electronic device that has two main parts: an internal portion composed of an array of microelectrodes inserted into the spiraling turns of the cochlea and an external portion that receives, processes, and transmits speech sounds to the internal portion via an ear level attachment. The FDA (Food and Drug Administration) has approved the surgery in babies 12 months of age, or younger in some cases (because the cochlea is essentially full-sized at birth). Increasingly, bilateral implants are recommended (over unilateral) to improve binaural processing and sound localization. Team evaluation of potential implant candidates assesses the child's medical and developmental status, and the family's expectations and ability to follow through with the intensive process of auditory (re)habilitation. Many children show remarkably positive outcomes, becoming competent oral–aural communicators and functioning well in mainstreamed school settings. Children with additional disabilities can be quite successful cochlear implant candidates or users, but the ultimate prognosis may be more guarded. School speech therapists, as well as those in private agencies, should be supported by collaboration with hospital-to-school liaison staff on the cochlear implant team. Many children and adults who make good use of cochlear implants also continue to use and benefit from Cued Speech and/or American Sign Language (ASL) communication, following a bilingual–bicultural approach. Of importance to the primary care clinician, case reports of post–implant site infections and meningitis warrant vigilance about maintaining immunization schedules and prompt treatment of ear infections in these children.
- **Communication options**
  - Oral–aural (spoken) communication entails intensive instruction and practice with speech, listening, and speech-reading skills and maximizes the child's use of his or her residual or restored hearing. Children who have milder hearing losses or a more successful experience with hearing aids or cochlear implants tend to acquire spoken language more easily. Some oral communication methods emphasize listening without use of visual cues or signs, whereas others represent an eclectic mix of approaches.

- Cued Speech is a system of hand shapes and hand positions ("cues") that assist in speech-reading. The hand cues visually represent specific sounds or phonemes that, when used during conversation, can remove the ambiguity between sounds that look alike on the lips, for example, /p/ and /b/, as in "pen" versus "Ben." Even deaf individuals who are proficient speech-readers may comprehend only about 40%–50% of what is said and rely on the context of the conversation to extract meaning. Cued Speech can help children with hearing loss grasp important phonemic distinctions, an important foundation for emerging literacy.
- ASL is considered the native or natural language of the Deaf Community in the United States. ASL uses hands, arms, facial expression, body position, and movement to convey meaning, with unique grammatical rules that are visually based and therefore quite different from English. Many hearing parents, teachers, and others learning ASL as a second language may use Pidgin Signed English that uses ASL signs, paired with spoken English. ASL is not a global or universal signed language, but rather, it is unique to most of North America and actually has its historical, linguistic roots in French Sign Language.
- **Education and psychoeducational evaluation.** With such wide individual differences among children, there is no one-size-fits-all educational program. School programs differ in the communication options that they offer. They also differ in the extent to which children are mainstreamed or congregated.
  - Children who are deaf or hard of hearing (DHH) may be included within a regular classroom, perhaps using a notetaker, and/or a Cued Speech, Signed English, or ASL interpreter to better understand and communicate with the teacher and classmates. ASL and spoken or written English are both languages of direct instruction in bilingual–bicultural academic programs.
  - Many students use assistive listening devices, such as an FM system, in which the teacher wears a microphone that transmits speech sounds directly to the child's hearing aid.
  - Computer-assisted real time captioning and voice-recognition software for teachers is becoming a popular option for DHH high school and college students to follow along during class, and also study the printed transcript of a lecture.
  - Psychological or psychoeducational evaluation of deaf children should be done by a clinician who is knowledgeable about developmental, educational, linguistic, and cultural issues associated with deafness, and fluent in the child's primary communication mode, or highly experienced in working with interpreters. Tests of reasoning and problem-solving using visual patterns and pictures are usually the most appropriate way to measure intelligence in children who are deaf. Verbal question-and-answer tests may be useful to assess proficiency with conceptualizing problems and articulating solutions in English, keeping in mind that the child's exposure to English language–based concepts and culture may be limited. For children with hearing loss, struggles with English speech or literacy *cannot* be ascribed to low intelligence. On the other hand, children with deafness, especially those who have other neurologic compromise, can also have developmental and learning disabilities, including language-processing disorders. Teachers and caregivers may mistakenly assume that a child's problems with learning, language, memory, attention, or emotional self-regulation occur "just because of his or her deafness." These children should be evaluated by a psychologist who is familiar with "typically developing" deaf children, who can assess whether the presenting concerns are consistent with deafness, per se, or represent an additional, potentially treatable, neurodevelopmental condition.
- **Community building and social support.** Parents need to understand that there are a variety of choices, but no "one right way" to raise a deaf child. However, parents should be forewarned that some professionals, other parents, books, and media will strongly advocate for one or another "right way." Parents are likely to need professional support to learn about and select communication options and educational programs for their child. The bibliography lists contact information for agencies and support groups that help parents make these decisions.
- **Mental health.** In general, the same parenting attitudes and skills that promote mental health, strong self-esteem, and prosocial behavior in all children are also associated with positive adjustment among children who are deaf or hard of hearing. Specifically, a supportive, warm family environment is associated with better social skills and happier mood in the child. The presence of harsh, critical, aggressive, or lax and inconsistent parenting is associated with children's aggressive and rule-breaking behavior. Establishing strong social support networks for deaf and hard of hearing children and adolescents is crucial to healthy development. Healthy and appropriate use of social

media, text messaging, and videophones have been crucial in avoiding social isolation, particularly for those with more severe degrees of hearing loss.

* **Ongoing role of the primary care practitioner:** Create and provide a compassionate and conscientious "medical (or health care) home" for children with hearing loss and their parents. Fostering a realistic, but hopeful sense of the future and awareness of the many available resources is critical in energizing parents for the challenges ahead. Timely referrals to and care coordination with subspecialists, as above, can streamline the diagnostic and treatment planning process. Maintain a "whole child" perspective, addressing the child's unique temperament, interests, aspirations, and general health surveillance, along with knowledgeable management of audiologic and communication issues.

VI. CLINICAL PEARLS AND PITFALLS

* A baby is never too young to test hearing. If a parent or grandparent raises concern about hearing in a child, refer the family to a pediatric audiologist as soon as possible.
* Early identification of hearing loss can radically improve developmental outcome. Engage the family as soon as possible with local early intervention or DHH educational services. Consider interdisciplinary team evaluation to clarify diagnosis and treatment.
* Think "eyes," not just "ears," when thinking about deaf children. They will learn about their world through their eyes, as much or more than hearing children do, whether they communicate using speech-reading or sign, or both. Screen and monitor visual acuity.
* Terminology in this field can be tricky. Many individuals take offense at the clinical term "hearing impaired" (often because of the view that the signing Deaf Community represents a healthy, linguistic minority, rather than a disability group), whereas others do not like "hearing loss" when the condition has been present from birth. Thus, it is best to simply ask parents or older patients what words they use to describe themselves or their children.
* Parent-to-parent support is vitally important as the parents of a child with hearing loss are coming to terms with the diagnosis and exploring treatment options, which can be confusing and controversial. Reliable, unbiased national parent resources, as well as local parent networks, exist in many regions. Forewarn parents that some professionals, agencies, books, and other parents may be strongly biased toward the view that there is only "one right way" to raise, educate, and communicate with a child who is deaf. Try to provide parents with a more balanced view, such as is represented in the bibliography that follows.

Bibliography

FOR PARENTS AND CLINICIANS

Bodner-Johnson B, Sass-Lehrer M, eds. *The Young Deaf or Hard of Hearing Child: A Family-Centered Approach to Early Education*. Baltimore, MD: Paul H. Brookes Publishing; 2003.

Candlish PM. *Not Deaf Enough: Raising a Child Who is Hard of Hearing With Hugs and Humor*. Washington, DC: Alexander Graham Bell Association; 1996.

Dorros C, Kurtzer-White E, Ahlgren M, Simon P, Vohr B. Medical home for children with hearing loss: physician perspectives and practices. *Pediatrics*. 2007;120:288-294.

Medwid DJ, Chapman WD. *Kid Friendly Parenting with Deaf and Hard of Hearing Children*. Washington, DC: Gallaudet University Press; 1995.

Schwartz S, ed. *Choices in Deafness: A Parents' Guide to Communication Options*. 3rd ed. Bethesda, MD: Woodbine House; 2007.

Young N, Kirk KI. *Pediatric Cochlear Implantation: Learning and the Brain*. New York, NY: Springer Science+Business Media LLC; 2016.

WEB SITES

Alexander Graham Bell Association. www.agbell.org.

American Academy of Audiology. www.audiology.org.

American Society for Deaf Children. www.deafchildren.org.

Boy's Town Institute: Omaha, NB. www.babyhearing.org (English and Spanish).

Clerc Center and Boston Children's Hospital collaborative curriculum module program: Setting Language in Motion. http://www.gallaudet.edu/clerc-center-sites/setting-language-in-motion.html.

Deaf Education Enhancement: Michigan State University. www.deafed.net.

Early Hearing Detection and Intervention (from Centers for Disease Control). http://www.cdc.gov/ncbddd/ehdi (English and Spanish).

Family Voices. www.familyvoices.org.

Hands and Voices. www.handsandvoices.org (Parent-to-Parent Support).

Helen Keller National Center for Deaf-Blind Youth and Adults. www.hknc.org/.

Laurent Clerc National Center (Gallaudet University). www.clerccenter.gallaudet.edu/.
National Association of the Deaf. www.nad.org.
National Center for Hearing Assessment and Management (Utah). www.infanthearing.org.
National Dissemination Center for Children with Disabilities (formerly the National Information Clearinghouse for Handicapped Children and Youth). www.nichcy.org *The "State Resources Sheets" are an invaluable list of agencies in every state that provide parent support and governmental oversight of services related to hearing loss.*
Self Help for Hard of Hearing People, Hearing Loss Association of America. www.shhh.org.

CHAPTER 56

Incarceration of Parents

Stephanie Blenner

I. **DESCRIPTION OF THE ISSUE.** Parental incarceration is an experience shared by a significant number of children in the United States. Having a parent incarcerated can affect family structure and functioning, as well as a child's behavior and development. Pediatric clinicians have the opportunity to help support children and families affected by a parent's incarceration.
   A. **Epidemiology**
   - It is estimated that approximately 2.6 million US children are affected by parental incarceration.
   - In the 2011–2012 National Survey of Children's Health, 6.9% of children had experienced the incarceration of a custodial parent.
   B. **Terminology.** Parents may be confined in jails or prisons. Jails are local or county facilities that typically house inmates serving shorter sentences or awaiting transfer to prison. Prisons are state or federal institutions where inmates serve longer sentences; prisons are often located distant to communities where offenders' families live.
   C. **Characteristics of incarcerated parents.** The majority of parents are fathers, although maternal incarceration is increasing more rapidly. African American fathers compose the largest percentage of those incarcerated, whereas inmate mothers are more likely to be white. Many inmates have their own childhood histories involving risk factors such as parental substance use, foster care involvement, abuse, and family members who were also involved with the criminal justice system. Drug offenses, often accompanied by chronic substance abuse, are a common reason for incarceration. Almost half of inmates lived with their children before arrest; this percentage is higher for parents in local or county jails or when the mother is incarcerated. Most inmate parents maintain some contact with their children during incarceration.
   D. **Affected children.** The majority of affected children are 14 years or younger. African American children are 6.5 times more likely and Hispanic children 2.5 times more likely than white children to have a parent in prison. Like their parents, children often have multiple risks that may potentially affect their developmental outcome.

II. **IMPACT OF PARENTAL INCARCERATION**
   A. **Custodial status.** The child's custodial status during a parent's incarceration varies depending on whether it is the father or the mother who is incarcerated. Most children with an incarcerated father are cared for by their biologic mother. When the mother is incarcerated, children typically are cared for by relatives, often a grandparent. Involvement with the child welfare system is more likely when the mother is incarcerated.
   B. **Socioeconomic consequences.** Affected children often grow up in impoverished households and are affected by additional incarceration-related financial strains. More than half of inmates report having provided primary financial support for their children before incarceration. Not only does the household lose the parent's income during incarceration but also relatives caring for the children may incur additional substantial cost trying to maintain the parent–child relationship through visitation or phone contact. Recurring costs can include transportation to distant facilities, food and lodging, commissary deposits for prisoners, and collect phone calls. A history of incarceration may also be stigmatizing, making postrelease employment difficult.
   C. **Behavior.** Studies based on caregiver report have identified a range of child behavioral responses to a parent's incarceration. Common reactions include sadness, withdrawal, and acting-out behavior. Boys more typically display externalizing behaviors, whereas girls are more likely to manifest internalizing behaviors. Social support is critical, with children who have lower levels of support demonstrating more behavioral difficulties. Children who are less hopeful, after accounting for stress and social support, also have more behavioral difficulties.
   D. **Development.** There has been limited study of the impact of parental incarceration on a child's development. Younger children and those experiencing maternal incarceration may be particularly vulnerable to developing a pattern of insecure caregiver

attachment, with subsequent developmental consequences. In one study of children 2.5–7.5 years of age experiencing maternal incarceration, almost half scored at or below 84 on the Stanford–Binet Intelligence Scale. Poorer cognitive outcomes were associated with higher caregiver risk status and mediated by the family environment.

E. **Longitudinal effects.** An often-asked question by both professionals and caregivers concerns the long-term impact of a parent's incarceration. Both biologic and social mechanisms, including unmet heath care needs particularly around mental health, may contribute to increased risk of adverse health outcomes. In longitudinal studies, parental incarceration has been found to be associated with depression, alcohol use, and delinquency in the teenage years. In several studies, these associations were partly or fully attenuated after controlling for familial and social risk factors other than incarceration.

III. MANAGEMENT

A. **Identify affected families.** Caregivers may not readily share a parent's incarceration with pediatric clinicians, although most caregivers report not doing so because they were not asked. Effective screening can be incorporated into standard care by inquiring about household composition and changes at each visit. For example, *"Have there been any changes in your family or in who is living at home?"* Using nonjudgmental language and focusing on a willingness to help support the child and family will help facilitate disclosure.

B. **Provide developmentally appropriate information.**
- Caregivers may need guidance in how to talk with children about incarceration. In what has been called a "conspiracy of silence," many children are not told about the incarceration or are given other reasons for a parent's absence such as being told that the parent is at work, at school, or traveling. It is important to provide developmentally appropriate, truthful demystification to help the child understand the situation, emphasizing that the circumstances are not the child's fault. In the absence of such information, children will often invent their own explanation that may differ significantly from reality. Solicit questions from children and clarify misinformation. "Bibliotherapy" (see Bibliography) can often be helpful.
- The age of the child will determine the details included in the explanation. When dealing with younger children, the caregiver may simply explain that the parent needs to be away but is safe and misses the child very much. As children get older, additional explanation about what a prison/jail is and why the parent is there may be appropriate depending on the specifics of each case. With school-aged children, it is also critical to discuss with whom, under what circumstances, and how a child would share information about the parent's situation.
- Contact with the incarcerated parent is frequently a concern for caregivers. When in the child's best interest, visitation, telephone contact, or letters can help support the parent–child relationship. Some facilities have programs in which inmates tape-record themselves reading a child's favorite bedtime book to share with the child. When bringing a child to visit a correctional facility, the caregiver should be prepared with childcare items, toys, and snacks. Younger children should visit only if rested and healthy. School-aged children will benefit from a detailed explanation of what to expect. For example, previsit screening procedures, what type of contact is allowed, how long will the visit last, and when will the child see the parent again.

C. **Address co-occurring developmental and behavioral problems.** Developmental, behavioral, or emotional concerns should be identified and the child and/or family referred for appropriate intervention.

D. **Support caregiver and cultivate protective factors.** Family/caregiver stress may be decreased by referring eligible families for financial support, legal advocacy or housing, energy, and childcare assistance. A child's social support can be enhanced by involvement with after-school programs, athletics, or religious or civic groups. Some communities have targeted programs for children dealing with parental incarceration or for grandparents raising grandchildren.

Recognize that incarceration often is a cycle and that children and families may need support at each stage—arrest, confinement, and reintegration.

Bibliography

FOR PROFESSIONALS AND CAREGIVERS

Sesame Street Communities Coping with Incarceration. Online and app. includes video and print resources for caregivers and families to use with young children dealing with parental incarceration.

The Center for Children of Incarcerated Parents. www.e-ccip.org.

The National Resource Center on Children and Families of the Incarcerated. nrccfi.camden. rutgers.edu.

FOR CHILDREN
Brisson P. *Mama Loves Me From Away*. Honesdale, PA: Boyds Mills Press; 2004. (Ages 7 and up).
Growing Up On 21st Street, Northeast Washington, DC: A Memoir by Bryant Mayo, Ages 10–18, June 2015.
Hodgkins K, Bergen S. *My Mom Went to Jail*. Madison, WI: The Rainbow Project; 1997. (Written at two levels: right pages for preschoolers; left pages for children 6–10 years).
McGuckie CJ. *What Is Jail, Mommy?* Centennial, CO: Lifevest Publishing; 2006. (Ages 4–8). www.whatisjailmommy.com.

CHAPTER 57

Intellectual Disability: Evaluation and Management

Nicole Baumer | David L. Coulter

I. **DESCRIPTION OF THE PROBLEM.** Intellectual disability (previously termed "mental retardation") is characterized by significant limitations both in intellectual functioning and in adaptive behavior and skills (communication, social, self-care) with onset during the developmental period, usually before age 18 years.

  A. **Definitions.** The definition of intellectual disability has been formalized by the American Association on Intellectual and Developmental Disabilities (AAIDD), as well as in the *Diagnostic and Statistical Manual of Mental Disorders, Fifth Edition (DSM-5)*.

  Significant limitation in intellectual functioning means an IQ (intelligence quotient) score that is more than approximately two standard deviations below the mean (usually less than 70–75), considering the standard error of measurement for the specific IQ test used.

  Significant limitation in adaptive behavior means an adaptive behavior score that is more than approximately two standard deviations below the mean, considering the standard error of measurement for the specific adaptive behavior test used.

  Classification of individuals with intellectual disability as mild, moderate, severe, and profound should not be based on IQ score. The AAIDD bases severity classification on type and intensity of supports and services needed by the individual. The classification of intellectual disability was also revised in the most recent edition of the DSM-5 to be based on adaptive skill needs, rather than on IQ score.

  B. **Etiology.** Intellectual disability may be the end result of *one or more* of the following categories of risk.

   1. **Biomedical.** These are factors that have had a deleterious impact on the child's central nervous system (e.g., genetic and metabolic disorders, environmental toxins, infections, epilepsy, prematurity/neonatal brain injury).

   2. **Social/environmental.** Inadequacies in the social and/or family environment (e.g., inadequate stimulation, social unresponsiveness, extreme poverty, trauma, or maternal substance abuse) can diminish cognitive and social growth and functioning and can lead to intellectual disability.

   3. **Educational.** The availability and quality of educational and early intensive training programs can affect intellectual development and influence whether or not a child functions in the range of intellectual disability.

   4. **Interactions between risk factors.** In any given case, multiple risk factors may be present and may interact at different ages or stages of development. This concept reflects the transactional approach to human development, in which reciprocal interactions between individuals and their environment influence the developmental outcome. Some risk factors may be more significant (principal or primary cause of intellectual disability), and others may be less significant (contributing or secondary cause), but the interaction between them is almost always important. For example, a child with phenylketonuria (a biomedical risk factor) may function at a lower level because of both environmental deprivation (a social risk factor) and poor parental compliance with the prescribed diet (a behavioral risk factor).

II. **DIAGNOSTIC EVALUATION**

  A. **Signs and symptoms.** Intellectual disability should be suspected in any child who is significantly below the normative developmental milestones for his or her age. Many (but not all) children diagnosed with global developmental delay will eventually meet the criteria for a diagnosis of intellectual disability, depending on etiology of developmental delay. Stability of intellectual functioning is increased after age 6 years; therefore, repeated assessments of young children are required. It should also be noted that children with an *established* risk (e.g., Down syndrome) are very likely to have intellectual disability.

B. Etiologic evaluation

1. An understanding of the etiology of intellectual disability begins with a **complete medical and psychosocial history** and a **complete physical and neurologic examination.** This preliminary assessment results in a list of possible causes or differential diagnosis, which should include consideration of any and all potential risk factors.

2. The differential diagnosis should be thought of as a set of **hypotheses about the etiology** so that the subsequent workup is designed to test the most reasonable hypotheses. Table 57-1 is designed to help the primary care clinician design an appropriate workup based on the most likely hypotheses in a particular case. This table lists a series of possible hypotheses based on whether the potential risk occurred prenatally, perinatally, or postnatally.

3. **There is no single diagnostic workup that is appropriate to all cases.** In some cases, the workup will be very simple (as in chromosomal analysis when Down syndrome is suspected). In most cases, however, the etiology will not be obvious, and a careful workup will be needed. Such an evaluation, however, will result in identification of the principal or primary cause of intellectual disability in only about one-third of cases. Because new diagnostic measures for intellectual disability are emerging rapidly, the etiologic evaluation in "idiopathic" cases should be considered an ongoing process that can take advantage of the newest techniques and research.

   Most clinicians recommend the following studies for evaluation of the child with intellectual disability. These tests should be considered if/when specific features do not suggest more specific or directed testing (such as FISH/karyotype if features of Down syndrome.)

   a. **High-resolution chromosomal analysis and fragile X studies** are recommended because not all chromosomal abnormalities lead to obvious physical signs (diagnostic yield approximately 5%–6%).

   b. **Chromosomal microarray** (genomic hybridization) studies are recommended, preferably using the newest and most sensitive versions available (additional diagnostic yield 5%–10%).

   c. *Methyl CpG binding protein 2 (MeCP2) testing* is recommended by many specialists because the spectrum of conditions associated with this gene is now recognized to be broader than just classic Rett syndrome (e.g., the *MeCP2* duplication syndrome that is associated with autism in boys).

   d. **Radiologic imaging of the brain** is recommended especially if brain injury or structural abnormality is suspected, if history of seizure, focal neurologic examination, or if unrevealing genetic evaluation. MRI (magnetic resonance imaging) is preferred (diagnostic yield 48.5%–65.5%) to CT (computed tomography) (diagnostic yield 30%).

   e. **Metabolic screening** for amino acid and organic acid disorders has a low diagnostic yield but may identify potentially treatable disorders and so is recommended when genetic studies and neuroimaging are unrevealing or when there are certain symptoms suggestive such as episodic symptoms, regression or deterioration, prolonged recovery from acute illness, feeding intolerance, vomiting, growth concerns, physical examination findings, or a history of parental consanguinity or family history.

C. Conveying the diagnosis. Primary care clinicians are often present when the diagnosis is first made. Unfortunately, parents often have unpleasant memories about how the diagnosis was first conveyed to them. To avoid this and to help ensure that the diagnosis is conveyed sensitively, clinicians can follow these guidelines:

1. **Listen to what the parents say about the child.** This will give the clinician a sense of their level of sophistication, understanding, and emotional acceptance of the child's problems.

2. **Ask the parents about which particular aspects of their child's problems are of greatest concern for the family.** This will help to address the issues *most important to them.*

3. **Review the results of the evaluation in a way that is easily understandable and unambiguous.** Avoid technical jargon and overly complex explanations. Assess parental understanding by asking them to rehearse how they will explain their child's problem to a family member.

4. Parents will be all too eager to assume the responsibility and guilt for their child's problem. **Consistent and persistent reassurance that the condition was not their fault is always indicated.**

Table 57-1 • HYPOTHESES AND STRATEGIES FOR DETERMINING ETIOLOGY OF INTELLECTUAL DISABILITY

Hypothesis	Possible Strategies
Prenatal Onset	
Chromosomal disorder	Extended physical examination (including growth/measurements, assessment of dysmorphology)
	Referral to geneticist, neurologist, or other specialist as needed
	Karyotype, chromosomal microarray, and fragile X study; consider *MeCP2* or other specific genetic testing, gene panel testing, or in some cases whole exome sequencing
	Extended family history and examination of relatives
Inborn error of metabolism	Screening for amino acids and organic acids
	Quantitation of amino acids in blood, urine, and/or CSF (cerebro-spinal fluid)
	Analysis of organic acids by GC–MS (gas chromatography–mass spectrometry) or other methods
	Blood levels of lactate, pyruvate, carnitine, and long-chain fatty acids
	Arterial ammonia and gases
	Assays of specific enzymes; consider mitochondrial genome studies; consider CSF neurotransmitter analysis
	Biopsies of specific tissue for light and electron microscopic study and biochemical analysis
Developmental disorder of brain formation	CT (computed tomography) or MRI (magnetic resonance imaging) scan of brain
Environmental influences	Growth charts
	Placental pathology
	Maternal history and physical examination of mother
	Toxicologic screening of mother at prenatal visits and of child at birth
	Referral to clinical geneticist
	Review maternal records (prenatal care, labor, and delivery)
Perinatal Onset	Review birth and neonatal records
Postnatal Onset	
Head injuries	Detailed medical history
	Skull X-rays, CT, or MRI scan (for evidence of sequelae)
Infections	Detailed medical history
Demyelinating disorders	CT or MRI scan; CSF analysis
Degenerative disorders	CT or MRI scan
	Electroencephalography
	Assays of specific enzymes
	Genetic and metabolic evaluation
Seizure disorders	Electroencephalography

Table 57-1 • HYPOTHESES AND STRATEGIES FOR DETERMINING ETIOLOGY OF INTELLECTUAL DISABILITY (CONTINUED)

Hypothesis	Possible Strategies
Toxic–metabolic disorders	See "Inborn error of metabolism"
	Toxicologic studies
	Heavy metal assays
Malnutrition	Body measurements
	Detailed nutritional history
	Family history of nutrition
Environmental	Detailed social history
	Psychological evaluation
	Observation in new environment

5. The clinician should respect the parents' preference for using an alternative term to "intellectual disability" (such as "special needs" child). However, it may be useful for them to understand that their child meets the diagnostic criteria for intellectual disability when such a designation provides eligibility for important supports and services.

III. MANAGEMENT OF INTELLECTUAL DIAGNOSIS

A. General clinical issues

1. Primary care issues include **health supervision, immunizations, nutrition and growth, gynecologic care, and sex education, and sometimes management of co-occurring behavioral, neurodevelopmental, or mental health conditions.** Some children with intellectual disability also have other problems that may require referral to a specialist (e.g., neurologist, developmental and behavioral pediatrician, psychiatrist, orthopedist, or physiatrist). The primary care clinician should work collaboratively with the family and with any specialists involved in the child's care.

2. The primary care clinician should closely monitor the **academic progress of the child** with intellectual disability. A young child (age <3 years) should be referred for early intervention services as soon as a developmental problem is identified (often before the diagnosis of intellectual disability is actually made). An older child should be referred to the public school system to ensure that a comprehensive evaluation is done and an appropriate individualized education program is developed.

3. As the child gets older, the clinician will need to anticipate concerns about the **transition to adult living**: guardianship, living arrangements, vocation and employment, relationships and sexuality, and family planning, among others.

4. The primary care clinician understands better than most specialists that the child with intellectual disability belongs to a family that may be extended and/or nontraditional. Improving the child's quality of life requires improving the family's quality of life. Particular attention should be paid to helping siblings of the child with intellectual disability understand and accept their role, which may become prominent during adulthood (as their parents age).

B. Co-occurring medical, behavioral, and neurodevelopmental/mental health conditions

1. **Medical conditions.** Individuals with intellectual disability have a higher frequency of health conditions such as cerebral palsy, feeding dysfunction, liver dysfunction, seizures, sleep issues, and pica. There is also a higher frequency of sensory impairments such as vision or hearing impairment. Clinicians should assess for these as part of the evaluation and management of individuals with intellectual disability.

2. **Behavioral challenges.** Behavioral challenges such as aggression, self-injury, disruptive behaviors, rumination, elopement, property destruction, and other behaviors may be seen in individuals with intellectual disability. When assessing behavioral disorders, it is important to assess for underlying medical/health-related causes that may be occult, given communication barriers. For example, it is

important to consider epilepsy, possible thyroid dysfunction, and sources of pain or infection. Evaluation includes careful history including assessment of potential medication side effects, a comprehensive physical examination, and sometimes laboratory testing when clinical suspicions arise or when there are increased risks of medical issues such as celiac disease or hypothyroidism in a child with Down syndrome. The clinician should formulate a diagnostic hypothesis before prescribing a treatment.

The behavior of the child with intellectual disability may serve as a means of communication or may represent an attempt to control or alter the environment to avoid demands. Understanding the motivation underlying the behavior begins with functional behavioral analysis and is best conducted as part of a comprehensive behavioral diagnostic process. Behavioral problems may then be reduced or eliminated as the child is taught appropriate replacement behaviors that can serve the same function. Steps needed to develop a diagnosis and treatment plan for children with intellectual disability and behavioral problems are outlined in Table 57-2. Treatment of behavioral problems may require changes in the child's environment, including behavioral interventions, medical interventions, or use of psychoactive medications, or any combination of the three. Interventions for children with intellectual disability and behavioral problems should be accompanied by careful follow-up. The behavioral response to the treatment plan should receive careful scrutiny.

3. **Co-occurring neurodevelopmental/mental health disorders.** Neurodevelopmental conditions including autism spectrum disorder, attention-deficit/hyperactivity disorder, communication impairment, repetitive/stereotypic movement disorders, or mental health disorders such as depression or anxiety occur more frequently (5%–10%) in individuals with intellectual disability. Specialized behavioral questionnaires can be helpful to diagnose and monitor behavioral problems over time. It is frequently of benefit to use two or more inventories and to have more than one caregiver complete the instrument, such as parent and teacher, to gain information regarding symptoms in more than one setting. In some cases, strict diagnostic criteria for psychiatric disorders may not be met because of a number of features related to intellectual disability (cognitive or communication deficits), and clinicians may recommend empiric trial-and-error interventions, including with psychotropic pharmacologic treatments. In addition, the diagnosis may need to be reconsidered in light of the response to treatment.

C. **Psychoactive medications.** Given the vast number of psychoactive medications on the market, it is wise to be familiar with one or two drugs in each of the major classes of medications. This is generally sufficient to allow the clinician the flexibility to make appropriate choices between treatments. Classes of drugs that are commonly used include anticonvulsants, antidepressants, stimulants, and atypical neuroleptics. The general points in Table 57-2 should be noted when considering the use of psychotropic medication in children with intellectual disabilities. The general indications for use of many of these medications are included in Table 57-3. Children taking psychoactive medication may require periodic screening for drug levels, side effects, and behavioral changes, depending on the medication used.

D. **Conveying the prognosis.** The primary care clinician should help the family to prepare for the future. This requires an understanding of the child's prognosis for functioning as an adult. In general, pediatric clinicians tend to *underestimate* the level at which adults with intellectual disability can function in the community. The clinician must achieve the delicate balance of not giving overly optimistic predictions of the

---

Table 57-2 • CLINICAL CONSIDERATIONS WHEN USING PSYCHOPHARMACOLOGY IN CHILDREN WITH INTELLECTUAL DISABILITIES AND BEHAVIORAL PROBLEMS

The diagnosis should guide treatment. Attempt to establish a psychiatric diagnosis using standard or modified criteria.
The more severe the behavior or the degree of intellectual disabilities, the more likely that the problem is of biological and/or psychiatric origin and will respond to appropriate medical treatment.
Treat multiple diagnoses with a single medication if possible.
Develop specific treatment goals, and monitor treatment with predetermined methodology.
The end point in a trial of medication is remission of symptoms or intolerable side effects.

Table 57-3 • BEHAVIORAL SYMPTOMS SUGGESTING POTENTIAL EMPIRIC TREATMENT

Sleep	Melatonin, alpha agonists, antihistamines, antidepressants
Impulsivity, hyperactivity, inattention	Stimulant, nonstimulant (atomoxetine), alpha agonists
Mood swings, depression, anxiety, obsessive–compulsive behavior	Antidepressants, anticonvulsants, mood stabilizers, atypical neuroleptics
Irritability, aggression, self-injurious behaviors	Alpha agonists, Atypical neuroleptics
Stereotypic behavior, repetitive behaviors	Sometimes SSRIs (note: pharmacological treatment may not be indicated or effective)

SSRIs, selective serotonin reuptake inhibitors.

child's potential capabilities (thereby engendering intense disappointment over time) and not underestimating his or her long-term potential (thereby creating a negative self-fulfilling prophecy). The clinician should ensure, over time, that the family accepts the prognosis, incorporates it into the family planning (e.g., for guardianship and financial trusts), and has realistic expectations for the child's future.

Specialists may support interface with community providers and schools regarding how best to intervene to promote optimal outcomes.

Bibliography

FOR PARENTS

FOR PROFESSIONALS

Every state has a government agency responsible for providing services to people with intellectual disability, but available services may be limited by state-specific policy and budgetary factors. http://www.gottransition.org/.
The Arc is the largest organization for parents of children with intellectual disability. Many local Arcs have parent support groups as well as case advocacy and specific supports and services. Their Web site (www.thearc.org) has much useful information for parents and families.

FOR PROFESSIONALS

ASSOCIATIONS

The American Association on Intellectual and Developmental Disabilities conducts workshops and publishes journals and books on intellectual disability. Their Web site (www.aaidd.org) is a useful source for professionals seeking further information.
The Association of University Centers on Disability coordinates a network of regional training and service programs. Their Web site (www.aucd.org) also has information on current policy perspectives relating to intellectual and other developmental disabilities.

PUBLICATIONS

Accardo PJ. *Capute and Accardo's Neurodevelopmental Disabilities in Infancy and Childhood*. 3rd ed. Baltimore, MD: Paul H. Brookes; 2008.
American Psychiatric Association. *Diagnostic and Statistical Manual of Mental Disorders, Fifth Edition (DSM-5)*. Washington DC: American Psychiatric Association; 2013.
Betz CL, Nehring WM. *Promoting Health Care Transitions for Adolescents With Special Health Care Needs and Disabilities*. Baltimore, MD: Paul H. Brookes; 2007.
Critical Issues in Intellectual and Developmental Disabilities: Contemporary Research, Practice, and Policy, AAIDD 2016.
Dykens EM, Hodapp RM, Finucane BM. *Genetics and Mental Retardation Syndromes: A New Look at Behavior and Interventions*. Baltimore, MD: Paul H Brookes; 2000.
Fletcher RJ, Barnhill J, Cooper S-A. *Diagnostic Manual—Intellectual Disability 2 (DM-ID): A Textbook of Diagnosis of Mental Disorders in Persons with Intellectual Disability*. New York: Kingston; 2017.
Michelson DJ, Shevell MI, Sherr EH, et al. Evidence report: genetic and metabolic testing on children with global developmental delay: report of the Quality Standards Subcommittee of the American Academy of Neurology and the Practice Committee of the Child Neurology Society. *Neurology*. 2011;77(17):1629-1635.
Rubin IL, Crocker AC, eds. *Medical Care for Children and Adults With Developmental Disabilities*. 2nd ed. Baltimore, MD: Paul H. Brookes; 2006.

Schalock RL, Borthwick-Duffy SA, Bradley VJ, et al. *Intellectual Disability: Definition, Classification and Systems of Supports*. 11th ed. Washington, DC: American Association on Intellectual and Developmental Disabilities; 2010. [See especially Chapter 6 on Etiology and Chapter 10 on Prevention].

Shevell M, ed. *Neurodevelopmental Disabilities: Clinical and Scientific Foundations*. London: Mac Keith Press; 2009.

CHAPTER 58

Language Delays

Heidi M. Feldman | Julie N. Youssef

I. DEFINITIONS

- **Language** is a distinctly human method for structured, symbolic communication.
  - **Expressive language** refers to the ability to generate symbolic output. Typically, this output is speech but may be signs, gestures, or pictures.
  - **Receptive language** refers to the ability to understand (i.e., extract meaning from) the language output of others. Receptive language encompasses auditory (listening comprehension) and visual skills (e.g., understanding visual schedules, sign language comprehension, reading for meaning).
- **Speech** is the usual output of the language system and requires coordination of breath with oral motor mechanisms.
- **Language delay** is defined as development of language skills that is slower than expected for age but follows the usual pattern of development.
- **Language disorders** represent deficiencies in the ability to express or understand information through symbolic means. Disorders may affect one or more aspects of language, including the phonologic system (rules of sound production), morphosyntax (grammar), semantics (meaning), or pragmatics (social aspects of speech, such as intonation and conversational turn-taking).
- **Speech disorders** represent difficulties with perception or production of speech sounds, including difficulties with articulation, coordination of breath and oral motor movements, planning and execution of speech sounds, speech intelligibility, rate, rhythm, vocal quality, and/or fluidity.

II. TYPICAL STAGES OF LANGUAGE AND SPEECH DEVELOPMENT

- Language development results from a complex interplay of biological capabilities and environmental stimulation. Infants acquire language through listening to and interacting with speakers in their environment. Infants and young toddlers do not learn language from television or computer programs. Developmental milestones characterize the typical ordering and timing of skill development in language and speech. However, vast individual differences can be found for many milestones. It is important to understand when a child is performing outside of that "normal" range in the context of substantial variation.
- Prelinguistic stage: Table 58-1 summarizes communication milestones that develop in the first year of life. Vocalizations during the first 6 months of life (cooing, monosyllabic and polysyllabic babbling) are biologically programmed; they are universal across cultures and occur even in infants who are deaf. By the latter half of the first year of life, a hearing infant's vocalizations begin to reflect the vocal repertoire of his or her caregivers, with selective refinement of some sounds (the guttural "ch" for Germanic and Semitic speakers, the rolling "r" in Spanish, etc.), and the pruning away of other sounds. At this age, vocalizations begin to dwindle in an infant with congenital deafness. Children approaching age 12 months know that they can signify a desired object by pointing to it rather than reaching for it.
- One-word stage: Table 58-2 summarizes stages of language development. By age 12 months, normal infants begin to grasp the notion that an arbitrary set of sounds symbolically *represent* a specific object or action; the arbitrary sound "milk" not only results in the child getting fed a sweet, white liquid, but the sound "milk" also *means* milk. This ability to represent objects or actions in symbolic form constitutes the central feature of language. Initial vocabulary development is slow and erratic, with an approximate rate of one to two words per week. Early vocabulary is often comprised consonant–vowel repetitions (e.g., ba-ba for bottle, wa-wa for water) or consonant–vowel–consonant duplications (e.g., wuf-wuf for dog). Words may disappear from the vocabulary as new words enter. Words may be used in very restricted settings (e.g., shoe only for the child's shoe) or more broadly than adult use (e.g., doggy for dogs, cats, horses, and cows).
- Two-word stage: Typically, by age 24 months, the vocabulary size reaches 50 and two-word utterances appear. Vocabulary then expands rapidly, at an approximate rate of one to two words per day. Vocabulary gradually diversifies to include verbs, adjectives (such as color), adverbs, and pronouns.

Table 58-1 • COMMUNICATIVE MILESTONES IN THE FIRST YEAR OF LIFE

Age	Receptive Skills	Expressive Skills
Newborn	• Attends to voice • Regards face	• Cries
3 mo	• Smiles when spoken to	• Differentiates cry • Coos (makes vowel-like musical sounds) • Coos reciprocally with an adult
6 mo	• Turns when name is called	• Begins to babble (adds consonants)
9 mo	• Stops when told "No" • Learns routines, such as "Wave bye-bye"	• Points to wants or to interesting objects or actions • Says "ma-ma" or "da-da" nonspecifically
12 mo	• Follows simple commands with gestures	• Says "ma-ma" or "da-da" specifically • Jargons (strings of babble that sound like speech, but no words) • Says first words

Table 58-2 • STAGES OF LANGUAGE DEVELOPMENT

Age Range	Receptive Skills	Expressive Skills
15–18 mo	• Points to body parts • Follows single command without gesture	• Acquires words slowly • Uses simple and idiosyncratic forms • Participates in conversations
18–24 mo	• Understands sentences	• Exhibits a vocabulary of ≥50 words • Learns new vocabulary items easily • Uses two-word phrases
24–36 mo	• Follows two- and three-step commands • Answers "wh-questions"	• Uses short sentences • Uses increasing complex grammar, such as negation, questions
36–48 mo	• Understands plurals, pronouns, and possessives • Understands questions of "who," "why," and "how many"	• Combines three to four words in a sentence • Uses conjunctions
48–60 mo	• Understands concepts, such as same/different	• Uses mature grammar at near-adult levels • Constructs narrative discourse, such as retells stories, makes explanations

- Grammatical development: The ability to produce short complete sentences typically is present by age 36 months. Children learn negation (e.g., "I no do it" and then "I didn't do it") and complex sentences (e.g., "He fell 'cus he was running"). The ability to respond to common "wh" questions (who, what, when, where, and why) typically is developed by 48 months.
- Phonologic development: Young children simplify adult speech with phonologic processes. Table 58-3 lists these phonologic processes and the age at which they disappear, indicating maturation.
- Speech development: Speech matures up to age 7–8 years. Usually, children are fully intelligible by kindergarten entry even though they may be immature in the production of specific sounds, such as r, l, sh, ch, and consonant clusters. Table 58-4 lists the ages by which consonant sounds typically are mature.

Table 58-3 • EXAMPLES OF PHONOLOGIC PROCESSES AND THE AGES THAT THE PROCESS IS ELIMINATED

Process	Description	Example	Age of Elimination (y)
Final consonant deletion	Deletion of the final consonant of a word	*bu* for *bus*	3.3
Fronting	Sound made in the back of the mouth (velar) is replaced with a sound made in the front of the mouth (e.g., alveolar)	*tar* for *car*; *date* for *gate*	3.6
Cluster reduction	Consonant cluster is simplified into a single consonant	*top* for *stop*	4.0
Weak syllable deletion	Unstressed syllable in a word is deleted	*nana* for *banana*	4.0
Gliding	Liquid (/r/, /l/) is replaced with a glide (/w/, /j/)	*wabbit* for *rabbit*	5.0
Stopping voiceless/ th/	A fricative is replaced with a stop sound	*ting* for *thing*	5.0

Table 58-4 • AGE AT WHICH SELECTED CONSONANT SOUNDS ARE ACQUIRED

Speech Sounds	Age at Which 50% of Children Accurately Produce Sound	Age at Which 90% of Children Accurately Produce Sound
p, m, h, n, w, b	1.6	3.0
k, g, d, t, ng	2.0	4.0
f, y	2.6	4.0
r, l, s	3.0	6.0
ch, sh, z	3.6	7.0
J	4.0	7.0
v	4.0	8.0
voiceless th (thing)	4.6	7.0

III. LANGUAGE AND SPEECH DELAYS AND DISORDERS

A. **Misconceptions about the implications of language and speech delays.** People often have misconceptions about whether to be concerned about delays in speech and language development. Watchful waiting in the following situations is not appropriate.
   - Male sex is *not* associated with clinically significant delays in language, sufficient to reach a positive result on screening tests. At the same time, boys are more likely to have conditions associated with language disorders, such as autism spectrum disorder (ASD). Therefore, an early language delay in a boy should prompt evaluation and if necessary, treatment.
   - Bilingual upbringing *does not* cause speech or language delay. The bilingual child may intermix the vocabularies of both languages, but total vocabulary size and length of utterance should be equivalent to those of a child reared in a monolingual environment. Children exposed to two or more languages with delays may have a language disorder. If a child is experiencing language delay, it is not necessary to

suspend bilingual exposure in an effort to make the learning easier. Bilingualism confers several short- and long-term advantages, including ability to interact with individuals from other cultures and to obtain employment where speaking multiple language is required.

- Birth order or having an older sibling who "talks for the child" does *not* cause speech or language delay. Having a twin also does not delay language development.
- Chronic otitis media with effusion is *not* the cause of developmental delays in language, cognition, academic skills, or behavioral functioning. Tympanostomy tube placement for chronic otitis media does not change these outcomes in children with chronic otitis media. Chronic otitis media is more prevalent in situations that also put language learning at risk, including poverty, crowding, limited breastfeeding, and parental smoking.

B. Language and/or speech delay. Delayed development of language and/or speech is common, occurring in 10%–15% of preschool children, depending on definitions. Children may present with isolated language delay, isolated speech delay, or both. Approximately half of those delayed at age 2 years have caught up to peers by age 3 years and often are called "late bloomers." A delay becomes a disorder if it persists to school age; limits learning, communication, and/or social functions; is different from the typical pattern of development; or is very severe. Among US children 3–5 years of age, issues of speech and language are the most common reasons for referral to special education services (Fig. 58-1).

1. Primary language disorder
- Language disorder may occur in the absence of other developmental delays or disorders. In this case, the condition may be known as primary language impairment (PLI), developmental language disorder, or specific language impairment. PLI is clinically heterogeneous and may involve some combination of phonologic development (speech sound production), semantics (meaning), syntax (sentence structure), and pragmatics (use of language as a tool for social interchange). Children with PLI typically present with delayed emergence of single words, phrases, and sentences. Comprehension often appears relatively spared, at least initially. Speech skills also may be impaired.
- Primary language disorder clusters in families, suggesting a strong genetic contribution. Linkage studies have identified several loci in PLI. However, heritability estimates are moderate. Amount of caregiver speech to children is associated with rate of language development. These findings suggest an important environmental contribution to early language development.
- Children with PLI generally have a good prognosis for basic functional language and communication. Residual problems may be subtle, revealed only on testing. These children are at increased risk for language-based learning disabilities, such as delays in the learning to read.

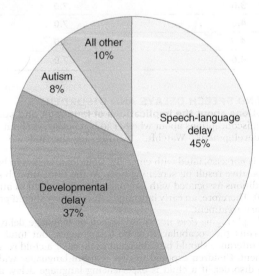

Figure 58-1 Primary eligibility criteria for special education services in children aged 3–5 years, based on US Department of Education data from 2015.

Table 58-5 • SECONDARY CAUSES OF DISORDERS OF LANGUAGE AND SPEECH

Factors	Psychosocial	Hearing	Brain Structure and Function	Oral Mechanisms
Usual circum-stances	Warm relation-ships, frequent parent–child communication	Intact hearing	Normal cogni-tion, normal brain structures	Normal oral mechanisms
High risk factors for language disorder	Strained rela-tionships, limited child-directed speech	Mild to profound sensory-neural hearing loss	Genetic disor-ders; neuro-logic disorders; intellectual dis-ability; autism	Abnormal structure or function
Examples of high risk	Raised in orphanage, child abuse or neglect, parents with limited education	Congenital deaf-ness or hard of hearing, acquired deaf-ness or hard of hearing	Fragile X, tuber-ous sclerosis, stroke, Landau–Kleffner seizure disorder	Cleft palate, velopharyn-geal insufficiency, Spastic oral movements

    2. **Secondary language disorders**
- Language disorders may occur as one facet of another disorder (e.g., ASD, Down syndrome). Table 58-5 shows requirements for normal language learning and conditions associated with secondary language disorders.
- Prognosis for children with secondary language disorders is a function of the nature and severity of the primary disability and the effectiveness of treatment.

  C. Speech disorders
    1. **Speech sound disorders.** Speech sound disorders include articulation disorders, i.e., the persistent or severe failure to produce speech sounds accurately. They also include motor-speech disorders due to neurological damage that affect the motor control of speech muscles (dysarthria, common in children with cerebral palsy) or motor programming of speech movements (childhood apraxia of speech).
    2. **Voice and resonance disorders.** Voice disorders are characterized by abnormal pitch, loudness, or quality of the speech sounds produced by the larynx. They may be transient, as with laryngitis, or persistent, as with laryngeal nodules.
    3. **Fluency disorders.** Fluency refers to continuity, smoothness, rate, and effort of producing speech. Developmental dysfluency is common in children aged 3–4 years and is characterized by disruption of the flow of speech because of repetition of whole words and phrases. Stuttering, the most common fluency disorder, is an interruption in the flow of speaking by repetitions (sounds and syllables as well as words and phrases), sound prolongations, blocks, interjections, and revisions, which affect the rate and rhythm of speech. Cluttering is a breakdown in fluency and clarity because of rapid and/or irregular speech rate that leads to deletion or collapse of syllables.

IV. MAKING THE DIAGNOSIS
  A. Evaluation in primary care settings. Parents may express concerns regarding "delayed speech." The practitioner must determine whether language or speech is delayed. In contrast, the practitioner may be concerned whereas parents, unfamiliar with developmental milestones, are not. The pattern of speech and language delay, coupled with an appraisal of development in other domains (fine motor, adaptive, play, personal/social), often suggests a specific developmental diagnosis. A child's failure to reach speech and language milestones as expected may be a "red flag" or warning, indicating a speech and language development problem. "Red flags" are noted at ages where 90% of typically developing children have achieved a developmental milestone. Red flags for language delay are listed in Table 58-6.
    1. **History.** A well-taken developmental history is the most important diagnostic tool. The language history should encompass receptive and expressive skills in auditory and visual language (such as use of gestures). It is important to review the birth history and prenatal/perinatal complications, including teratogenic in utero

Table 58-6 • RED FLAGS FOR SPEECH LANGUAGE DELAY

By 6 mo	• Does not laugh and/or vocalize • Does not respond to sounds
By 9 mo	• Does not respond to name • Does not babble
By 12 mo	• Does not point to objects or use gestures such as waving or shaking head • Does not say "ma-ma" or "da-da" specifically
By 15 mo	• Does not say any words other than "ma-ma" or "da-da"
By 18 mo	• Does not use at least five words spontaneously and consistently • Does not follow simple directions without gesture
By 24 mo	• Has a vocabulary less than 50 words • Does not combine two words together • Has limited interest in social interactions
By 36 mo	• Does not follow simple directions without gesture • Strangers or unfamiliar adults have difficulty understanding most of what the child is saying • Cannot create simple three-word novel sentences spontaneously • Does not participate in reciprocal conversation

exposures (tobacco, alcohol, prescription and illicit drugs). Risk factors for hearing loss, including use of ototoxic medications, should be reviewed. The developmental history should also cover general cognitive development (tool use, self-care skills), motor development, and personal–social development (social interaction with caregivers and peers, play, and atypical behaviors such as insistence on routines or stereotypies). A careful review of the child's adaptive functioning can give clues as to whether the language delay occurs in isolation or is part of global developmental delays. Information about the child's home language and degree of exposure to English can help to ascertain whether delays reflect lack of exposure or a true concern.

2. **Family and social history.** Important aspects of the family medical history to review include family members with language delays, learning differences, childhood hearing loss or deafness, and other conditions associated with language or speech disorders, such as autism. An important part of the history to review is the social history. The parents' level of educational achievement may be associated with the quantity and quality of language in the home. Also pertinent is physical deprivation (poverty, malnutrition) and social deprivation (inadequate linguistic stimulation, emotional stress, neglect), as these factors have adverse effects on speech development.

3. **Physical examination.** During the physical examination, key observations directly relating to the stage of language and speech development include the child's attention to speech in the room; ability to follow instructions with or without gestures; and production of gestures, signs, sounds or speech. Elements of the physical examination pertinent to identifying causes of language delay are listed in Table 58-7.

B. **Primary care office screening and evaluation of language or speech delay**
   • The American Academy of Pediatrics (AAP) recommends that all children be screened for developmental delays and disabilities during regular well-child visits using a validated screening tool at 9 months, 18 months, and 24 or 30 months. Formal screening is also recommended whenever the parent or practitioner has a developmental concern. Appropriate instruments include Parents' Evaluation of Developmental Status (http://www.pedstest.com/) and the Ages and Stages Questionnaires, Third Edition (http://agesandstages.com/products-services/asq3/), used in children aged 1 month to 5.5 years. Can be completed in 10–15 minutes and scored in 2–3 minutes.
   • In addition to broad developmental screening at 9, 18, and 24 or 30 months, the AAP recommends that all children be assessed with an *ASD-specific* screening measure at 18 and 24 months of age. One of the AAP-recommended tools, the Modified Checklist for Autism in Toddlers, Revised with Follow-up (M-CHAT-R/F) is a useful screening tool for atypicality (see Chapter 5).

Table 58-7 • PHYSICAL EXAMINATION FINDINGS IN THE EVALUATION OF YOUNG CHILDREN WITH SPEECH OR LANGUAGE DELAY SUGGESTIVE OF SPECIFIC ETIOLOGY

Physical Examination Findings	Possible Etiology or Associated Condition
Lack of eye contact, stereotyped repetitive motor mannerisms, social impairments	Autism spectrum disorder (see Chapter 28)
Spasticity, hyperreflexia, clonus, contractures, dysarthria, aphasia	Cerebral palsy
Bifid uvula, submucosal cleft, velopharyngeal insufficiency	Cleft lip, palate
Chorioretinitis	Congenital toxoplasmosis, congenital cytomegalovirus
Enlarged pinna, long narrow facies, prognathism, macroorchidism	Fragile X syndrome
Deformities of external ear canal, auricle	Hearing loss
Café-au lait spots	Neurofibromatosis
Short stature, obesity, hypogonadism	Prader–Willi syndrome
Excessive rapid growth, acromegalic features, high-arched palate	Sotos syndrome
Hypopigmented spots, adenoma sebaceum, shagreen patches	Tuberous sclerosis
Cleft palate, cardiac anomalies, dysmorphic facies	Velocardiofacial syndrome (22q11.2 deletion syndrome)
White forelock, cutaneous hypopigmentation, hypertelorism, heterochromia	Waardenburg syndrome
Oral hypotonia, drooling, inability to protrude tongue or show teeth on demand	Neurological or neuromotor disorders

1. *Parent-report* language-specific screeners or assessments that can be used in the primary care evaluation
   - MacArthur-Bates Communicative Development Inventory—Used in children 8–37 months. Takes caregivers 20–40 minutes to complete and professionals 10–15 minutes to score.
   - Language Development Survey—Uses caregivers' report of the child's vocabulary to identify language delays in children aged 18–35 months. Can be completed in 10 minutes and only requires fifth grade reading skills.
2. Language-specific assessments that require at least some *direct observation* of children
   - The Capute Scales (http://www.brookespublishing.com/resource-center/screening-and-assessment/the-capute-scales/) comprise two scales: Clinical Adaptive Test and the Clinical Linguistic and Auditory Milestone Scale. Used in children from birth to 36 months of age. Generates age equivalents and developmental quotients for each scale.
   - Communication and Symbolic Behavior Scales Developmental Profile (CSBS DP) Infant Toddler Checklist (http://brookespublishing.com/wp-content/uploads/2012/06/csbs-dp-itc.pdf): Used in children aged 6–24 months. Tallies raw

scores in seven clusters (Emotion and Eye Gaze, Communication, Gestures, Sounds, Words, Understanding, and Object Use) and three composites (Social, Speech, and Symbolic).

C. Evaluation of delay or disorder

1. **Hearing.** Office-based hearing screening procedures used by clinicians are prone to yield false-negative results or are inappropriate for the very young child. All children with speech or language delay should have their hearing tested by a certified audiologist, regardless of the parents or clinician's subjective impression of how well the child hears.

2. **Formal developmental testing.** Language, cognitive, and behavioral function should be assessed. It is important to understand the child's overall cognitive level and to determine if child language skills are commensurate with child cognitive level. Atypical behaviors and concerns should be elicited and identified, including presence of repetitive behaviors and restricted interests, stereotyped motor mannerisms, sensory sensitivities, and social impairments.

3. **Laboratory tests.** Laboratory tests may be warranted, depending on the history and physical examination. Genetic testing (Fragile X analysis, chromosomal microarray) and in some cases metabolic testing are recommended for children with language delays in the context of ASD or global developmental delays. Blood lead level and a complete blood count should be obtained to rule out lead toxicity (in children who mouth nonfood items) and anemia, respectively, both of which are associated with expressive language delay. EEG (electroencephalogram) is appropriate for children with staring spells, seizures, or suspicions of Landau–Kleffner syndrome (epileptic aphasia). Brain imaging should be obtained for asymmetric neurologic examinations and developmental regression.

D. Referral. If the screening reveals an isolated delay or concern in speech or language, then referral to a speech-language pathologist for further evaluation and treatment is appropriate. If other developmental or behavioral issues are identified, the primary care clinician can refer children for further diagnostic testing with a pediatric subspecialist, such as developmental and behavioral pediatrician, child neurologist, or child psychologist. If these subspecialists are not available or the delay in consulting them is long, the primary care clinician can also refer the child and family for further assessment and treatment through the local early intervention clinician (typically administered via a state-designated county department), or special education program (usually requiring the family to request in writing an evaluation at the local school). If the results are negative, reassurance or enhanced monitoring may be appropriate; if the results are positive, developmental intervention can be implemented in a timely fashion.

V. ANTICIPATORY GUIDANCE FOR LANGUAGE DELAYS AND DISORDERS

A. Primary goals. The primary goal of management is to promote optimal development of language, while minimizing frustration for the child and parents. Table 58-8 offers suggestions for parents to provide a linguistically enriched environment.

B. Information for the primary care clinician

* Amount of verbal input that parents provide is correlated with the child's rate of development. Encourage parents to interact with their child.
* Do not rush to judgment. Parents do not want either false reassurance ("Don't worry, your child will grow out of it") or needless anxiety ("He or she will never be able to...").
* On the other hand, do not procrastinate once the outcome seems clear. If there is a speech or language delay or disorder, this finding should be explained to the parents in a straightforward yet compassionate manner. ("Why didn't our doctor tell us before now?" is a common complaint). Above all, listen to the family. ("We tried to tell our doctor there was a problem, but the doctor wouldn't listen to us" is another equally common complaint.)
* Following identification of a speech-language disorder or any other developmental disorder, the primary care clinician coordinates ongoing care across all the diverse providers within the health care system and community, ensuring that the consultants who are involved have appropriately explained the issues, and regularly monitors the child and the family's progress. This responsibility is part of the primary care medical home.
* With the explosion of information available on the Internet, many specific resources and support groups may be available for children with developmental disorders. Clinicians should help family evaluate the quality of the information and resources. High-quality Web sites are listed below.
* Connecting the family to other parents of similarly affected children is a source of great strength and comfort to most families.

Table 58-8 • RECOMMENDATIONS FOR PARENTS AND CAREGIVERS TO ENCOURAGE SPEECH AND LANGUAGE DEVELOPMENT

1. Talk to your child frequently and directly. Talking to other adults in the room is not as helpful. The television is not a good method to teach language.
2. Narrate what your child is doing. This approach is called child-directed speech. If your child is playing with a toy, eating a food, or noticing people or objects, talk about that interest. Narrate your day as you shop, play at the park, or bathe or dress her. ("Look at the bright red apples!" "The girl kicked the ball." "Put your arm in the shirt." "Now we are washing your belly.")
3. When describing items or events, present words in many different sentences. Each repetition is an opportunity to learn the word. If your child is playing with a car you might say, "You have a car. Look at that blue car. That car goes fast. Can you make the car go vroom?"
4. Respond to your child. Expand on what the child says. If he or she says "banana" or part of the word ("nana") while pointing at a piece of fruit, you might say, "You want that banana. Here is the yellow banana. This banana is for you." Every time you repeat the word, you reinforce learning.
5. Use facial expressions and gestures to add interest and information to spoken language.
6. Encourage your child to speak. Ask questions. Offer choices. Do not withhold what your child wants to the point of frustration or tantrum. Your child may not say the word, but if you repeat it, he or she may learn to understand the word.
7. Model correct speech. If your child pronounces a word incorrectly, simply say it correctly, without repeating the incorrect pronunciation. This approach exposes his or her to the correct pronunciation of that word.
8. If family members have different primary languages, speak to the child in whichever language you feel most comfortable. Grandparents may use one language with a child, for instance, and parents another. Being exposed to multiple languages does not cause language delays.
9. Share books with your child. When reading books to him or her, use different voices and add drama if you can. If he or she is not interested in the words of the book, talk about the pictures. Let your child hold the book and turn the pages. Make the interaction fun for both of you.
10. Explore your local library. Most libraries have story time for young children. Ask the librarian to help you choose books that your child might like.
11. Playing with other children may motivate your child to speak. Consider play dates, nursery school, or day care.

C. Treatment

- **Speech-language therapy** is indicated for delays and disorders and typically is play-based with specific goals. Speech-language therapy is often integrated into other developmental services.
  - Infants and toddlers up to age 36 months may be served in a home or community-based program.
  - Enrollment in a special education program administered by the child's school district is often the best option for children of age 36 months or older because a classroom setting will provide not just language instruction but practical experience in the use of language in a social setting.
- **Parent education and participation** (especially through preschool age) is critical to leverage the intervention time with the therapist and to allow the child to generalize new skills into everyday situations.
- **Sign language** is commonly used for children with severe speech and language delays (Down syndrome, intellectual disability). Parents can be assured with confidence that signing does not delay speech. On the contrary, sign language exposure may actually promote oral language development. Therapy for the child with hearing loss will vary, depending on the degree of hearing loss, but may include some combination of orally based speech therapy plus signing, as well as amplification or cochlear implantation.
- **Picture Exchange communication System (PECS)** may be used in the education of children with ASD who have failed other conventional and behavioral speech-language therapy.
- **Augmentative communication devices** (picture boards, electronic communication devices) are also widely available for children with persistent, severe deficits of speech and language due to cognitive or motor impairment.

Bibliography

FOR PARENTS

WEB SITES

Babyhearing.org. https://www.babyhearing.org/.

National Center For Hearing Assessment and Management (NCHAM) Infant hearing http://www.infanthearing.org/.

National Institute on Deafness and Other Communication Disorders (NIDCD) Fact Sheet: "Your Baby's Hearing and Communicative Development Checklist" https://www.nidcd.nih.gov/sites/default/files/Documents/health/hearing/NIDCD-Hearing-Development-Checklist.pdf.

BOOKS

Agin MC, Geng LF, Nicholl MJ. *The Late Talker: What to Do If Your Child Isn't Talking Yet.* New York: St. Martin's Press; 2004.

Eichten PI. *Help Me Talk: A Parent's Guide to Speech and Language Stimulation Techniques for Children 1 to 3 Years.* Glen Allen, VA: Pi Communication Materials; 2000.

Hulit LM, Fahey KR, Howard MR. *Born to Talk: An Introduction to Speech and Language Development.* Upper Saddle River, New Jersey: Pearson; 2015.

FOR PROFESSIONALS

WEB SITES

American Speech-Language Hearing Association. http://www.asha.org/ce/.

Information about developmental milestones available on the CDC's "Learn the Signs. Act Early" Web site: https://www.cdc.gov/ncbddd/actearly/index.html.

The American Academy of Pediatrics Bright Futures. www.brightfutures.org.

BOOKS

Batshaw ML, Roizen NJ, Lotrecchiano GR. *Children With Disabilities.* Baltimore: Paul H. Brookes Publishing; 2013.

Beukelman DR, Mirenda P, Beukelman DR. *Augmentative and Alternative Communication: Supporting Children and Adults With Complex Communication Needs.* Baltimore: Paul H. Brookes Publishing; 2013.

CHAPTER 59

Learning Disability

Marilyn Augustyn | Maryanne Wolf

I. **DESCRIPTION OF THE PROBLEM.** According to the National Center for Education Studies, more than 13% of all public-school students in the United States receive special education services, and among them, 35% had specific learning disabilities (LDs). LDs and school failure are complex issues that challenge traditional methods of pediatric evaluation and management. Although learning problems are of obvious multidisciplinary concern, the primary care clinician plays a vital role in clarifying the reasons for school failure, including an LD, and facilitating appropriate evaluation and intervention.

A. **Reasons for school failure.** A wide variety of causes may contribute to a child's failure in school. A simple classification scheme identifies **intrinsic** or child-related causes (e.g., specific LDs, attention deficits) and **extrinsic** or environmental-related causes relating to either the home (e.g., parental separation or divorce) or the school setting (e.g., poor instruction, challenged school system). In most cases, school failure is not due to a single factor but rather the result of a **complex interaction of child-, home-, and school-related variables**. By federal guidelines there are 14 qualifying diagnoses: autism, developmental delay, deaf-blindness, deafness, emotional disturbance, hearing impairment, intellectual disability, multiple disabilities, orthopedic impairment, other health impairment, speech or language impairment, traumatic brain injury, visual impairment including blindness, and specific LD.

B. **Specific causes**

1. **Learning disabilities.** As defined by federal legislation: *Specific learning disability means a disorder in one or more of the basic psychological processes involved in understanding or in using language, spoken or written, which may manifest itself in an imperfect ability to listen, think, speak, read, write, spell, or to do mathematical calculations.*

   The term includes conditions such as perceptual disabilities, brain injury, minimal brain dysfunction, dyslexia, and developmental aphasia. The term does not include children who have problems that are primarily the result of visual, hearing, or motor disabilities; intellectual disability; emotional disturbance; or environmental, cultural, or economic disadvantage. Family, genetic, cognitive, and neuroanatomical factors are all implicated as etiologies for LDs.

   The great majority of youth with LDs have underlying weaknesses in written language functions that include difficulties in learning to read, write, and spell. These include both the 5%–10% of the population with diagnosed dyslexia and children with reading disabilities (RDs) that are due to environmental factors such as inadequate instruction, dual language learners, or poor language enrichment and development.

   In previous decades, LDs and RDs were characterized by a **discrepancy between ability (as measured by intelligence tests) and actual academic achievement**. In recent years, the discrepancy definition has been rejected by most researchers in the RD fields who emphasize the need for services for children with reading failure regardless of intelligence tests, which can be skewed by environmental factors such as socioeconomic status. Consequently, recent federal legislation adds a response to intervention (RTI) component to the evaluation of an LD. The expectation is that students in Tier 1 will receive high-quality, scientifically based instruction (that is, with evidence from empirically based studies), differentiated to meet their needs, and are screened on a periodic basis to identify struggling learners who need additional support. Tier 2 consists of students not making adequate progress in the core curriculum, who are then provided with increasingly intensive instruction matched to their needs on the basis of levels of performance and rates of progress. In most states, the eligibility of a child for special education and related services is considered when a child has not succeeded in Tiers 1 or 2 and is considered appropriate for the Tier 3 level of RTI. Such a child has been in Tier 2 for a predetermined amount of time and an evaluation is given, after which a meeting is called to determine eligibility for special education services.

In addition, and by contrast, weaknesses in other higher-order cognitive functions (the putative metacognitive skills) have been increasingly recognized among children with nonverbal LDs. Such children may have difficulties with reasoning, memory, or focusing their attention and have been described as "passive learners" because of their difficulties with selecting strategies for problem solving.

2. **Attention deficits.** There exists significant overlap among children with LD, RD, and attention-deficit/hyperactivity disorder (ADHD) (see Chapter27). From a clinical standpoint, distinguishing between children with an intrinsic deficit of attention and those with attention deficits secondary to other developmental and behavioral dysfunctions (e.g., language impairment, dyslexia, depression) is often difficult, but important to discern. For example, some children with RD can appear to manifest attentional issues that are due more to their avoidance of reading, whereas others may have comorbid conditions that exacerbate both attention and reading issues.

3. **Intellectual disability.** Mild intellectual disability is often not identified until children are confronted with the cognitive demands of school. At that time, a slow learning rate and ultimate acquisition of academic skills up to the fifth- or sixth-grade level is typically seen.

4. **Sensory impairment.** Hearing loss results in a significant educational handicap because language acquisition and communication skills are impaired. Such students typically experience difficulties in reading, arithmetic reasoning, and problem solving. They may exhibit classroom maladjustment, behavioral problems, and social immaturity. The prognosis directly relates to the age at which identification occurs. In comparison, visually impaired children usually fare better within the classroom and those who experience school failure tend to have additional handicaps.

5. **Emotional illness.** From 30% to 80% of emotionally disturbed students have problems with academic achievement and classroom behavior. Emotional problems such as low self-esteem and poor self-image often exacerbate school failure brought on by other causes, such as LD or ADHD.

6. **Chronic illness/other health impairment.** From 25% to 33% of chronically ill students have problems with academic achievement. Possible adverse influences on school performance include limited alertness or stamina, chronic pain, medication side effects, absenteeism, emotional maladjustment, low intelligence (primarily children with certain neurologic disorders), the inferior quality of alternative classroom placement, and inappropriate or unrealistic expectations by teachers and parents. In addition, certain chronic diseases (e.g., epilepsy, cerebral palsy, myelomeningocele) are associated with an increased incidence of LD.

7. **Temperamental dysfunction.** The temperamentally "difficult" student may become easily frustrated and angry when confronted with material not easily mastered. The initial reluctance to participate and tendency to withdraw of the "slow-to-warm-up" child may be misinterpreted as anxiety or as a limited capacity for learning. Although the temperamentally "easy" student usually fares well, problems may arise when expectations for behavior markedly differ between home and school. For example, a student's mild intensity of reaction to situations or stimuli may be misinterpreted within the classroom as a lack of interest or motivation.

8. **Family dysfunction and social problems.** Family issues that contribute to school failure include parental separation and divorce, child abuse and neglect, the illness or death of an immediate family member, parental psychopathology, early parenthood, substance abuse, community violence, and poverty.

9. **Ineffective schooling.** School *processes* are more important determinants of students' performance than features such as whether schools are public or private, class size, the age and spaciousness of school buildings, and student–teacher ratio. Rather, the school's academic emphasis, expectations for attainment, amount of homework, teachers' actions during lessons, use of group instruction, and the use of rewards and praise have major influences on students' performance. Aspects of the school's social environment (such as the amount of praise offered to children) may be particularly important for children from disadvantaged homes in which less emphasis is placed on academic attainment and standards for classroom behavior. Knowledge of the relationships between school effectiveness and school achievement has important implications for assessing and promoting both individual student performance and public policy.

II. MAKING THE DIAGNOSIS

A. **Psychoeducational evaluation.** Under the Individuals with Disabilities Education Improvement Act of 2004, no single procedure is used as the sole criterion for determining an appropriate educational program for a child. Further, the child must be assessed in all areas related to the suspected disability. These areas include, where appropriate, health, vision, hearing, social and emotional status, general intelligence, academic performance, communicative status, and motor abilities. Specifically:

1. Individual psychological evaluation, including general intelligence
2. Social history based on interviews with parents and the student
3. Academic history with interviews or reports from past teachers
4. Physical examination, including specific assessments that relate to vision, hearing, and health
5. Classroom observation of the student in his or her current educational setting
6. Achievement educational evaluation specifically pinpointing the areas of deficit or suspected disability including, but not limited to, educational achievement, academic needs, learning strengths and needs, and vocational assessments

There is increasing emphasis on the establishment of discrete profiles of LDs and RDs that can be used to target forms of intervention. For example, whereas some RDs involved the failure to establish the correspondences between letters and sounds, others involved an ability to gain the fluency necessary to read with comprehension. Differential diagnosis increases the likelihood of success by targeting forms of RD and LD with appropriate, evidence-based interventions, rather than the frequently mistaken use of whatever intervention the school or teacher has available.

The following might also be considered.

* Functional behavioral assessment to describe the relationship between a skill or performance problem and variables that contribute to its occurrence
* Bilingual assessment for students with limited English proficiency
* Speech and language evaluations
* Physical and/or occupational evaluations

B. Pediatric evaluation. If psychoeducational evaluation has already identified the reasons for a student's school failure (e.g., LD or mild intellectual disability), the goal of pediatric evaluation is to exclude medical problems as contributors to poor classroom performance. In addition, the primary care clinician's familiarity with the child and family may be helpful in identifying social or emotional factors that further impair school performance. For the child with newly recognized school failure, the pediatric clinician must identify conditions such as sensory impairment or chronic illness, while searching for medical, neurophysiologic, and psychological correlates of other conditions such as LD, intellectual disability, and emotional illness. Possible components of the evaluation of children with school failure include the following.

C. History. Important historic information should be sought from parents, teachers, and the child. Review of the student's perinatal and medical history, developmental milestones, past and present behavior, and family and social history may yield findings with possible implications for school failure (Table 59-1).

D. Key clinical questions

* *"Which subjects are particularly difficult for the child?"* The pattern of delays may suggest a specific etiology; for example, children with an LD typically have discrete difficulties in selected subjects, whereas students with mild cognitive impairment have more pervasive academic delays.
* *"How does the child behave in the classroom?"* Classroom behavior may suggest ADHD, poor self-image, or conduct disorder. It is important to ascertain whether such aberrant behavior may be the consequence of a particular learning weakness such as reading, rather than an actual conduct disorder.
* *"How many days has the child missed school?"* Poor school attendance may be due to chronic illness, school phobia, or poor motivation due to LD.
* *"Has past testing been performed?"* Past educational or psychological testing may have identified causes of a child's school failure.
* *"What special services has the child received?"* Responses to different instructional techniques ("diagnostic teaching") may suggest reasons for school failure.

E. Physical examination. The physical examination has a limited, but important, role in the evaluation of children with school failure. Certain specific aspects deserve special emphasis such as characteristics of genetic syndromes and neurodermal syndromes.

F. Mental status examination. Simple projective techniques may suggest emotional issues such as depression, anxiety, or poor self-image as the cause or, even more likely, the consequence of school failure. Examples include the following:

1. *"If you had three wishes, what would they be?"*

Table 59-1 • THE ROLE OF HISTORY IN THE EVALUATION OF SCHOOL LEARNING PROBLEMS

Aspect	Findings Suggestive of Learning Disorders
School Functioning	
Academic achievement	Discrete delays in select subject (e.g., language) Adequate early performance, with difficulties emerging later (e.g., mathematics, writing)
Classroom behavior	Long-standing, pervasive problems with inattention, impulsivity, overactivity Disorganization and poor strategy formation Depression, moodiness
Attendance	Excessive absenteeism School avoidance
Past psychoeducational testing	Discrepancy between cognitive abilities and academic achievement
Special education services received	Response to "diagnostic teaching"
Perinatal history	Clusters of adverse events Maternal alcohol or drug intake
Medical history	Recurrent and/or persistent otitis media Iron deficiency anemia Lead poisoning Seizures Frequent injuries Chronic medication use
Development	Delayed or disordered language acquisition and communication skills Subtle delays in select milestones Uneven pattern of skills and interests
Behavioral history	Long-standing, pervasive problems with attention span, impulsivity, acting out, overactivity Sadness Poor self-esteem
Family history	Learning problems School failure among first-degree relatives
Social history	Child abuse or neglect Other stressors

From Dworkin PH. School learning problems and developmental differences. In: McInerny TK, Adam HM, Campbell DE, et al. eds. *Textbook of Pediatric Care.* 1st ed. Elk Grove Village, IL: American Academy of Pediatrics; 2009:1149-1155.

2. *"If you could make three changes in your life, what would they be?"* The sad or anxious child may be unwilling to offer wishes or hope for changes in family or school circumstances.

3. *"Draw a picture of your family"* may suggest concerns with family composition or reveal anxiety or uncertainty regarding the child's status within the family.

G. **Laboratory studies.** No laboratory studies are routinely indicated in the assessment of school failure (except perhaps screening for lead poisoning). Rather, tests should be performed based on specific indications. In the future, genetic studies may prove useful in establishing a profile for specific forms of dyslexia, which has a strong genetic basis. Now, it is very important to have information on any familial history of dyslexia or other LDS.

III. **MANAGEMENT.** For LDs, mild cognitive impairment, and other common causes of school failure, research indicates the earlier the intervention, the better the outcome. Nonetheless, a variety of important primary care roles are both feasible and important in the management of school failure.

A. Specific medical intervention is the most traditional of pediatric roles. Examples include the following:
   1. **The treatment of underlying medical conditions,** such as asthma or a seizure disorder, that influence school performance
   2. **Pharmacologic management** of ADHD
B. Counseling is a traditional mode of pediatric intervention. Aspects may include the following:
   1. Clarification of a student's strengths and weaknesses and demystification of any diagnosis such as LD and cognitive impairment.
   2. Anticipatory guidance regarding commonly encountered school difficulties and the consequences of school failure (e.g., low self-esteem).
   3. Alleviation of guilt and anxiety. One of the most important contributions of the pediatric clinician in cases of dyslexia is the assurance to parent and child that dyslexia involves a different organization of the brain for language but has nothing to do with intelligence. Many children (and their parents, peers, and teachers) mistakenly believe the failure to learn to read easily reflects a lack of intelligence. This false belief leads to multiple negative sequelae in children who are in fact intellectually adept and often gifted in some areas.
   4. Explaining the legal rights of students and families.
   5. Guidance regarding the lack of effectiveness of nontraditional treatment strategies (e.g., dietary manipulation, optometric training).
   6. Offering advice regarding specific behavior management strategies, such as time-out and positive reinforcement.
   7. Recommending educational and advocacy organizations to families such as the International Dyslexia Society (www.interdys.org), the Learning Disabilities Association of America (www.ldaamerica.org), the Dyslexia Foundation, the National Center for Learning Disabilities (www.ncld.org), and the National Institute of Neurological Disorders and Stroke (www.ninds.nih.gov).
C. The primary care clinician can assume an active role in monitoring the progress of children with learning problems. Office visits provide important opportunities to monitor self-esteem, search for signs of depression, and offer encouragement and praise for progress.

Bibliography

FOR PARENTS

Great Schools. www.greatschools.org.

Learning Disabilities Association of America. www.ldanatl.org.

Wolf M. *Proust and the Squid*: The Story and Science of the Reading Brain. NY: HarperCollins; 2008.

FOR PROFESSIONALS

Handler SM, Fierson WM, Section on Ophthalmology; Council on Children with Disabilities; American Academy of Ophthalmology; American Association for Pediatric Ophthalmology and Strabismus; American Association of Certified Orthoptists. Learning disabilities, dyslexia, and vision. *Pediatrics*. 2011;127(3):e818-e856.

Lovett M, Fritters J, Wolf M, Morris R, Early intervention for children at risk for reading disabilities: The impact of grade at intervention and individual differences on intervention outcomes. *J Educ Psych*. 2017;109(7):889-914.

Prince E, Ring H. Causes of learning disability and epilepsy: a review. *Curr Opin Neurol*. 2011;24(2):154-158.

Rimrodt SL, Lipkin PH. Learning disabilities and school failure. *Pediatr Rev*. 2011;32(8): 315-324.

CHAPTER **60**

Lying, Cheating, and Stealing

Nerissa S. Bauer | Martin T. Stein

I. DESCRIPTION OF THE PROBLEM. The significance of three related behaviors in children—lying, stealing, and cheating—can be identified in the context of developmental tasks. Imagination and symbolic thinking in the preschool child followed by the formation of a conscience, understanding the cause and effect, and self-esteem in a school-aged child determine and modulate the meaning of these behaviors. Every child lies and cheats at some time, and many children steal something before adolescence. The challenge for the pediatric clinician is to unravel the significance of these events for an individual child—to clarify a normal developmental experience from disruptive, developmentally inappropriate misbehavior. These behaviors may be grouped under the general term "disruptive behavior disorders," but may be a component of other conditions in the *Diagnostic and Statistical Manual of Mental Disorders, Fifth Edition (DSM-5)*: disorders such as oppositional defiant disorder, conduct disorder, and attention-deficit/hyperactivity disorder (ADHD), especially if untreated or if it goes undiagnosed in its earliest stages.

A. Epidemiology
   1. These behaviors are seen occasionally in all children. A precise prevalence is unknown for the normal population.
   2. Estimate of gender difference: three to four times more common in boys.
   3. When occurring frequently in association with aggressive behaviors and affecting adversely development and function:
      a. Oppositional defiant disorder: 2%–16%
      b. Conduct disorder: 6%–16% (males); 2%–9% (females)
      c. Significant stealing: 5%
   4. Risk factors: inappropriate parental response to or unrealistic expectations for behavior, family disharmony, coercive discipline, difficult temperament, excessive exposure to violence (in home, community, television, movies), and cognitive deficiency.

B. Familial transmission. Both environmental and genetic components are found in the most severe forms when there is consideration of a disruptive behavior disorder.

C. Etiology/contributing factors
   1. **Environmental.** The child's immediate environment may be a contributing factor. When a preschool child expresses a developmentally appropriate "untruth," parental overreaction (e.g., expression of guilt or excessive discipline) may contribute to repetition of the behavior. Situational stress may come from school (recent change in grade, new school, bullying, or victimization), home (parental unemployment, poor housing conditions, parental illness, exposure to violence), or community (child abduction, natural disaster, violence in media).
   2. **Developmental.** Temperament, activity level, attention, and self-regulation may in some children be associated with excessive lying, stealing, and cheating. Both behavioral inhibition or low self-regulation and the "difficult child" may predispose to these behaviors, especially in the context of a parent or teacher whose own temperament is not adaptable to the child.

   Characteristics of a developmental stage clarify many behaviors. In the 3- and 4-year-olds, an active imagination can generate "tall tales" or "white lies." They reflect developmentally appropriate processing of events. Young children often have a difficult time distinguishing between fantasy and reality during the toddler and preschool years. Young children cope with stressful situations by reflection—how a child wishes things were or how they should be. In school-aged children, there is an awareness of societal expectations and the gradual emergence of a conscience (usually by the age of 8 years) with the cognitive and emotional maturity to differentiate a truth from an untruth. Clinicians should be mindful that it is around this developmental time frame that children are increasingly able to maintain consistency in subsequent statements when lying and thus may escape detection. Cheating behavior develops with age and has been documented as early as preschool age in laboratory experiments (such as when asking children between 3 and 5 years of age not to peek at a toy while left alone in a room). It is seen occasionally in the school-aged children and more often in middle school. Winning games and academic success in school may overcome the child's sense of what is right and desire to be part of a team. Before the age of 7 years, children will often "bend" rules to win board games and not have a true understanding that rules are not to be broken. However, as children transition from late childhood to early adolescence, cheating behavior decreases. As children age, executive function (e.g., self-regulation, planning, attentional flexibility, inhibitory control) influences children's decision to cheat and the tactics used to cover up the behavior. Children with inhibitory control and working memory choose to cheat less often; yet if a child decides to cheat, children with more attentional flexibility and planning may use more sophisticated tactics.

Stealing may begin with a toddler/preschool child whose actions are guided by egocentrism and who does not understand that taking something that does not belong to him or her is wrong. "What's mine is mine" and "What's yours is mine" is reflective of the typical mind-set of these young children. In school-aged children, isolated stealing is usually an impulsive act. At this age and in middle school, stealing may develop out from the child's desire for possessions or a result of attention seeking or revenge. It may reflect poor parental role modeling or ill-defined rules/boundaries. Collectively, lying, cheating, and stealing can be present in varying degrees among children as they age; however, illegal rule-breaking behavior (e.g., vandalism, setting fires) is rarely observed among typically developing children and should be a cause for concern and further workup for clinically significant levels of psychopathology.

3. **Parenting and other role models.** Considering the frequency of lying, stealing, and cheating during early development, the parental response to an event is a critical factor. Each of these behaviors is a potential opportunity to teach a child about his or her role in society—a preschool child who steals a candy bar, a school-aged child who lies about a grade, or a middle school youth who cheats on an examination. The manner in which parents, teachers, and other adults respond to these events is important. In addition, the way parents live their own lives models significant behaviors for children each day.

4. **Organic.** Neurobehavioral disorders may be associated with poor self-regulation and lead to excessive lying, cheating, and stealing. It may be seen in children and youth with oppositional behaviors as a component of depression, anxiety, or conduct disorder. Genetic disorders and fetal drug exposure (e.g., fetal alcohol syndrome) may predispose to repetitive and chronic lying, cheating, or stealing.

II. **MAKING THE DIAGNOSIS.** The assessment should take place in a supportive environment that allows for a thorough history and physical examination, review of pertinent supporting documents (i.e., teacher narratives, past psychoeducational testing), and time to address specific parental concerns. The pediatric clinician should (1) distinguish if the misbehavior is normal in terms of the child's overall cognitive development or abnormal; (2) evaluate potential risk or protective factors that may be contributing or can readily extinguish the misbehavior; and (3) provide guidance to parents that encompass both preventive and practical parenting strategies to be used "in the moment."

A. **Signs and symptoms.** Parents and clinicians usually (or eventually) know when a child has lied, cheated, or stolen something. The recognition of these behaviors begins the process of a behavioral diagnosis. An isolated symptom in the absence of other behavior problems or developmental delay suggests that the behavior may be consistent with normal developmental expectations. First and foremost, the pediatric clinician should obtain an understanding of the misbehavior in concrete terms, using the ABC framework.

1. Antecedent to misbehavior (any triggers or patterns)

2. Behavior (concrete, discrete behavior)

3. Consequence (parental response to misbehavior)

Pediatric clinicians who rely on this type of behavioral history taking framework will find it easier to understand the parent's perspective of the misbehavior and be better prepared to counsel the family on management. If parents have limited insight into the issue, asking the parent to describe the last time the misbehavior of concern occurred can help the clinician gather the necessary information.

In addition to the specifics of the behavior, assessment should also include the following:

• Developmental milestones with an emphasis on language, cognitive capacity, and social interactions. Developmental mastery at specific stages is protective against persistent disruptive behaviors.

- Family role modeling and parental response to behaviors.
- Experience with peers in context of social role models; peer pressure.
- Educational achievement, including family and child's expectation for performance.
- Low self-esteem.

B. Differential diagnosis. When the behaviors cannot be explained in the context of normal developmental stages, consider more pervasive type of disorders. Lying, cheating, and stealing may be associated with a specific behavioral disorder, including oppositional defiant disorder, conduct disorder, ADHD, anxiety, depression, posttraumatic stress disorder, an adjustment disorder, or pervasive developmental delay. Or it may be reflective of a child's lower cognitive functioning. These behaviors may reflect aggression manifested by words or actions that seem intended to harm another person or oneself. Lying, for example, is seen in bullying behavior and stealing may be a part of retaliatory or reactive behavior.

C. History: key clinical questions. Start with an inventory of possible risk and protective factors.

1. **Individual risk factors.** Prenatal history (exposure to drugs, alcohol, cigarettes, lead), birth history (resuscitative events or prolonged neonatal intensive care unit experience), quality of early attachment experiences, temperament (poor adaptability, distractible, intense reaction to change), immature social skills, vulnerable peer groups, developmental regression.

2. **Familial and relational risk factors.** Poor temperament match between the parent and the child, ineffective parenting practices, marital conflicts, parental separation, divorce, domestic violence, family history of psychopathology (e.g., alcoholism, depression), especially in parents, child abuse/neglect.

3. **Community factors.** Neighborhood and media violence exposure, availability of firearms, neighborhood-level socioeconomic status.

4. **Protective factors/patient strengths.** Strong and stable social support in home or community, child's special talents, academic success, complementary temperament of child and parents, parental warmth and sensitivity to child.

5. **For the family**
   - *Has there been any major change or other stress in the life of the child or family?* Lying, cheating, or stealing may manifest as a new behavior after a significant shift in the child's life and may affect the ability to cope with a new situation or event. Assess the different environments—home: parental conflict, birth of a new sibling; school: change in school or poor adjustment to new academic level, problems with friends or bullying; community: exposure to negative role model, unstable parental employment.
   - *How often does the behavior occur?* If it happens infrequently, examine the circumstances immediately preceding, during, and following the event. *Does it occur only in certain settings?* Assess patterns in the behavior, including an increased intensity or severity. If the behavior is chronic, consider depression, anxiety, conduct disorder.
   - *How do the parents respond to the behavior?*

6. **For the child** (it may be helpful to separate the child from the parent.)
   - *What happened immediately before the event?*
   - *What were you feeling when you....?* Assess motivation and insight.
   - *How did you feel afterward?* Regret or remorse reflects moral development. Lack of remorse may indicate a conduct disorder.
   - *How do you feel about it now?*
   - *What makes you angry? What helps you to calm down?*
   - *How do you think you could have handled the situation differently?*

D. Behavioral observation. Observational data in the office may be helpful in assessment. Observe the child's interactions with the parent, with you, and during self-play. Note parental warmth and sensitivity toward the child, as well as affect of the parent. Parental mental health issues or ineffective and inconsistent parenting can inhibit/contribute to a parent's ability to adequately respond to a child. For instance, disruptive behaviors are more likely in children whose primary caregiver is depressed or in parents who model aggressive conflict resolution skills. A clinical assessment of temperament as well as activity level, impulsivity, affect, cognitive functioning, and social responses should be recorded. Observed behaviors should be interpreted in the context of the child's developmental stage.

E. Tests. To determine the contextual aspect of the behaviors, a daily behavioral diary (following the ABC framework) is useful. For a 1- to 2-week period, request a recording of the antecedents to the behavior (what was going on), the behavior (what the child did or said), and the consequences (what happened after the event). Clues to specific diagnoses associated with these behaviors will surface during a comprehensive behavioral–developmental and family history. In specific situations, behavioral questionnaires or psychoeducational testing may define the problem with greater precision.

III. MANAGEMENT

A. Information for the family. Educating the family is the initial step toward effective collaboration with the pediatric clinician. When addressing negative behavioral issues, begin the discussion by pointing out the patient's and family's strengths. Guide parents to an understanding of how these qualities support a positive outcome. Framing the behavior in context of developmental principles should lead to an understanding of the behavior and insight into the child's temperament, motivation, and responses to the environment. Discuss the child and family vulnerabilities that may be associated with the behaviors.

B. Helpful behavioral management tips for the family

1. **Prevention.** Parents can be taught positive parenting strategies that focus on building a trusting relationship with the child that promotes a child's self-esteem, healthy conscience, and open parent–child communication.

   * Praise the child's efforts early and often. Remind parents to foster positive self-esteem by encouraging the child to try things and focus on the process and not the end product. Children who receive immediate and specific praise for small steps in the right direction when learning new or complex behaviors will more likely internalize these pronouncements and feel good about their actions. They will come to readily understand parental expectations between acceptable, desired behaviors and less desired ones.

   * Have realistic expectations of the child's behavior. Clinicians can help promote an understanding of normal child development and abilities during well-child visits.

   * Parents can jumpstart a young child's healthy development of emotional self-regulation and empathy by commenting on the child's feelings during toddlerhood/preschool age. Children can be taught to express their emotions in verbal ways, rather than outwardly showing frustration or other negative emotions. These children will more likely be able to articulate their feelings more freely. When parents validate a child's emotions, the development of empathy and compassion is fostered.

   * Role model acceptable behavior. Parents are their children's first teachers—this includes modeling appropriate verbal and nonverbal behavior.

   * Reward appropriate behavior with low-cost or no-cost rewards (such as extra story at bedtime, snuggle time with a parent, going to the park) and/or social reinforcers (such as hugs, kisses, and specific and immediate praise).

2. **Capitalize on teachable moments**

   a. **Lying.** Consider the context in which it occurs and do not accuse or label the child as a "liar." The 3- to 4-year-old child processes experience with magical, egocentric thinking; the preschool child is in the early stage of understanding right from wrong. By 8 or 9 years of age, the conscience is more developed and becomes an internal moral guide. Help parents to use this knowledge to respond to their child. After an episode of lying, discuss the reasons for the behavior in an open manner. Reassure the child you will always love him or her. Reassurance can help ease a child's anxieties and help him or her share feelings and reasons for lying. Parents should be counseled to not set up a child for lying. If a parent wants the child to "confess" or admit to a known misbehavior, he or she should be advised to bring up the issue upfront rather than start the conversation as an open-ended question. For instance, if a child misbehaved at school and the teacher contacted the parent, the parent should openly discuss this with the child, rather than leading off with a question as the child may not openly admit to any wrong-doings—leading to parental frustration.

   b. **Stealing.** A clear explanation about possessions and the concept of ownership should be given to the child. Firm limits and logical consequences should be in place. Modeling appropriate behavior and instituting consistent discipline in response, such as "let us return the toy back to Johnnie" or "let us go say sorry and pay for the candy" should be used. Do not overreact because this may frighten the child. Parents should begin to talk about ownership, sharing, and asking for what he or she wants as early as toddler age. If stealing is repetitive, seek additional help.

    c. **Cheating.** Parents can talk about how cheating hurts other people's feelings and ask the child if there is a better solution. Approach the child in a gentle manner and refrain from harsh punishment. Explain consequences in a calm, matter-of-fact way. If cheating is repetitive, closer examination into reasons for cheating should be performed (e.g., low self-esteem, learning disabilities, low impulse control) and/or seek additional help.

C. Anticipatory guidance

    1. Ineffective parenting styles can be addressed in the context of helping to prevent ongoing escalations of disruptive behavior.

    2. Exposure to violence in the media should be decreased because it reduces restraints on aggressive behavior, desensitizes the response to viewing violence, and distorts a child's emerging understanding about appropriate conflict resolution.

    3. Availability of firearms, especially when in the home of a child with significant disruptive behaviors, should be discussed. Options for the removal or proper storage to ensure safety of the individual should be outlined.

D. Treatment. If a neurobehavioral condition is discovered, the intervention should be based on the specific diagnosis (i.e., conduct disorder depression, obsessive–compulsive disorder, anxiety, ADHD).

E. Criteria for referral

    1. When lying, cheating, or stealing is frequent and not responsive to education and behavior management, consider referral to a mental health professional.

    2. Domestic violence or child abuse should be reported to an appropriate agency as mandated by law.

    3. Ongoing parent–child conflicts, a significant temperament mismatch, or underlying psychopathology should be managed concurrently with a mental health professional.

    4. Social issues such as parental unemployment and lack of adequate childcare may be addressed by referral to a social worker or case manager involved with a community-based organization.

Bibliography

FOR PARENTS

Brazelton TB, Sparrow JD. *Touchpoints: Three to Six: Your Child's Emotional and Behavioral Development*. 2nd ed. Cambridge, MA: Perseus Books; 2006.

Pruitt DB, ed. *Your Child: What Every Parent Needs to Know About Childhood Development from Birth to Preadolescence*. New York, NY: Harper Collins; 1998.

Spock B, Needlman R. *Dr. Spock's Baby and Child Care*. 9th ed. New York, NY: Simon & Schuster Adult Publishing Group, Pocket Books; 2011.

Webster-Stratton C. *The Incredible Years: A Troubleshooting Guide for Parents of Children Aged 2–8 Years*. Seattle, WA: The Incredible Years; 2005.

FOR PROFESSIONALS

Ding XP, Omrin DS, Evans AD, Fu G, Chen G, Lee K. Elementary school children's cheating behavior and its cognitive correlates. *J Exp Child Psychol*. 2014;121:85-95.

Dixon SD, Stein MT. *Encounters with Children: Pediatric Behavior and Development*. 4th ed. Philadelphia, PA: Mosby Elsevier; 2006.

Evans AD, Lee K. Emergence of lying in very young children. *Dev Psychol*. 2013;49(10):1958-1963.

Odgers CL, Caspi A, Russell MA, Sampson RJ, Arsenault L, Moffitt TE. Supportive parenting mediates widening neighborhood socioeconomic disparities in children's antisocial behavior from ages 5 to 12. *Dev Psychopathol*. 2012;24(3):705-721.

CHAPTER 61

Masturbation

Ilgi Ertem | Bahar Bingoler Pekcici

I. **DESCRIPTION OF THE PROBLEM.** The World Health Organization (WHO) defines sexual health as the "integration of the somatic, emotional, intellectual, and social aspects of sexual being, in ways that are positively enriching and that enhance personality, communication, and love." The clinician should view childhood sexuality as an integral part of child development as are physical health, growth, and other developmental domains. It is within this framework that the clinician should address parental concern with masturbation, one of the early manifestations of the sexual development of the child.

- The term *masturbation* is derived from the Latin words for "hand" (*manus*) and "defilement" (*stupratio*). It is defined as a deliberate self-stimulation that results in sexual arousal.
- At least since the time of Hippocrates (400 BC), masturbation has evoked negative attitudes within societies. For example, during the 18th century, two-thirds of all human illnesses were attributed to masturbation. Various treatment regimens, such as disciplining the patient, mechanical preventions, cautery of genitals, clitorectomy, and castration, were established and practiced until the mid-20th century. It is still true that parents' and teachers' responses to sexual behavior in children are largely influenced by cultural patterns. Some societies condone and encourage self-stimulation during childhood; others condemn it. In general, Western societies take a more restrictive view of masturbation. Childhood masturbation is not included as a specific psychiatric disorder in the *Diagnostic and Statistical Manual of Mental Disorders (5th edition)*. The WHO places excessive childhood masturbation under "Other specified behavioral and emotional disorders with onset usually occurring in childhood and adolescence" in the *International Statistical Classification System of Diseases and Related Health Problems 10th edition (ICD-10)*.

A. **Epidemiology.** Masturbation is universal and may start as early as infancy. Normative studies of sexual behavior have shown that approximately 16% of children aged 2–5 years of both sexes masturbate with their hand, and that almost all boys and 25% of girls have masturbated to the point of orgasm by 15 years of age.

B. **Environmental, developmental, and transactional factors in etiology.** Masturbatory activity has been observed in the male fetus in utero. In the first months of life, infants of both sexes learn to experience the sensations associated with diapering and the cleansing of genitals. A developmental progression toward adult erotic responsiveness proceeds from these early pleasurable sensations. This includes the differentiation and appreciation of genitals, inclusion of sexual parts in the body concept, "exhibitionism" to test adult reactions, mastery of a variety of self-elicited sensations, and the integration of sexual function into the emerging self-concept.

C. **Signs and symptoms.** Masturbatory activity in older children may resemble that of adults and involves handling or rubbing of genitals, sweating, flushing, tachypnea, and muscular contractions. Masturbatory activity in infants and toddlers typically does not involve handling of the genitals and may therefore make the diagnosis difficult. More typically masturbation in infants involves stereotyped posturing of the lower extremities; pressing and rubbing on the perineum or suprapubic area; leaning the suprapubic region on a firm edge; stiffening of the lower extremities; rocking movements in various positions; and symptoms of sexual arousal including sweating, brief bouts of crying, intermittent grunting, irregular breathing, facial flushing, and diaphoresis. These episodes may last from a few seconds to several hours. At any age, there should be no alteration of consciousness; the child should stop when distracted.

II. **MAKING THE DIAGNOSIS**

A. **Differential diagnosis**

1. **Masturbatory actions may be misdiagnosed as seizures** because of the abrupt onset of the episodes, the tonic posturing, facial flushing, irregular breathing, and the child's preoccupation. During masturbation, there may also be blank stares or tremulous movements. The child may resume his or her previous play or activity

after the event or may appear drowsy and fall asleep, mimicking children in the postictal phase. Tonic posturing with crossing of the thighs has been reported to occur as early as 3 months of age. Masturbatory activity in children has been associated with unnecessary investigations for organic disease such as seizures, epilepsy, paroxysmal dystonia, carcinoid syndrome, or urinary tract infections. The symptoms of masturbation also have been confused with abdominal pain or the "retentive" posturing that occurs in children who withhold stool. This is manifested as episodic tightening of the buttock and thighs, often accompanied by facial flushing and grunting.

   2. **The clinician should consider the diagnosis of sexual abuse** in children with compulsive masturbation, especially if accompanied by other sexualized behaviors. The term compulsive or excessive masturbation has not been well defined. The following uncommon sexualized behaviors should alert the clinician to the possibility of sexual abuse: obsessive masturbation with or without pleasure and with decreased interest in other activities, masturbation causing pain, using objects against own or other child's genitals/anus, attempting to make an adult touch the child's genitals or touching a child/adult's genitals using hand or mouth, inserting tongue in mouth when kissing.

B. **History: key clinical questions.** A thorough history is the key to an appropriate diagnosis and effective management. Because masturbation is not harmful, it should be considered a problem only when it causes distress to the child, parental anxiety, or social condemnation.

   1. *"Tell me what you've noticed about your child's touching his or her genitals. Where does this happen? In school? At home?"* This elicits the method the child uses and the frequency and the context in which the child engages in masturbation and other sexualized behaviors.

   2. Parents have different thoughts and feelings when their children touch their own genitals. *"Can you tell me how it is for you? What do you do when this happens?"* The meaning of masturbatory behavior to the parents and their responses to the behavior should be understood.

   3. *"When you respond like that, how do you think he or she feels?"* The parents' perceptions of the consequences of their responses and the outcome of the behavior are important.

   4. Are there any significant stressors for family and/or child, and/or developmental delays?

C. **Physical examination.** Clinical circumstances may dictate exploration of a more pathologic interpretation of the masturbatory behaviors. It should be noted that masturbation and physical illness can co-occur. Masturbation may begin with genital irritation or discomfort due to rashes, diaper dermatitis, urinary tract or parasitic infections. If the behavior is especially compulsive or of acute onset, consider the possibility of sexual abuse. A child who has been sexually abused may have physical findings suggestive of or consistent with genital trauma. Also, children may insert objects in their genitalia during sex play. Therefore, the anus, genitalia, and perineum should be examined as part of a general physical examination.

D. **Tests.** Laboratory tests are almost never required during a workup for masturbation. However, causes of irritation such as pinworm infestations or urinary tract infections will require appropriate diagnosis and treatment. Home-video recordings have been shown to be effective in the evaluation of paroxysmal events in children. The widespread availability of home-video recordings may provide the opportunity to examine in detail the child's activity and may prevent the use of unnecessary investigations and referrals.

III. **MANAGEMENT**

A. **Anticipatory guidance.** A clinician who, from the beginning of a relationship with parents, is open to discussing issues of sexuality is more likely to receive questions about sexual development, behaviors, and problems as the child grows older. Parents are less likely to be anxious, confused, or scornful of masturbatory behavior in their child if they have been told in advance that this behavior is normal, universal, and healthy. Such anticipatory guidance should be offered early in life, when infants begin to explore their bodies. During a review of developmental milestones or during a genital examination, parents can be asked in a matter-of-fact manner whether their child has discovered his or her genitals and whether he or she plays with them. Parental feelings and attitudes can then be explored and information on how they would react to the situation can be obtained.

B. **When masturbation is viewed as a problem behavior**
- The clinician should not simply dismiss parental concerns about the issue by flatly stating that "masturbation is normal." Rather he or she should attempt to understand the level of parental discomfort and the social and psychological consequences of the behavior for the child, with the goals of alleviating parental anxiety and diminishing feelings of fear, anxiety, guilt, and shame in the child.
- A detailed history will not only establish the diagnosis but also give the parents a chance to discuss their fears and worries. Examples of parental concerns include the fear that their child has an organic disease, has been sexually abused, is experiencing conflict with a family member or teacher/caretaker, will develop promiscuity, or will be mentally handicapped. The masturbatory behavior may evoke a parent's own conflicts about sexuality, and the parent may withdraw attention and/or affection from the child. In the majority of cases, after such concerns and attitudes are explored, reassurance will be sufficient.
- Parents should be advised not to overreact to the child's behavior. It should be emphasized that punishing and scolding can be harmful to the child's self-esteem and long-term sexual development.
- Parents can tell their preschool child that masturbation is a private behavior that is best not done in public (e.g., *"There are some things that we do around other people. This is one of the things that we do in private"*).
- Behavioral modification techniques, such as positive reinforcement, have been helpful in cases of compulsive masturbation (especially in children with mental retardation).

C. **Criteria for referral.** Refer to developmental and behavioral pediatric specialist if:
- appropriate counseling by the clinician elicits complaints by the parents that the **child is in psychologic distress;**
- **unusual manifestations or excessive masturbation impedes self-esteem** and adaptive functioning of the child and/or cause social problems;
- **other family or interpersonal pathology** is recognized by the clinician to contribute to the problem;
- there are accompanying **developmental/behavioral or affective disturbances** in the child.

  Refer to child neurology specialist if: history or physical examination indicates diagnostic workup for seizures or paroxysmal movement disorders.

  Refer to child abuse specialist if: history or physical examination indicates diagnostic workup for child abuse.

Bibliography

FOR PARENTS

American Academy of Pediatrics. https://www.healthychildren.org/English/ages-stages/preschool/Pages/Talking-to-Your-Young-Child-About-Sex.aspx.

University of Michigan, C.S. Mott Children's Hospital. Your Child-Parenting Guides and Resources. https://www.mottchildren.org/posts/your-child/masturbation-and-young-children.

FOR PROFESSIONALS

Friedrich WN, Grambsch P, Broughton D, et al. Normative sexual behavior in children. *Pediatrics.* 1991;88:456-464.

Kellogg ND; the AAP Committee on Child Abuse and Neglect. Clinical report—the evaluation of sexual behaviors in children. *Pediatrics.* 2009;124:992-998.

Mallants C, Casteels K. Practical approach to childhood masturbation—a review. *Eur J Pediatr.* 2008;167:1111-1117.

Martin KA. Making sense of children's sexual behavior in child care: an analysis of adult responses in special investigation reports. *Child Abuse Negl.* 2014;38(10):1636-1646.

Strachan E, Staples B. Masturbation. *Pediatr Rev.* 2012;33(4):190-191.

CHAPTER **62**

Digital Media

Jenny S. Radesky

I. DESCRIPTION OF THE ISSUE. Digital media such as TV, videos, computers, video games, the Internet, social media, and mobile devices (e.g., smartphones, tablets, and their applications, "apps") have exhibited their fastest evolution over the past 10 years, since the introduction of the iPhone in 2007. The idea of "screen time" has become outdated as screen-based activities vary from Skyping to taking photos to first-person shooter games, and new technologies such as virtual assistants and virtual reality are introduced. Pediatric providers can assume that the majority of their patients regularly use digital media: studies have shown that over 90% of 1-year-olds have used a mobile device, approximately 75% of teenagers own a smartphone, 24% of which describe themselves as "constantly connected" to the Internet, and 50% feeling "addicted" to their phones. The increasing mobility, individualization, ease of access, and gamification of child play and social connection have completely changed the ways in which children interact with computers and media and at the same time make it more difficult for parents to keep track of what media children are using. This poses challenges for maintaining balance between the healthy behaviors and routines known to protect child health, and the potential risks and benefits of plugged-in time.

Here are some overarching concepts to keep in mind when discussing media use with families:

- Digital media and technological change are at sometimes polarizing topics, about which parents often feel judged. Keep conversation family-centered by asking about the particular ways each family uses media and how it fits into their child-rearing goals and value systems. By acknowledging how challenging it is for any adult to keep up with the new forms of media being constantly introduced, providers can normalize the "overwhelm" that many parents feel.
- Media plays many important functions in families: keeping children busy and calm, providing entertainment or knowledge, being a stress reliever, or a source of social support. If providers and families want to change media habits, other behaviors that serve these same functions will need to be adopted.
- Parent technology use should be part of the conversation. Unplugged time recommendations apply to all household members, and children learn a lot through parental role modeling of healthy (or maladaptive) media habits.
- Media is thought to influence children's health and development through many mechanisms, including (1) social learning (e.g., observing and copying); (2) acting as a "superpeer" that inflates the importance of certain values or behaviors; (3) as a direct source of information (or misinformation on the Internet); (4) and through distraction from (e.g., multitasking during homework) or displacement of other important activities (e.g., sleep, play, physical activity, mealtime conversation). It is crucial for children to build awareness of how media influences them, and to learn how to use media as a tool that suits their values and goals rather than feel controlled by it.

II. AREAS OF CONCERN. Parents are not always familiar with the following areas of concern, which may act as helpful talking points when trying to motivate media habit changes.

A. Early childhood development. Infants and toddlers watch about 1 hour/day of media, although lower-income infants/toddlers watch, on average, 2 or more hours/day. Most toddlers have used a mobile device, and a study from a low-income clinic showed that 75% of preschoolers owned their own tablet. Heavy or inappropriate (i.e., adult-oriented, violent) media use in early childhood has been linked with language delays, behavioral problems, executive functioning deficits, and poor school readiness. This may be due to decreases in parent–child interaction that occur during media use (even background TV), poorer sleep, and less reading and play—the primary means by which children's brains are wired to learn at these ages.

It is important to counsel parents that, although touch screens and interactive apps are marketed as "educational," the vast majority of children's apps are not evidence-based, teach only basic skills, and have no input from developmental experts. Moreover, the interactive features and "bells and whistles" of interactive media may distract children from the educational content and don't challenge children to use their executive functions of planning and carrying out tasks. Although children may appear highly focused on apps and touch screens, it's the interactive features that are doing the work of sustaining the child's attention, not the child's brain.

B. Violence. Violence and aggression—often in humorous or fantasy contexts—are extremely common in children's programming. Graphic and gratuitous violence is frequently found in video games, to which younger children now have access through YouTube gamer videos. Dozens of studies have found links between media violence exposure and child externalizing behavior, aggression, desensitization, and lower empathy. One randomized controlled trial found that preschoolers whose media content was changed from fantasy violence (e.g., *Power Rangers*) to prosocial, educational programming (e.g., *Arthur, Sesame Street)* showed significant improvements in social and emotional skills. Thus, changing content may be a more actionable step for many families, and the Common Sense Media Web site is a good guide for finding replacement content.

Exposure to real-life community or worldwide violence through social media, news, or streaming video is a new source of stress for children, which has not been studied. When terrorist attacks or natural disasters occur, the American Academy of Pediatrics (AAP) usually releases guidance for how parents can discuss disturbing content or images children may encounter through media.

C. Commercialism and privacy. An enormous amount of money is spent on advertising to children and teens each year in the United States. Advertising to children younger than 8 years is especially problematic because they do not understand the difference between programming and commercials, or that commercials do not always tell the truth. Children exposed to advertising request more toys, fast food, and junk food. Because mobile advertising (on social media, games, on apps, etc.) is more tailored to the child's prior behavior and embedded within the user interface, it may be more difficult for children to discern from actual content, so parents and teachers may need to pay extra attention to teaching children to recognize when they are being manipulated. Moreover, children don't usually understand digital privacy and are often not aware that their data are being collected and used by Web sites, apps, or tech companies.

D. Obesity. There is very strong evidence of associations between digital media use and overweight/obesity risk, starting at age 2 years. The AAP now recommends a 1-hour limit for entertainment media use for children whose weight status is a concern, based on newer research suggesting the increase in obesity risk starts above 1–1.5 hours/day. It is easier to start such time limits in early childhood, before children become accustomed to several hours of TV or videos per day. Mechanisms include (1) the effects of food advertising; (2) eating with the TV on inhibits satiety cues; and (3) lower sleep duration and quality.

E. Sleep. From infancy to adolescence, media use behaviors are associated with poorer sleep. Infants exposed to TV have a longer sleep latency and shorter sleep duration, particularly with evening exposure. Toddlers and school-aged children who watch media in the evenings or view arousing (e.g., violent) content take longer to fall asleep, have more awakenings, and have shorter overall sleep duration. Tweens and teens having a mobile device in their bedroom and evening media use are associated with the same negative sleep outcomes.

F. High risk behaviors. Children and teens who view media depicting high-risk behaviors such as sex, drinking alcohol, and drug use are significantly more likely to take part in these behaviors. The Internet and social media are a primary means by which teens gather information about sex and other illicit activities, particularly if their parents do not regularly monitor their media use or talk with them about health or social behaviors. For example, teens with eating disorders have access to a wide range of pro-anorexia and pro-bulimia Web sites and social media feeds, where they can learn new ways of hiding their condition or consuming fewer calories.

G. Social media and mental health. The relationship between adolescent mental health and social media use is complicated, which some studies suggest is U-shaped: people with good mental health tend to have moderate amounts of active, positive social media engagement, whereas those with mental health concerns have excessive, negative social media use, or none at all. Although Internet addiction is not recognized by the DSM-5 as an official psychiatric diagnosis (as it is in some Asian countries), most clinicians have encountered older children with problematic media habits, which often co-occur with ADHD, mood disorders, school failure, social difficulties, or circadian rhythm disorders.

In addition, as parents and schools have become more aware of cyberbullying and its impact on teens' mental health, providers may want to discuss it during psychosocial screening at well-child visits. When cyberbullying or problematic media use are identified, parents and adolescents can be directed to the Common Sense Media Web site or https://www.stopbullying.gov/cyberbullying/index.html for additional information and action-oriented resources.

H. Areas of benefit. When discussing media with families, it may be helpful to frame the conversation in terms of using media as a tool, highlighting a few examples of how media has been used in positive ways:

- Starting around age 2.5 years, children can learn literacy, math, science, and social skills from viewing high-quality programming such as Public Broadcasting Service or Sesame Workshop shows, videos, or apps.
- Mobile devices and computers can help support children who learn differently, for example, by providing dictation software or audiobooks for children with dyslexia; visual schedules and organizers for children with autism or ADHD; or story-based social–emotional learning (e.g., *Daniel Tiger's Neighborhood*) for young children with behavioral difficulties.
- When used appropriately, social media can increase adolescents' civic engagement as well as their social connection with other children with similar experiences. For example, children with chronic illnesses such as cystic fibrosis benefit from connecting virtually when they cannot do so in person. LGBTQ (lesbian, gay, bisexual, transgender, and queer) youth who do not have local support groups have also been shown to benefit from social support via social media.
- Emerging research suggests that virtual experiences with people from different backgrounds or viewpoints may increase tolerance.

III. ADVICE AND GUIDANCE FOR FAMILIES

- Rather than using a one-size-fits-all set of media guidance, the AAP recommends that families develop and individualize house rules to meet their distinct needs. Parents who report that they spoke with their child's provider about media are more likely to follow AAP guidelines; unfortunately, only about 20% of US parents do so. These conversations can be supplemented with resources such as Common Sense Media, which is constantly updated to address the changing media landscape.
- Media guidance can be integrated into any anticipatory guidance conversations. To list a few examples, sleep hygiene in infants and toddlers; family meals without the TV on; child development and the range of play opportunities children have; safety (online and while driving); and school (media multitasking during homework, use of iPads in school)—all involve media in some way. Parents report wanting to hear media guidance from early ages, starting in infancy, so that they can be more aware about how to establish healthy media habits.
- When discussing media use with families, pediatric providers can show parents the AAP Family Media Use Plan, which lists a range of different healthy media use behavior choices families can choose for children of different ages. Rather than telling families what not to do, the Media Use Plan asks parents to think about values and health goals—for example, how meals, physical activity, sleep, reading, and parent–child emotional connection fit into the family's typical day—and how to change media use behaviors to meet these goals.
- Creating a Family Media Use Plan emphasizes the importance of managing media proactively, rather than reactively responding to parent stress, child demands or emotional distress, peer pressure, or other family dynamics (not to mention the mobile device notifications and the design features that tend to suck our attention in!).
- When media use has become problematic in childhood or adolescence, encourage parents to:
  - change content to more educational and prosocial content, including PBS/Sesame Workshop for younger children, or recommendations from Common Sense Media for older children;
  - find other activities that are motivating, engaging, or calming for the child, and replace some media time each day with those activities;
  - establish screen-free zones (e.g., bedrooms, car) and times of day (e.g., mealtimes, play time), to be enforced for all family members (including parents, whose role modeling plays an important part);
  - charge all mobile devices in the kitchen or out of bedrooms overnight, and establish a curfew 1 hour before bed;
  - use media together more with children—whether through a family movie night, playing video games, Skyping with family members, or discovering new creative apps or

Web sites. Children learn more from media this way, parents find it easier to monitor what their children are viewing, and resulting conversations about media content help build digital literacy and tech-savviness in children and parents. These conversations also set the stage for children feeling safe coming to their parents to talk about uncomfortable online experiences such as cyberbullying.

- If parents seek ways to track or filter their child's mobile device, Internet, and social media use, Common Sense Media has a helpful guide: https://www.commonsensemedia.org/blog/everything-you-need-to-know-about-parental-controls.
- For older children, providers can screen for problematic Internet use and Internet gaming disorder using validated tools, such as the Internet Gaming Disorder scale (https://www.researchgate.net/publication/270652917_The_Internet_Gaming_Disorder_Scale) and the Problematic and Risky Internet Use Screening Scale (http://mediad.public-broadcasting.net/p/kplu/files/201502/PRIUSS_scale_and_guidelines.pdf).

Bibliography

FOR PROFESSIONALS AND PARENTS

ORGANIZATIONS

American Academy of Pediatrics, Council on Communications and Media. http://cocm.blogspot.com/.

American Academy of Pediatrics, HealthyChildren.org (has many articles for parents about media www.healthychildren.org and the AAP Media Use Plan: https://www.healthychildren.org/English/media/Pages/default.aspx).

Common Sense Media. www.commonsensemedia.org.

Center on Media and Child Health. www.cmch.tv.

Center for Media Literacy. www.medialit.org.

Joan Ganz Cooney Center at Sesame Workshop. http://www.joanganzcooneycenter.org/.

Pew Center for Internet Research. http://www.pewinternet.org/.

PUBLICATIONS

Moreno MA, Jelenchick L, Cox E, Young H, Christakis DA. Problematic internet use among US youth: a systematic review. *Arch Pediatr Adolesc Med*. 2011;165(9):797-805.

Radesky JS, Christakis DA. Increased screen time: implications for early childhood development and behavior. *Pediatr Clin North Am*. 2016;63(5):827-839.

Radesky J, Christakis D, Hill D, et al. Media and young minds. *Pediatrics*. 2016;138(5).

Selkie EM, Fales JL, Moreno MA. Cyberbullying prevalence among US middle and high school–aged adolescents: a systematic review and quality assessment. *J Adolesc Health*. 2016;58(2):125-133.

CHAPTER **63**

Military Families and Deployment

Molinda M. Chartrand

I. DESCRIPTION

A. Military deployment. Deployment is the short-term assignment of military service members to a duty location other than the one to which they are assigned. Deployments may be planned or unexpected, to a combat or noncombat zone, and can last from 1 to 18 months. Typical deployments last 12–15 months. One thing that all deployments have in common is the separation of service members from their family. Both active duty and reserve military members experience deployment. These deployments may have significant repercussions for every member of the military family.

B. Military culture. The military, in the broadest sense, encompasses everyone that wears a military uniform as well as his or her family members. This includes both active duty (full-time) military service members and the reserve/guard component members. In general, the military community tends to be close-knit and supportive. On top of shared day-to-day and life experiences, there are strong core values for each service (Army, Air Force, Navy, and Marines) that help to bring a sense of purpose and meaning through difficult times. Among those are patriotism, duty, honor, and courage.

Military families routinely face many stressors such as frequent moves, separation from extended family support systems, and significant job-related hazards. They are typically resilient to these various challenges. The factors that contribute to military family resilience are not different from those for civilian families; that is, the health, mental health, and functioning of the mother, the father, and the family contribute to the development and well-being of children.

II. DEMOGRAPHICS

A. Active duty members. In 2015, there were 1.3 million active duty military members in the Army, Air Force, Navy, and Marines. They are accompanied by 641,639 spouses and more than 1.0 million children (0–5 years: 42%; 6–11 years: 32%; 12–18 years: 22%). They typically live on or near a military base and have relatively easy access to a wide variety of military support services including family-readiness center, military family life consultants, mental health care providers, spousal support groups, and childcare.

B. Reserve members. In 2015, the reserve component had more than 820 thousand members, 374,000 spouses, and 687,000 children (0–5 years: 30.5%; 6–11 years: 30–9%; 12–18 years: 27.5%). Service members and their families who are serving in the reserves face unique challenges. These "citizen soldiers" are rarely located near a large military base and as a result have limited access to military-specific resources that are related to deployment. These service members and their families often receive their medical care in the civilian community from clinicians who may not be aware of military unique circumstances or the impact of deployments on families.

III. DEPLOYMENT

A. Emotional cycle of deployment. Every family handles deployments differently. For some families, deployment is a part of the "military lifestyle"; they are resilient and able to cope with minor hiccups. For other families, deployment can be a catastrophe. A family's response to deployment can be complicated and is not limited just to the time of separation. The emotional cycle of deployment (Fig. 63-1) is a typical and predictable pattern of emotional response when a military member is deployed. The cycle can provide a guide for intervention. The framework divides deployment into five phases: predeployment, deployment, sustainment, redeployment, and postdeployment. Each stage is characterized by a defined set of emotional changes and different stressors.

- During **predeployment,** the family has been notified that the family member is leaving. Family members may not know where, and it may also be short notice. Accompanied by this notification is an immediate anticipation of loss that is balanced by denial. Military service members often spend long hours away from the family training and getting affairs in order. There can be a mental/physical distancing. Emotional stress may lead to arguments and saying things you wish you had not on the part of everyone.

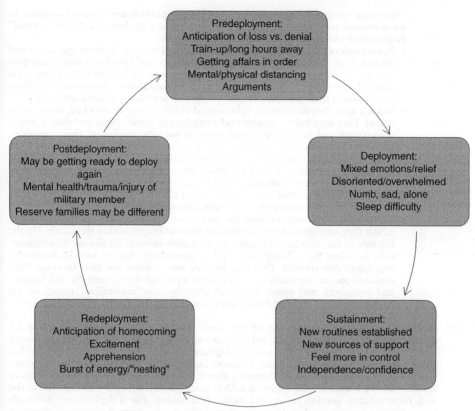

Figure 63-1 The emotional cycle of deployment. Adapted from Logan KL. Emotional cycle of deployment. *Proceedings*. 1987:43-47.

- With **deployment,** there can be mixed emotions, even a sense of relief. The remaining parent can feel overwhelmed with new duties. There may be difficulty with sleep.
- After some time, the family members enter the **sustainment** phase. They settle into new routines, and new sources of support are found (may be more difficult for reserve families). There also may be a sense of independence and confidence.
- With **redeployment** home of the service member, the anticipation of homecoming is a new emotional whirlwind: excitement, apprehension.
- Finally, the member has returned home in the **postdeployment phase:** There is the joy of having him or her home safe and sound, but there is a loss of independence, disruption of routines, and the challenge of reintegrating the military member back into the family. Because of the recent trend toward back-to-back deployments, some have begun to speak of deployment as a "spiral" rather than a "cycle" because there is never a return to normal life.
    B. **Risk factors during deployment.** Research conducted during the first Gulf War and the current conflicts has identified certain characteristics that can place a family at greater risk for adverse response to deployment. They are as follows:
    - Young and recently married (<5 years), lower-ranking soldier families
    - Younger children (<5 years old)
    - Families that have experienced multiple deployments
    - Families with prior mental health stresses and families that were not functioning well before deployment for any reason
    - Reserve/guard families
        1. **Typical child responses during deployment.** In general, children take their emotional cues from their parents. If their parent is anxious, irritable, or frightened, young children will respond and mirror these emotions. Children cope best when the adults in their life can be supportive and available. All family members will

experience emotions during the cycles of deployment that are a normal response to an abnormal situation that is unique to the military deployment. Some "normal" responses of children to deployment are as follows:

- **Preschoolers.** They may be clingy and irritable. They may be more aggressive and act out. They may have more somatic complaints and have fears about their parents or others leaving. They may also seem to regress behaviorally—potty accidents, thumb-sucking, baby talk, or refusing to sleep alone. When service members return home, their preschooler may be shy and fearful or talkative and clingy.
- **School age.** Despite support, school-aged children may be shocked, angry, or in denial. They may have a greater understanding of world events and their military parent's job and so may be fearful for their parent's well-being. These emotions may manifest with angry outburst, lots of "what if" types of questions, and limit testing. Sleep disturbances are common. Children of reserve/guard families may have a sense of isolation and loneliness because they may be the only child in their neighborhood/community who is experiencing a deployment. When the service member returns home, school-aged children will be excited and crave their parent's attention or they may still have some anger at being left.
- **Teenagers.** For teenagers, deployment can be a time of personal growth during which they take on additional roles and responsibilities within the family. On the flip side, it can also be a difficult time that adds stress to an already developmentally turbulent time. Teens may become emotionally distant, moody, depressed, angry, and disrespectful. They may become very worried and anxious about their deployed parent, especially in the setting of a combat deployment. School, friends, and homework may suffer. Teens can often become "parentified," taking on the deployed parent's roles and responsibilities, which can create a challenging transition at homecoming.

IV. **EPIDEMIOLOGY.** Since the start of the conflicts in Iraq and Afghanistan, almost 2.5 million military members have served at least one deployment, with 34% having served more than one deployment. The wars in Afghanistan and Iraq are the longest combat operations since Vietnam War. Many stressors face these Operation Enduring Freedom/Operation Iraqi Freedom troops. Currently, almost 2 million children are living in military families during a time of war. A pivotal RAND study published in 2016 found that, in the end, most military families return to baseline functioning after a deployment. Although most military families and children weather deployments, some detrimental effects of military deployments are as follows.

A. **Impact on military members**
- Since 2003, tens of thousands of service members have been injured, and thousands have died in military service.
- Early in the current conflicts, one in five service members met screening criteria for posttraumatic stress disorder (PTSD) 1 year after return, and injured soldiers have higher rates. More soldiers screen positive for PTSD at 7 months than at 1 month, indicating that the posttraumatic effects may be delayed.
- As troops have experienced more repeated deployments and predeployment preparation activities, there is no overall significant effect of deployment on psychological or behavioral outcomes for service members. However, deployed service members who experienced deployment trauma did show a persistent increase in their depression, PTSD, and anxiety symptoms relative to their predeployment levels.
- Estimates of depression in returning troops vary widely but range from 3% to 25%. National Guard members and Reservists screen positive for mental health concerns at slightly higher rates than active duty members.

B. **Impact on the military spouse.** Military spouses are more likely to experience depression during a spousal deployment as well as lower marital satisfaction and the perception of less social support than civilian wives.

When husband and wife perceive an upcoming deployment in positive terms, spousal relationships are also more positive.

Couples report less marital satisfaction.

Social support predicts a positive mental health outcome for wives and children of deployed fathers.

When a service member experienced physical trauma during deployment, spouses showed persistent increase in depression, PTSD, and anxiety symptoms.

C. **Impact on children in military families.** Children with a deployed father are at risk for the following:
- More behavioral problems.
- Higher levels of depression and anxiety.

- Twofold increase in rates of child neglect during combat deployments.
- Negative effects on social–emotional function at school.
- In adolescent boys, longer deployments (>180 days in the past 3 years) are associated with decreased academic performance, independence, and responsibility.

    Adolescents with a deployed parent had higher heart rates, systolic blood pressures, and higher self-perceived stress.

    Approximately 30,000 United States children have experienced the return of an injured parent or the death of a parent. The impact of living with a parent who may be suffering with PTSD, other mental health disorder, or significant physical injury is unclear.

V. SUPPORTING MILITARY FAMILIES. The most important step in supporting military families is identifying them in your practice. Screen your families for military involvement and deployment history. Some questions that will help you support military families are as follows.

A. If you have a military family in your practice:
- Active duty or reserve component?
- Where is the family in the "cycle of deployment"?
- Ask about possibility of deployment.
- Obtain a deployment history—how many previous deployments have happened, how did the family function? What was easy and what was hard?
- Screen for predeployment risk factors.

B. If a family member is deployed:
- Ask about his or her job, where is he or she, how often he or she is able to communicate?
- Are there worries about the service member's safety?
- How are the nondeployed spouse and the children doing? Screen for typical responses to deployment and provide reassurance when typical responses occur.
- Is there support in the area—families, friends, community, and military base? Become knowledgeable about available community resources.

C. If a family member has been deployed and has returned:
- Ask about the reunification adjustment, how is everyone reconnecting?
- How is the service member doing? Any concerning behaviors?

D. Provide routine support for military families that are doing well. Make them aware of available resources. If a child is having extremely disruptive behaviors, the symptoms last longer than 2 weeks, or threats of injury to themselves or others occur, a referral for mental health care provider is warranted.

Bibliography

FOR PARENTS

Military Child Education Coalition. www.militarychild.org. The Military Child Education Coalition is a nonprofit organization that identifies the challenges facing the highly mobile military child, increases awareness of these challenges in military and educational communities, and initiates and implements programs to meet these challenges.

Military One Source. http://www.militaryonesource.mil/ or call 1800-342-9647. Military One Source is provided by the Department of Defense at no cost to active duty, guard, and reserve (regardless of activation status) and their families to help with childcare, personal finance, emotional support during deployments, relocation information, and resources needed for special circumstances. The service is available by phone, online, and face-to-face through private counseling sessions in the local community. Highly qualified, master's degree–prepared consultants provide the service.

NMFA—Operation Purple Camps. http://www.militaryfamily.org/kids-operation-purple/camps/. The goal of these free summer camps is to bring together youth who are experiencing some stage of a deployment and the stress that goes along with it. Operation Purple camps give children the coping skills and support networks of peers to better handle life's ups and downs.

Talk Listen Connect. http://www.sesameworkshop.org/what-we-do/our-initiatives/military-families/. Talk, Listen, Connect is a multiphase, bilingual, multimedia initiative that guides families through multiple challenges, such as deployments, homecomings, and changes that occur when a parent comes home.

Tragedy Assistance Program for Survivors. www.taps.org or call 800-959-TAPS. The Tragedy Assistance Program for Survivors, Inc. is a nonprofit Veteran Service Organization offering hope, healing, comfort, and care to thousands of American armed forces families each year who experience the death of a loved one.

Zero to Three—Coming Together Around Military Families. https://www.zerotothree.org/our-work/military-family-projects. Military Projects at Zero to Three has launched Coming Together

Around Military Families, a program aimed at strengthening the resilience of young children and their families who are experiencing deployment and separation.

FOR KIDS

Ferguson-Cohen M. *Daddy, You're My Hero! Mommy, You're My Hero!* 2005. (For kids ages 4–8)

La Greca AM, Sevin SW, Sevin EL. Helping Children Cope with the Challenges of War and Terrorism. (Kids ages 7–12). 7–Dippity. Entire Book is available for download: www.7-dippity.com/other/UWA_war_book.pdf Supplement (for using with school classes or groups): www.7-dippity.com/other/Supplement.pdf.

Robertson R. *Deployment Journal for Kids*. St. Paul, MN: Elva Resa Publishers; 2005.

Spinelli E, Graef R. *While You Are Away*. New York, NY: Hyperion Books for Children; 2004. [Picture book for children whose parents are deployed; ages 4–8]

FOR TEENS

Sherman MD, Sherman DM. My Story: Blogs by Four Military Teens is a series of blogs by four military teens that highlights their feelings and experiences before, during, and after parental deployment. www.seedsofhopebooks.com.

FOR PROFESSIONALS

American Academy of Pediatrics (AAP) Deployment and Military Medical Home Resources site. https://www.aap.org/en-us/advocacy-and-policy/aap-health-initiatives/Pages/Deployment-and-Military.aspx.

Caring for America's children military youth in a time of war. *Pediatr Rev*. 2009;30:e42-e48.

Meadows SO, Tanielian T, Karney B, et al. *The Deployment Life Study: Longitudinal Analysis of Military Families Across the Deployment Cycle*. Santa Monica, CA: RAND Corporation; 2016. https://www.rand.org/pubs/research_reports/RR1388.html. Also available in print form.

Nicosia N, Wong E, Shier V, Massachi S, Datar A. Parental deployment, adolescent academic and social-behavioral maladjustment, and parental psychological well-being in military families. *Public Health Rep*. 2017;132(1):93-105.

Zero to Three—Coming Together Around Military Families. https://www.zerotothree.org/our-work/military-family-projects.

CHAPTER 64

Motor Delays

Ana Carolina Sanchez | Peter A. Blasco

I. DESCRIPTION OF THE PROBLEM. Delayed motor milestones are the highest-ranked concern of parents with children aged between 6 and 12 months. Related complaints include vague references to tone abnormalities ("too stiff" or "too weak"), perceived structural abnormalities (most commonly the legs or feet), or an awkward/clumsy gait in the ambulating child. Early identification of motor delays is crucial to allow prompt referral for appropriate developmental interventions, diagnostic evaluations, and management. In some cases, the early initiation of treatment can slow down disease progression and improve outcome.

A. Epidemiology
- The prevalence of significant motor delays in the general pediatric population is not established. By statistical definition, 2%–3% of infants will fall outside the range of normal motor milestone attainment. A minority of these milestone-delayed children (15%–20%) will prove to have a significant neuromotor diagnosis, most commonly cerebral palsy or a birth defect, rarely some progressive nervous system or muscle disease.
- Early motor delays in the remainder of children often represent a marker for subtle neurologic dysfunction, which manifests itself more definitively in later childhood as troublesome awkwardness (now referred to diagnostically as *developmental coordination disorder*), attention deficit syndromes, and/or specific learning disabilities.

II. MAKING THE DIAGNOSIS
A. Evaluation. The clinician should organize data gathered from the history, physical examination, and neurodevelopmental examination into three domains: motor developmental milestones, the classic neurologic examination, and markers of cerebral neuromotor maturation (primitive reflexes and postural reactions).

1. **Motor milestones** are extracted from the developmental history as well as from observations during the neurodevelopmental examination. As recommended by the AAP policy statement in 2006, all children should receive periodic developmental surveillance at every well-child visit and screening at the 9-, 18-, 30-, or 48-month visit by using a standardized tool.

    At the recommended screening visits the following motor skills should be observed (Tables 64-1 and 64-2). The absence of skills typically acquired at an earlier age signifies delay.

2. **Neurologic examination.** Motor milestones are purely measures of function and do not consider the *quality* of a child's movement. The motor portion of the **neurologic examination** includes assessments of tone (passive resistance), strength (active resistance), deep tendon reflexes, and coordination plus observations of station and gait. The best clues often come from observation, not handling.

    a. **Tone.** Spontaneous postures (e.g., frog legs seen with hypotonia or scissoring with spasticity) provide visual clues to tone abnormalities.

    b. **Strength.** Spontaneous or prompted motor activities (e.g., weight bearing in sitting or standing) require adequate strength. A classic example is the Gower sign (arising from floor sitting to standing using the hands to "walk up" one's legs), which indicates pelvic girdle and quadriceps muscular weakness.

    c. **Station** refers to the posture assumed in sitting or standing and should be viewed from anterior, lateral, and posterior perspectives, looking for body alignment.

    d. **Gait** refers to walking and is examined in progress. Initially, the toddler walks on a wide base, slightly crouched, with the arms abducted and elevated a bit. Forward progression is more staccato than smooth. Movements gradually become more fluid, the base narrows, and arm swing evolves, leading to an adult pattern of walking by the age of 3 years.

3. **Primitive reflexes** are movement patterns that develop during the last trimester of gestation and gradually disappear between 3 and 6 months after birth. Each requires a specific sensory stimulus to generate the stereotyped motor response.

Table 64-1 • GROSS MOTOR DEVELOPMENT TIMETABLE

Prone	
Head up	1 mo
Chest up	2 mo
Up on elbows	3 mo
Up on hands	4 mo
Rolling	
Front to back	3–5 mo
Back to front	4–5 mo
Sitting	
Sit with support ("tripod" sitting)	5 mo
Sit without support	7 mo
Get up to sit (unassisted)	8 mo
Walking	
Pull to stand	8–9 mo
Cruise	9–10 mo
Walk with two hands held	10 mo
Walk with one hand held	11 mo
Walk alone	12 mo
Run (stiff-legged)	15 mo
Walk up stairs (with rail)	21 mo
Jump in place	24 mo
Pedal tricycle	30 mo
Walk up stairs, alternating feet Broad jumps	3 y
Walks up and down stairs, alternating feet Hops on one foot	4 y
Skips by alternating feet Tandem walks backward	5 y
Rides a bicycle	6 y

The Moro, tonic labyrinthine, asymmetric tonic neck, and positive support reflexes are the most clinically useful. Normal babies and infants demonstrate these postures inconsistently and transiently, whereas those with neurologic dysfunction show stronger and more sustained primitive reflex posturing. Although primitive reflexes are somewhat tricky to gauge, even in expert hands, the clinician should keep attuned to the following four factors:

  a. **Some form of primitive reflex response** should be clearly elicitable in the newborn through ages 2–3 months.
  b. **Symmetry of response** is important, especially with the Moro.
  c. **An obligatory primitive reflex is abnormal at any time.** This is the situation where the child remains "stuck" in the primitive reflex posture as long as the stimulus is imposed and breaks free only when the stimulus is removed.
  d. Visible primitive reflexes **should no longer be present after ages 6–8 months.**
4. **Postural reactions** consist of countermovements, which are much less stereotyped than the primitive reflexes and involve a complex interplay of cerebral and cerebellar cortical adjustments to a barrage of proprioceptive, visual, and vestibular sensory inputs. They are not present at birth but sequentially develop between ages 2 and 10 months. Postural reactions are sought in each of the three major categories: righting, protection, and equilibrium. Although easy to elicit in the normal infant, they are markedly slower in their appearance in the baby with nervous system injury.

Red flag findings in the evaluation of a child with neuromotor delay warrant expedited referral or close observation with a time-definite follow-up plan. Red flags needing prompt referral include elevated creatine kinase levels greater than three times normal values in boys and girls (myopathy), fasciculations (lower motor neuron disorder), dysmorphism, organomegaly, signs of heart failure, joint contracture (glycogen storage disease), abnormalities on brain MRI (neurosurgery

Table 64-2 • FINE MOTOR DEVELOPMENT TIMETABLE

Retain ring (rattle)	1 mo
Hands unfisted	3 mo
Reach	3–4 mo
Hands to midline	3–4 mo
Transfer	5 mo
Takes a 1-inch cube	5–6 mo
Takes pellet (crude grasp)	6–7 mo
Immature pincer	7–8 mo
Mature pincer	10 mo
Release	12 mo
Scribbles Drinks from a cup	15 mo
Tower of four cubes Feeds self with spoon	18 mo
Tower of six cubes Turns pages of a book Removes clothing	24 mo
Tower of eight cubes Imitates vertical stroke with crayon Copies a circle	36 mo
Copies a cross Draws an individual with four body parts	48 mo
Copies a square Draws an individual with six body parts Tripod pencil grasp Print letters	60 mo

consultation), respiratory insufficiency or generalized weakness due to risk of respiratory failure, loss of motor milestones (neurodegenerative disorder), and motor delays present during minor acute illness (mitochondrial disorders).

B. Classification of motor impairments

1. **Static central nervous system (CNS) disorders** indicate some type of nonprogressive brain damage. The insult may have arisen during early fetal development, resulting in a CNS anomaly. Alternatively, a brain developing in a normal fashion can be damaged before, during, or after birth by a wide variety of infectious, traumatic, and other insults. When a motor impairment is due to a brain anomaly or a static lesion that occurs before cerebral maturation is complete (roughly age 16 years), the neuromotor disorder is referred to as *cerebral palsy*. This group represents the largest number of children with disabling motor problems.

2. **Progressive diseases** of the brain, spinal cord, peripheral nerves, or muscles produce motor impairment that worsens with time (e.g., Duchenne muscular dystrophy, Werdnig–Hoffman spinal muscular atrophy, nervous system tumors). Children with progressive conditions initially experience a period of normal or near-normal development. Evidence of a progressive disease is determined by careful history and/or by repeated examinations over time. The fraction of all motor-impaired children with progressive diseases is small. Uncovering the specific diagnosis helps one anticipate the rate of progression, provides other prognostic information, and forms the basis for accurate genetic counseling.

3. **Spinal cord and peripheral nerve disorders** are almost all static conditions. The exceptions are rare instances of an intrinsic spinal cord tumor, progressive extrinsic compression syndromes, and rare neurogenetic degenerations primarily involving spinal cord tracts or peripheral nerves (e.g., the *hereditary motor and sensory neuropathies*). The largest single group in this category consists of children with myelodysplasia.

4. **Structural defects** refer to conditions in which an anatomical structure is missing or deformed (e.g., a limb deficiency) or in which the support tissues for nerves and muscles are inadequate (e.g., connective tissue defects, abnormal bones). On the mildest end of the spectrum, there exist a wide variety of fairly common orthopedic deformities, which may or may not affect early motor milestones (club feet, developmental hip dysplasia, etc.). More severe disorders in this category include osteogenesis imperfecta and some varieties of childhood arthritis.

III. **MANAGEMENT.** Ensuring an accurate primary diagnosis is fundamental to determining therapy. Neuroimaging, other neurodiagnostic studies, and/or metabolic and genetic tests may be needed. Direct treatment for the child with a motor disability falls into five categories: (1) counseling and support for the child and family, (2) hands-on therapy, (3) assistive devices, (4) medication, and (5) surgery. A multidisciplinary subspecialty team should be consulted to provide state-of-the-art diagnostic evaluation, treatment services, and counseling. Professionals skilled in different disciplines need to work together and *in concert with the parents.* The primary clinician's roles include seeing to the patient's general health, monitoring overall development, helping the child and family to cope with many stresses (especially at anniversary and transition times), promoting the child's self-esteem and long-term adaptation to disability, and helping parents keep the multitude of subspecialty inputs in perspective.

Bibliography

FOR PARENTS

Geralis E. *Children With Cerebral Palsy: A Parent's Guide*. 2nd ed. Bethesda, MD: Woodbine House; 1998.

FOR PROFESSIONALS PUBLICATIONS

Nortitz GH, Murphy NA; Neuromotor Screening Expert Panel. Motor delays: early identification and evaluation. *Pediatrics*. 2013;131(6). Available from: www.pediatrics.org/cgi/content/full/131/6/e2016.

Rosenbaum PL, Rosenbloom L. *Cerebral Palsy: From Diagnosis to Adult Life*. London: Mac Keith Press; 2012.

WEB SITES

Child Muscle Weakness. childmuscleweakness.org.

Exceptional Parent. www.eParent.com.

Muscular Dystrophy-Diagnosis tools. https://www.cdc.gov/ncbddd/musculardystrophy/diagnostic-tool.html.

Pathways Awareness Foundation. www.pathwaysawareness.org.

Physical Developmental Delay: What to Look For. http://motordelay.aap.org.

CHAPTER 65

Neglect

Howard Dubowitz

I. **DESCRIPTION OF THE PROBLEM.** Child neglect is usually defined as **parental omissions in care, resulting in actual or potential harm to a child**. Child Protective Services (CPS) typically requires evidence of harm, unless the risks are serious (such as when very young children are left home alone). Some states exclude situations attributed to poverty.

An alternative and broader view of neglect is from a child's perspective, defining neglect as **occurring when a child's basic needs are not adequately met**. Basic needs include adequate health care, food, clothing, shelter, supervision/protection, emotional support, education, and nurturance. However, it is often difficult to establish at what point any of these needs are "adequately" met and thresholds may be rather arbitrary. Usually, the "neglect" label is applied to clearly worrisome circumstances. Less serious circumstances may still require intervention, perhaps without labeling them as "neglect."

There are several advantages to this child-focused definition. It fits with the broad goal of ensuring children's health and safety. It is less blaming and more constructive. It draws attention to other contributors to the problem (discussed later) aside from parents and encourages a broader range of interventions. Clearly, many neglect situations may require intervention (e.g., a child with failure to thrive due to an inadequate diet) but may not warrant or meet criteria for CPS involvement. Practitioners, however, need to be aware of the laws and regulations in their area and factor these into their practice.

A. **Epidemiology.** Neglect is the most common form of child maltreatment, involved in about three-quarters of all cases reported annually to CPS. It was a factor in approximately 80% of the estimated 1670 deaths due to child maltreatment in 2015; 7.3% were due to medical neglect. Because of ambiguity in diagnostic criteria and underreporting, accurate prevalence data are impossible to determine. One study in 2010 identified 30.6 cases of neglect per 1000 (or 2,251,600) children in the US population, but it is likely that these are very conservative estimates, as neglect is a problem that mostly occurs "behind closed doors."

B. **Manifestations of possible neglect.** Aside from direct observation, the possibility of neglect should be considered in the following circumstances, especially if a child is harmed, or at risk of significant harm:
   - Noncompliance (nonadherence) with health care recommendations
   - Delay or failure in obtaining medical, mental health, or dental care
   - Hunger, failure to thrive, and morbid obesity that is not being addressed
   - Drug-exposed newborns and older children
   - Exposure to hazards in the home: ingestions, recurrent injuries, exposure of children with pulmonary disease to second-hand smoke, access to guns, and exposure to intimate partner (or domestic) violence
   - Exposure to hazards outside the home: failure to use car seat belt, and not wearing bike helmet
   - Emotional concerns (e.g., excessive quietness or apathy in a toddler), behavior issues (e.g., withdrawal), learning problems (especially if not being addressed), and extreme risk-taking behavior (*may* reflect inadequate nurturance, affection, or supervision)
   - Poor hygiene
   - Inadequate clothing, given the weather
   - Educational needs not being met
   - Abandonment
   - Homelessness

C. **Etiology.** There are often multiple *and* interacting contributors to child neglect, including the following:
   - *Child*: disability, chronic illness, prematurity, challenging behaviors
   - *Parent:* depression, substance abuse, low IQ, limited nurturing as a child
   - *Family:* intimate partner violence, father uninvolved, many children in the family

- *Community*: social isolation, violence, lack of treatment or support programs, medical professional not adequately explaining treatment plan or missing opportunities to address problems such as parental depression and food insecurity
- *Society:* poverty, lack of health insurance

D. General principles for assessing possible neglect. The heterogeneity of neglect precludes specifying how to assess for the array of possible circumstances. Instead, the following general principles and questions serve as a guide.

- Given the complexity and possible ramifications of determining that a child is being neglected, an interdisciplinary assessment is ideal, including input from professionals involved with the family.
- Verbal children should be separately interviewed, at an appropriate developmental level. Possible questions include: *"Who do you go to if you're feeling sad? Who helps you if you have a problem? What happens when you feel sick?"*
- Do the circumstances indicate that the child's need(s) is not being adequately met? Is there evidence of actual harm? Is there evidence of potential harm and on what basis?
- What is the nature of the neglect?
- Is there a pattern of neglect? Are there indications of other forms of neglect, or abuse? Has there been prior CPS involvement?
- A child's safety is a paramount concern. What is the risk of imminent harm, and of what severity?
- What is contributing to the neglect? Consider factors listed under the section "C. Etiology".
- What strengths/resources are there? This is as important as identifying problems. They are often the hook or handle one has to work with to be effective.
  - Child (e.g., the child wants to play sports, requiring better health)
  - Parent (e.g., the parent wants to keep the child out of the hospital)
  - Family (e.g., other family members willing to help)
  - Professionals (e.g., a caring physician or nurse who conveys interest in helping)
  - Community (e.g., programs for parents, families)
- What interventions have been tried, with what results? Knowing the nature of the interventions can be useful, including from the parent's perspective. What has the pediatric clinician done to address the problem?
- Assess the possibility of other children in the household also being neglected.
- What is the prognosis? Is the family motivated to improve the circumstances and accept help, or resistant? Are suitable resources, formal and informal, available?

E. General principles for addressing child neglect

- Convey concerns to family, kindly but forthrightly. Avoid blaming.
- Be empathic and state interest in helping, or suggest another pediatric clinician.
- Address contributory factors, prioritizing those most important and amenable to being remedied (e.g., recommending treatment for a mother's depression). Parents may need their problems addressed to enable them to adequately care for their children. Parent training programs can be helpful.
- Begin with least intrusive approach, usually not CPS.
- Establish specific objectives (e.g., diabetes will be adequately controlled), with measurable outcomes (e.g., urine dipsticks, hemoglobin A1c). Similarly, advice should be specific and limited to a few reasonable steps. A written and signed contract can be very helpful—a copy for the parent and one for the medical chart.
- Engage the family in developing the plan; solicit their input and agreement.
- Build on strengths; there are always some, providing a valuable way to engage parents who may be reluctant to do so.
- Encourage positive family functioning.
- Be innovative and consider resources, such as using pots and pans for play. Encouraging reading can promote both literacy and intimacy.
- Encourage informal supports (i.e., family, friends; encourage fathers to participate in office visits). This is where most people get their support, not from professionals.
- Consider support available through a family's religious affiliation.
- Consider need for concrete services (e.g., Medical Assistance, Temporary Assistance to Needy Families [TANF], Food Stamps).
- Consider children's specific needs, given what is known about the possible outcomes of neglect. Too often, maltreated children do not receive direct services.
- Be knowledgeable about community resources, and facilitate appropriate referrals.

- Consider the need to involve CPS, particularly when moderate or serious harm is involved and when less intrusive interventions have failed. Present the referral as a necessary effort to clarify what is occurring and what might be needed, and how to help the child and family. Most states have developed an alternative response system—especially for neglect. This approach focuses on supporting families to do better, rather than on investigating what was done wrong. It attempts to be conciliatory and constructive, rather than punitive. Most importantly, it prioritizes the crux of the issue: addressing the needs of children and families.
- Provide support, follow up, review of progress, and adjust the plan if needed.
- Recognize that neglect often requires long-term intervention with ongoing support and monitoring.
- Try ensuring continuity of care as the primary health care provider.

F. Preventing child neglect: a role for pediatric clinicians. Instead of addressing the consequences of child neglect, it would be far preferable to help prevent the problem. There are several ways that clinicians can do so. In addition to helping prevent child neglect and abuse, these strategies can enhance family functioning; support parents; and help promote children's health, development, and safety.

The social history offers an opportunity to learn what is happening within the family and there are brief questionnaires that can screen for specific problems, such as depression, intimate partner violence, and substance abuse. Often these problems are well masked and go undetected. Astute observation is a critical tool, noting the appearance and behavior of parent(s) and child and their interaction. In addition to noting problems (e.g., parent appears high on drugs), efforts should be made to identify strengths. The Safe Environment for Every Kid model is an evidence-based approach for preventing neglect, applicable to pediatric primary care.

For children with chronic diseases, health education and extra support help ensure adequate care. Anticipatory guidance aims to ensure children's safety and well-being. Clinicians' support, monitoring, and counseling are useful ways to help families to take adequate care of their children. Encouraging fathers to come in for routine visits and engaging them may increase their involvement in their children's lives. At times, referrals to other professionals and agencies are necessary; helping a family obtain appropriate services is another valuable role that pediatric clinicians play. At the broader level, advocacy for policies and programs that support families is also important for addressing problems that contribute to the neglect of children.

Bibliography

CDC Preventing Child Abuse and Neglect. https://www.cdc.gov/violenceprevention/childabuseand-neglect/index.html.

Dubowitz H. Neglect in children. *Pediatr Ann.* 2013;42(4):73-77.

Dubowitz H. The safe environment for every kid model: promotion of children's health, development, and safety, and prevention of child neglect. *Pediatr Ann.* 2014;43(11):e271-e277.

Proctor LJ, Dubowitz H. Child neglect: challenges and controversies. In: Korbin J, Krugman R, eds. *Handbook of Child Maltreatment.* New York: Springer Science; 2013.

CHAPTER 66

Night Terrors and Nightmares

Mandeep Rana | Barry Zuckerman

I. DESCRIPTION OF THE PROBLEM. Nightmares and night terrors are the most common physical events or experiences occurring predominantly during sleep and along with other rare events called parasomnias. Parasomnias are classified as (1) non–rapid eye movement (NREM)–related parasomnias, (2) rapid eye movement (REM)–related parasomnias, and (3) other parasomnias.

A. NREM-related parasomnias (also known as disorders of arousal). These complex behaviors occur during partial arousal from slow-wave deep sleep. More often they emerge in first third or first half of typical sleep period, 1–1.5 hours after sleep onset when slow-wave sleep is most prominent. The patient is neither awake nor fully asleep. It may be difficult to awaken the child and, when awakened, is often confused. There is usually no memory for these episodes. Most episodes are brief but may last as long as 30–40 minutes in some children. These may be accompanied by sleep talking and shouting.

1. **Epidemiology.** Most commonly seen in children between 2–12 years. These typically resolve by puberty but may persist in adolescence or adulthood.

   Risk factors include positive family history, sleep deprivation, irregular sleep schedule, illness, fever, stress, anxiety, and sleeping in different environment. Conditions fragmenting sleep, such as sleep apnea and periodic leg movements of sleep (PLMS), may bring on these behaviors.

2. **Clinical subtypes**
   a. **Sleep/night terrors** is the most common NREM parasomnia usually occurring 15–60 minutes after going to sleep, with prevalence of approximately 18%. Children bolt upright from sleep screaming with a glassy-eyed stare, appearing fearful and unresponsive to external stimuli. Running during the event is uncommon. Autonomic features with tachycardia, tachypnea, flushing of skin, mydriasis, and increased muscle tone may occur. These events occur while the child is in NREM sleep and not actually awake. This physical event does not contain any images that accompany nightmares, so there is no description in response to parents' questions about what they are dreaming about. Children remain asleep, or if parents woke them, they easily return to sleep. It is parents who sometimes have trouble returning to sleep because they are upset by the event.
   b. **Sleepwalking.** Prevalence is approximately 7%. It typically begins as a confusional arousal. It can also begin with child immediately leaving bed and walking or even bolting from bed and running. Behaviors can be simple and non–goal-directed or agitated and violent. Ambulation may terminate in parent's bed, couch, or inappropriate places such as closet. They are at risk from falls, lacerations, and even hypothermia.
   c. **Sleep talking**—life time prevalence is 50%. Parents rarely bring this problem to clinicians' attention; many times, it's a source of amusement.
   d. **Confusional arousals**—common in infants and toddlers. It usually starts with some movements, sitting up, moaning, and progressing to crying, often in association with thrashing in the bed or crib. An infant may be described as crying inconsolably and appearing confused, with eyes open or closed. Holding, cuddling, usually do not provide reassurance; instead child often resists and may become more agitated. Parents' inability to comfort their child, who appears to be in great distress, is often a concern to them.

3. **Differential diagnosis**—nightmares, nocturnal panic attacks, nocturnal seizures, hypnic headaches.

4. **Diagnosis is dependent on description of event and history including** how soon after sleep onset it occurred. Occurrence during nap raises suspicion of seizures. Children with frequent NREM parasomnias should be screened for comorbid sleep disorders. Polysomnography should only be performed if there is a suspicion for sleep-disordered breathing, loud snoring, periodic limb movement disorder, or imitating seizure.

Table 66-1 • COMPARISONS OF NIGHTMARES AND NIGHT TERRORS

Characteristic	Night Terror, Sleepwalking, Confusional Arousal	Nightmare
Stage of sleep	NREM—N3 (deep sleep)	REM
Time of sleep period	Usually within first third of night	More common during second half of night
Stereotypy	Low	Low
Amnesia for event	Yes	No
Postevent confusion	Yes	No

5. **Treatment**
   a. The primary goal is to reassure parents regarding the benign and self-limiting nature of these events. Management also involves demystification of disorders of arousal especially differentiating night terrors from nightmares (Table 66-1). Parents often misunderstand the problem and fear that intensity of arousal reflects psychological distress. When parents know that there is nothing wrong with their child, they can usually tolerate periodic episodes.
   b. Child safety is of paramount concern. The child should not sleep on the upper level of bunk bed; obstructions should be removed from the room. For sleepwalking, door gates and high locks may need to be installed on doors and windows, or security system alerting parents that door or window has been opened. For adolescent's impact of alcohol use, sleep restriction and irregular sleep wake schedule should be discussed when they move out of home.
   c. Sleep extension and schedule regularization: scheduled awakening 15–30 minutes before usual time of arousal when events are frequent. The child needs to open his or her eyes and at least mumble a response before being allowed to return to sleep.
   d. Medications: No medications are FDA-approved for treatment of disorders of arousal but if events are frequent or extreme referral to a specialist is indicated for further evaluation and possible medication.
B. **REM-related parasomnias**
   1. **Clinical subtypes. Nightmares** are common, occurring in 60%–75% of children, beginning as young as 2.5 years. Nightmares are vivid dreams with intense feelings of terror that awaken a child from sleep. Children can usually give a detailed description of the dream. These commonly occur in the latter half of the night. While infrequent nightmares are normal, frequent nightmares associated with daytime problems interfering with normal functioning need further evaluation.
   2. **Treatment.** Although children may know that a nightmare is a dream, they remain frightened nevertheless.
      a. Parents need to accept child's fear and not dismiss it as "just bad dream."
      b. Parents should comfort and stay with the child until child's distress has abated.
      c. Most importantly children's fears of nightmares represent magical thinking for young children; it's real. However, children's magical thinking extends to the power of their parents who can reassure their child that wherever the monster is, parents will protect them from the monster hunting them. For children beyond the age of magical thinking usually past 5 years, parents should discuss the nightmares and explain what nightmares are in the comforting light of the day.
C. **Other parasomnias** include sleep enuresis, sleep-related hallucinations, exploding head syndrome, and REM behavior disorder.

Bibliography

FOR PROFESSIONALS

AAP. *Guide to Your Child's Sleep*. Chicago, IL: AAP Press; 2000.

Armstrong KH, Kohler WC, Lilly CM. The young and the restless: a pediatrician's guide to managing sleep problems. *Contemp Pediatr*. 2009;26:28-35.

Laberge L, Tremblay RE, Vitaro F, et al. Development of parasomnias from childhood to early adolescence. *Pediatrics*. 2000;106:67-74.

Leuck L, Buelner M. *My Monster Mama Loves Me So*. New York, NY:Harper Collins; 1999.

Parasomnias. *International Classification of Sleep Disorders*. 3rd ed. Darien, IL: American Academy of Sleep Medicine; 2014:225-278.

Sheldon SH, Ferber R, Kryger MH, Gozal D. *Principles and Practices of Pediatric Sleep Medicine*. 2nd ed. Philadelphia, PA: Elsevier Saunders; 2014.

Zucconi M, Ferini-Strambi L. NREM parasomnias: arousal disorders and differentiation from nocturnal frontal lobe epilepsy. *Clin Neurophysiol*. 2000;111(suppl 2):S129-S135.

FOR PARENTS

Moon R. *Sleep What Every Parent Needs to Know*; 2013.

CHAPTER 67

Oppositional Defiant Disorder

Ross W. Greene

I. DESCRIPTION OF THE PROBLEM. Many children go through phases of varying levels of oppositional behavior, including noncompliance, angry outbursts, arguing, and disobedience. These behaviors are particularly common during the toddler years (when skills such as language and locomotion emerge). Oppositional behavior becomes a concern when it is intense, persistent, and pervasive and when it affects a child's family, social, and/or academic functioning to a significant degree. Pediatric clinicians—who are often the first to hear about a child's oppositional behavior—can play a crucial role in helping caregivers understand and handle such behavior. Assessment of whether a child's behavior meets a diagnostic threshold is not necessarily of paramount importance: If caregivers are concerned by the frequency or severity of a child's oppositional behavior, there is need for additional discussion, information gathering, and possibly help.

Current estimates suggest a prevalence approximating 3% of all children aged 6–18 years, and a lifetime prevalence approximating 10%.

II. DIAGNOSTIC CRITERIA. The *Diagnostic and Statistical Manual of Mental Disorders, Fifth Edition (DSM-5)* provides specific criteria for this diagnosis, which includes at least four symptoms from any of three categories—angry and irritable mood; argumentative and defiant behavior; or vindictiveness—and occurs with at least one individual who is not a sibling. The behavior needs to cause significant problems at work, school, or home and occurs on its own, rather than as part of the course of another mental health problem. The symptoms also must last at least 6 months.

III. DIFFERENTIAL DIAGNOSIS. Although oppositional defiant disorder (ODD) shares a number of characteristics with conduct disorder (CD), ODD can be distinguished from CD by the absence of severe forms of antisocial behavior, such as physical assault, destruction of property, theft, and other serious violations of societal norms. When the youth's pattern of behavior meets the criteria for both ODD and CD, the diagnosis of CD takes precedence. A diagnosis that found its way into the 2013 DSM—disruptive mood dysregulation disorder—also shares a number of characteristics with ODD but appears to represent a more severe variant of oppositional behavior with a stronger mood component.

IV. COMORBIDITY. ODD is a highly comorbid disorder. Research suggests that the vast majority of youth meeting criteria for ODD also meet criteria for at least one comorbid disorder. The most common comorbidities are attention-deficit/hyperactivity disorder (ADHD, characterized by hyperactivity, impulsiveness, and/or inattention), mood disorders (characterized by irritability and depression), anxiety disorders (excessive nervousness and worry, sometimes more generalized and other times in response to specific stimuli), and learning disabilities. Because oppositionality almost always occurs in the context of frustration, it may well be that the characteristics of these other disorders increase the likelihood of oppositional responses. In other words, hyperactivity, impulsiveness, irritability, anxiety, and learning inefficiencies can make it difficult for a child to meet certain expectations (e.g., complying with adult directives, completing homework), thereby increasing the likelihood of an oppositional response.

V. KEY CLINICAL QUESTIONS

- *What expectations is the child having difficulty meeting that precipitate oppositional behavior? Under what conditions do oppositional episodes occur?*
- *If oppositional behavior occurs in the context of completing academic tasks, has there been a formal evaluation of cognitive and academic functioning?*
- *Is the child hyperactive, impulsive, and/or inattentive? Does the child have any difficulty expressing himself/herself in words or understanding what is being said by others? Would you describe the child as cranky, grouchy, grumpy, and/or irritable? Would you describe your child as anxious, nervous, worried, and/or scared? Is your child a very concrete, literal, rigid, inflexible, black-and-white thinker? Does your child have friends? If not, what have you observed about his/her interactions with other kids that may explain this?*
- *What discipline strategies are currently being tried? Are these strategies making things better or worse?*

VI. MANAGEMENT. As noted earlier, pediatric clinicians are often the first to hear of a child's oppositional behavior and can play an essential role in helping caregivers understand such behavior and access clinical resources. It is never sufficient to reassure concerned caregivers that a child will outgrow oppositional behavior, that the oppositional behavior is attributable to a child's gender (boys will be boys), or to place the blame on passive, permissive, inconsistent, noncontingent parenting practices (most parents of oppositional youth have well-behaved siblings). Because of time constraints, medical clinicians often play the crucial role of triaging oppositional behavior and ensuring that parents are pointed in the right direction.

A. Medication. There are no medications to address the specific behaviors associated with ODD. As such, clinical practice guidelines recommend that psychosocial interventions for the child and family are the first-line treatments for ODD. However, there are medications to address some of the disorders and behaviors that are often comorbid with (and may contribute to the development of) ODD. Medications for ADHD, including stimulants (e.g., methylphenidate and amphetamine formulations) and alpha-adrenergic agonists (e.g., clonidine and guanfacine) have been noted to reduce comorbid oppositional behaviors along with the primary symptoms of inattention, hyperactivity, and impulsivity. Medications for depression and anxiety may also reduce the behaviors associated with ODD. Of course, medication cannot be expected to solve many of the problems that may precipitate oppositional episodes.

There are several evidence-based psychosocial treatment approaches for ODD.

B. Parent management training. Parent management training (PMT) is focused primarily on reducing oppositional behavior through use of contingent rewards and punishments and has long been considered the standard of care for ODD. Parents are helped to identify undesirable behaviors (which will be consistently and contingently punished) and desired replacement behaviors (which will be rewarded). This evidence-based intervention helps parents closely monitor a child's behavior through use of a record-keeping system (stickers, points, and the like), which also determines when rewards are dispensed and punishments are administered. Parents receiving PMT also typically receive training in the use of positive attending and time-out procedures.

C. Collaborative and Proactive Solutions. In Collaborative and Proactive Solutions (CPS)—formerly known as Collaborative Problem Solving—parents are helped to focus on identifying and solving the problems that are causing challenging behaviors. Thus, the CPS model is oriented toward the specific *conditions* in which challenging behaviors occur (rather than on the behaviors themselves). Identifying these problems is facilitated by the use of an instrument called the *Assessment of Lagging Skills and Unsolved Problems* (see Fig. 67-1). Unsolved problems are the specific expectations a child is having difficulty meeting reliably. Once the unsolved problems are identified and prioritized and caregivers are viewing the child's difficulties as the by-product of lagging cognitive skills (rather than inept parenting practices or poor motivation), parents and kids are taught and coached to solve problems collaboratively and proactively. This involves three steps: in the Empathy step, caregivers gather information from the child about his or her concern, perspective, or point of view on a given unsolved problem; in the Define Adult Concerns step, caregivers enter their concerns into consideration; and in the Invitation step, kids and caregivers collaborate on solutions that are mutually satisfactory and realistic. CPS is also an evidence-based treatment; research shows that reductions in oppositional behavior through use of CPS is equivalent to reductions found in PMT.

D. Anger management training. Another psychosocial intervention with evidence of effectiveness for the treatment of ODD is anger management training, in which children learn strategies to increase their awareness of feelings (particularly anger) and techniques to express anger in socially appropriate ways.

VII. COURSE OF THE DISORDER. Approximately two-thirds of children with a diagnosis of ODD no longer meet diagnostic criteria for the disorder at 3-year follow-up. This, or course, does not mean that oppositional behavior has completely remitted. Earlier age at onset of oppositional symptoms conveys a poorer prognosis, and preschool children with oppositionality are at greater risk for the development of other psychiatric disorders several years later. An estimated one-third of children with ODD progress to CD; the risk of progression is higher with comorbid ADHD.

If oppositional behavior persists, children are at heightened risk for a wide range of psychiatric disorders in adulthood (e.g., substance abuse, major depression, antisocial

ALSUP ASSESSMENT OF LAGGING SKILLS & UNSOLVED PROBLEMS

Collaborative & Proactive Solutions
THIS IS HOW PROBLEMS GET SOLVED

CHILD'S NAME _____   DATE _____

INSTRUCTIONS: The ALSUP is intended for use as a discussion guide rather than as a freestanding check-list or rating scale. It should be used to identify specific lagging skills and unsolved problems that pertain to a particular child or adolescent.

If a lagging skill applies, check it off and then (before moving on to the next lagging skill) identify the specific expectations the child is having difficulty meeting in association with that lagging skill (unsolved problems). A non-exhaustive list of sample unsolved problems is shown at the bottom of the page.

LAGGING SKILLS	UNSOLVED PROBLEMS
❑ Difficulty handling transitions, shifting from one mindset or task to another	
❑ Difficulty doing things in a logical sequence or prescribed order	
❑ Difficulty persisting on challenging or tedious tasks	
❑ Poor sense of time	
❑ Difficulty maintaining focus	
❑ Difficulty considering the likely outcomes or consequences of actions (impulsive)	
❑ Difficulty considering a range of solutions to a problem	
❑ Difficulty expressing concerns, needs, or thoughts in words	
❑ Difficulty managing emotional response to frustration so as to think rationally	
❑ Chronic irritability and/or anxiety significantly impede capacity for problem-solving or heighten frustration	
❑ Difficulty seeing "grays"/concrete, literal, black & white, thinking	
❑ Difficulty deviating from rules, routine	
❑ Difficulty handling unpredictability, ambiguity, uncertainty, novelty	
❑ Difficulty shifting from original idea, plan, or solution	
❑ Difficulty taking into account situational factors that would suggest the need to adjust a plan of action	
❑ Inflexible, inaccurate interpretations/cognitive distortions or biases (e.g., "Everyone's out to get me," "Nobody likes me," "You always blame me, "It's not fair," "I'm stupid")	
❑ Difficulty attending to or accurately interpreting social cues/ poor perception of social nuances	
❑ Difficulty starting conversations, entering groups, connecting with people/lacking other basic social skills	
❑ Difficulty seeking attention in appropriate ways	
❑ Difficulty appreciating how his/her behavior is affecting others	
❑ Difficulty empathizing with others, appreciating another person's perspective or point of view	
❑ Difficulty appreciating how s/he is coming across or being perceived by others	
❑ Sensory/motor difficulties	

UNSOLVED PROBLEMS GUIDE:
Unsolved problems are the specific expectations a child is having difficulty meeting. Unsolved problems should be free of maladaptive behavior; free of adult theories and explanations; "split" (not "clumped"); and specific.

HOME EXAMPLES
* Difficulty getting out of bed in the morning in time to get to school
* Difficulty getting started on or completing homework (specify assignment)
* Difficulty ending the video game to get ready for bed at night
* Difficulty coming indoors for dinner when playing outside
* Difficulty agreeing with brother about what TV show to watch after school
* Difficulty with the feelings of seams in socks
* Difficulty brushing teeth before bedtime

SCHOOL EXAMPLES
* Difficulty moving from choice time to math
* Difficulty sitting next to Kyle during circle time
* Difficulty raising hand during social studies discussions
* Difficulty getting started on project on tectonic plates in geography
* Difficulty standing in line for lunch

REV 060417

Lives in the Balance
FOSTERING COLLABORATION • TRANSFORMING LIVES • INSPIRING CHANGE

livesinthebalance.org

Figure 67-1 Assessment of lagging skills and unsolved problems. Courtesy of Ross Greene, MD, used with permission.

personality disorder) as well as many other adverse outcomes such as suicidal behavior, delinquency, educational difficulties, unemployment, and teenage pregnancy. The disruptive disorders often trigger a chain of adverse events (e.g., parental hostility, peer rejection) that heighten the risk for additional adverse events (e.g., conflict with authority, deviant peers) extending through adolescence and into adulthood.

Bibliography

American Academy of Child and Adolescent Psychiatry. Practice parameters for the assessment and treatment of children and adolescents with oppositional defiant disorder. *J Am Acad Child Adolesc Psychiatry*. 2007;46:126-141.

Eyberg SM, Nelson MM, Boggs SR. Evidence-based psychosocial treatments for children and adolescents with disruptive behavior. *J Clin Child Adolesc Psychol*. 2008;37(1):215-237.

Ipser J, Stein DJ. Systematic review of pharmacotherapy of disruptive behavior disorders in children and adolescents. *Psychopharmacology*. 2007;191:127-140.

Ollendick TH, Greene RW, Fraire MG, et al. Parent management training (PMT) and collaborative & proactive solutions (CPS) in the treatment of oppositional defiant disorder in youth: a randomized control trial. *J Child Adoles Psychol*. 2015.

PARENT MANAGEMENT TRAINING PROGRAMS
Incredible Years. www.incredibleyears.com.
Parent—Child Interaction Therapy. http://www.pcit.org.
Triple P-Positive Parenting Program. http://www.triplep.net.

COLLABORATIVE & PROACTIVE SOLUTIONS
Lives in the Balance. www.livesinthebalance.org.

CHAPTER 68

Picky Eating

Megan H. Pesch | Julie Lumeng

I. DESCRIPTION OF THE PROBLEM. Picky eating occurs on a continuum, and there is no clear cutoff for when it becomes problematic. Parental perception that their child's unwillingness to eat familiar foods or sample new foods is outside the range of normal is probably the major reason for seeking medical advice. Therefore, the best definition of picky eating incorporates parental concern: *an unwillingness to eat familiar foods or try new foods, severe enough to interfere with daily routines to an extent that is problematic to the parent, child, or parent–child relationship.*

A. Epidemiology
- Although the prevalence is hard to pin down because there is no strict definition, 36% of toddlers are described as "picky eaters." In addition, 54% are not always hungry at mealtime, 33% do not seem to enjoy mealtimes, 34% have strong food preferences, 26% frequently refuse to eat, 21% request specific foods and then refuse them, and 42% try to end a meal after a few bites. Nearly two-thirds of parents report one or more problems in eating with their toddler.
- Children who are picky eaters more often have negative temperamental traits and are more often behaviorally inhibited (shy) and anxious. Greater parent negative affect has also been associated with picky eating, pointing toward the dyadic nature of feeding difficulties.
- The most commonly rejected foods are vegetables, and picky eaters have lower dietary variety but no significant difference in overall nutrient intake.
- Picky eating in childhood has been associated with male sex, higher socioeconomic status, lower maternal age, and fewer children in the family. The relationship between picky eating and child weight status is unclear. Picky eating has been associated with a higher risk of being underweight but also being overweight. Other studies have found no association at all. Having been breastfed and having a mother who eats more fruits and vegetables have been linked with being less picky. Being picky has not been associated with race, having medical problems, or food allergies.
- The prevalence of picky eating increases over infancy and toddlerhood, from 19% at 4–6 months of age to 50% at 19–24 months of age. There is significant continuity in pickiness during this age range. Pickiness seems to continue to increase to 3 years of age but thereafter seems to decline to about 20% by 8 years of age. If children are still described as picky after about 8–9 years of age, they are likely to continue to be picky.
- There seems to be a critical period during which children will expand the repertoire of liked foods in their diet that closes around 4 years of age. After 4 years of age, parents continue to introduce new foods, but the number of new foods children try that they learn to like does not continue to increase in the same way it did before 4 years of age.

B. Evolutionary framework. Picky eating seems to increase as children gain mobility. Some theorize that children are "wired" for pickiness to protect them from eating potentially poisonous substances in the environment. Children who are inherently reluctant to eat an unfamiliar food, or to eat a variety of foods, will not "wander into the bush and eat a poison berry."

C. Developmental framework. The increase in prevalence of picky eating during the toddler and preschool years coincides with a developmentally normative increase in autonomy around all activities including eating. As a matter of fact, 7- to 9-month-old infants refusing a bottle or being fed food in a spoon, even in the face of hunger, is one of the earliest autonomy asserting behaviors; the solution is to let the child hold the bottle or provide finger foods. As self-feeding progresses, children develop the ability to assert their preferences in food selection, making them more likely to reject foods that are unappealing to them. Picky eating is one of numerous acts of autonomy and not one of disobedience or rebellion. This early experience is an opportunity to highlight and prepare parents for their infants soon to grow skills in independence in many areas.

D. Etiology

- People reject foods because they (1) dislike the sensory characteristics (flavor, smell, texture, or appearance); (2) have a fear of negative consequences (e.g., it causes stomach upset upon eating); or (3) are disgusted by the food (due to contamination or the thought of where it came from), which does not begin until 7–8 years of age.
- Pickiness runs in families: about two-thirds of the variability in pickiness is explained by genetics. However, "nurture" (child caregiving practices) can modify "nature."

II. MAKING THE DIAGNOSIS

A. History: key clinical questions

1. *"Tell me which foods he/she won't eat."* A pattern of refusal, such as only refusing milk products or certain textures, raises the question of food allergies/intolerances or oral hypersensitivity.
2. *"Tell me what he/she ate yesterday, starting with breakfast."* A diet history can give a flavor to how picky the child is and opens a discussion about what foods are presented to the child, how, and what is done when the child rejects them.
3. *"What do you do when he/she rejects a food at dinner? What sort of rules do you have in your house around eating?"* Obtaining a history that the child is required to remain at the table until his or her plate is clean, or that the child is coerced to eat a particular food, is important. Neither of these methods has been shown to result in a long-term improvement in picky eating, and both likely simply add stress and negativity to the family mealtime.
4. *"What worries you the most about your child's eating?"* Frequently, parents are concerned the child has a growth or vitamin deficiency. Reassurance that the child is growing adequately (try showing the parent a growth chart) is often helpful, as is demystifying the behavior by describing how common it is (see prevalence data mentioned earlier) and the theories as to why it is present (see section "B. Evolutionary framework"). Recommending a multivitamin with iron (and supplemental fiber if needed) often assuages a great deal of parental concern about limited vegetable intake. Today, the risk of obesity is greater than the risk of malnutrition and in some studies, less pickiness is linked with higher weight status. Therefore, some degree of pickiness, within reason, may have benefits.
5. *"Is there anyone else in your family who is a picky eater?"* This question (to which the answer is nearly universally "yes") often opens the door to talking about the natural course of picky eating and may provide some insight into why the parent views the behavior as so problematic.

B. Physical examination and laboratory testing.
Careful measurement of weight and height, with plotting on the appropriate growth chart, is important. If growth deficiency is present, a different approach should be taken, which includes an exhaustive history with directed laboratory testing. If the child's diet is particularly restricted in iron-rich foods, testing for iron deficiency anemia is warranted. Children should also be screened by history and physical examination for constipation. The picky eater's diet is often low in fiber, and constipation can result in abdominal discomfort that only worsens the eating behavior.

C. Differential diagnosis

- Lactose intolerance or food allergies can present with refusal of specific types of foods.
- Gastroesophageal reflux disease, as evidenced by frequent vomiting or pain after eating, can result in problematic eating behavior.
- Children can present with oral hypersensitivity, the etiology of which is not always clear. These children respond negatively to oral stimuli and have difficulty with textured foods.
- Escalating negative affect in the caregiver and child, or an unusually strong focus on the issue, may signal an interactional problem. Picky eating may be the presenting complaint of a larger relationship problem that may benefit from an appropriate mental health referral.
- Unrealistic parental expectations about the quantity and range of food that a child will eat may be present. Expecting the child to eat every food presented at the dinner table every evening (including spicy or bitter flavors) may be a goal that cannot be met by all children.
- Limitation of resources. The family may not have adequate financial resources to supply a range of palatable foods at each meal. Parents may be concerned that the child's picky eating, in combination with limited choice, is affecting the child's health.

Table 68-1 • STRATEGIES TO SUGGEST TO PARENTS TO REDUCE PICKY EATING

Strategy	Comments
Functional analysis. What are the properties of the foods the child likes?	If child likes food with a particular temperature or texture, try expanding the repertoire of foods with similar kind of foods first.
Mealtime atmosphere. Calm, pleasant meals can improve willingness to try new foods. Food tastes better when it is eaten in a positive social context.	Children who are prone to anxiety or overstimulation may benefit from a calm eating atmosphere.
Social cues. Modeling eating a food by a parent is helpful, but peers are more powerful.	If child has the opportunity to eat meals with other children (such as in preschool), this may be an opportunity to expand the child's repertoire of foods.
Positive reinforcement. Parents should not provide material, verbal, or food rewards for eating, and children should never be punished for refusal to try a new food.	When children are given a reward (dessert) for eating a food (a vegetable), they eventually learn to like the food they were rewarded for eating (the vegetable) less over time (not the desired goal).
Repeated exposure. Increased familiarity results in increased liking, and foods typically must be introduced 10 times before they are accepted. Less than 10% of parents offer a food to a child this many times before giving up based on the impression that the child does not like it.	If the family wishes for the child to accept a vegetable, choose a generally mild, palatable vegetable to be served at dinner repeatedly.
Encouraging a child to try a bite. The "try one bite" rule has been shown to result in an increased willingness to try other new foods over time. It may be due to decreasing the expectation of disliking the target food.	If the child has a difficult temperament, however, and requiring the child to take a bite is disruptive to mealtime, this method should be abandoned.
Providing information. For older children, providing information about a food's flavor will increase willingness to try the food.	If younger children do not grasp the meaning of "flavor words" (i.e., sweet, salty, sour), or have not yet developed a vocabulary of "food words," this method may not be effective.
Combining foods. Combining a nonpreferred food (a meat) with a preferred food (ketchup) may be helpful—even in seemingly illogical combinations.	If a child wants to dip carrot sticks in soup, and this increases his willingness to eat the carrots, this should be accepted (in lieu of disallowing it because it is "bad manners").
Compromise. Allowing children to compromise on parent request to try a food (i.e., trying the vegetable without the sauce) may be more supportive of a child's autonomy around eating than demanding compliance.	Supporting a child's agency in eating may lead to better self-regulation of intake and decreased eating beyond satiety.

- Children with autism spectrum disorders are commonly picky eaters.
- Children with avoidant/restrictive food intake disorder can present as extreme picky eaters, often with weight loss and malnutrition.

III. **MANAGEMENT.** A thorough history is essential to clearly define the problem. The mainstay of management is to demystify for parents that picky eating is, in most cases, a behavior that worsens during the toddler and preschool years and then begins to improve through the early elementary years unless it becomes fixed as part of parent–child conflict. In other cases, it can be seen as a personality trait. Either way, there is rarely a medical indication for intervention. Behavioral interventions should be recommended only when parents are eager to put effort into modifying the behavior. Interventions must be benign and simple and should never be continued if they result in increased stress or discord at mealtimes. Some strategies that could be suggested to parents to reduce picky eating are listed in Table 68-1.

   A. **Clinical pearls and pitfalls.** Parents who are concerned about a child's picky eating may be articulating the eating as the problem, when it is really a discrete symptom of an overarching concern: a difficult temperament. Although picky eating occurs on a continuum and is a "normal" behavior, parental concerns should not be minimized. Helping the parent to understand the child's temperamental qualities, and how the picky eating is a symptom of them, will likely be most helpful in the long term in the parent–child relationship.

Bibliography

FOR PARENTS

American Academy of Pediatrics. "How to Please a Fussy Eater" from HealthyChildren.org. Updated 11/21/2015. https://www.healthychildren.org/English/healthy-living/nutrition/Pages/How-To-Please-Fussy-Eaters.aspx.

Ellyn Satter has published several books for parents and professionals about childhood eating and feeding behavior, and maintains a Web site. http://www.ellynsatter.com/.

Muth ND, Sampson S. *The Picky Eater Project: 6 Weeks to Happier, Healthier Family Mealtimes*. American Academy of Pediatrics; 2016.

FOR PROFESSIONALS

Dietz W, Birch LL. *Eating Behaviors of the Young Child: Prenatal and Postnatal Influences for Healthy Eating*. Elk Grove Village, IL: American Academy of Pediatrics; 2007.

Dovey TM, Staples PA, Gibson EL, et al. Food neophobia and "picky/fussy" eating in children: a review. *Appetite*. 2008;50(2–3):181-193.

Walton K, et al. Time to re-think picky eating? A relational approach to understanding picky eating. *Int J Behav Nutr Phys Act*. 2017;14:62.

CHAPTER 69

Posttraumatic Stress, Child Victimization, and Exposure to Trauma

Neena McConnico | Betsy McAlister Groves | Lisa R. Fortuna

I. DESCRIPTION OF PROBLEM. Child victimization and exposure to trauma is a serious public health problem, affecting millions of children in the United States and internationally, with significant impact on their short and long-term physical health, social–emotional development, and cognitive functioning. Traumatic experiences may include exposure to death, threatened death, actual or threatened serious injury, actual or threatened sexual violence as well as experiences of child maltreatment, sudden loss of a parent, exposure to domestic violence, medical trauma/illness, accidents/serious injury, exposure to disasters, war-related trauma, and forced displacement.

A. Epidemiology. In a national telephone survey, researchers found that more than 60% of children were exposed to violence within the past year. Thirty-eight percent experienced multiple victimizations within the past year; more than one-third of respondents had witnessed violence against another person in their lifetime. Ten percent of adolescents had witnessed a shooting in their lifetime.

Out of 3.4 million reports of suspected child abuse/neglect to child protection services in the United States, 683,000 children were found to be victims of child abuse or neglect in 2015; children younger than 1 year have the highest rate of victimization. Seven million children live in homes where there is domestic violence with children younger than 6 years disproportionately represented in the population of children who are exposed to domestic violence. The two most commonly reported traumatic events were traumatic loss/separation/bereavement and domestic violence.

The severity of trauma exposure and parental trauma-related distress are positively related to posttraumatic stress disorder (PTSD) symptoms in children. A child's temperament and prior exposure to trauma, as well as a range of risk and protective factors, including the kind of support the child has at home and from other adults, may also influence whether a child will experience ongoing difficulties following a traumatic event. These findings suggest that identifying traumatic exposures, family distress, and ways of coping (both adaptive and less adaptive) are important to evaluate in addition to child trauma symptoms.

B. Etiology/contributing factors. Children who suffer from traumatic stress can develop reactions that affect their functioning long after the traumatic event has ended and can be three to four times more likely to have depression and/or anxiety at a later age. Symptoms can vary according to developmental stage. For instance, an infant or toddler may lose previously acquired skills, such as toileting or language skills, while a teen might exhibit unusually reckless, aggressive, or self-destructive behavior including substance use. Short-term symptoms in children can include sleep difficulties, avoidance of reminders of the event, somatic symptoms, hyperarousal, helplessness, and fear, even if the child is not immediately in danger. Studies suggest that young children are particularly vulnerable to the impact of violence or other traumatic experiences, and that chronic exposure may affect brain development and self-regulatory processes. In addition, children younger than 4 years are particularly vulnerable to threats that involve the safety (or perceived safety) of their caregivers. Witnessing domestic violence and/or other victimization of the caregiver are important risk factors for the development of posttraumatic stress in children.

Social support can mitigate the severity of PTSD in children and adults following traumatic events. However, in adolescents with previous early childhood adversity, more severe level of violence exposure, comorbid anxiety, depression symptoms, substance abuse, and limited coping strategies, social support may not be enough to mitigate the effects of trauma. In those cases, medical and psychotherapy intervention are important in addition to providing environmental and social supports. Because there are symptoms common to both PTSD and attention deficit hyperactivity disorder

(ADHD)—difficulty concentrating, disorganization, hyperactivity, restlessness, and difficulty sleeping—children either need to be distinguished or may have both. When evaluating for ADHD, it is important to screen for a history of potentially traumatic experiences, to rule out trauma as the cause for dysregulated behavior. Symptoms that emerge as part of a posttraumatic situation with longer than a month's duration and a negative impact on functioning should be further evaluated for PTSD diagnosis.

The impact of trauma and victimization can be mitigated by protective factors that enhance and build resilience. Positive, healthy, nurturing relationship with significant adults is the most important protective factor to help children heal and thrive in the aftermath of trauma. Not all trauma exposure results in PTSD or poor functioning in children. Only a thorough assessment and diagnostic evaluation that includes a biopsychosocial approach can help differentiate between diagnoses and identify posttraumatic symptoms and risk factors.

C. Identifying children and adolescents affected by trauma. Primary care clinicians should inquire about violence in the lives of all children to consider trauma exposure as a possibility or contributing factor for behaviors of concern. Because many families feel comfortable with their child's primary care clinician, they may be more likely to disclose violence exposure and seek help from them compared with other providers.

Although assessing for child symptoms is necessary, the pediatric provider should also consider the child's primary caregiver. Given the essential role of the attachment relationship in helping children heal, it is important to assess both the child and caregiver for potential risks and protective factors that can serve as a buffer to mitigate the negative effects of trauma exposure. Positive, nurturing relationships with significant adults are the single most important factor to buffer negative effects of trauma exposure and promote healing; therefore, determining the quality of this relationship and identifying ways to strengthen, enhance, and maintain this relationship is paramount. Early and timely intervention is critical to promote an optimal healthy developmental trajectory. When screening for possible traumatic experiences, the pediatric provider should follow the given steps:

1. Assess for strengths and needs.
2. Assess for environmental supports that can help stabilize the child and family.
3. Assess the quality of the caregiver–child relationship.

Medical practitioners can incorporate questions about trauma and violence exposure into interviews with families and caregivers. Questions may be prefaced by a statement that assures the family members that they are not being singled out for this line of questioning and that the provider considers the topic of violence to be within the scope of problems to be addressed in a medical visit. By doing so, the provider has communicated that violence and exposure to trauma are risks to the child's well-being and are a legitimate focus of concern during the clinical visit.

There are many ways to ask about trauma. Some practitioners prefer to use open-ended questions; others use structured tools that screen for trauma exposure. The decision about the best way to get this information is dependent on the patient population, the workflow of the practice, the preference of the clinician, and the comfort of the families who are seen in the practice.

Examples of open-ended questions:
- "I know that there is a lot of violence in our world these days. I have begun to ask all of my patients about their experiences with violence and other stressors. I would like to ask you a few questions."
  - "Since the last visit, has your child experienced any event or circumstance that has affected or been distressing to them?"
  - "Are you ever worried about your child's safety?"
  - "Has your child seen frightening things?"

The following standardized instruments can be used to assess trauma exposure, symptoms, and overall functioning for children and their caregivers (Table 69-1).

D. Practice guidelines for practitioners. If there are disclosures of trauma or violent experiences, the clinician should elicit basic information from both the child and the parent, if possible, and address the following:
- Assess for safety.
- Assess the child's symptoms and functioning.
- Assess the parent's reaction and functioning.
- Provide education about common reactions or behaviors associated with trauma.
  Depending on the pediatric clinician's assessment and family preference:
- Make a referral for further assessment and/or treatment.
- Schedule a follow-up appointment for 2–3 weeks later.

Table 69-1 • SCREENING AND ASSESSMENT TOOLS

Measure	Description	Age	Cost/Proprietary
Trauma Exposure			
Traumatic events screening inventory—parent report revised (TESI-PRR)	Assesses traumatic events exposure and impacts among children	0–6 y	Freely accessible
UCLA-PTSD RI (posttraumatic stress disorder reaction index)	20-item questionnaire that assesses exposure to traumatic events and potential impacts of traumatic events	Child: 7–12 y Youth: 13 y and above	Behavioral health innovations https://www.reactionindex.com/index.php/
Trauma Symptoms			
Trauma symptom checklist for children (TSCC)	Standardized instrument that assesses trauma symptoms in children across eight clinical scales	8–16 y	Psychological assessment resources http://www4.parinc.com
Trauma symptom checklist for young children (TSCYC)	Caregiver questionnaire assessing trauma symptoms in young children across eight clinical scales	3–12 y	Psychological assessment resources http://www4.parinc.com
Child behavior checklist (CBCL)	Standardized measure that assesses internalizing and externalizing behavior across eight clinical scales	1.5–5 y 6–18 y	Achenbach system of empirically based assessment (ASEBA) http://www.aseba.org/
Early childhood screening assessment	Assesses emotional and behavioral development in young children and maternal distress	18 mo–5 y	Freely accessible
Caregiver Functioning and Exposure to Trauma			
Parenting stress index (PSI)	Standardized norm-referenced caregiver report assessing parental distress, parent–child dysfunctional interaction, and difficult child	1–12 y	PAR https://www.parinc.com/
Edinburgh maternal depression scale	10 item self-report measure that screens women for depression	Adult	Freely accessible
Pediatric intake form (family psychosocial screen)	Screens for parental depression, substance use, domestic violence, parental history of abuse, and social supports	Adult	Freely accessible

Referrals should be made to mental health specialists who have expertise treating children who have experienced trauma. If the case involves domestic violence, the adult victim may be referred to a domestic violence program. Evidence-based interventions that have demonstrated positive outcomes and effectiveness treating children and adolescents exposed to trauma include Child Parent Psychotherapy (CPP), Attachment-Regulation and Competence (ARC), and Trauma-Focused Cognitive Behavioral Therapy (TF-CBT).

Bibliography

RESOURCES

American Academy of Pediatrics. The medical home approach to identifying and responding to trauma; 2014. https://www.aap.org/en-us/Documents/ttb_medicalhomeapproach.pdf.

American Academy of Pediatrics. Adverse childhood experiences and the lifeline consequences of trauma; 2014. https://www.aap.org/en-us/Documents/ttb_aces_consequences.pdf.

Bair-Merritt MH, Blackstone M, Feudtner C. Physical health outcomes of childhood exposure to intimate partner violence: a systematic review. *Pediatrics*. 2006;117:e278-e290. doi:10.1542/peds.2005-1473.

Child Welfare Information Gateway. *Child Maltreatment 2015: Summary of Key Findings*. Washington, DC: U.S. Department of Health and Human Services, Children's Bureau; 2017.

Cohen JA, Kelleher KJ, Mannarino AP. Identifying, treating, and referring traumatized children: the role of pediatric providers. *Arch Pediatr Adolesc Med*. 2008;162(5): 447-452.

Committee on Psychosocial Aspects of Child and Family Health; Committee on Early Childhood, Adoption, and Dependent Care, and Section on Developmental and Behavioral Pediatrics; Garner AS, Shonkoff JP, Siegel BS, et al. Early childhood adversity, toxic stress, and the role of the pediatrician: translating developmental science into lifelong health. *Pediatrics*. 2012;129:e224; originally published online December 26, 2011. doi:10.1542/peds.2011-2662.

Preer G, Groves BM. The pediatrician's role in patient and family recovery after child abuse. *Pediatr Ann*. 2012;41:12.

CHAPTER 70

Prematurity: Follow-Up

Douglas L. Vanderbilt | Kelly Schifsky

I. **DESCRIPTION OF THE PROBLEM.** Infants born before the 37th week of gestation are at risk for chronic medical, neurodevelopmental, and behavioral problems. Different problems unfold over the various stages of development with the high-risk constellation never "going away." The shorter the gestation and the greater number of medical complications and biopsychosocial risk factors, the higher the risk and need for close primary care surveillance to assess need for early intervention developmental services and monitoring of infant and caregiver mental health.

A. **Epidemiology**
   - Approximately 9.6% of all births are preterm (less than 37 weeks' gestation), with 8% being moderately preterm (32–36 weeks' gestation) and the remaining 1.6% being very preterm (less than 32 weeks' gestation).
   - While the incidence of prematurity has been stable over the last decade, mortality for these groups have declined dramatically.
      - Survival rate for infants born greater than 22 weeks' gestation has improved (e.g., 22–24 weeks, 39%; 25–27 weeks, 81% in one NICHD study).
      - Medical advances including more aggressive delivery room resuscitation, surfactant use, antenatal corticosteroid utilization, improved ventilatory techniques, and nutritional management have led to improved survival rates for all preterm infants.
   - Despite the gains, high rates of disability exist for infants born extremely preterm (less than 28 weeks) increasing down to the limit of viability.
   - Any preterm infant remains at increased risk for future neurodevelopmental, psychological, and behavioral and functional impairments (Table 70-1).
   - Multiples births, often premature, have increased owing to popularity of in vitro fertilization.

B. **Risk factors for developmental and behavioral problems.** Risk of developmental and behavioral outcomes increases with decreasing gestational age (GA). Risk factors for follow-up programs mandating especially close developmental screening and assessment include the following:
   - Birth weight (BW) < 1500 g or GA at birth < 32 weeks, or
   - BW > 1500 g or GA > 32 weeks and one of the following:
      - Cardiorespiratory depression at birth
      - Apgar <5 at 3 minutes
      - Prolonged hypoxia, acidemia, hypoglycemia, and/or hypotension requiring pressors
      - Persistent apnea requiring medication
      - Oxygen support for >28 days and X-ray findings consistent with chronic lung disease
      - Extracorporeal membrane oxygenation intervention
      - Persistent pulmonary hypertension of the newborn
      - Seizure activity
      - Intracranial pathology: intracranial hemorrhage, periventricular leukomalacia, cerebral thrombosis, cerebral infarction, developmental central nervous system (CNS) abnormality
      - Other neurologic insults: hypoxic ischemic encephalopathy, kernicterus, sepsis, CNS infection

   Biological risk alone does not determine outcome. Rather, it is the interaction of those risks with social and environmental factors that best predicts long-term functioning. At the core of this intersection of the biopsychosocial interaction is the infant–caregiver relationship. Often these social risks contributed to the preterm birth and continue to influence outcomes.

   Optimal infant development occurs within the context of a secure infant–caregiver relationship. A caregiver who is responsive and sensitive to an infant's emotional, physical, and personal needs provides an opportunity for that infant to optimize their

Table 70-1 • DEVELOPMENTAL AND BEHAVIORAL RISK. PRIMARY CARE PROVIDERS MUST CLOSELY MONITOR FOR THE FOLLOWING MORBIDITIES SEEN AT HIGHER RATES IN PREMATURITY

Neurodevelopmental	Psychological and Behavioral	Functional Disabilities
Fine motor deficits	Attention-deficit/hyperactivity disorder	Motor coordination
Gross motor deficits	Difficulty with peer interactions	Social skills
Cerebral palsy	Bullying	Executive functioning
Vision and hearing loss	Anxiety/depression	
	Autism spectrum disorder	

neurodevelopmental outcomes. However, the characteristics, needs, and fragility of preterm infants serve as a stressor to a parent's ability to engage in a sensitive and responsive way to their infant's needs. Parents of infants born premature and who spent time in the neonatal intensive care unit (NICU) are at greater risk for depression and traumatic stress. These conditions place additional stress on this relationship, with the potential to negatively impact developmental outcomes. While follow-up clinicians are unable to change the preexisting biological insult sustained by the infant, they are in a unique position to improve a child's neurodevelopmental and behavioral outcomes by supporting the infant–caregiver relationship by strengthening the caregivers through attending to their mental health and enhancing social and resource supports.

II. EVALUATION

   A. **Common health problems of the premature infant.** Because chronic medical problems and developmental and behavioral difficulties are inextricably linked, comprehensive management of these problems will enhance the likelihood of optimal outcomes. A secure caregiver–infant relationship is critical for not only optimal developmental and behavioral outcomes, but medical outcomes as well. Infants of mothers with higher levels of depression and traumatic stress are at an increased risk for difficulties with feeding, weight gain, and appropriate utilization of the health care system. Thus, the clinician must closely monitor the below-mentioned potential health challenges while also monitoring and supporting the mental health of infant and caregiver.

   1. **Neurologic.** Maintain seizure control through use of anticonvulsant medications in consultation with a pediatric neurologist. Anticonvulsants for neonatal seizures often are weaned through growth during the first year of life.

      Many premature infants leave the NICU with retinopathy of prematurity that is not fully resolved. Strabismus and myopia are more common among premature infants. Ensure follow-up by a pediatric ophthalmologist or optometrist.

   2. **Audiologic.** All infants should undergo a newborn hearing screen by 1 month of age. Those who fail this screening should undergo an audiologic evaluation by 3 months of age. Infants with confirmed hearing loss should receive appropriate intervention by no later than 6 months of age. Auditory brainstem response (ABR) is the only appropriate screening technique for use in the NICU. NICU infants who fail ABR testing should be directly referred to pediatric audiologist. Infants with syndromes associated with hearing loss, hyperbilirubinemia requiring exchange transfusion, congenital infection, or other medical risks should be screened more frequently (see Chapter 55).

   3. **Respiratory.** In concert with pediatric pulmonologists, optimize pulmonary function with airway management, medications, supplemental oxygen, or ventilator support. Annual influenza vaccine and respiratory syncytial virus prophylaxis for eligible infants are also important to ensure developmental progress. Consideration of child care arrangements should be made with a thought to respiratory vulnerability.

   B. **Growth and feeding.** Premature infants may come home from the hospital with feeding problems: tube dependency, inadequate caloric intake, or volume intolerance due to cardiopulmonary or gastrointestinal disease. Good nutrition is critical for optimal developmental gain. Premature infants should remain on special care formulas through the first year. Attention should be paid to appropriate weight gain, caloric density of the formula, daily caloric intake, and feeding mechanics and relationship. Key questions to ask the family include the following:

   • *How do you feel about your child's feeding patterns?*
   • *Do you think it is easy to feed your child?*

- *How long does it take to feed your child?*
- *Does your child have difficulty sucking or swallowing?*

Growth patterns should be monitored over time using standard growth charts. For premature infants, measurements can be plotted on special growth charts for premature infants, or, after age adjustment (chronological age in weeks minus number of weeks premature), they can be plotted on a regular growth chart up to 2 years of age.

1. Growth trends

  a. Dropping growth percentiles or moving further below the fifth percentile. This may be secondary to medical, nutritional, family dynamic, or neurologic factors. Further investigation is warranted.

  b. Catch-up growth or forward movement across percentiles. Catch-up growth may begin slowly and continue over the first 2 years of life.

  c. Growth parallel to the fifth percentile. The child may continue to be small or catch up in future years. This pattern is often seen following extreme low BW and/or intrauterine growth restriction.

  d. Rapid head growth. Catch-up head growth is a good sign. However, when head circumference crosses percentiles more rapidly than length or weight, head ultrasound evaluation for hydrocephalus should be considered. Benign enlargement of the subarachnoid space is usually a benign and transient condition. Babies with grade III–IV intraventricular hemorrhage may have late-onset hydrocephalus requiring a shunt.

  e. Head growth lagging behind other parameters. This is a concerning sign, often associated with global developmental delays.

C. Behavior and development

  1. History: key clinical questions

   • *"How does your baby regulate his/her feeding, sleeping, and crying levels?"* Premature babies may be especially passive or irritable due to central nervous system (CNS) injury, interruption of typical gestational maturation, or the prolonged hospital experience. Infants with CNS injury manifest the same problems as all other infants (e.g., colic, night wakening, temper tantrums), but they tend to be more intense or prolonged.

   • *"How do you feel about caring for your premature infant and supporting his/her physical and emotional needs?"* Having a premature infant can lead to increased levels of stress, anxiety, and depression, which, in turn, can make it more difficult for parents to feel emotionally capable of meeting their infants needs and/or lead to more negative views of caring for a perceived "fragile" infant.

   • *"How worried are you about your child?"* It is sometimes difficult for parents to modify their perception of the child from "fragile" to "healthy." It may take a prolonged period for the child to achieve medical stability and even longer to change parental representations of their child as vulnerable. Common pediatric illnesses may be overinterpreted as evidence of continuing vulnerability (see Chapter 55).

   • *"Does your child seem either stiff or floppy?"* Hypotonia with compensation with extensor posturing is fairly common among premature infants and usually resolves. Persistent hypertonia may be a sign of cerebral palsy. Initial hypotonia may evolve over several months into hypertonia.

   • *"Does your child have any unusual movement patterns?"* Dragging the legs along in crawling, body rolling (instead of crawling), or seat scooting may be manifestations of neuromotor abnormalities. Early hand preference is abnormal and may indicate injury to subcortical white matter or the corticospinal tract contralateral to the less used upper extremity. In such a case, a head imaging (MRI) study is indicated.

  2. Assessment. Although developmental screening is recommended for all children, careful and regular assessment is even more important for premature children.

   Experts have suggested comprehensive primary care with attention to vision, hearing, growth, and developmental assessments for those with very low BW. Despite this, there are no current national guidelines for formal developmental screening and/or assessment specific for premature infants owing to the wide risk categories and reimbursement challenges to this care. The following represents an ideal care flow:

   • Infants should be discharged from the NICU into the care of a primary care clinician familiar with the care of preterm infants. This clinician will serve as the medical home for well-child care and coordinating referrals to subspecialists as necessary.

     • Most screening and assessment tests recommend correction until 2 years of age. If the child is not achieving corrected age skills for, referral is warranted.

- Upon discharge from the NICU, eligible infants should be referred to a High-Risk Infant Follow-up (HRIF) clinic and/or to the appropriate Early Intervention (EI) services based on risk and/or delays.
  - Within the HRIF clinic, a multidisciplinary team can assess the infant's fine and gross motor, language, cognitive, and social/emotional development with the use of standardized tools.
  - Assessments of nutritional status, feeding, sensory regulation, infant mental health, and need for family supportive services should all be included.
  - This multidisciplinary team should further ensure that infants not meeting developmental milestones for corrected GA are connected to EI services.
- When a child turns 3 years of age, they become eligible for evaluation for special education services through the local public school district. Evaluation domains that help to determine eligibility for an Individualized Educational Plan and for special education services include, but are not limited to, the following:
  - Cognitive functioning (IQ), language development, preacademic skills, social interaction/communication
- Premature infants should be followed closely during their school-age years for the following:
  - Learning disabilities, externalizing symptoms of attention-deficit/hyperactivity disorder (ADHD), internalizing symptoms of anxiety and depression
- In adolescence, ongoing monitoring for specific learning disorders, ADHD, and anxiety/depression should continue.
- Increased risk-taking behavior may be present and should be routinely screened for using standardized screens. As premature infants continue to survive into thriving adults, many adult clinicians are now caring for conditions that were once thought to be "childhood" conditions. Owing to this shift, it is critical that primary care clinicians begin to develop a transition plan for their patients that ensures they develop in their own understanding of their health care needs, can advocate for future needs, and becomes established with an adult health care team.

D. Psychosocial issues

1. **Family dynamics and stress.** Shortened gestation interrupts the normal psychological preparation for life with a newborn. The long, uncertain intensive care experience can be traumatic for parents. Parents take home an infant who is often different than originally expected and possibly having higher caregiving demands medically and with self-regulation. As a result, caregivers of premature infants are at a greater risk for depression and anxiety symptoms. Standard mental health screening tools may be used to gain more concrete information regarding caregiver's emotions and mental health and to catch families at risk for depression and/or posttraumatic stress disorder. Screening for mental health should be consistent in the NICU and into infancy. An early "decompression visit" for the parents is helpful to process the NICU experience and connect with needed supportive resources. Linking at-risk families to counseling services is critical to support their mental health. Family support groups may also be helpful for families to further discuss their emotions after NICU discharge.

III. CLINICAL PEARLS AND PITFALLS

- Beware of overwhelming the family with services or appointments. Prioritization and coordination of services as well as shared decision-making will decrease family stress and ensure better overall compliance and satisfaction.
- Do not assume that an infant will outgrow any identified risk. Appropriate evaluation and correction for the degree of prematurity should allow the clinician to make an informed judgment about the infant's status.
- Comprehensive follow-up includes support of the infant–caregiver relationship. Clinicians must screen for caregiver mental health and refer to counseling services when warranted.

Bibliography

FOR PARENTS

WEB SITES

American Academy of Pediatrics. www.healthychildrehttps://www.healthychildren.org/English/ages-stages/baby/preemie/Pages/Health-Issues-of-Premature-Babies.aspx.

March of Dimes. www.marchofdimes.org/peristats/.

Premature Baby. kidshealth.org/parent/growth/growing/preemies.html.

PUBLICATIONS

Linden DW, Paroli ET, Doron MW. Preemies—Second Edition: The Essential Guide for Parents of Premature Babies, Pocket; 2010.

Madden SL. *The Preemie Parents' Companion: The Essential Guide to Caring for Your Premature Baby in the Hospital, at Home, and Through the First Years*. Boston, MA: Harvard Common Press; 2000.

Zaichkin J. *Understanding the NICU: What Parents of Preemies and Other Hospitalized Newborns Need to Know*. Elk Grove Village, IL: American Academy of Pediatrics; 2016.

FOR PROFESSIONALS

Brodsky D, Ouellette MA. *Primary Care of the Premature Infant*. Philadelphia, PA: Saunders; 2008.

Doyle LW, et al. Long term follow up of high risk children: who,why and how? *BMC Pediatr.* 2014;14:279.

Guralnick MJ. Preventive interventions for preterm children: effectiveness and developmental mechanisms. *J Dev Behav Pediatr.* 2012;33(4):352-364.

Joint Committee on Infant Hearing. Year 2007 position statement: principles and guidelines for early hearing detection and intervention programs. *Pediatrics.* 2007;120(4).

Stephens ES. Neurodevelopmental outcome of the premature infant. *Pediatric Clin N Am.* 2009;56:631-646.

Vanderbilt D, Gleason M. Mental health concerns of the premature infant through the lifespan. *Pediatric Clin N Am.* 2011;58:815-832.

Wang CJ, et al. Quality-of-Care indicators for the neurodevelopmental follow-up of very low birth weight children: results of an expert panel process. *Pediatrics.* 2006;117(6):2080-2092.

CHAPTER **71**

School Readiness

Margot Kaplan-Sanoff | Jaime Wildman Peterson

I. **DESCRIPTION OF THE PROBLEM.** *School readiness* is the term used to describe those characteristics that are considered prerequisites for a child to be ready to succeed in a school setting. Early school readiness predicts later academic achievement; research demonstrates that a vocabulary gap at age 3 years predicted language scores in third grade. Third-grade language and reading proficiency is important because it is a predictor of high school graduation, and it is at third grade that the curriculum transitions from "learning to read" to "reading to learn." Yet lack of *universal* early childhood education systems often places the burden of school preparation on parents and caregivers. Additionally, there are emotional concerns for both parents ("unfamiliar people will be judging my child and, by extension, my parenting") and children ("can I meet the challenges of the BIG school?"). Table 71-1 lists the criteria most often identified as necessary for academic success in kindergarten or first grade and lists suggestions for how parents can support school readiness with their child. There are a number of social, emotional, motoric, cognitive, and linguistic factors to consider when assessing school readiness.

A. **Ability to master new experiences.** The ability to grapple with and master new experiences defines the initial task of school success. Children are asked to listen and relate to unfamiliar adults, follow specific rules, interact with a large group of children, and manage daily tasks by themselves. Children who, when confronted with new experiences, can build on familiar experiences will quickly gain mastery of the new situations required by school, such as getting their lunch in the cafeteria. On the other hand, children who are easily overwhelmed, who panic at new experiences, and who are unable to bring knowledge of the familiar to bear on new demands may have a difficult time. Each new piece of learning disorients them, and they are unable to understand how to manage successfully in school.

B. **Lack of experience.** Some children simply lack the experience of being in a group of children of their own age. Others may lack access to books and learning materials in their homes. Because of the enormous burdens of poverty, family trauma and stress, inappropriately low expectations for preacademic development, or diverse cultural backgrounds, these children are unfamiliar with the tasks required for success in school (such as waiting in line, sharing materials, taking turns, or following verbal directions).

C. **Ability to tolerate separations from primary caregivers.** The relationships that children develop with teachers are different from their relationships with parents and extended family. Children are expected to establish and maintain the teacher's attention in a large group through socially acceptable ways such as waiting to be called on, or holding up their hands to answer a question or make a request.

D. **Independence in most activities of daily living.** Separated from primary caregivers, children are required to be independent in caregiving functions such as eating, toileting, napping, dressing, and taking care of their possessions.

E. **Executive function and the ability to control impulses.** Executive function refers to the skills that children develop to help them order and coordinate their thoughts and behavior, process information in a coherent way, hold relevant details in their short-term memory, avoid distractions, and focus on the task at hand (see Chapter 46). Children should have the self-control to sit in a circle without bothering other children, attend to adults for a limited amount of time (5–10 minutes), and listen to and follow adult directions, some of which might be delivered from the other side of a busy room.

F. **Appropriate play skills.** Early school success is dependent, in part, on the child's ability to get along with peers, manage in a group, and engage in developmentally appropriate play. Children should be able to play with other children without resorting to hitting, biting, or yelling to resolve conflicts. They should be able to manage the give-and-take of peer relationships, both within a structured play activity such as a board game and in fantasy play. Children should also be able to differentiate fantasy play and stories from reality. Opportunities to engage in sustained, mature play can foster strong executive function and self-regulation skills.

Table 71-1 • SCHOOL READINESS SKILLS

Expected Developmental Skills for Kindergarten and 1st Grade	Before Kindergarten Parents Should
Social Skills	
Kindergarten Begins to share with others Plays cooperative with peers Starts to follow rules Able to recognize authority Manages bathroom needs **First grade** Works cooperatively with groups of children	Establish routines (bedtime) Consistent discipline Preschool enrollment Peer play opportunities *(play groups, library story time)*
Emotional and Self-regulation Skills	
Kindergarten Pays attention for 5–10 min of adult-directed tasks Separates from parents without being upset Begins to control oneself Listens to stories without interrupting **First grade** Same as above	Play games: Red Light, Green Light, Simon Says, etc. Prepare for separation Read for 20 min every day
Motor Skills	
Kindergarten Draws a person Prints name Cuts with scissors Traces basic shapes Buttons shirts, pants, and coats and zips up zippers **First grade** Copies letters and numerals	Outside activity *(run, bike)* Encourage drawing and painting Do art projects Be patient, allow self-dressing Practice buttons and zippers
Cognitive Skills	
Kindergarten Recognizes rhyming sounds Shows understanding of general times of day Looks at pictures and then tells stories Identifies some alphabet letters Recognizes some common sight words such as "stop" Sorts and labels similar objects by color, size, and shape Recognizes groups of one, two, three, four, and five objects Counts 20 objects **First grade** Prints many uppercase and lowercase letters Identifies numerals 1 to 20 Demonstrates conservation of mass, length, and volume Knows address and birth date Reads simple sight words Reads emergent texts	Clap and rhyme together Ask open-ended questions Read for 20 min every day. Look for letters and shapes in daily life Compare objects, measure and use tools, match socks Group and sort toys Puzzles with shapes and colors Count together (# of trees)
Language and Communication Skills	
Kindergarten Speaks understandably Talks in complete sentences of five to six words Identifies rhyming words **First grade** Speaks in more complex sentences Uses words/phrases from conversation to respond to questions	Talk and sing to your child Ask open-ended questions Give the child time to answer

G. Mental health concerns. There is growing awareness of mental health concerns in young children. From 9.5% to 14.2% of children younger than 6 years have emotional problems serious enough to hurt their ability to function, including anxiety or behavioral disorders and depression. Early stresses, including child abuse or neglect, domestic or community violence, extreme poverty and food insecurity, and parental mental health concerns and/or substance abuse, can prime neurobiological stress systems to become hyperresponsive to adversity. Known as "toxic stress," these early stressors interfere with developing brain circuits and pose a serious threat to young children not only by undermining their emotional well-being but also by impairing early learning, exploration and curiosity, and school readiness.

H. Developmental delays. Specific cognitive or learning problems, receptive or expressive language delays, and visual motor or sensory integration problems may make it difficult for a child to succeed in a regular school classroom. Yet these are the very children who benefit most from a more formal learning environment. They should be evaluated by the school department and placed in the least restrictive learning environment within the school, perhaps in a transitional classroom or a resource room program with a significant portion of their school day spent in a regular classroom. Children who do not possess sufficient school readiness skills will not benefit from "another year" at home or in childcare waiting to be ready for school. At 3 years of age, they are legally eligible for public school services and should be provided with specific educational placement because of either developmental delays or social–emotional concerns such as parental social determinants of health, depending on the regulations of the individual state's Department of Education.

II. **MAKING THE DIAGNOSIS.** The skills and tips for parents listed in Table 71-1 constitute the "how" of school readiness. Such specific cognitive and motor tasks (e.g., knowing the ABCs, printing one's name, using a computer mouse, or cutting with scissors) are highly idiosyncratic milestones and do not automatically correlate to the actual tasks of school learning. For example, knowing the alphabet by singing the ABC song is a far less powerful predictor of reading success than is the child's understanding of the power and function of the written word. Additionally, kindergarten teachers report that social and emotional skills such as the ability to control impulses, understand language, and engage in age-appropriate play are more important for successful learning than the discrete cognitive skills such as counting or letter recognition.

A. History taking. Involving both parents and child in a developmental history taking can provide the clinician with a great deal of information pertinent to the issue of school readiness. This activity can have particular significance when considering the 3- or 4-year-old well-child visit as a "transition/school readiness" check to determine how well the child is acquiring the skills (Table 71-1) needed to succeed in kindergarten. Input from the childcare provider can add an additional perspective to the diagnosis. The following clinical inquiries can be used to guide the discussion and trigger the need for additional information:

1. *"Has the child achieved age-appropriate developmental skills in language, cognitive, social, and motor development?"*
2. *"How does the child respond to unusual events at home or in childcare such as a substitute provider or a change in the daily routine?"*
3. *"Has the child had any preschool or group care experience? How has she/he done in these settings? Were there any learning or behavior concerns?"*
4. *"Does the child play cooperatively with peers? Or does the child consistently choose to play alone or with younger children?"*
5. *"Does the child cling to behaviors more appropriate for a younger child (e.g., continual thumb-sucking, frequent toileting accidents, tantrums)?"*
6. *"Can the child identify colors, shapes, letters, and numbers?"*
7. *"Is the child's speech understandable and can he/she converse with the clinician about everyday topics of interest?"*
8. *"Does the child sit and listen to stories and look at picture books by himself/herself?"*

B. Issues within the family. In some situations, children's behavior and development might be hampered by patterns within the family such as domestic conflict, alcohol or substance abuse, parental depression, financial concerns and food insecurity, crisis within the extended families, and loss and grief. In other families, developmental expectations might be based on gender, birth order, or learning problems within the family. Inappropriate family expectations for school success or differences between family members about school readiness should be discussed. Concerns about family functioning and support systems should be identified and addressed:

1. *"Have there been any changes within the family such as a move, change in employment, unemployment, separation or divorce, deployment, deportation, illness or death within extended family or friends? Have you noticed any changes in your child's behavior as a result?"*
2. *"All couples have their ups and downs. Would you say that currently your relationship is up, down, or in the middle? How do you and your partner resolve conflicts?"*

3. *"How is your health and the health of family members? Has that changed recently?"*
4. *"What was your experience in school? Were you happy and successful in school or was it a difficult experience for you? For the child's father/mother?"*

C. Physical examination. During the routine physical examination, place emphasis on handedness; coordination of gross, visual motor, and fine motor activities; and the presence or absence of excessive overflow movements. Examine the child's vision, hearing, dentition, neurologic status, sensory integration, and neurodevelopmental maturation. A quick informal assessment of multiple domains is to ask the child, *"Can you draw me a picture of your family?"* The clinician will quickly be able to assess the child's receptive language, willingness to follow directions, fine motor skills to hold the pen/pencil properly, his or her handedness and sustained attention to the task. Any concerns should prompt a formal screening with an age-appropriate screen (see Chapter 5).

D. Developmental assessment. Unfortunately, there are currently few good developmental screening tests that are predictive of school success. Most instruments available to the pediatric clinician are not equipped to detect subtle learning disabilities or a more complicated diagnosis. If assessment is warranted because of parental, school, or pediatric concern, a referral should be made, either to the school district for an evaluation, or to an independent specialist such as a developmental and behavioral pediatrician, neuropsychologist, or learning disabilities specialist.

III. MANAGEMENT

A. Children with specific learning or developmental problems. Children with identified learning problems should be referred for a complete evaluation by the school department or by an independent evaluator. Pediatric clinics should have referral information easily available to help parents navigate the evaluation process and assist with future referrals for assessment, treatment, or therapeutic interventions. Under federal law, children with special learning needs are required to receive appropriate services within "the least restrictive environment." Parents may opt to provide additional independent services such as speech or sensory integration therapy if these are not provided in the child's individual education plan. Clinicians should monitor the child's progress carefully to determine the accessibility and effectiveness of the particular therapy or educational plan. For children with identified problems, school entry can be a particularly challenging time for parents who may have been able to deny a child's learning problems during the preschool period. Parents often look to clinicians for projections about their child's future, thus it is important to provide realistic, but hopeful, parameters for families with commitment to follow the child's progress with them.

B. Behavioral issues. School placement for children who present with acting out, impulsive behaviors, or extremely shy, inhibited behaviors should be carefully considered. Parents and clinicians must be vigilant in addressing the issues behind the labeling so that the label does not become a self-fulfilling prophecy for the child. Some school settings are a bad fit for these children. Because of overcrowding, inadequate teaching, or the overwhelming needs of the larger school population, withdrawn or inhibited children who cause no trouble can be ignored as attention goes to more aggressive or demanding children. Similarly, disruptive children or those with impulse control problems can be quickly identified as difficult students even if they are quite bright. Not surprisingly, kindergarten teachers report that it is easiest to help children to develop their academic skills and hardest to make an impact in developing their self-regulation skills.

C. Low-income and minority students. Low-income and minority students are more likely to enter school behind than their more advantaged peers. The children at highest risk for poor school readiness are children living in poverty, "English language learners", and those with mothers with low maternal educational backgrounds. Pediatric providers have universal access to these children before formal school entry and can help parents provide positive early learning opportunities to offset the later achievement gap. Providers can encourage parents to talk, read, and sing with their child in their home language regardless of their own literacy level; model book sharing and reading at different development stages; encourage participation in local play groups or library story times; and provide resources on local childcare. Before age 3 years, providers should discuss the benefits of preschool and encourage enrollment in high-quality preschool programs, as many families qualify for subsidized state or federally funded HeadStart programs, but may face long waitlists. Priority is given to low-income children with special needs including mild language delays.

D. Is the school ready for the child? The new Common Core kindergarten standards (2014) are driven by an increased focus on mastery of English language arts and math skills such as reading and counting rather than an as introduction to learning, time for socialization, and pretend play. Yet only modest gains have been reported from this more rigorous academic approach. In fact, research continues to indicate that incorporating play and pretend play into classroom settings improves children's executive function and self-regulation skills.

Perhaps the most challenging task for clinicians is to help families negotiate school entrance when the school does not have appropriate options for children with particular special needs. Although schools are required to educate all children within the least restrictive environment, they are often unable to provide carefully planned learning experiences for children with significant emotional or technological needs. Some schools cannot provide the developmentally appropriate experiences needed by children who have experienced trauma such as extreme poverty, child abuse, domestic violence, or parental depression and substance abuse. Finally, many schools do not have the resources to cope with the increasing linguistic demands of children who have recently immigrated to this country. Clinicians have tremendous untapped power to advocate on behalf of these children. Clinicians need to join voices with the families to persuade schools to provide appropriate educational experiences for all children. Clinicians should review initial and annual "Individual Education Plans" with parents to ensure they understand the goals for their child and how to support them both at school and home. If outlined services are not being provided, clinicians can contact the school district directly, help the parent write a letter, or refer the family to local support services.

E. **Waiting another year.** School entrance deadlines are arbitrarily set, based as much on demographics and finances (how many young children are in the upcoming kindergarten cohort and does the school have the space and teaching resources to provide for them if the cutoff date is June or November?) as they are on best practice. There is no magic age when all children are optimally ready for school. It is important to support parents of babies born in late summer or early fall as they think through the options available to them and their child. Transitional kindergarten has emerged with strong evidence as an alternative for this cohort as opposed to remaining in preschool or at home for another year. Providers can help parents consider the best option for their child:

1. *"Is transitional kindergarten offered by the school or school district?"*
2. *"Will there be appropriate social and learning peers in the preschool for the child?"*
3. *"Will there be adequate new challenges in the preschool for the child?"*
4. *"Are the child's physical appearance and social skills in line with the proposed preschool placement?"* This may differ for boys and girls.
5. *"Do both parents agree with the decision to retain the child in preschool?"*
6. *"Does the preschool program agree with the parents' decision to retain the child for another year?"*
7. *"What is the community norm? Do many parents hold back their 'fall' children?"*
8. *"What does the child expect to happen? Will the child perceive staying in preschool as a failure if everyone else goes on to transitional kindergarten or kindergarten?"*
9. *"If needed, will supplemental interventions and extra support such as speech therapy be provided?"*

If the parents decide to send the child on to elementary school:

1. *"What options might be available now for preparing the child for school entry?"*
2. Parents can ask for the upcoming class list and arrange for their child to spend time with a few children who will be in the same class. Seeing familiar faces when entering a new school can be extremely reassuring, especially to shy or slow-to-warm-up children.
3. *"Does the school have options for additional support for the child such as a transitional classroom, a second year of kindergarten if warranted, resource room support, or after school programming?"*

If the child begins to have serious problems in school, it is important to acknowledge the placement mistake early on, rather than continuing to push the child ahead in the hope that he or she will catch up. It is much easier to retain a child for a second year in kindergarten or first grade than it is to repeat the fourth grade where serious learning problems may prevent the child from keeping up. Many parents report that their young or immature children do all right in the first half of the school year when much of the work is reviewed, but that they encounter significant and disheartening failure during the second half of the school year as teachers push children to master the required curriculum. Because school learning and success are so closely related to lifelong self-esteem, initial placement decisions should be taken seriously and careful thought be given to possible retention if the child is struggling in kindergarten or first grade.

Bibliography

FOR PARENTS

Pianta R, Kraft-Sayre M. *Successful Kindergarten Transition: Your Guide to Connecting Children, Families, & Schools*. Baltimore, MD: Paul H. Brookes Pub Co; 2003.

FOR CHILDREN

Cohen M, Hoban L. *Will I Have a Friend?* New York, NY: Aladin Paperbacks; 1986.

Davis K. *Kindergarten Rocks!* New York, NY: Harcourt Children's Books; 2005.

McGhee A. *Countdown to Kindergarten*. New York, NY: Harcourt Children's Books; 2002.

Silicon Valley Community Foundation. *Video Series: Kindergarten Readiness Guide—Tools and Tips to Help Children Succeed in Kindergarten*. https://www.youtube.com/watch?v=38MNjl60iOI&index=1&list=PLHGt6gSkGo7dreyqmf23NxsKGQ7oe_zsD.

Wing N, Durrell J. *The Night Before Kindergarten*. New York, NY: Grosset & Dunlap; 2001.

FOR PROFESSIONALS

American Academy of Pediatrics Policy. *The Inappropriate Use of School Readiness Tests*. http://www.aap.org/policy/00694.html.

Council on early childhood, Council on school health. The pediatrician's role in optimizing school readiness. *Pediatrics*. 2016;138(3).

Hagan JF, Shaw SJ, Duncan PM, eds. *Bright Futures: Guidelines for Health Supervision of Infants, Children, and Adolescents*. 3rd ed. Elk Grove Village, IL: American Academy of Pediatrics; 2008.

Hart B, Risley TR. The early catastrophe: the 30 million word gap by age 3. *American Educator*. 2003;27(1):4-9.

Shonkoff JP, Garner AS. The lifelong effects of early childhood adversity and toxic stress. *Pediatrics*. 2012;129(1):e232-e246.

U.S. Department of Education. *Talk, Read and Sing Together Everyday: Tip Sheets for Families, Caregivers and Early Learning Educators*. https://www.ed.gov/early-learning/talk-read-sing.

CHAPTER 72

Selective Mutism

Naomi Steiner

I. DESCRIPTION OF THE PROBLEM. According to the DSM-5, selective mutism is an **anxiety disorder** characterized by the following:

- A child's inability to speak in certain social settings (such as childcare, school) where speaking is expected, despite speaking in other, usually more familiar settings (such as at home). This disturbance affects the child's daily function.
- Onset **usually before age 5 years**, although it may not come to clinical attention until school entry.
- **Lasting for at least 1 month** (not including the first month of school or childcare, during which many children may be shy or reluctant to speak).

A. Epidemiology
- Limited research reports a **prevalence of 0.4%–0.7%** children in the general population.
- Around **70% of these children also have another anxiety-related disorder, with social phobia being the most frequent.**
- Girls outnumber boys 2 to 1.
- Although selective mutism usually lasts for only a few months, it may persist longer and may even continue for several years.

B. Etiology/contributing factors
1. **Genetic predisposition.** There is often a first-degree family history of social anxiety (38%) and social phobia (37%).
2. **Speech and language delays** are present in around 30% (most commonly expressive language and phonologic disorders) of the children with selective mutism.
3. **Bilingualism.** Immigrant children who are unfamiliar with or uncomfortable in a new language may refuse to speak to strangers in their new environment; this behavior should not be misdiagnosed as selective mutism. However, a prolonged silent phase should be seen as a potential red flag when selective mutism and language delay are being considered.
4. **No research has associated selective mutism with abuse, neglect, or trauma.**

II. MAKING THE DIAGNOSIS. Initial screenings are simple, involving some observation and a few questions. The classic sign of selective mutism is that the child talks well within the home but not outside in social settings.

A. Behavioral observations
- Symptoms of withdrawal in unfamiliar situations are difficulty with eye contact, avoidance of social interaction, stiff body language, blank facial expression, using only gestures to communicate in the office, etc.
- Marked contrast between selected environments and **the home situation**, where parents often report a very chatty child. Clinicians may want to view a videotape of the child at home to be reassured that the child's language and social communication in a comfortable environment is normal.
- Shy children will "button up" and not speak for a few hours or days but will eventually start speaking. A shy child can function. Those with selected mutism will not speak for a prolonged period, causing significant and prolonged social dysfunction.

B. History: key clinical questions
- *"How was your child as an infant or toddler?"*
- *"How is he/she at school? Or birthday parties?"*
- *"How is he/she at home?"*
- *"Is there anybody in your family with selective mutism, anxiety, panic attacks, extreme shyness, or other emotional issues?"*

C. Differential diagnosis. In the past, selective mutism was sometimes misunderstood as a strong-willed and manipulative child *refusing* to speak (as in oppositional defiant disorder), as opposed to a child conditioned by a true fear of speaking. Selective mutism should be distinguished from speech disturbances that are **better accounted for by a communication disorder such as phonologic disorder** or developmental language disorder. Individuals with autism spectrum disorder or intellectual disability may have problems in social communication and be unable to speak appropriately in social situations. However, in contrast, in selective mutism the child has an established capacity to speak in some social situations, for example, typically at home.

D. Tests

1. **Audiogram**—as with any speech and language disorder, it is always prudent to assure normal hearing.
2. **Speech and language evaluation** is often indicated as 30%–40% of children with selective mutism also have some speech and language delay. This may be very difficult to obtain as the stress of the testing situation may preclude optimal testing in which case a videotape may suffice.

III. MANAGEMENT

A. Early diagnosis and rapid referral is essential for the child with selective mutism. Children with selective mutism do not necessarily outgrow their disability. Many may start to speak a little, whereas others spend years growing up without speaking. If these children do not learn to cope, they may remain significantly impaired compared with their unaffected peers. The overall goal is **to treat the anxiety rather than force the child to speak**.

1. **Team approach.** The family, school, and therapist should work together to develop an individualized plan to **reduce anxiety, reduce pressure to speak, and increase self-esteem**. Education of the teaching team is critical, as constraining the child to speak can lead to the child withdrawing more and speaking less. Consistent, supportive relationships outside the home are the mainstay of achieving these goals.
2. **Behavioral therapy** is increasingly recognized as the first-line approach for treatment of selective mutism, frequently with a cognitive approach for older children. It is extremely important that the child be referred to an experienced clinician who will work closely with the family and the school. Often weekly appointments will be necessary with "homework" to achieve progress. Group therapy can be very effective. The therapist will use techniques such as contingency and stimulus fading (where the child requires less and less prompting to speak out loud in a given situation), positive reinforcement, systematic desensitization (or gradual exposure therapy, offers situations where the child is able to practice speaking), extinction (where refusing to speak is ignored), modeling (even using videotapes), and social problem-solving.
3. **Other psychological approaches** such as family therapy, self-modeling, relaxation training (e.g., learning breathing techniques), and social skills groups can also be helpful in adjunct to the behavioral approach.
4. **Medication in combination with therapy** is used in the most chronic cases. Selective serotonin reuptake inhibitors have been shown to have a positive effect as they lower the anxiety threshold.

Bibliography

FOR PARENTS

American Speech Language Hearing Association. http://www.asha.org/Practice-Portal/Clinical-Topics/Selective-Mutism/.

Selective Mutism. www.selectivemutism.org.

FOR PROFESSIONALS

Kristensen H. Selective mutism and comorbidity with developmental disorder/delay, anxiety disorder, and elimination disorder. *J Am Acad Child Adolesc Psychiatry*. 2000;39:249-256.

Manassis K, Oerbeck B, Overgaard KR. The use of medication in selective mutism: a systematic review. *Eur Child Adolesc Psychiatry*. 2015;6:1-8.

Viana AG, Beidel DC, Rabian B. Selective mutism: a review and integration of the last 15 years. *Clin Psychol Rev*. 2009;29:57-67. doi:10.1016/j.cpr.2008.09.009.

Wong P. Selective mutism: a review of etiology, comorbidities, and treatment. *Psychiatry (Edgmont)*. 2010;7(3):23-31.

CHAPTER 73

Sensory Processing Difficulties

Neelkamal S. Soares

I. **DESCRIPTION OF THE PROBLEM.** Sensory processing refers to the way the brain detects, registers, organizes, modulates, and responds to sensory stimuli, both from the environment (external) and body processes (internal). The term "sensory processing" has recently replaced "sensory integration," as the latter more appropriately describes the neurologic process that occurs at a cellular level and the theoretical underpinnings of symptoms, whereas the former refers to the clinical symptoms and presentation. Alterations in sensory processing leading to overstimulation or understimulation in response to sensory stimuli are termed sensory processing difficulties (SPDs). The term "sensory processing disorder" was first used in the 1970s by clinicians but has not been included in either *Diagnostic and Statistical Manual of Mental Disorders- 5th edition* (DSM-5) or International Classification of Diseases, 10th Edition. (ICD-10), and the American Academy of Pediatrics (AAP) recommends that sensory processing disorder generally should not be diagnosed. Although these recommendations are acknowledged, SPD is included in this chapter because occupational therapists, parents, media, and other professionals use it and it is likely to be brought to the attention of primary care clinicians.

II. **EPIDEMIOLOGY.** Prevalence estimates for SPD have been difficult to determine because of the lack of standardized diagnostic guidelines and methods. A study of 730 parent perceptions from one suburban school district yielded a prevalence of sensory processing disorders between 5.3% and 13.7% consistent with the range from other studies whether by parent report or by direct assessment. Studies have also been conducted in specific clinical populations, with small cohorts, including 95% rate among children with autism spectrum disorder (ASD) and 44%–64% of children with developmental and/or behavioral concerns depending on the criteria applied.

Clinicians report higher incidence of SPD in boys than in girls. In twin studies, concordance rates were higher among monozygotic than dizygotic pairs, with a greater heritable influence for tactile difficulties compared with auditory difficulties.

III. **ETIOLOGY/CONTRIBUTING FACTORS.** Although there is no definitive etiology underlying SPDs, several contributing factors are thought to be implicated: temperament, autonomic nervous system responses, and neurophysiology. There is emerging neurophysiological information that looks at correlates but no definitive etiology.

Risk factors. Studies have found that some medical conditions are risk factors for SPD, including low birthweight, prematurity, intrauterine exposure to maternal medications, and psychosocial risk factors such as ethnic minority, living with a single parent, higher parenting stress, and low socioeconomic status.

IV. **FEATURES OF SPD.** There are three distinct patterns of SPD, which have been grouped in the following classification:
- Sensory modulation
- Sensory-based motor
- Sensory discrimination

A. **Sensory modulation disorder.** Sensory modulation is the process of grading and regulating one's response to sensory input. Impairment in regulating the degree, intensity, and nature of responses to sensory input results in impact on daily roles and routines. Depending on the "mismatch" between the magnitude of the child's response with the perceived stimulus, there are three types of SMDs:
1. Sensory overresponsivity
2. Sensory underresponsivity
3. Sensory seeking

Table 73-1 outlines the behavioral manifestation of this self-regulation in these different types of sensory modulation disorders (SMDs).

B. **Sensory discrimination disorder.** Sensory discrimination disorder is characterized by inappropriate qualitative processing of one or more sensory modalities. Some impacts are felt in visual discrimination (affecting pattern recognition and visuospatial skills), auditory discrimination (affecting sound discrimination, which can affect language processing), and tactile discrimination (which can affect stereognosis and graphesthesia).

Table 73-1 • BEHAVIORAL REGULATION IN CHILDREN WITH DIFFERENT TYPES OF SENSORY MODULATION DISORDER

	Sensory Overresponsivity	Sensory Underresponsivity	Sensory Seeking
Arousal	Usually high arousal	Usually decreased arousal	Arousal may be heightened, but labile
Attention	Inability to focus, easily distractible	Inattentive, has a latency to concentrate, lack of awareness of novelty	Poorly modulated attention
Affect	Predominantly negative affect—often in "fight or flight" state	Restricted or flat affect—may appear sad or emotionally unavailable	Affect is variable, but may become overexcited with excess sensory input
Action	Impulsive reaction—may seem aggressive	Passive—may observe other children, but not engage in active peer play	Action is geared primarily to gaining sensation, may be impulsive and take excess risks

Somatosensory discrimination involves the proprioceptive and vestibular system and is responsible for movement planning and postural awareness and stability. This contributes to the sensory-based motor disorders (below).

C. **Sensory-based motor disorders.** There are two types of sensory-based motor disorders: **dyspraxia** and **postural**; both are thought to be more related to a deficit in sensory processing than motor impairment.

Dyspraxia is an inability to formulate, plan, and execute unfamiliar complex motor acts. This generally does not affect a commonly practiced, familiar task (self-dressing, etc.). These children can appear clumsy or accident-prone and tend to avoid unfamiliar gross and fine motor actions. They may demonstrate poor timing, grading, and accuracy of movement and may struggle to learn new motor tasks or generalize a skill to new situations. Children with dyspraxia may have low self-esteem, have low frustration tolerance, prefer sedentary or language-based activities, and tend to be creative in activities that do not require much motor planning.

Postural disorders are characterized by difficulty in moving, stabilizing, and adjusting posture. It is often associated with mild hypotonia, poor bilateral coordination, and poor equilibrium reactions. They are associated with poor processing of vestibular and proprioceptive input (see above). An example is a child who is unable to maintain proper seated posture while working on bimanual tasks (writing, coloring) in a classroom environment. Postural disorders often occur in combination with sensory modulation and discrimination disorders or dyspraxia.

V. **MAKING THE DIAGNOSIS.** SPD is not a discrete medical diagnosis, and the AAP does not recommend considering it so, without consideration of some of the comorbid risk factors listed above. Although SPD can be seen in isolation, it is often diagnosed by occupational therapists and some psychologists. Different disciplines approach diagnostics differently, leading to confusion in families. Clinicians need to be familiar with the diagnostic approaches used by medical and allied professionals.

A. **History.** The first step in exploring SPD is to identify the relevant symptoms of concern to families and/or other providers (childcare, educational). Some examples of symptoms are provided in Table 73-1. All the sensory systems can be involved in SPD, either singularly or in combination including tactile, auditory, visual, vestibular, proprioceptive, olfactory, and gustatory. The clinical expression can be varied from general symptoms, such as poor self-regulation of arousal, attention, and affect, to specific system symptoms and can affect developmental domains (cognitive, motor) and functional abilities exhibited through behavior and emotion.

The next step is determining if, and how, symptoms are interfering with daily functioning across a variety of developmental, behavioral, and interpersonal domains. Other developmental and behavioral disorders will need to be considered, which may take precedence over a stand-alone consideration of SPD.

Information should be elicited from targeted history from caregivers and other respondents using questions such as the following:

General:

- *"Was the child unusually fussy, difficult to console, or easily startled as an infant?"*
- *"Does the child have sensory preferences or avoidances? Are these preferences consistent?"*
- *"Does the child overreact (or underreact) to specific situations? Does the child express an appropriate range of affect in response to sensory input?"*

  Specific:
- *"Is the child over- or undersensitive to clothing (e.g., refusal to wear certain fabrics or types of clothes; not notice wearing shoes on the wrong foot)?"*
- *"Does the child avoid or strongly dislike of baths, haircuts, or nail cutting?"*
- *"Does the child use an inappropriate amount of force when handling objects, writing, or touching siblings or pets?"*
- *"Is the child clumsy, fall frequently, bump into furniture or people, or have trouble judging the position of their body in relation to the surrounding space?"*

The clinician should remember that symptoms will vary based on the age and developmental stage of the child, the environmental context, and the expectations of the caregivers.

In infancy, these children often do not cuddle, are fussy, and have problematic sleep patterns. As children get older and more independent in activities of daily living, they resist or have inappropriate behavioral responses to sensory stimuli. Problematic behaviors may be variable and contextual (certain locations, times of day) and depend on the degree of stimuli (a problem when others touch the child but not vice versa).

Impact of these symptoms on daily life can be gleaned from the developmental history, where caregivers generally report normal to low normal acquisition of developmental milestones. If present, delays may be seen in gross motor domain with posture, mildly late walking, and limited flexibility in the utilization of new skills. Socialization with peers or siblings can be affected by sensory responses and occasionally a child may be delayed in acquisition of adaptive/self-care skills. Generally, language and cognitive domains are not impaired. Learning can be affected if the child cannot sustain attention in the class setting because of being overwhelmed or distracted by environmental stimuli.

Impact of the SPD symptoms on family functioning can be gauged from history of reduced attempts to make community trips as a family, parental stress, and reduced parental perceived competence.

- B. **Measures.** Some instruments developed to measure sensory symptoms include the following:
  1. **Sensory Profile-2** (Dunn, 2014)
  2. **Sensory Processing Measure** (Parham et al., 2010)
  3. **De Gangi-Berk Test of Sensory Integration** (DeGangi and Berk, 2013)
  4. **Sensory Integration and Praxis Test** (Ayres, 1989)

     Additionally, therapists will often collect subjective data of the strengths and limitations of a child, including observations in naturalistic (home and school) settings to complement the objective data from the measures above.
- C. **Multidisciplinary evaluation.** Apart from an occupational therapy evaluation for SPD, evaluations to rule out comorbid learning or behavioral disorders may require a multidisciplinary team evaluation involving special educators, psychologists, and medical professionals

     These may be conducted concurrently or sequentially depending on resources available in any particular clinical setting.

VI. **DIFFERENTIAL DIAGNOSIS.** Children with other disabilities can also have symptoms associated with SPDs. Many children, especially when younger, experience symptoms of SPD. Examples include tactile (picky about clothing, tags, fingernail trimming, and teeth brushing), oral (food texture, taste, temperature), and auditory (loud sounds such as fireworks, machinery). However, these generally do not progress toward impairing functioning in daily living, are intermittent, and are outgrown, although they can be a source of distress for children and families.

It is widely understood that SPDs can occur in several neurodevelopmental disorders, which can also modulate symptoms. Some examples are as follows:

- A. **ASD.** Although sensory features were in the original Kanner's description of autism in the 1940s, they were not considered essential criteria until the most recent edition (DSM-5) under the restricted repetitive patterns of behaviors, interests, or activities as hyper- or hyporeactivity to sensory input or unusual interests in the sensory environment.
- B. Fetal alcohol spectrum disorder
- C. Fragile X syndrome

D. Affective disorders
E. Attention deficit hyperactivity disorder

Additionally, specific sensory-based motor disorders should be differentiated from DSM-5 neurodevelopmental disorders such as developmental coordination disorder and other neurologic disorders with motor symptoms (cerebral palsy, cerebellar, and brain stem disorders). SMDs should be differentiated from behavioral disorders such as stereotypic movement disorder.

VII. MANAGEMENT

A. Caregiver education. Caregivers and educators who work with children who demonstrate SPD need help and guidance on strategies to assist the child. The clinician, occupational therapist, and behavior specialist can all provide guidance in this regard. Goals for this education:

- To recognize stimuli triggers and the child's responses to the stimuli
- To be prepared to adjust the situation or help the child cope with the situation to reduce distress
- To support the child's self-esteem and social participation

Caregivers and educators are important collaborators in assisting a child with SPD, as they are most familiar with the child in naturalistic environments. They can implement strategies devised by occupational therapists and can share data with clinicians to aid in the diagnostic process.

Key information that can help formulate the management plan include the following:

- The nature of the physical and social environment the child is exposed to
- The potential triggers in the environment or activity that the child is engaging in
- The child's innate (temperament) characteristics and style of learning and interacting

Caregivers need to be taught about autonomic signs and behavioral signals of increased arousal, distress, and impending behavioral responses so that they can effectively and promptly intervene with appropriate strategies. The ultimate goal is to allow families the opportunity to organize daily routines that are sustainable and meaningful for all family members and for learning environments to provide the child optimal opportunities for social participation and self-regulation, while building competence and working on developmental skills.

B. Direct intervention. Many clinicians can be involved in interventions for children with SPD; primary among them are not only occupational therapists (with training or experience in sensory integration strategies) but also behavior therapists, psychologists, or special educators.

Direct intervention usually occurs in a clinic environment, is intermittent, and is delivered by the clinician, whereas indirect interventions occur in home, school, or other naturalistic environments and are delivered by caregivers, educators, and other childcare workers (under the direction of clinician recommendations).

According to sensory integration theory, providing sensory-rich inputs is supposed to improve the integration of sensory information by the nervous system. However, there is no standard protocol for implementing treatments and there is a lack of empirical support for their benefit, at least in children with identified developmental disorders. Treatments can be costly, are generally not covered by insurance (although some overlap with developmental disorders allows therapists to bill for specific activities), and can involve a significant time commitment from families, which may conflict with time and resources for other empirically based treatments.

Interventions range from passive modalities (wearing a weighted vest or blanket, brushing, and massage, using therapy balls) to more active (e.g., jumping on a trampoline, climbing on monkey-bars) activities, and target hyper- or hyposensitivities. A "sensory diet" is a menu of activities and items that families can select from on a daily basis to stimulate the child with SPD.

The AAP recommends that clinicians working with families who choose to follow sensory-based treatments should monitor their efficacy, help families define "end points" for achieving intended results, and prioritize treatments that affect the child's daily functioning while being aware of the cost of pursuing the treatments.

Bibliography

BOOKS FOR PARENTS

Dunn W. *Living Sensationally: Understanding Your Senses.* 1st ed. Philadelphia, PA: Jessica Kingsley Publishers; 2009.

Kranowitz CS. *The Out of Sync Child: Recognizing and Coping With Sensory Integrative Dysfunction.* Revised ed. New York, NY: Perigee; 2006.

Miller LG, Fuller DA. *Sensational Kids: Hope and Help for Children with SPD*. Revised ed. New York, NY: Perigee; 2014.

BOOKS FOR CHILDREN

Harding JHH, Padgett D. *Ellie Bean the Drama Queen: A Children's Book about Sensory Processing Disorder*. Arlington, TX: Sensory World; 2011.

Veenendall J. *Why Does Izzy Cover Her Ears? Dealing with Sensory Overload*. 1st ed. Shawnee Mission, KS: Autism Asperger Publishing Company; 2009.

WEB SITES

Star Institute for Sensory Processing Disorder. Formed in 2016 from two merged organizations SPD Foundation and STAR Center, it provides information regarding treatment, education, and research for children, adolescents, and adults with SPD. http://www.spdfoundation.net/.

FOR PROFESSIONALS

Ahn RR, Miller LJ, Milberger S, McIntosh DN. Prevalence of parents' perceptions of sensory processing disorders among kindergarten children. *Am J Occup Ther*. 2004;58(3):287-293.

American Academy of Pediatrics Section on Complementary and Integrative Disabilities and Council on Children With Disabilities. Sensory integration therapies for children with developmental and behavioral disorders. *Pediatrics*. 2012;129(6):1186-1189.

Barton EE, Reichow B, Schnitz A, Smith IC, Sherlock D. A systematic review of sensory-based treatments for children with disabilities. *Res Dev Disabil*. 2015;37:64-80.

Gourley L, Wind C, Henninger EM, Chinitz S. Sensory processing difficulties, behavioral problems, and parental stress in a clinical population of young children. *J Child Fam Stud*. 2013;22(7):912-921.

McCormick C, Hepburn S, Young GS, Rogers SJ. Sensory symptoms in children with autism spectrum disorder, other developmental disorders and typical development: a longitudinal study. *Autism*. 2016;20(5):572-579.

Owen JP, Marco EJ, Desai S, et al. Abnormal white matter microstructure in children with sensory processing disorders. *NeuroImage Clin*. 2013;2(1):844-853.

BOOKS

Bundy AC, Lane SJ, Murray EA, eds. *Sensory Integration: Theory and Practice*. 2nd ed. Philadelphia: FA Davis Co.; 2002.

Williamson GG, Anzalone ME. *Sensory Integration and Self-regulation in Infants and Toddlers: Helping Young Children to Interact with Their Environments*. Washington, DC: Zero-to-Three; 2001.

CHAPTER 74

Sex and the Adolescent

Melissa T. Nass | Linda M. Grant

I. DESCRIPTION OF THE ISSUE. The expression of human sexuality is a complex interplay of biologic, psychological, interpersonal, and social factors—each with varying importance as the child grows up. In fact, sexual development begins long before puberty and involves much more than basic reproductive physiology. Intimacy, reciprocity, self-esteem, body image, gender identity, attraction, and pleasure are fundamentals of human sexuality that develop over the course of a lifetime. However, the enormous cognitive and emotional changes that occur during adolescence, coupled with the teen's newly discovered ability to engage in sexual activity, make adolescence a precarious time for sexual health and wellness. The "adolescent visit" presents a ripe opportunity for the pediatric clinician to move beyond a simple "risk reduction" dialogue with the teen to one that promotes healthy sexual behavior and responsible decision-making.

A. Epidemiology. There is no one profile of adolescent sexuality. Trends in coital initiation and continuation of sexual activity reflect differing ethnic, cultural, and sex-specific rates.

1. **Sexual activity.** Among US high school students surveyed using the CDC's Youth Risk Behavior Surveillance System (YRBSS) in 2015:
   - 41% had ever had sexual intercourse.
   - 30% had had sexual intercourse during the previous 3 months, and of these:
     - 43% did not use a condom the last time they had sex.
     - 14% did not use any method to prevent pregnancy.
     - 21% had drunk alcohol or used drugs before last sexual intercourse.
   - On average, young people in the United States have sex for the first time at about age 17 years.
   - Teen sex is increasingly likely to be described as wanted.

2. **Teen pregnancy.** The United States has one of the highest rates of teenage pregnancy of any industrialized country.
   - Nearly 230,000 babies were born to teen girls aged 15–19 years in 2015.
   - In 2011, about 553,000 US women aged 15–19 years became pregnant. Seventy percent of teen pregnancies occurred among the oldest teens (18- to 19-year-olds).

3. **Sexually transmitted diseases/infections**
   - Only 10% of all students have ever been tested for human immunodeficiency virus (HIV).
   - Young people (aged 13–24 years) accounted for an estimated 22% of all new HIV diagnoses in the United States in 2015.
   - Half of the nearly 20 million new sexually transmitted diseases (STDs) reported each year are among young people, between the ages of 15–24 years.
   - Human papillomavirus (HPV) is the most common sexually transmitted infection (STI).
   - HPV infections account for more than two-thirds of STIs diagnosed among 15- to 24-year-olds each year.
   - Chlamydia is the next most common STI diagnosed among 15- to 24-year-olds, accounting for nearly 20% of diagnoses each year. Genital herpes, gonorrhea, and trichomoniasis together account for about 11% of diagnoses. HIV, syphilis, and hepatitis B are estimated to account for less than 1% of diagnoses.

4. **Contraceptive use**
   - The proportion of US females aged 15–19 years who used contraceptives the first time they had sex has increased from 48% in 1982 to 79% in 2011–2013.
   - Adolescents who report having had sex at age 14 years or younger are less likely than those who initiated sex later to have used a contraceptive method at first sex, and they take longer to begin using contraceptives.
   - The condom is the contraceptive method most commonly used at first intercourse.

- In 2012, 4.3% of female contraceptive users aged 15–19 years used a long-acting reversible contraceptive method (intrauterine device [IUD] or implant) in the last month.
- In 2006–2010, 14% of sexually experienced females aged 15–19 years had ever used emergency contraception.

5. Intimate partner violence
- Among high school students who date, 21% of females and 10% of males experience physical and/or sexual dating violence.
- Among adult victims of rape/physical violence and/or stalking by an intimate partner, 22% of women and 10% of men first experience some sort of dating violence between the ages of 11 and 17 years.

6. LGBTQ. Lesbian, gay, bisexual, transgender, and questioning (LGBTQ) adolescents have higher rates of attempted and completed suicide, violence victimization, substance abuse, and human immunodeficiency virus (HIV) risk. Most have an awareness of their orientation by the age of 9 or 10 years.
- Three percent of females and eight percent of males aged 18–19 years in 2006–2008 reported their sexual orientation as lesbian/gay or bisexual. During the same period, 12% of females and 4% of males aged 18–19 years reported same-sex sexual behaviors (see Chapter 52).

B. Understanding teen sexual behavior in a developmental framework. The transition from childhood to adulthood is not a continuous, synchronous process. Furthermore, adolescents are a diverse group and display wide variation of biologic, psychological, and emotional growth—"a 15-year-old, is not a 15-year-old." Although these two factors present challenges when working with teens, the clinician must consider adolescent sexual behavior in the context of the adolescent's normative developmental framework. This makes it easier for him or her to identify the adolescent's strengths and vulnerabilities and counsel without judgment.

C. Developing secondary sexual characteristics. At puberty, the teen faces a changing body and bewildering emotions, often fueled by hormonal surges. Early adolescence is characterized by:
- a preoccupation with self and pubertal changes,
- uncertainty about appearance and attractiveness,
- frequent comparison with one's own body and those of other adolescents, and
- a tendency to magnify one's own personal situation.

Adolescents are often uncomfortable with their changing physical identity. Developing a positive self-image and personal comfort with body parts and bodily functions are important for healthy sexual development. The pediatric clinician can support this by respecting the teen's modesty and need for privacy when doing a physical examination and by using anatomically correct language when discussing body parts and bodily functions.

1. Developing a separate identity. The adolescent must develop an identity separate from the family. As adolescents separate from the family, they develop "replacement relationships" with their peers. The mid-adolescent will have little interest in his parents, intense involvement in his or her subculture, and conformity with peer values. Social networking platforms provide an obvious venue to support these developmental tasks. By understanding sexual behavior as a rite of passage that distinguishes oneself from the family and appreciating the importance of the social network for teens, it is understandable why teens may engage in high-risk online "sexting,"—the act of sending sexually explicit messages or photographs.

2. Developing intimate relationships. Developing the capacity for intimate and meaningful mutual relationships is an ongoing task of adolescence. Early relationships may involve physical intimacy as a means of comparison and experimentation. Fleeting relationships and same-sex exploration are not uncommon. Later, with the addition of formal operational thinking, emotional intimacy and reciprocity can be incorporated into relationships. The clinician can address this important developmental task by discussing mutuality, respect, and reciprocity directly and by screening for intimate partner violence.

3. Developing the ability to think abstractly. Concrete operational thinking dominates early adolescence and mid-adolescence. Therefore, young adolescents are incapable of fully understanding the ramifications of their actions. This limitation, coupled with a sense of infallibility and invulnerability, and an inability to delay gratification, increases sexual risk taking.

Formal operational thinking, developed later in adolescence, allows teens to generate a more appropriate decision-making tree and to develop abstract thinking on moral values. Clinicians should be mindful to use concrete language with discussing sexuality with young adolescents, reserving abstract discussion for more mature teens.

4. **Sexual orientation.** Children have a sense of their sexual orientation at an early age. Gay teens have the same developmental tasks as heterosexual teens but may not have access to positive support systems that allow for fine-tuning the learning tasks of dating and loving (see Chapter 52).

5. **Special needs.** Children with cognitive and/or physical disabilities have the same sexual feelings and sexual developmental needs as their nondisabled peers. Additionally, adolescents with physical disabilities are as sexually experienced as their typically developing peers. However, most adolescents with physical and developmental disabilities report that they lack knowledge on parenthood, birth control, and STIs. Discussions and/or planning for these needs with parents should be an integral part of medical home management.

II. THE CLINICAL VISIT

A. **History.** The sexual history should be approached with the teen fully clothed and sitting at eye level with the provider.

B. **Confidentiality.** The key to engaging adolescents is creating a trusting, confidential, nonjudgmental, and honest atmosphere. For adolescents to talk about their sexual behaviors with the primary care clinician, they must be assured that their disclosure will not compromise their relationships with their family, friends, or the community. Adolescents often resist medical visits because they fear that their information will be shared with their parent. It is important to establish with them that what is said will be confidential and equally important is to inform them of any qualifying parameters.

Lay the parameters with the teen and the parent in the examination room together; for example, *"With all of my adolescent patients, I ask the parent to step out of the room (and into the waiting room where they can't eavesdrop!). This allows you to talk to me in private. Anything discussed will be kept confidential, unless it is a life-threatening situation or a situation of abuse—like physical or sexual abuse—then I need to get another grown-up involved. But we can talk about your body, your mood, your friends, sex, sexuality, smoking, drinking, drugs—all of those things are safe to talk about here."*

Note: clinicians should be aware of their state's statutes regarding mature and emancipated minors.

The sexual history is a part of a larger social history that screens for all risk behaviors while also assessing the strengths of the teen. The goal of a sexual history is to determine if there has been sexual activity and, if so, the degree of health or emotional risk involved. Questioning needs to be direct and comprehensive. The clinician should make no a priori assumptions about the sexual activity, practices, or sexual orientation of any adolescent.

C. **Identity versus behavior.** It is important to ask questions about sexual orientation and gender identity during the sexual history because attraction and identity are two important and wholly different components of healthy sexual development. The clinician has an important opportunity to validate the experience of LGBTQ youth, assess for support systems, and identify risk of depression, bullying, substance abuse, and physical abuse. However, he or she should not assume sexual orientation or gender identity predict sexual practices. Screening and sexual health counseling should be based on sexual behaviors—not identity.

- The clinician should use the gender-neutral pronouns "they" and "them" and should follow the patient's lead when discussing sexual partners and romantic relationships.
- The clinician should use neutral terms such as "sexual partner"; he or she should avoid using terms such as "boyfriend" or "girlfriend," which are gender specific and imply a relationship.

D. **Key clinical questions**

1. *"Have you ever had sex in your whole entire life?"*

   This is a much more concrete question than the frequently asked, "Are you sexually active?" which implies ongoing, frequent behavior and does not capture sexual behavior that may have occurred in the past. This first question is easier for young teens to answer truthfully.

2. *Have you ever done more than kissing?*

   This question addresses behaviors that the teen might not consider "sex" but still pose a risk such as oral or anal sex. More directly, the provider could ask, *"Have you ever had oral sex or anal sex?"*

3. *Have you ever used a condom or barrier method?* Followed by, *"Have you ever not used a condom or barrier method?"*

These questions more accurately assess risk than the frequently asked, "Do you use condoms?"

4. *"How many partners have you had in the last 2 months? What about the last 6 months? How about in your entire life?"*

Asking the question in this graduated manner, makes it easier for the teen to disclose.

5. *"Who talks with you about sex? What do they tell you?"*
6. *"Do you have any questions about sex that you would like to ask me?"*
7. *"If you wanted to have sex but didn't want to get pregnant/get an STI, what should you do?"*
8. *"How old were you when you first had intercourse?"*
9. *"What made you decide to have sex?"*
10. *"Have you ever been pregnant? What happened to the pregnancy?"* or *"Have you gotten someone pregnant?"*
11. *"Are your partners boys, girls, or both?"*
12. *Are you attracted to boys, girls, both, or neither?"*
13. *"Is sex an enjoyable experience for you?"*
14. *Do you think of yourself as a male, female, or something else?*
15. *"What do you know about the different methods of birth control?"*
16. *"How do you feel about not being sexually active?"*
17. *"Have you ever 'sexted'?"*
18. *Tell me something that your partner does to show you they care about you. Has your partner ever slapped, hit, or threatened you? Have you ever been in a relationship that was violent?*
19. *"Has anyone ever forced you to have sex?"*

E. **Physical examination.** It is prudent to ask about the patient's comfort level and request for a chaperone.

"Now I am going to do a full physical examination, including a check of your genitals/ private parts. Some patients feel more comfortable with a nurse/chaperone in the room. Would you like me to ask a nurse to chaperone the examination?"

1. **Pelvic examination: necessary or not?** Current guidelines suggest that adolescents do not require cervical cancer screening until the age of 21 years. Before then, the need to perform a pelvic examination will depend on the gynecological symptoms, history, and the availability of newer urine or self-swab tests for STI screening. It is also important to note that a pelvic examination is no longer required before the initiation of contraception.

   • A pelvic examination is rarely indicated in an adolescent who is *not* sexually active. Variables to consider include the patient's request and the nature of the gynecologic complaint. For the non–sexually active adolescent with a gynecologic complaint, external visualization and bimanual rectal palpation and/or pelvic ultrasound may be adequate.

   • Developing a positive attitude toward pelvic examinations begins with the first. Involve the adolescent so that she feels in control of the process. Each step should be anticipated so that there are no surprises. For example, she can be asked if she wants to look at her cervix and external genitalia in a handheld mirror. She should also be told that the examination will be stopped if she feels pain and she should describe any discomfort.

2. **Male genital examination.** The male genital examination is an important part of the adolescent visit but may also be anxiety provoking for the teen. After age 10 years, the male should be examined while standing, and it is helpful and educational to describe anatomic findings as a diversion during the examination. It is not necessary to comment on an erection unless the adolescent seems particularly embarrassed by it.

3. **Screening.** The "CDC Sexually Transmitted Disease Guidelines" remains an excellent resource for STI screening recommendations for adolescents. Below is a summary of the most recent (2015) recommendations for STI screening.

   • Routine screening for *Chlamydia trachomatis and Neisseria gonorrhoeae* of all sexually active females aged ≤25 years is recommended annually.

   • Evidence is insufficient to recommend routine screening for *C. trachomatis* in sexually active young men based on feasibility, efficacy, and cost-effectiveness. However, screening of sexually active young men should be considered in clinical settings associated with high prevalence of chlamydia.

- HIV screening should be offered to all adolescents 13 years and older and offered annually to young men having sex with men (YMSM).
- Guidelines from USPSTF and the American Congress of Obstetricians and Gynecologists (ACOG) recommend that cervical cancer screening begin at age 21 years.
- Syphilis serology with confirmatory testing should be offered annually to all YMSM.
- Screening for urethral infection with *N. gonorrhea* and *C. trachomatis* in men who have insertive intercourse should be offered annually.
- Screening for rectal infection with *N. gonorrhea* and *C. trachomatis* in young men who have receptive anal intercourse should be offered annually.
- Screening for pharyngeal infection with *N. gonorrhea* in men who have had receptive oral intercourse should be offered annually.

The above recommendations are *guidelines*; clinicians should also consider local disease prevalence when screening. Additionally, special populations such as pregnant adolescents, HIV-infected teens, or incarcerated youth may require additional screening.

III. MANAGEMENT

A. Prevention. Updated recommendations by the Advisory Committee on Immunization Practices (ACIP) in 2016 include support for a two-dose schedule for HPV vaccination in patients less than 15 years of age. For persons initiating vaccination on or after their 15th birthday, the recommended immunization schedule is three doses of HPV vaccine. The second dose should be administered 1–2 months after the first dose, and the third dose should be administered 6 months after the first dose (0, 1–2, 6 month schedule). ACIP also recommends vaccination for females through age 26 years and for males through age 21 years who were not adequately vaccinated previously. For children with a history of sexual abuse or assault, ACIP recommends routine HPV vaccination beginning at age 9 years. ACIP recommends vaccination of YMSM through age 26 years, for those who were not adequately vaccinated previously.

B. Anticipatory guidance. Because human sexual development is a process that begins at birth, the pediatric visit provides numerous opportunities for the clinician to influence the healthy sexual development of children. Thoughtful, knowledgeable, and developmentally appropriate parental guidance in early childhood allow for a more natural dialogue about sexual issues at puberty. See Tables 74-1 and 74-2 for examples of appropriate anticipatory guidance as they relate to sexual development from infancy onward.

C. Addressing adolescent sexuality. The primary goals of sexual health counseling are to promote a healthy sexual attitude and to decrease sexual risk behaviors.

The clinician must avoid scare tactics and should provide medically accurate, evidence-based information for the teen patient. Interactive counseling approaches such as high-intensity behavioral counseling and motivational interviewing have been found to be effective risk-reduction techniques when counseling teens.

D. Parent involvement. While the sexual history and counseling typically occurs in private with the adolescent and without parental involvement, some teens could benefit from involving a parent or other adult in discussions on sexual health. In these instances, the provider should offer to facilitate a discussion with the parent while maintaining the confidentiality of the teen at all costs.

Helping parents to understand the predictable tasks of adolescent sexual development is important to help parents understand their child better.

E. Agency and consent. Whether it is "saying no" or requesting that a partner use a condom, all adolescents need to hear that it is their right with whom, when, and how they express their sexuality. The clinician should help them understand that sex should never be something that is "done" to them. The practitioner can role-play situations to assist these concepts. For example, he or she can strategize empowered constructive responses to typical lines, such as "It doesn't feel as good with a rubber" or "If you really loved me you'd do it with me".

F. Sexuality and a partner. Involving a partner in the visit can help to facilitate joint sexual decision-making and may improve compliance with safer sexual practices.

G. Promoting barrier methods. If an adolescent is sexually active, condom use or barrier methods should be promoted at every opportunity, no matter what the nature of the office visit. Clearly stating that the condom/barrier must be in place during any genital contact is important—many teens begin with, but remove the condom during sex. Discussing the use of lubrication with condoms is one way to promote their use and address sexual pleasure.

Table 74-1 • PREADOLESCENT SEXUALITY ANTICIPATORY GUIDANCE

Age	Sexuality Issues and Development	Parental Concerns	Areas of Anticipatory Guidance
Prenatal	Fetuses have been shown to suck their fingers in utero	"I don't care if it's a boy or girl as long as it's healthy"	Sex stereotyping: expectations for male–female differences in behavior are present even before birth. Awareness of this allows for later dialogue about expressions of individuality.
		"If it's a boy, what about circumcision?"	Discussing circumcision provides an introduction to discussing sexually related topics.
		"Should I breast feed?"	Breastfeeding discussions help emphasize importance of body contact. It is also important to stress importance of paternal body contact, cuddling, stroking.
2 wk	Temperament	"When I change the baby, his wee-wee stands up. Am I stimulating him too much?"	Use appropriate genitalia names (penis, vagina, clitoris) during the examination. This facilitates discussions as child ages Infants and children enjoy and respond to touch but not with the same sexual/erotic context as adults. It is unlikely that normal touching is ever overstimulating at this age.
2 mo	Bonding	"I feel sexually aroused when I nurse."	Parents (both father and mother) may have erotic sensations and dreams about their child, especially in the first few months. This is normal. (Acting on one's fantasies with a child is not.)
		"My wife and I don't have a relationship like we used to."	The postpartum period is often a stressful time in a previously happy relationship. The clinician may be the only medical provider involved with the family at this point and can help the parents recognize and deal with the changes a new baby brings, including changes in sexual activity.
4–6 mo	Genital play initiation; body exploration	"My son plays with his penis when I change his diaper."	Exploration of the body (toes, fingers, genitalia) is a normal aspect of human development. Self-pleasuring (thumb-sucking, genital manipulation) is a natural extension of this. Masturbation continues throughout life. Start discussions early.
9–12 mo	Avoidance of stigmatization	"I'm afraid to let my daughter go without a diaper at the beach because she plays with herself."	As with other social behaviors (e.g., eating, play), sexuality and its expression must be shaped into a social context. This is a process that starts at this age and proceeds gradually to ages 3–4 y. Shame, doubt, and confusion result from inappropriate expectations.
12–15 mo	Sex-stereotyped play	"I bought my son a doll, but he only wants to play with trucks."	Most parents would like their daughters to achieve to their abilities and sons to be empathetic and caring. Responding to the child's individuality rather than trying to alter sex-specific behaviors is the appropriate path to this goal.

Table 74-1 • PREADOLESCENT SEXUALITY ANTICIPATORY GUIDANCE   (CONTINUED)

Age	Sexuality Issues and Development	Parental Concerns	Areas of Anticipatory Guidance
18 mo	Toilet training	"I want her out of diapers before this baby is born."	Toilet training should be initiated on the child's schedule of readiness, not the parents'.
2–3 y	Anatomical comparisons	"He's asking questions. What should I say?"	Simple but accurate explanations are best. If a child wants to know more and if the answer is straightforward, he will generally ask more. Pregnancy is a fascination; sibling births provide opportunities to discuss reproduction as well as feelings. Toddlers are very much aware of the anatomical similarities with the same-sex parent and the contrasts with the opposite-sex parent. They identify their concept of gender role in this manner.
	Relationships	"My son saw my husband and I having sex. Is that bad for him?"	If intercourse is explained as a way that mothers and fathers have of showing affection and love, there is no psychological trauma for the child who interrupts his parents *in flagrante delicto*. Parents should initiate discussions of privacy and closed doors.
3–4 y	Family flirtation	"My daughter flirts with my husband. Is this normal?"	Family members are the child's source of learning about human relationships. This is a time of magical thinking when children imagine marrying their opposite-sex parent. At this time children can begin to understand parental love for each other as different from a parent's love for a child.
	Sex play with peers	"I found my 4-year-old daughter with the 4-year-old neighbor boy without any clothes."	Sex play between children of the same or opposite sexes continues through childhood without harm, as long as adults remain calm when they discover their children in these games. Children at this age can begin to understand the difference between such play with same-age children and such play with adults or older children.
4–6 y	Sexual appropriateness	"When can I teach my child about good and bad touching?"	Children at this age can understand that their bodies are their own, that sex play between adults and children is not appropriate, and that children have a right to say "no" to an adult's touching if it makes them feel funny or uncomfortable or if they don't understand what's happening.
	Modesty	"My son and daughter share a room. Is this a problem?"	The beginnings of privacy were taught with early body exploration. No matter how relaxed a child's family has been about bodies, the child's natural modesty at this age should be respected.

(continued)

Table 74-1 • PREADOLESCENT SEXUALITY ANTICIPATORY GUIDANCE (CONTINUED)

Age	Sexuality Issues and Development	Parental Concerns	Areas of Anticipatory Guidance
6–10 y	Intimacy	"I've taken showers with my daughter since she was an infant. Should I stop this?"	Each family needs to decide what they are comfortable with and to discuss it. As long as feelings can be discussed openly, there should be no conflict or feelings of rejection if parent–child bathing is discontinued. There are many other comfortable ways for families to show affection. Children and parents sometimes find it comfortable to acknowledge that fantasies are common and are not a problem unless acted upon.
	Fantasy versus reality	"My 9-year-old son seems to have a crush on a 14-year-old neighbor boy. I'm concerned he might be gay."	Same-sex crushes are a normal part of development for both males and females and help consolidate gender identity. Discussion helps both child and parent appreciate normal development. Most who will continue with same-sex experiences recognize their homosexuality at this age.
	Out-of-home influences increase	"I won't let him watch the Playboy channel on cable so he goes next door and watches it."	Media influences are so pervasive that isolated censorship generally does not work. Open discussion of sexual themes in movies, magazines, and songs can help parents open conversations about attitudes that they are not comfortable with and this allows their children to express their viewpoints.
	Sex education	"When should I be having the 'birds and the bees' talk?" I am concerned about Internet safety"	Puberty is occurring at an earlier age. The average 8-year-old is developmentally able to understand simple explanations about sexual activity. Parents should be encouraged to initiate this discussion. New technologies supporting networking have broadened sexual risk taking. It is important to begin *discussions of the risks of cyber sharing of personal information.*

H. Abstinence as a healthy choice. An adolescent needs to hear that abstaining from sexual activity is normal and is becoming increasingly common, and that masturbation and noncoital petting are acceptable ways to relieve sexual tensions safely. Oral and anal sex, with its risk of STIs, is not abstinence.

Teens who are choosing abstinence still need to know about pregnancy and STI risk reduction. *"It sounds like you are not interested in having sex right now. If that changes, it is important for you to know how to prevent pregnancy and STIs."*

I. Contraceptive choice. The American Academy of Pediatrics (AAP) and ACOG have recommended long-acting reversible contraception (LARC) such as the IUD or intradermal implant as the first-line contraceptive for teens. These methods are recommended for teens for many reasons including their efficacy, privacy, reversibility, and side effect profile.

Teens should be counseled about and offered LARC as a contraceptive option among others. However, the adolescent is often the best judge of which method will work best for her. The pediatrician must provide objective information and dispel common myths while avoiding coercive practices.

Both boys and girls should be counseled on the availability of emergency contraception.

Table 74-2 • ANTICIPATORY GUIDANCE FOR ADOLESCENT SEXUALITY

Age	Sexual Areas of Concern	Risk Factors	Anticipatory Guidance
Early adolescence, early puberty: 10–12 y	Pubertal changes	Self-image	Gynecomastia is normal in adolescent males as is breast asynchrony in females. Such body disproportions distort adolescents' image of themselves. Early maturers, particularly females, need special guidance to avoid low self-esteem and premature sexual advances.
		Hormonal influences	Masturbation is a normal behavior that relieves sexual tension. Fantasies are normal while masturbating. Masturbation is a choice—teens can choose to do it or not.
	Children with developmental disabilities		Issues of sexuality are as important to children and adolescents with disabilities as they are to other children and adolescents. Providing clinical supervision to children and adolescents with disabilities includes helping them understand their changing, maturing bodies and the choices available to them.
Late puberty: 12–14 y	Initiation of sexual activity without intimacy	Concrete thought. Cannot perceive long-range implications of current actions	Discussions of sexual choices should emphasize that it is all right to say "no"; discussions regarding contraceptive use need to emphasize more immediate as well as long-term benefits (e.g., in addition to pregnancy prevention, oral contraceptives may relieve dysmenorrhea).
Mid-adolescence: 14–17 y	Intimacy related to sexual romanticism rather than genuine commitment	Looks to peer group for support as he or she separates from family	Parents should be encouraged to continue sexual dialogue begun in latency. They should know their own values (what sex is for; who it is for; what makes it enjoyable; what makes it exploitive). Parental values should be shared with opinions, rather than judgments. Parents should respect teens' decisions. Discussions about sexting and cyber relationships are especially important at this age.
	Sporadic or absent use of birth control; sexual experimentation	Formal operational thinking, variably applied	Teens begin to understand future implications of current actions; they know that use of birth control will protect from unwanted pregnancy, condoms will protect from STDs. Adolescents at this age may believe that oral sex is not as big a deal as sexual intercourse and is safe.
		Risk taking and sense of omnipotence	Risk taking should be discussed. Once a young woman risks unprotected intercourse without becoming pregnant, she is likely to risk it again. Other risk behaviors such as drunk driving and drug use may have a negative interactive effect on sexual decision-making.
Late adolescence: 17–21 y	Intimacy involves commitment	Family conflicts resolving as independence established Comfort with bodies and gender identity	Teen begins to plan for future, including marriage and family. Relationships involve a mutual reciprocity. Counseling involves understanding of female sexual response and couple's discussions of feelings.

Adapted from Grant L, Efstratios D. Adolescent sexuality. *Pediatr Clin North Am.* 1988;5(6):1271-1289.
STDs, sexually transmitted diseases.

J. "Teachable moments" in daily life. Broadcast and written media offer frequent examples of sexual subject matter. News events cover stories on sexual assault and controversies over gay, lesbian, and transgender issues. Rock stars use explicit language in their lyrics, and actors have explicit love scenes. Parents and clinicians should be encouraged to use these examples to initiate conversations with their children and patients around these experiences.

K. Sexually healthy environment. Adolescents may need an impetus to begin discussions of sexual issues. Availability of factual sexual information in the waiting room (e.g., posters, pamphlets, books, or fact sheets) will alert the adolescent that it is acceptable to raise these issues.

L. School-based teaching. School health curricula consider many adolescent behavioral issues, including sexuality. Condom availability and distribution programs, for example, have been incorporated into some health programs and have been shown to support sexual responsibility. Ideally, the pediatrician can advocate for these services in his or her school system and help dispel the myths that open discussions of sexuality contribute to sexual risk taking. The AAP strongly supports comprehensive sexual education.

M. Clinical pearls and pitfalls
- The pediatric clinician must come to terms with his or her own sexual biases. A clinician who is uncomfortable with gender issues or explicit sexual questions cannot effectively counsel. If he or she is unwilling (or unable) to discuss sexuality issues objectively, he or she should have appropriate referral sources so that patients are not denied information. Alternatively, this practitioner should not see adolescent patients.
- Teenagers need guidance, not directives. A practitioner should express his or her opinions in a nonjudgmental way and allow adolescents the legitimacy of their own opinions. *"I don't judge and I won't be disappointed. My job is to listen and give you honest feedback about safety."*
- The clinician should not assume that all sexual relationships are heterosexual. Providing literature in the waiting room on gay, lesbian, and bisexual health issues signals that he or she is comfortable in discussing same-sex experiences.
- The parent–clinician relationship needs to be renegotiated before puberty so that parents understand confidentiality issues and the partnership; that is, values belong in the family—parents need reassurance that the adolescent/practitioner relationship is value-neutral and that safety is the main concern of the practitioner. *"My job is to give you medically accurate information so you can make safe and healthy choices. It is you parent's job to teach you about your family's values."*
- Sexuality is not a joking matter. Too often, adults deal with their own discomfort about sex by making jokes. Discussions with adolescents should always be serious but not somber.

Bibliography

FOR PARENTS AND ADOLESCENTS
BOOKS
Bell R. *Changing Bodies, Changing Lives: A Book for Teens on Sex and Relationships.* Expanded Third Edition. New York: Random House; 1998. For 8th grade and up.
Harris R. *It's Perfectly Normal: Changing Bodies, Growing Up, Sex and Sexual Health.* Cambridge, MA: Candlewick Press; 2009. For 9–12 year olds with chapter on Internet safety.

WEB SITES
https://www.cdc.gov/std/tg2015/tg-2015-print.pdf
SIECUS (Sexuality, information and education council of the United States), excellent resource for accurate information for both parents and teens; includes numerous Web sites. www.siecus.org. Accessed June 4, 2010.

FOR PROFESSIONALS
Gavin L, MacKay A, Brown K, et al. Sexual and reproductive health of persons aged 10–24 years—United States, 2002–2007. *MMWR Surveill Summ.* 2009;58(SS-6):1-58.
Hoff T, Greene L, Davis J. *National Survey of Adolescents and Young Adults: Sexual Health, Knowledge, Attitudes and Experiences.* Menlo Park, CA: Henry Kaiser Family Foundation; 2003.
Murphy NA, Elias ER. Sexuality of children and adolescents with developmental disabilities. *Pediatrics.* 2006;118(1):398-403.

CHAPTER 75

Sibling Rivalry

Robert Needlman

I. **DESCRIPTION OF THE PROBLEM.** The destructive power of sibling rivalry features prominently in the Old Testament and the formative epics of many cultures. These days, sibling conflicts routinely generate high levels of verbal aggression, sometimes rising to physical fighting or actual physical abuse. Conflict-ridden sibling relationships predict depression or other internalizing disorders in adolescence, independent of the parent–child relationship. On the bright side, cooperative play, negotiation, and friendly competition between siblings enhance social skills. Positive sibling support decreases acting-out behaviors. Affection between siblings can blunt the deleterious effects of stress. Parents care deeply about their children getting along. Sibling relationships are often life's most enduring, and filial solidarity often provides crucial social support.

A. **Epidemiology**
- In the United States, about 80% of children grow up with siblings (single children are more common in urban areas). In childhood, sibs spend on average 13% of their waking time together, often more time than with anyone other than with their parents.
- Following the birth of a sibling, some degree of upset and behavioral regression (e.g., bed-wetting) is expected. One-third of children also show developmental gains after a sibling's birth, such as increased self-care and language sophistication.
- Among younger siblings, negative interactions occur on average eight times per hour, including struggles over toys, hitting or pushing, teasing, name-calling, and verbal threats. The rate decreases with age.
- Violent acts occur in 49%–68% of sibling pairs, with boy–girl pairs having the most, and girl–girl pairs the least. In one study, 40% of children had hit a sibling with an object.
- Older siblings are more likely to engage in verbal (as opposed to physical) antagonism. However, in most surveys the frequency of positive sibling interactions is greater still. Girl siblings are often closer during the teen years; boy siblings are often closer before or after their teens.

B. **Etiology/contributing factors**
1. **Loss of exclusive relationship.** Children with the closest relationships to their mothers may show the greatest upset after the birth of a sibling. In contrast, a close relationship with the father may be protective.
2. **Spacing of siblings.** Siblings spaced about 2 years apart may experience the most intense rivalries, perhaps because the older child must cope with sharing the mother's attention at a time when separation is particularly difficult. Twins, in contrast, seem less prone to rivalry, as do children born 3 or more years apart.
3. **Temperament and developmental differences.** Siblings with very different behavioral styles may irritate each other or simply not develop common interests. Behavioral disorders (e.g., attention-deficit/hyperactivity disorder) are associated with sibling conflict. Children with developmental disabilities evoke disparate responses in siblings, either pride and protectiveness or intense resentment.
4. **Role uncertainty.** Older children are often required to take leadership or managerial roles vis-à-vis their younger siblings. At other times, the children may be expected to play together as equals, with no designated boss. Moving back and forth between these quite different relationships generates friction.
5. **Family organization and parenting.** High levels of family chaos as well as harsh or emotionally cold parental discipline foster sibling conflict.
6. **Favoritism and fairness.** Parental favoritism, real or perceived, exacerbates sibling conflicts and fosters anxiety, depression, and acting out in the nonfavored child. In contrast, a belief in parental fairness reduces jealousy.

II. **MAKING THE DIAGNOSIS**
A. **Signs and symptoms.** Sibling fighting may be the chief complaint, or its concerns may emerge during the assessment of other problems, such as aggression, school failure, or acting out. Naughty behavior and mild regression after the birth of a new baby

are expected; withdrawn, listless behavior signals more serious psychological strain. Jealousy may also underlie perfectionism, obsessive worries ("What if the baby gets hurt?"), or overly grown-up (parentified) behavior. It is safe to assume that ambivalent feelings exist whether or not they are apparent.

B. History: key clinical questions

1. *[to the child]* *"Tell me about your brother(s) and sister(s)."* Most children find this question nonthreatening. Invite the child to draw a picture of everyone in the family doing something (a functional family drawing). "What do they like to do together? When do they get mad at each other?"

2. *[to the child]* *"What happens when you and ... fight?"* To get beyond generalizations, ask about specific, recent events. Elicit a play-by-play account, focusing on the antecedents, behaviors, and consequences. "What were you doing before the fight began? How did it start? What did your mom/dad do? How did it end? Is that how it usually goes?"

3. *[to the parent]* *"How have you handled sibling fights in the past?"* Before offering advice, find out what the parent has already tried.

4. *"Tell me about your children."* Listen for typecasting ("my independent one; my peacemaker"), stereotyping ("She's always the first to get into an argument"), and siblings with special problems or accomplishments. How does the parent–child relationship vary among the siblings?

5. *"Where does everyone in the family sleep?"* Conflicts may be greater in families in which privacy and personal possessions are not respected.

6. *"How did your child respond to the birth of his/her younger siblings?"* Jealousy may not arise until the older child realizes the baby is staying; or until the baby becomes more interactive around 4 months; or begins to take the older child's toys around a year.

7. *"Tell me the history of your family, from the start."* When the child was born were the parents beginning careers and trying to make ends meet? What was life like in the family with the addition of each child? External changes—for example, a promotion, a move, and death of a grandparent—can greatly affect a child's experience growing up, exacerbating differential treatment by parents and thus sibling jealousy.

8. *"In your family, how are arguments usually settled?"* Sibling conflicts tend to be more violent in the context of marital hostility. Children may fight either in response to built-up anger and tension or to draw attention away from simmering marital conflicts. Where sibling conflict is part of a larger pattern of dysfunction, family intervention may be necessary.

III. MANAGEMENT

A. Primary goals

1. **Insight.** Parents may respond with greater empathy, less anger, and more firmness if they recognize in themselves the strong emotions that drive sibling conflicts. To encourage this perspective taking, ask parents how they would feel if their spouse brought home a second husband/wife one day and wanted everyone to live happily together.

2. **Reasonable expectations.** Parents need reasonable expectations for sibling coexistence. Ambivalence is normal; friction may be inevitable. Draw attention to the positive aspects of the relationship (e.g., loyalty). It may not be reasonable to expect an older sibling to take on a supervisory or custodial role if the behavior of the younger sibling is challenging.

3. **Appropriate intervention.** Parents may need to step in to prevent physical harm. Young siblings left to their own devices fight more, at times viciously. Older siblings may be better able to work out their differences on their own. A parent who always comes in on the side of one child (the identified victim) may be inadvertently fueling future attacks. Parents should intervene as much as they have to, but no more.

B. Specific strategies

1. **Let older siblings help.** With a new baby in the house, a toddler (male or female child) may benefit from having a baby doll to take care of (or drop head first). Advise parents to involve the older child, such as by saying, "The baby is crying! What do you think? Should we try getting a new diaper?"

2. **Avoid comparisons and labels.** Sensitize parents to listen for typecasting statements ("my problem child"). Even positive labels such as "my good listener" or "my little helper" can lead the child to misbehave to assert his or her individuality or can imply to the other children that they are not expected to show those positive qualities.

3. **Fairness, not equivalence.** Parents should explain that everyone in the family is different and everyone needs different things. Children do not get the same thing, but they each get what they need. It helps to refer to fairness: "I pay attention to you when you need me, but right now your sister needs my attention."

4. **State principles.** The perception of parental unfairness fuels sibling resentment. To demonstrate fairness, parents need to set forth principles and refer to them when making their judgments. For example, it is a good principle that every child has the right to privacy in his or her own room or space; siblings have to go away, if asked.

5. **Separate young children.** For siblings, playing together is a privilege, not a right. Let children try to work out their differences but step in and separate the combatants before fighting breaks out. This may mean time-outs for both children, either in opposite corners or in separate rooms.

6. **Challenge the victim/aggressor roles.** Although it is true that an older child may consistently dominate a younger one, often the "innocent victim" is actually needling the other sibling to the point of explosion and then basking in parental sympathy while watching the rival being punished.

C. **Follow-up/backup strategies.** Schedule repeated visits to reinforce new patterns of parenting. In particular, after parents limit their intervention, sibling conflicts may temporarily increase. Have parents role-play management strategies (e.g., praising a child's behavior without commenting on the general goodness of the child or making covert sibling comparisons). The following features should suggest referral for subspecialist care.

1. **Multiproblem children.** When sibling jealousy accompanies other problems, such as oppositionality to parents or teachers, aggression toward nonsibling peers, or school failure, the problem is unlikely to resolve without attention to the whole picture.

2. **Multiproblem families.** Parental anger, violence, disorganization, depression, or disengagement may require family or individual therapy, or legal assistance; the sibling relationship may improve as a result.

3. **Physical abuse.** A pattern of repeated injury inflicted by one sibling against another signals a family emergency. The risk of psychological damage is high to both the aggressor and the victim. Parents need to establish the family as a zone of safety, if not tranquility. If they cannot, then more intensive intervention is called for.

Bibliography

FOR PARENTS

Faber A, Mazlish E. *Siblings Without Rivalry: How to Help Your Children Live Together So You Can Live Too*. New York, NY: Avon Books; 1988. (An excellent guide designed to help parents understand their children's behavior and make the necessary changes in their own. It presents sound principles using wonderfully clear examples. The cartoon scenarios are particularly helpful).

Reit S. *Sibling Rivalry*. New York, NY: Ballantine Books; 1985 (A good review of the subject, written for parents, full of useful information).

WEB SITES

KidsHealth. http://kidshealth.org/parent/emotions/feelings/sibling_rivalry.html.

University of Michigan. http://www.med.umich.edu/yourchild/topics/sibriv.htm.

FOR PROFESSIONALS

Dirks MA, Persram R, Recchia HE, Howe N. Sibling relationships as sources of risk and resilience in the development and maintenance of internalizing and externalizing problems during childhood and adolescence. *Clin Psychol Rev*. 2015;42:145-155.

Dunn J. *Sisters and Brothers*. Cambridge, MA: Harvard University Press; 1985 (Dunn has carried out some of the best and most relevant longitudinal research on siblings, well summarized here).

Newman J. Conflict and friendship in sibling relationships: a review. *Child Study J*. 1994;24(2):119-152 (A thorough review of decades of studies).

CHAPTER 76

Sleep Problems

Judith A. Owens

I. DESCRIPTION OF THE PROBLEM.
Sleep problems constitute one of the most frequent parental complaints in pediatric practice.

- Childhood *sleeplessness,* insufficient or disturbed sleep, in its many forms, clearly is a common parental concern.
- In contrast, the relationship between **sleepiness** and its many manifestations is less frequently recognized by parents but is nonetheless a significant clinical concern. A wealth of empirical evidence from several lines of research clearly indicates that children and adolescents experience significant daytime sleepiness as a result of inadequate or disturbed sleep, and that significant performance impairments and mood dysfunction, as well as behavior, academic, and health problems in childhood, are associated with that daytime sleepiness.

A. Epidemiology
1. 25% of all children experience a sleep problem at some point during childhood, ranging from short-term situational difficulties in falling asleep to night wakings to more chronic and persistent sleep disorders.
2. Although many sleep problems in infants and children are transient and self-limited, the common wisdom that children "grow out of" sleep problems is not an accurate perception. Certain intrinsic and extrinsic risk factors (e.g., difficult temperament, maternal depression, family stress) may predispose a given child to develop a more chronic sleep disturbance.
3. Sleep problems are a **significant source of distress** for families. It may be, for example, a primary reason for caregiver stress in families with children who have chronic medical illnesses or severe neurodevelopmental delays.
4. The impact of childhood sleep problems is intensified by their direct relationship to **the quality and quantity of parents' sleep**, particularly if disrupted sleep results in parental daytime fatigue and mood disturbances, which impact negatively on the quality of parenting.
5. Vulnerable populations, such as children who are at high risk for developmental and behavioral problems because of poverty, parental substance abuse and mental illness, or violence in the home, may be even more likely to experience "double jeopardy" as a result of sleep problems.

B. Etiology/contributing factors
1. **Child variables** include temperament and behavioral style, individual variations in circadian preference, cognitive and language **delays**, and the presence of comorbid medical and psychiatric conditions.
2. **Parental variables** include parenting and discipline styles, parents' education level and knowledge of child development, mental health issues such as maternal depression, family stress, and quality and quantity of parents' sleep.
3. **Environmental variables** include the physical environment (space, noise, perceived environmental threats to safety, room and bed sharing, televisions in the bedroom), family composition (number, ages, and health status of siblings and extended family members), and lifestyle issues (parental work status, competing priorities for time).
4. **Cultural and family context,** for example, cosleeping of infants and parents, is a common and accepted practice in many ethnic groups (including African Americans, Hispanics, and Southeast Asians) both in their countries of origin and in the United States. Therefore, the developmental goal of independent "self-soothing" in infants at bedtime and after night wakings may not be shared by all families.
5. **Specific medical conditions** that may have an increased risk of sleep problems include the following:
   - Asthma and allergies
   - Headaches
   - Neurologic disorders and rheumatologic conditions

- Children with anxiety and affective disorders are particularly vulnerable to sleep problems. Studies of children with major depressive disorder, for example, have reported a prevalence of insomnia of up to 75% and sleep-onset delay in one-third of depressed adolescents. Use of psychotropic medications in these children may have significant negative effects on sleep.
- Significant sleep problems occur in 30%–80% of children with severe mental retardation and in at least 50% of children with less severe cognitive impairment. Similar estimates in children with autism/pervasive developmental delay are in the 50%–70% range.

II. MAKING THE DIAGNOSIS

A. Sleep physiology

1. **The framework or architecture of sleep** is based on recognition of two distinct sleep stages. These stages are defined by distinct polysomnographic (or "overnight sleep study") features of EEG patterns, eye movement, and muscle tone.
   - **REM sleep** (rapid eye movement or "dream" sleep). REM sleep (20%–25% of total) is characterized by high levels of cortical activity and low or absent muscle tone.
   - **Non-REM sleep** (75%–80% of sleep in healthy young adults). Non-REM sleep is further divided into:
     - **Stage 1** sleep (2%–5%), which occurs at the sleep–wake transition and is often referred to as "light sleep"
     - **Stage 2** sleep (45%–55%), which is usually considered the initiation of "true" sleep and is characterized by bursts of rhythmic rapid EEG activity and high-amplitude slow-wave spikes
     - **Stages 3** sleep (3%–23%), which are otherwise known as "deep" sleep, "slow-wave sleep," or "delta sleep," during which the highest arousal threshold (most difficult to awaken) also occurs

2. **Cycling of stages**
   - Non-REM and REM sleep alternate throughout the night in cycles of about 90–110 minutes in adults (50 minutes in infancy and gradually lengthening through childhood to adult levels).
   - Brief arousals normally followed by a rapid return to sleep often occur at the end of each sleep cycle (4–6 times per night in adults; 7–10 times per night in infants).
   - The relative proportion of REM and non-REM sleep per cycle changes across the night, such that slow-wave sleep predominates in the first third of the night and REM sleep in the last third.

3. **Two-process sleep system.** Sleep and wakefulness are regulated by two basic highly coupled processes operating simultaneously:
   - The **sleep homeostatic process,** which primarily regulates the length and depth of sleep. The homeostatic "pressure" for sleep builds in a linear fashion, as awake time increases in duration and is gradually dissipated during the nocturnal sleep period. The homeostatic sleep drive also builds more quickly in young children (thus necessitating a daytime sleep period or "nap") and slows during adolescence.
   - **Endogenous circadian rhythms** ("biological time clock"), which influence the internal organization of sleep and the timing and duration of daily sleep–wake cycles. **Circadian** clocks are now known to be present in virtually every cell in the body and thus govern many other physiologic systems (e.g., cardiovascular, gastrointestinal, respiratory) in addition to sleep–wake cycles. Circadian rhythms are also synchronized to the 24-hour day cycle by environmental cues, the most powerful of which is the light–dark cycle that influences melatonin secretion by the pineal gland.

4. **Duration of sleep**
   a. **Newborns**
      - Newborns sleep approximately 16–20 hours per day, in 1- to 4-hour sleep periods, followed by 1- to 2-hour awake periods.
      - Sleep–wake cycles are largely dependent on hunger and satiety. Sleep amounts during the day approximately equal the amount of nighttime sleep.
   b. **Infants**
      - Sleep duration recommendations for optimal health at 4–12 months are 12–16 hours/24 hours on a regular basis (including naps).
      - Sleep periods last about 3–4 hours during the first 3 months and extend to 6–8 hours at 4–6 months.

- By 9 months, 70%–80% infants "sleep through the night" (*sleep consolidation*).
- **Day/night differentiation** develops between 6 and 12 weeks and nocturnal sleep periods become increasingly longer.
- The ability to **regulate sleep or control internal states of arousal in order to fall asleep** at bedtime and to fall back asleep during the night begins to develop in the first 12 weeks of life.
- Most infants nap between 2 and 4 hours divided as 2 naps per day.
- Issues of attachment and social interaction also play an important role in shaping sleep behaviors in infants. Transitional objects, such as a pacifier or a blanket, and bedtime routines become more important as infancy progresses.

c. **Toddlers**
- Sleep duration recommendations for optimal health at 1–2 years are 11–14 hours/24 hours on a regular basis (including naps).
- Most give up a second nap by 18 months and generally nap 1.5–3.5 hours as 1 nap per day.
- The peak of separation anxiety at 9–18 months is often associated with increased night wakings.

d. **Preschoolers**
- Sleep duration recommendations for optimal health at 3–5 years are 10–13 hours/24 hours on a regular basis (including naps).
- Most children give up napping by 5 years.
- Difficulties falling asleep and night wakings (15%–30%) are still common in this age group, in many cases coexisting in the same child.

e. **Middle childhood (6–12 years)**
- Sleep duration recommendations for optimal health at 6–12 years are 9–12 hours/24 hours on a regular basis.
- Although it was previously believed that sleep problems are rare in middle childhood, recent studies have reported a high prevalence of significant parent-reported sleep problems in this age group.

f. **Adolescents (12–18 years)**
- Sleep duration recommendations for optimal health at 13 + years are 8–10 hours/24 hours on a regular basis.
- However, a number of studies have suggested that the average adolescent actually *gets* about 7 hours of sleep.

B. **Etiology**
- **Childhood insomnia (difficulty initiating and/or maintaining sleep).** "Insomnia" is a symptom and not a diagnosis. The causes of insomnia are varied and range from the medical (i.e., drug-related, pain-induced, associated with primary sleep disorders such as obstructive sleep apnea [OSA]) to the behavioral (i.e., associated with poor sleep hygiene or sleep-onset association disorder) and are often a combination of these factors. The most common causes of adolescent insomnia are listed next.

1. **Behavioral insomnia of childhood: sleep-onset association type.** The child has learned to fall asleep only under certain conditions or associations, such as being rocked or fed, and does not develop the ability to self-soothe. During the night, when the child experiences the type of brief arousal that normally occurs at the end of a sleep cycle (7–10 times per night in infants) or awakens for other reasons, he or she is not able to get back to sleep without those same conditions being present. Thus, the problem is one of prolonged night waking, resulting in insufficient sleep *that typically requires parental intervention*.

2. **Behavioral insomnia of childhood: limit-setting type.** This type of insomnia is typically characterized by difficulty falling asleep and bedtime resistance ("curtain calls") but may also be manifested in night wakings requiring parental intervention. Most commonly, this disorder develops from a parent's inability or unwillingness to set consistent bedtime rules and enforce a regular bedtime, often exacerbated by the child's oppositional behavior. In some cases, however, the child's resistance at bedtime is due to an underlying problem in falling asleep caused by other factors (e.g., medical conditions such as asthma or medication use, a sleep disorder such as restless legs, or anxiety) or a mismatch between the child's intrinsic circadian rhythm ("night owl") and parental expectations.

3. **Behavioral insomnia of childhood: excessive time in bed.** In some children, parental expectations regarding time in bed exceed the child's actual sleep needs. This situation may present as sleep-onset delay at the set bedtime, early morning waking before the desired wake time, or an extended period of wakefulness during

the night. In contrast to the other types of behavioral insomnia, night wakings are often characterized by relaxed wakefulness rather than distress and may not require parental intervention.

4. **Primary or "psychophysiologic" insomnia.** This type of difficulty initiating and/ or maintaining sleep is more common in older children and adolescents. In this disorder, the individual develops conditioned anxiety around falling or staying asleep, usually in combination with poor sleep habits, which leads to heightened arousal and which further compromises the ability to sleep. In terms of etiology, the "3P" model is often cited: predisposing factors (e.g., history of insomnia, mental health issues), precipitating factors (e.g., parental divorce, transition to a new school), and perpetuating factors (e.g., extending sleep or napping during the day, engaging in activities in bed other than sleeping).

5. **Sleep anxiety.** Nighttime fears are common and typically both normal and benign. Parental anxiety and family conflict may also play a role in exacerbating nighttime fears in children by increasing the level of emotional arousal in the child. Anxiety around sleep is characterized by fearful behaviors, such as crying, clinging, and leaving the bedroom to seek parental reassurance (at bedtime or in the middle of the night), and bedtime resistance, including refusal to go to bed, frequent "curtain calls," or requiring a parent to be present at bedtime. Some children may also experience frequent nightmares as part of the anxiety picture.

C. **Differential diagnosis**

1. **Insufficient sleep and inadequate sleep hygiene.** Chronic sleep loss resulting from voluntary sleep restriction (more common in adolescents) impacts on daytime functioning and causes excessive daytime sleepiness, which can be manifested in a number of ways in children and adolescents: falling asleep at unintended times, overactivity, and behavior problems. Inadequate sleep hygiene (unhealthy sleep habits) includes practices that increase arousal and/or are inconsistent with a regular sleep schedule.

   a. **Practices that increase arousal** include caffeine intake, evening electronic media use, and anxiety related to lying in bed worrying about falling asleep.

   b. **Practices that are inconsistent with a regular sleep schedule/sleep organization** include napping late in the day and inconsistent bedtimes and wake times.

2. **Circadian issues** may also play a role in some cases of bedtime struggles. When a relatively early bedtime coincides with the normal late-day circadian-mediated surge in alertness ("forbidden zone" or "second wind" phenomenon), a child may have significantly more difficulty settling, and this can result in bedtime resistance. Children with an "owl" circadian preference ("eveningness chronotype") for later sleep onset and wake times also tend to have a later forbidden zone and are thus particularly likely to have a settling problem if bedtime is set too early.

3. **Bedtime struggles** may be the result of a more global problem with **noncompliance,** including **oppositional defiant disorder (ODD)** or may be a feature of a more pervasive psychiatric problem.

4. Primarily medically based sleep problems such as **OSA and restless legs syndrome/periodic limb movement disorder (RLS/PLMD)** may present with bedtime resistance and/or night wakings and disturbed sleep.

D. **History: key clinical questions.** The clinical evaluation of a child presenting with a sleep problem involves a careful medical, mental health, and neurodevelopmental history to assess for potential underlying causes of sleep disturbances and to identify children at increased risk for sleep concerns, such as acute or chronic pain conditions, concomitant medication use, anxiety or depression, attention-deficit/hyperactivity disorder (ADHD), and autism spectrum disorder.

1. Current **sleep patterns,** including usual sleep duration and sleep–wake schedule, are often best assessed with a sleep diary, in which parents record daily sleep behaviors for an extended (at least 2 weeks) period.

2. A review of **sleep habits,** such as bedtime routines, daily caffeine intake, and the sleeping environment (temperature, noise level, etc.), may reveal environmental factors that contribute to the sleep problems.

3. Use of additional diagnostic tools such as an overnight in-lab **polysomnogram** are seldom warranted for routine evaluation of pediatric insomnia but may be appropriate if organic sleep disorders, such as OSA or PLMD, are suspected. Ancillary diagnostic tools also include actigraphy (a wristwatch-like device monitors body movement over a several-week period that in conjunction with a sleep diary can be used to approximate sleep–wake patterns in the home setting and confirm subjective reports) and home video recording of breathing (i.e., signs of OSA) or episodic nocturnal behavior (i.e., sleep terror versus nocturnal seizures).

III. MANAGEMENT. Successful treatment of pediatric sleep problems is highly dependent on identification of parental concerns, clarification of mutually acceptable treatment goals, active exploration of opportunities and obstacles, and ongoing communication of issues and concerns. Behavioral interventions coupled with basic healthy sleep habits education are the first line of treatment for childhood insomnia. Sedative/hypnotic medications are rarely needed and should never be the sole treatment strategy, especially in typically developing otherwise healthy children. Currently there are no FDA-approved medications for insomnia in the pediatric population. However, owing to the widespread use of over-the-counter melatonin for childhood insomnia in the community, the reader is directed to the consensus guidelines in the reference list.

  A. Behavioral insomnia of childhood: sleep-onset association type. The treatment approach typically involves a program of complete or partial withdrawal of parental intervention/assistance at sleep onset and during the night (systematic ignoring). It should be noted that these behavioral interventions have a considerable amount of empirical support regarding efficacy. In addition, several longitudinal studies have failed to demonstrate significant long-term negative effects on parent and child attachment, stress levels, and other developmental and social outcomes.

  1. The goal is to allow the infant or child to develop skills in self-soothing during the night, as well as at bedtime. In older infants and young children, the introduction of more appropriate sleep associations, which will be readily available to the child during the night (transitional objects such as a blanket or toy) in addition to positive reinforcement if developmentally appropriate (e.g., stickers for remaining in bed), are often beneficial.

  2. Unmodified extinction ("cry it out" approach) involves the caregiver putting the child to bed drowsy but still awake at the specified bedtime and ignoring protest behavior until the next morning. Studies have shown that this is a highly effective approach but is often poorly tolerated by caregivers.

  3. Graduated extinction ("Ferber method," "checking method") is a more gradual process of weaning the child from dependence on parental presence that utilizes periodic "check-ins" by the caregivers at fixed or successively longer time intervals during the sleep–wake transition to allow the child to fall asleep independently in-between check-ins. Once the child has acquired the ability to self-soothe, this will generalize to night wakings.

     In both types of approaches, caregivers must be consistent in applying behavioral techniques to avoid inadvertent intermittent reinforcement of bedtime resistance and/or night wakings; they should also be forewarned that crying and protest behavior frequently temporarily escalate at the beginning of treatment ("postextinction burst").

  B. Behavioral insomnia of childhood: limit-setting type. Successful treatment of limit-setting sleep disorder generally involves a combination of the following:
  • Decreased parental attention for bedtime-delaying behavior
  • Establishment of a consistent bedtime routine
  • Positive reinforcement (e.g., sticker charts) for appropriate behavior at bedtime
  • Bedtime fading (see below)

  C. Behavioral insomnia of childhood: excessive time in bed. The approach to this type of insomnia, whether manifested as delayed sleep onset, extended night waking, or early morning waking, involves calculating the amount of time the child typically spends asleep compared with time spent in bed (a sleep diary is very useful). The "sleep window" (bedtime and wake time) is then set to the actual time asleep (usually by delaying bedtime); extended sleep in the morning and longer daytime naps are to be avoided. Once the child is falling asleep easily, and/or consolidating nighttime sleep, the bedtime may be moved earlier gradually (in 15-minute increments every several days) to the target bedtime.

  D. Psychophysiologic insomnia. Treatment usually involves components of cognitive behavioral therapy for insomnia (CBT-I) such as educating the older child/adolescent about principles of sleep hygiene (e.g., regular sleep–wake schedule, avoidance of stimulants such as caffeine and nicotine, bedtime routine), instructing them to use the bed for sleep only and to get out of bed if unable to fall asleep (stimulus control), restricting time in bed to the actual time asleep (sleep restriction), and teaching relaxation techniques to reduce anxiety. Maladaptive cognitions about sleep, often characterized by "catastrophizing" ("if I can't get to sleep, I won't be able to wake up, I'll miss the test and fail the course"), are also addressed. CBT-I, especially in children/adolescents with mental health issues, is best conducted by a behavioral medicine provider with specialized sleep training.

E. Sleep anxiety. In general, strategies aimed at younger children more often involve parental reassurance, whereas older children typically benefit from an approach that includes teaching and positive reinforcement for independent coping skills.

- Use of security objects should be encouraged, as they can be comforting to the child.
- Television programs, and video and computer games that may be frightening or overstimulating, particularly just before bedtime, should be avoided. Also, electronics should be kept out of the bedroom.
- Many children may benefit from learning relaxation strategies, such as deep breathing or visual imagery, which can help a child relax at bedtime and fall asleep more easily.
- Bedtime pass. This is a behavioral strategy that involves giving the child a "pass card" at bedtime, which can then be used to get up once after lights out but must be handed in to caregivers. This technique is particularly useful for anxious children as a kind of "safety net." The child may also be incentivized by being rewarded in the morning for not using the pass during the night.

IV. CLINICAL PEARLS AND PITFALLS

- Because multiple sleep problems may coexist in the same child, it is always important to assess for additional nocturnal symptoms that may be indicative of a medically based sleep disorder, such as OSA (loud snoring, choking/gasping, sweating) or PLMD (restless sleep, repetitive kicking movements), even if the presenting complaint appears behaviorally based.
- All children presenting to pediatric clinicians with learning, attention, behavioral, or emotional concerns, especially ADHD, should be carefully assessed for underlying or comorbid sleep disorders as part of the routine evaluation. There is considerable overlap between the diagnostic features of ADHD (inattention, hyperactivity, impulsivity) and neurobehavioral deficits associated with any significant sleep problems in children. A number of primary sleep disorders, including OSA and RLS/PLMD, frequently include ADHD-like symptoms as part of their clinical presentation.
- Because parents of older children and adolescents, in particular, may not be aware of any existing sleep difficulties, it is also important to directly question the patient about sleep issues as well.

V. WHEN TO REFER. Referral to a sleep specialist for diagnosis and/or treatment should be considered under the following circumstances:

- Inadequate response or failure of adherence to behavioral interventions for insomnia
- Possible indications for pharmacologic treatment of insomnia
- Insomnia, mental health, and neurodevelopmental comorbidities
- Excessive daytime sleepiness not due to environmental sleep restriction
- "Unusual" episodic nocturnal sleep behaviors
- RLS symptoms not responsive to nonpharmacologic therapies (including iron supplementation)

Bibliography

FOR PARENTS

BOOKS

Ferber R. *Solve Your Child's Sleep Problems.* New, Revised and Expanded Edition. New York, NY: Simon & Schuster; 2006.

Weissbluth M. *Healthy Sleep Habits, Happy Child: A Step-by-Step Program for a Good Night's Sleep.* 4th ed. New York. Ballentine Books; 2015.

WEB SITES

American Academy of Sleep Medicine. www.aasmnet.org.

National Sleep Foundation. www.sleepfoundation.org.

Pediatric Sleep Council. www.babysleep.com/.

FOR PROFESSIONALS

Bruni O, Alonso-Alconada D, Besag F. Current role of melatonin in pediatric neurology: clinical recommendations. *Eur J Paediatr Neurol.* 2015;19:122-133.

Mindell J, Owens J. *A Clinical Guide to Pediatric Sleep: Diagnosis and Management of Sleep Problems in Children and Adolescents.* 3rd ed. Philadelphia, PA: Lippincott Williams & Wilkins; 2015.

Price A, Wake M, Ukoumunne O, Hiscock H. Five-year follow-up of harms and benefits of behavioral infant sleep intervention: randomized trial. *Pediatrics.* 2012;130(4).

Sheldon S, Ferber R, Kryger M, Gozal D. *Principles and Practices of Pediatric Sleep Medicine.* 2nd ed. Amsterdam; 2014.

CHAPTER 77

Speech Production Disorders

Kristine E. Strand

I. **SPEECH PRODUCTION DISORDERS.** Speech production disorders is an umbrella term for three categories of problems:
   A. **Speech sound disorders** (SSDs)—difficulty with the individual speech sounds and segments
   B. **Childhood apraxia of speech** (CAS)—difficulty with coordinated movements of speech
   C. **Stuttering** (disfluency)—difficulty with the flow speech production

II. **SPEECH SOUND DISORDERS**
   A. **Description of the problem.** The term "speech sound disorder" encompasses any combination of difficulties with speech perception, speech motor production, and phonological rules related to speech sounds and speech segments that adversely affect speech intelligibility. Historically, these disorders were referred to as articulation or phonological disorders. Currently, these terms are subtypes of SSDs. The term "articulation disorder" describes errors affecting the form of speech sounds (e.g., production of a lisp or sound substitution). The errors may arise from or be associated with physical difficulties such as cranial nerve damage, unrepaired cleft palate, laryngeal anomalies, dysarthria, or difficulties with respiratory control. The term "phonological disorder" describes disorders stemming from problems in the implicit knowledge of the rules for the phonological system (i.e., speech sounds, syllable structure, and stress and intonation patterns) of a language.

   Differences or variations in production of speech sounds that are attributable to dialect or non-English language influences are **not** considered SSDs.
   B. **Epidemiology**
      • An SSD is the most prevalent type of communication disorder among preschoolers, affecting approximately 10%–16% of children.
      • There is a higher prevalence of SSDs in boys than in girls during the preschool and early school years.
      • Approximately 75%–85% of preschoolers with SSDs also experience delays or disorders in language development.
      • An SSD in toddlers and preschoolers places a child at increased risk for later academic difficulties including specific reading disability/dyslexia during the school years.
      • Approximately 11%–15% of 6-year-old children with SSDs are also diagnosed with specific language impairment.
      • The most common speech sound errors involve the consonant sounds for the letters s, r, l, and th.
   C. **Familial transmission/genetics:** Drawing a direct connection between genes and SSDs is difficult although much research is currently under way in this area. It is likely that some SSDs have genetic influences that are most likely under the control of genetic networks, with broad effects on multiple cognitive processes including speech, language, and reading skills. Family histories of children with SSDs are often positive for speech and language disorders and for other learning problems in extended family members.
   D. **Organic etiologies**
      • Early recurrent periods of otitis media with effusion have been found to be a risk factor in about one-third of children with SSDs.
      • "Tongue thrust" or "tongue thrust swallow" refers to excessive anterior tongue movement during swallowing and a more anterior tongue position at rest. The impact of this oral muscle pattern on speech production is controversial, especially for the articulation of /s/ and /z/. Not all children who exhibit "tongue thrust" patterns develop a concomitant SSD. Everyone starts life with a tongue thrust swallowing pattern, but the pattern should be eliminated by the early school years.
      • Ankyloglossia ("tongue tie") refers to a restricted lingual frenum (frenulum). There is a small body of evidence to support the relationship between frenulum length and SSDs but only for children with moderate or severe levels of ankyloglossia (Ruffoli et al., 2005).

E. Natural history
- Speech sound development in children younger than 3 years of age is highly variable, however; general intelligibility is a good benchmark for typical development. In general, children are 100% intelligible to parents by 3 years and to unfamiliar listeners by 4 years, thus the "Rule of Fours":
  - 18-month-olds—approximately 25% intelligible
  - 2-year-olds—approximately 50% intelligible
  - 3-year-olds—approximately 75% intelligible
  - 4-year-olds—100% intelligible
- Babbling defined as the production of syllables (consonant + vowel), either the same syllable (e.g., ba-ba-ba) or varied syllable strings (e.g., ba-ga-da), is typically an established part of an infant's sound production by about 7–8 months of age.
- Infrequent vocalizations or feeding or swallowing problems may indicate oromotor problems that can predispose the infant to SSDs.
- See Table 77-1 for progression of consonant sound production.

F. Management. Signs and symptoms vary by age. See Table 77-2.
  1. History: key clinical questions
  - *"How well do you and others understand your child's speech, compared with the speech of other children of his or her age?"* Reduced intelligibility compared with peers is a strong indicator of a SSD.
  - *"When do you recall that your child was babbling regularly?"* Infants who have not established babbling production by 9–10 months of age is a strong indicator of delay in the motor processes underlying speech sound development. Reduced babbling in amount or variety may also suggest a hearing loss.
  - *"Has your child's speech changed much during the past 6 months?"* For children up to age 5 years, any response suggesting little change over time is a cause for concern.

Table 77-1 • MILESTONES OF CONSONANT PRODUCTION

By age 3 y	/p, m, h, n, w/
By age 4 y	/b, k, g, d, f, y/
By age 6 y	/t, ng, r, l/
By age 7 y	/ch, sh, j, v/
By age 8 y	/s, z, v/

Table 77-2 • SIGNS AND SYMPTOMS OF SPEECH SOUND DISORDERS

Any age	Speech is more difficult to understand than that of peers Teasing by others about speech (e.g., about a lisp) Shyness about speaking or excessive frustration when not understood
2 y or older	Intelligibility less than 50% Use of only four to five consonants (e.g., sounds represented by the letters *p, b, w, y, m*) and a limited number of vowels Consistent errors in the use of the sounds represented by the letters *p, b, m, n, h, w*, or any vowel sounds Consonants at the beginning of words are omitted (e.g., "ow" for "cow") One sound is used in the place of many others (e.g., *p* is used when *f, v, t*, or *k* is expected) The sounds *k* or *g* are used when *t* or *d* is expected (e.g., "ko" for "toe")
3 y or older	Intelligibility less than 75%
3.5 y or older	Consistent errors in the use of the sounds *f, v, k, g*, or *y* (e.g., "wu" for "you") Consistent errors that assume the following patterns: Consonants at the ends of words are omitted The sounds *t* or *d* are used when *k* or *g* is expected
4 y or older	Intelligibility less than 100%
5.5 y or older	Errors on two or more speech sounds that are obvious enough to call attention to the child's speech

- *"How do you and others respond to your child's poor speech? How does your child respond to any negative reactions?"* Teasing, frequent corrections, or requests to repeat can make the child frustrated or shy and withdrawn.
- *"Does your child have a history of problems with feeding or swallowing?"* This question addresses the possibility of developmental dysarthria or CAS as part of differential diagnosis.
- *"Do you ever think your child has day-to-day fluctuations or problems in hearing?"* This question addresses the potential for chronic or fluctuating hearing loss related to otitis media.

2. **Physical examination.** The physical examination can help rule out significant oral anomalies and screen for frank neurologic abnormalities, as well as provide information about the child's middle ear status.

3. **Referral.** The primary care clinician's principal goal in SSDs is appropriate referral as well as management of middle ear status. A licensed/certified speech-language pathologist can perform testing necessary for diagnosis of SSD.
   Criteria for referral:
   - Refer to a speech-language pathologist if the child's speech demonstrates any of the signs or symptoms mentioned in Table 77-2. Speech-language pathologists in early intervention programs or public school systems assess and treat children with all types of communication disorders.
   - Refer to a pediatric audiologist if the child has had recurrent episodes of otitis media and there is indication of delay in speech sound development.
   - Refer to the child's dentist if the child has a notable "tongue thrust," as this oral muscle position and swallowing pattern can cause certain types of malocclusion problems and/or altered patterns of facial development. Also refer to a speech-language pathologist if the child exhibits concomitant speech sound errors.
   - Even very young children at risk for SSDs will benefit from early efforts to stimulate vocal production and language development. Therefore, referral should be made as soon as any communication difficulty is suspected.

G. **Clinical pearls and pitfalls**
   - Remember the guidelines regarding intelligibility: A stranger should be able to understand about 50% of what a 2-year-old says, 75% of what a 3-year-old says, and 100% of what a 4-year-old says.
   - Tantrums or indications of extreme frustration from a child older than 3 years due to the parent's inability to understand the child's speech suggest a significant problem in speech or language development.
   - To avoid judging the child in terms of his or her own speech dialect, clinicians should ask parents to gauge how well the child is understood compared with peers.
   - Delays in referral not only can deprive the child of early treatment but can also result in increased parent–child conflict and possible later learning problems.

III. **CHILDHOOD APRAXIA OF SPEECH**
A. **Description of the Problem.** CAS as defined by the American Speech Language Hearing Association (ASHA) is a "neurological childhood (pediatric) speech sound disorder in which the precision and consistency of movements underlying speech are impaired in the absence of neuromuscular deficits (e.g., abnormal reflexes, abnormal tone). The core impairment in planning and/or programming spatiotemporal parameters of movement sequences results in errors in speech sound production and prosody."

The generally agreed on diagnostic term is CAS although terms including developmental apraxia of speech or developmental verbal dyspraxia are also found in the literature. At the present time there is no list of unique diagnostic features that differentiate CAS from other severe SSDs. However, there is some consensus that the disorder includes a complex mix of inconsistent errors on consonants and vowels in repeated productions of the same word or phrase; reduced intelligibility with increased length, rate, and linguistic complexity of speech production; and disturbances in prosody (intonation, tone, stress, and rhythm of connected speech).

The relative frequency of these features and other possible markers change with age, the severity of the disorder, and the complexity of the task. Thus speech production difficulty often diagnosed during the preschool years places children at risk for concomitant difficulty with expressive language development as well as the development of early literacy skills. Also, CAS is often part of a more generalized coordination disorder classified as developmental motor dyspraxia.

B. Epidemiology. Prevalence is not yet well established. One estimate based on referral data suggests overall prevalence of 1–2 cases in 1000 children, but these numbers vary widely most likely depending on specific etiology and comorbidity. Males are thought to outnumber females.

C. Familial transmission/genetics. Some recent research has identified a gene mutation associated with some cases of CAS. The gene *FOXP2* has been found in a multigenerational family in England and in at least one nonfamily member all of whom had severe speech production disorders. This gene mutation appears to affect speech motor/movement development; however, continuing research is needed in this area.

D. Organic etiologies. CAS is considered to be a neurologically based disorder, but as yet no one etiology has been determined to consistently result in CAS.

- CAS may occur in combination with other medical/developmental disorders/syndromes such as Down syndrome or autism spectrum disorder.
- Although CAS may exist in combination with dysarthria, the neural substrates of CAS differ from those underlying the several types of dysarthria.
- Most children with CAS have nothing in their prenatal, birth, or health history that suggests a possible organic cause.
- Most children with CAS have normal EEGs, MRIs, and basic neurologic examinations. Extended neurologic examinations including complex movement patterns may indicate more generalized motor movement dyspraxia.

E. Natural history

- The early speech development in children with suspected CAS often includes little babbling, cooing, or vocal play. They are often described by parents as being "very quiet, good babies". Babbling when it occurs is often late (beginning at 9–10 months) and with little variety in speech sounds.
- The onset of intelligible speech and expressive language is often delayed with many children not producing their first words until 2.5–3 years of age.
- Young children often have a restricted repertoire of speech sounds, i.e., consonants and vowels. They may be limited to the same syllable (e.g. /da/) or word in an attempt to communicate many different meanings resulting in what appears to be limited expressive vocabulary and causing increased frustration. The vocalizations of many children with CAS sound similar to children with hearing loss.
- Many young children with CAS are not successful in their attempts to imitate speech, especially early words.
- At all stages of development, children with CAS demonstrate higher receptive language skills than expressive language skills, which are constrained by their limited speech production abilities.
- For some children with a diagnosis of CAS even at middle school and beyond, their speech production continues to be more variable and less accurate than adult speech. Given continuing vowel errors some teenagers sound as though they have a language or dialect accent.

F. Management

1. Signs and symptoms

- *Unintelligible speech*: This is often a hallmark of CAS although it can also be observed in children with other severe SSDs. Many children with CAS have a restricted repertoire of different speech sounds and sound combinations. Some young children have only one or two vowel sounds they use and no consonants. Even when children have a larger speech sound repertoire, they tend to use the sounds inconsistently or omit them in words or phrases.
- *Vowel distortions*: Because of difficulty with nuanced and accurate tongue positioning, vowel distortions or use of a single neutral vowel is often an early marker of CAS.
- *Difficulty with speech movement patterns*: The central diagnostic characteristic of CAS is difficulty quickly and accurately sequencing and ordering the articulatory movements needed for intelligible connected speech. The earliest sign of this difficulty with articulatory movement is difficulty with syllable structure, which constitutes babbling. Even when children with CAS have a variety of speech sounds, they have difficulty putting the sounds and syllables together in the correct sequence to accurately produce more complex sequences in words, phrases, and sentences.
- *Inconsistency of speech production*: Even in imitation tasks, children with CAS often have difficulty repeating syllable sequences or words consistently and accurately. They may be able to produce a word accurately but then not be able to repeat it. Their articulatory movement patterns are inconsistent and as a result they may produce the same word with different error patterns in different speech contexts.

- *Difficulty with novel utterances*: Many children with CAS may produce some routine phrases, sing some simple songs, or repeat poems or movie dialogue with a much higher level of intelligibility than novel utterances. This can be an important CAS marker in many young children.
- *Unusual and atypical speech sound errors and patterns*: Children with CAS often do not follow the typical course of speech sound development. They often produce later developing sounds but have difficulty with earlier developing ones.

2. **History: key clinical questions.** Many of these questions are the same as those asked for SSDs because the history is often similar:
   - *"How well do you and others understand your child's speech, compared with the speech of other children of his or her age?"* Reduced intelligibility compared with peers is a strong indicator of some type of SSD including CAS.
   - *"At what age do you recall your child beginning to babble and what did it sound like?"* Infants who have not established babbling production by 9–10 months of age is a strong indicator of delay in the motor processes underlying speech sound development. Also, the babbling is limited to one or two different syllables (often /da/ or /ga/).
   - *"Has your child's speech changed much during the past 6 months?"* For children up to age 5 years, any response suggesting little change over time is a cause for concern.
   - *"Is your child frustrated when not able to be understood?"* Typically, children with CAS know they are having difficulty communicating and become increasingly frustrated in their multiple attempts to be understood.
   - *"Does your child have a history of problems with feeding or swallowing?"* This question addresses the possibility of developmental dysarthria or CAS as part of differential diagnosis.

3. **Physical examination.** The physical examination can include tasks to screen for general motor coordination development.

4. **Referral.** The primary care clinician's principal goal in CAS is early referral to a licensed/certified speech-language pathologist. A licensed/certified speech-language pathologist can perform testing necessary for diagnosis of CAS.
   Criteria for referral:
   - Refer to a speech-language pathologist if the child's speech demonstrates any of the signs or symptoms mentioned above. Speech-language pathologists in early intervention programs or public school systems assess and treat children with all types of communication disorders.
   - If the child is not babbling with a variety of syllables by 9–10 months, referral should be made for a speech and language evaluation. The child should also be referred for a complete audiologic assessment to rule out hearing loss.
   - Even very young children at risk for SSDs will benefit from early efforts to stimulate vocal production and language development. Therefore, referral should be made as soon as any communication difficulty is suspected.

5. **Clinical pearls and pitfalls**
   - Any child with reduced or delayed babbling should be referred at that point for a speech and language evaluation as well as an assessment for hearing. Waiting will only result in further delays in speech and language development with increasing frustration on the part of both parents and the child.
   - Remind parents not to require the child to produce a word clearly even though they may have done so once. One hallmark of CAS is inconsistency in accurate speech production.
   - Successful communication is key. Family and friends should respond to what the child is intending to communicate rather than requiring intelligible speech.

IV. STUTTERING

A. **Description of the problem.** Stuttering, the most common type of fluency disorder, is a disruption in speech production that is characterized by repetitions and prolongations of sounds, blockage of airflow, interjections, and revisions. Stuttering may also include secondary behaviors, physical tension, avoidance, and reduced communication.

The term *disfluency* is often used synonymously with *stuttering*, but it also may refer to the hesitations common in the speech of typical children learning to talk.

Both stuttering and SSD are problems of speech production—some aspects may have a motor component (comparable to articulation disorders) and others may have a language connection (phonological disorders). This comorbidity between SSD and stuttering may arise because of the child's limited capacity to manage several aspects of communication at the same time.

B. Epidemiology. The prevalence of stuttering is 1% among school-aged children, slightly lower in adults, and slightly higher in preschool children. Incidence statistics vary but are generally considered to be between 5%–10%. The difference between prevalence and incidence figures reflects the tendency for children who stutter to recover, usually before puberty. The male–female ratio among children younger than 6 years is about 2:1 and rises to 4:1 in adulthood, suggesting that females are more likely to recover. Recent studies have reported 30%–40% of children who stutter also have SSD. A child who stutters appears to be at higher risk for an SSD than a child in the general population.

C. Familial transmission/genetics. Parents who stutter are more likely to have children who stutter; this is especially so for women who stutter. A multifactorial (polygenic) model has been suggested to account for the transmission.

D. Organic/transactional etiologies
- Predispositions to stuttering include an inherited or acquired difficulty in speech motor coordination and a temperament, which reacts to stress with excess muscular tension and effort.
- Brain imaging studies of children who stutter suggest reduced gray matter volume in speech areas and abnormal white matter tracts in speech planning and speech motor areas.

E. Natural history. Stuttering usually appears between the ages of 18 months and 5 years. In 70% of children who begin to stutter (i.e., are dysfluent), early symptoms will resolve. Early onset of stuttering (between ages 2–3 years) is associated with more likely natural recovery than later onset.

In children who do not recover naturally, the signs and symptoms may worsen from (1) easy repetitions with minimal awareness to (2) rapid and physically tense repetitions with evidence of frustration to (3) blockages of speech, accompanying struggle behaviors, and avoidance of words and speaking situations.

A home or school environment that places high demands on a child's performance can contribute to stuttering. Examples of demands include a communication environment that pressures the child to speak more rapidly, articulately, or with more advanced language than the child is easily able to do. Stuttering may also be exacerbated by stressful but normal life events such as the birth of a sibling, separation from a parent, or a family move.

F. Management
1. **Signs and Symptoms. See Table 77-3.**
2. **History: key clinical questions**
   - *"How long have you been aware of your child's stuttering?"* If the child has stuttered for more than 6 months, suspect a potential chronic problem, particularly if it has not decreased in frequency or severity since onset.
   - *"How has the stuttering changed since it began?"* If there has been an increase in effort, emotion, or avoidance associated with stuttering, it is worsening.
   - *"What is your child's stuttering like at its worst?"* Many children who stutter will not stutter in the clinician's office; it is important to have the parents describe the signs and symptoms that have caused them concern.
   - *"Is the child bothered by his/her stuttering?"* If so, the child may soon react to his her stuttering with physical tension and struggle and should be referred.
3. **Screening.** Ask the child several direct questions (e.g., name, age, address) that are typically answered without substitution or circumlocution. This is likely to elicit stuttering or avoidance if child is a stutterer.
4. **Referral.** A licensed/certified speech-language pathologist can perform testing necessary for diagnosis of a stuttering disorder. It is important for the family to understand that the child is doing the best that he or she can in speaking, and the stuttering will only get worse if the family criticizes. Rather, the family should find ways to reduce stress and to verbalize their acceptance to the child.

   The primary care clinician's principal goal in stuttering is appropriate referral to a speech-language pathologist and to emphasize to the parents that they did not cause the problem.

   Criteria for referral:
   - If the child is stuttering with physical tension and/or is showing concern or frustration. The child should be referred immediately to a licensed/certified speech-language pathologist, preferably one who specializes in stuttering. The Stuttering Foundation Web site contains a referral list of clinicians experienced in the treatment of stuttering.
   - If disfluency continues over 2–3 months without appreciable lessening of the stuttering, referral should be made.

Table 77-3 • SIGNS AND SYMPTOMS OF NORMAL DISFLUENCY AND STUTTERING

	Normal Disfluency	Mild Stuttering	Severe Stuttering
Speech behavior	Occasional brief repetitions of sounds, syllables, or short words (li-like this)	Frequent long repetitions of sounds, syllables, or short words (li-li-li-like this). Occasional prolongations of sounds	Very frequent and often very long repetitions of sounds, syllables, or short words. Frequent sound prolongations and blockages
Other behavior	Occasional pauses, hesitations or fillers. Changing of words or thoughts	Repetitions and prolongations associated with blinking, looking away, and physical tension around mouth	More evidence of struggle, including pitch rise in voice. Extra words used as "starters"
When most noticeable	Comes and goes when child is excited, tired, sick, talking to inattentive listeners	Comes and goes in similar situations but is more often present than absent	Present in most speaking situations. More consistent
Child's reaction	Usually none apparent	May show a little concern or some frustration and embarrassment	Embarrassment, shame, and fear of speaking. Lack of eye contact when speaking
Parents' reaction	None to a great deal	Some concern, but not a great deal	Considerable degree of concern
Referral decision	Refer only if parents are quite concerned and are convinced their child is stuttering	Refer if continues for 6–8 wk or if parental concern justifies it	Refer as soon as possible

5. **Clinical pearls and pitfalls**
   - Most parents blame themselves. Reassure them that they didn't cause their child's stuttering, but they can play a big part in their child's ability to cope with it.
   - Most children will outgrow stuttering, especially if parents can reduce psychosocial pressures and increase acceptance of the child as he or she is now.
   - Parental attitudes that put a high premium on completely fluent speech probably interfere with recovery.
   - Effective programs for preschool children who stutter are intensive, involve the parents, and focus on natural, fluent speech. Intervention in the preschool years can eliminate stuttering.
   - Effective treatments for school-age children help the child speak more fluently and become confident about talking but do not aim for perfection.
   - Transient stuttering is sometimes associated with the use of medications for allergies, attention deficit disorders, and other childhood disorders.

Bibliography

SPEECH SOUNDS

FOR PROFESSIONALS

Bernthal JE, Bankson NW, Flpsen P Jr. *Articulation and Phonological Disorders*. Upper Saddle River, NJ: Pearson Education Inc; 2013.

Bleile KM. *The Manual of Speech Sound Disorders*. 3rd ed. Stamford, CT: Cengage Learning; 2015.

WEB SITES

American Speech-Language-Hearing Association. https://www.asha.org/public/.

APRAXIA

FOR PROFESSIONALS

Strode R, Chamberlain C. *The Source for Childhood Apraxia of Speech*. East Moline, IL: LinguiSystems; 2006.

FOR PARENTS

Lindsay L. *Speaking of Apraxia: A Parents' Guide to Childhood Apraxia of Speech*. Amazon; 2012.

WEB SITES

American Speech-Language-Hearing Association, American Speech-Language-Hearing Association. https://www.asha.org/public/.

www.apraxia-kids.org.

STUTTERING

WEB SITES

National Stuttering Association. www.nsastutter.org (This site is run by an organization of people who stutter and has information about support groups around the world and about NSA's annual conference.).

Stuttering Foundation. www.stutteringhelp.org (This site contains a list of things parents can do to help their child, a referral list of experienced clinicians for every state and many other countries, as well as an online store containing many inexpensive books and videos for parents and children who stutter.).

Stuttering Home Page. www.mnsu.edu/comdis/kuster/stutter.html (This site contains excellent resources for parents, children, and teens. There are support and discussion groups and a wealth of written material and links to other useful Web sites.).

FOR PARENTS

Conture E, Fraser J. *If Your Child Stutters: A Guide for Parents*. Memphis, TN: Stuttering Foundation; 2002.

FOR PROFESSIONALS

Bloodstein O, Ratner N. *A Handbook on Stuttering*. Chicago, IL: National Easter Seal Society for Crippled Children and Adults; 2008.

Guitar B. *Stuttering: An Integrated Approach to Its Nature and Treatment*. Baltimore, MD: Lippincott, Williams & Wilkins; 2006.

Guitar B, McCauley R. *Treatment of Stuttering*. Baltimore, MD: Lippincott, Williams & Wilkins; 2009.

Yairi E, Ambrose N. *Early Childhood Stuttering*. Austin, TX: PRO-ED; 2005.

CHAPTER **78**

Substance Use in Adolescence

Jessica Gray | Scott E. Hadland | Sarah M. Bagley

I. DESCRIPTION OF PROBLEM

- Alcohol use is consistently implicated in the top three leading causes of death among US teenagers, including unintentional injury fatalities (of which three-quarters are due to motor vehicle crashes), homicides, and suicides.
- Substance use is also associated with a wide range of serious problems, including school failure, respiratory diseases, high-risk sexual behaviors, transmission of human immunodeficiency virus and viral hepatitis, use of firearms, exposure to violence, and criminal justice system involvement.
- In addition to the potential immediate harms of alcohol and other drug use (AOD) early age of first use increases the risk of developing a substance use disorder (SUD) during later life.
- Alcohol and marijuana continue to be the most commonly used substances in adolescents. For the most recent trends, visit drugabuse.nida.gov.

A. Risk and protective factors associated with substance use during adolescence

1. **Risk factors**
   a. Individual: childhood history of experiencing or witnessing trauma, male gender, school failure, attention-deficit/hyperactivity disorder (ADHD) and learning disabilities, other co-occurring mental disorders, poor coping skills, nonconformity, and low religiousness.
   b. Family: genetic risks, family member who is actively abusing alcohol or other drugs, parent–child conflict, permissive or authoritarian parenting style, unstable parental relationships, or parental divorce.
   c. Community: widespread alcohol advertising, availability of other drugs, and substance-using peers.

2. **Protective factors**
   a. Individual: high self-esteem, internal locus of control, emotional well-being, resilient temperament, and school achievement.
   b. Community: use of evidence-based prevention programs, availability of after-school programs and mentoring, robust alcohol control policies, and lower alcohol outlet density.

II. MAKING THE DIAGNOSIS

A. Symptoms. Substance use in adolescence may not necessarily result in obvious symptoms detectable to a parent or clinician.

Symptoms: declining school performance; quitting extracurricular activities that were once enjoyable; isolation at home; increased confrontations with parents and siblings; labile mood; change in outward appearance and friendships; change in weight or eating habits; possession of drugs or drug paraphernalia; lying or covering-up behaviors; stealing from family members (missing cash, parental alcohol and medications, or other stolen property).

B. Differential diagnosis

- Mental health diagnoses (e.g., ADHD, depression, anxiety, bipolar disorder, posttraumatic stress disorder) or bullying at school.
- Metabolic disorders, neurologic diseases, and accidental poisoning.

C. History

1. **Screening.** The American Academy of Pediatrics (AAP) recommends screening for all adolescent patients. The following tools can be administered on paper, a computer, or in person.
   - CRAFFT is both a screening tool and brief assessment instrument. It is a mnemonic acronym for key words in each of the six questions and is a good way to quickly identify problems associated with substance use. "(1) *Have you ever ridden in a Car driven by someone (including yourself) who was "high" or had been using alcohol or drugs? (2) Do you ever use alcohol or drugs to Relax, feel better about yourself, or fit in? (3) Do you ever use alcohol or drugs while you are by yourself,*

or Alone? (4) Do you ever Forget things you did while using alcohol or drugs? (5) Do your Family or Friends ever tell you that you should cut down on your drinking or drug use? (6) Have you ever gotten into Trouble while you were using alcohol or drugs?"

- S2BI: Series of multiple choice questions validated to correlate with DSM-5 criteria for SUD:*"In the past year how many times have you used tobacco, alcohol, or marijuana?"* (Never, once or twice, monthly, weekly, or more). If positive, first questions are followed by the same questions for prescription drugs not prescribed to you, illegal drugs, inhalants, herbs or synthetic drugs.
- BSTAD: Brief Screener for Tobacco, Alcohol, and other Drugs asks: *"In the past year, on how many days have you had more than a few sips of alcohol, tobacco products or used marijuana?"*.

A positive screen (CRAFFT >2, S2BI any yes; and BSTAD any yes) should lead to a brief intervention including further assessment for an SUD and a follow-up plan.

D. Assessing severity of use. SUDs are diagnosed based on the Diagnostic and Statistical Manual of Mental Disorders, Fifth Edition (DSM-5) involving 11 criteria for SUD based on substance use occurring over 12 months:
- Taking larger amounts/over a longer period than intended
- Persistent desire or unsuccessful efforts to cut down
- Excess time spent in activities to obtain, use, or recover from substance use
- Cravings
- Failure to fulfill major role obligations at work, school, or home
- Continued use despite having persistent/recurrent social or interpersonal problems
- Social, occupational, or recreational activities given up
- Recurrent use in situations in which it is physically hazardous
- Continued use despite knowledge of having a persistent or recurrent physical or psychological problem
- Tolerance
- Withdrawal

If an individual has two to three criteria, SUD is classified as "mild"; four to five criteria, "moderate"; and six or more criteria, "severe."

Tolerance and withdrawal are included in the 11 criteria, but they in and of themselves do not indicate an SUD but demonstrate physical dependence. Early remission is considered for anyone with 3–12 months without applicable SUD criteria (excluding cravings). Sustained remission is similarly greater than 12 months of above.

E. Physical examination and laboratory testing. A targeted physical examination is indicated but is unlikely to yield significant findings in the absence of acute intoxication or withdrawal. Findings concerning for longer-term drug use include but are not limited to venous scarring (track marks), scars from skin picking, poor dentition, inflammation or erosions of nasal septum, wheezing, abdominal tenderness, or breast tissue development in males.

III. MANAGEMENT

A. The clinician through discussion with the youth will develop a treatment plan. See Table 78-1 for suggestions on staging therapeutic goals.

Most brief interventions include six key steps:
1. Ask permission to discuss the topic.
2. **Feedback.** Deliver feedback on the risks and/or negative consequences of substance use with the adolescent's own words whenever possible.
3. **Education.** Explain the health risks of alcohol and drugs.
4. **Recommendation.** Recommend that your patient use no alcohol and drugs for a specified period (e.g., 3 weeks) and make a plan to check back with the patient after the trial period.
5. **Negotiation.** If the patient refuses to quit completely, attempt to elicit any commitment to change.
6. **Agreement.** Ask for a brief written agreement that both of you will sign specifying the change and the period.
7. **Follow-up.** Make an appointment for a follow-up meeting to monitor success (or need for more intensive intervention).

B. Location of care. Location of care depends on severity of substance use, patient safety, family supports, and available community resources. Referral to specialty care will enable the patient to be directed to the appropriate level of care.

C. Pharmacotherapies. There are currently three SUDs for which we have pharmacotherapy: tobacco, alcohol, and opioid use disorder (OUD). Medications should be offered to patients regardless of treatment setting and have been shown to independently improve outcomes for decreasing and stopping use. Table 78-2 describes the methods.

Table 78-1 • STAGE-APPROPRIATE THERAPEUTIC GOALS FOR DRUG AND ALCOHOL USE (THIS MAY INCLUDE ROLE PLAYING DIFFERENT SITUATIONS)

Stage	Intervention Goal	Sample Language
Abstinence/no use	Positive reinforcement, anticipatory guidance	I am glad to hear that like most kids of your age you have never tried X. Avoiding alcohol, tobacco, and other drugs is one of the best ways to stay healthy.
Exposure/prior use	Education regarding risks	Can you tell me some of the risks of drinking alcohol? What do you plan to keep yourself safe?
Risky substance use	Risk reduction advice (e.g., driving/riding while impaired)	Can we role-play about what you could do if you need to drive home and have used alcohol? (Solutions can include calling parents, other trusted adult, older sibling.)
Risky substance use	Brief intervention (BI)	On the one hand, you use mj to relax and, on the other hand, you said that your grades were lower this semester and using mj was the reason.
Mild use disorder	BI, outpatient counseling, follow-up	My recommendation is for you to meet with our social worker and talk more about how substances may be affecting you. Can I make an appointment with him/her and then follow up with you in a couple of weeks?
Moderate/ severe use disorder	Referral to intensive treatment	Based on what we have talked about today, I think that you will need some help getting treatment for your substance use. I would recommend that you be seen by a specialist. What do you think about this?
Secondary abstinence	Positive reinforcement, support, follow-up	I know that you are working hard to stay sober and hope that you can be proud of the work that you are doing. Is there anything I can do to support your recovery?

mj, marijuana.

Table 78-2 • FDA-APPROVED MEDICATIONS FOR SUBSTANCE USE DISORDERS

Substance	Medications	Notes
Alcohol dependence	Naltrexone Acamprosate Disulfiram	Approved for age 18 y and over. Limited data for use for individuals younger than 18 y
Tobacco use	Nicotine replacement (patch, inhaler, nasal spray, gum, lozenges)	Nicotine replacement available OTC, covered by some insurance
	Bupropion Varenicline	Two FDA-approved medications for age 18+ y. Would consult with addiction specialist if considering off-label medication use
OUD	Buprenorphine	**Buprenorphine/naloxone** (sublingual tablet): safe, effective, can be prescribed by primary care after DEA waiver training. Approved for age 16+ y. In general, longer durations of treatment of buprenorphine appear more effective that short-term treatment
	Methadone	**Methadone** (liquid): restricted to specially licensed programs, in general do not accept age <18 y
	Naltrexone	**Naltrexone** (pill or long-acting injectable formulation): anyone can prescribe, approved for age >18 y, lacking comparative effectiveness data among youth

DEA, Drug Enforcement Agency; OTC, over the counter; OUD, opioid use disorder.

D. Drug testing. The AAP recommends that laboratory testing for alcohol or drugs *not* be performed on a conscious adolescent without his or her knowledge and consent. Interpretation of drug tests can be complicated, and clinicians should enlist the help of a toxicologist or addiction specialist to minimize the risks of misinterpretation such as false negatives or positives.

E. Recovery support services. For adolescents with an SUD, the pathway to recovery may also include nonprofessional support. This may include intensive school-based support such as dedicated recovery high schools or collegiate recovery programs, mutual support groups such as 12-step fellowship (e.g., Alcoholics Anonymous or Narcotics Anonymous) meetings. An adult guide or temporary sponsor may be needed to make meetings meaningful.

IV. CO-OCCURRING CONDITIONS WITH SUDS. Symptoms of a mental disorder may be subtle before initiation of substance use and/or may be a symptom of substance use. For example ADHD and SUD.
   • Given the risk-taking tendency and impulsivity of adolescents with ADHD, they may begin experimenting with tobacco, alcohol, and drugs at an earlier age compared with those without the disorder.
   • Children with ADHD are at elevated risk of developing an SUD later in life, and the presence of other co-occurring mental disorders raises the risk even higher.
   • Although adolescents with ADHD are at higher risk for SUD, appropriate pharmacologic treatment for ADHD does not increase that risk.
   • Consider using medications with less potential for illicit use (diversion) potential when there is concern for co-occurring disorder.

V. CLINICAL PEARLS AND PITFALLS
   1. Many youth do not think that use of AOD is a problem. It can be helpful to understand what your patient thinks would be risky to use and help provide age-appropriate education.
   2. Engaging the family is key. Ensuring that the teen has a safety plan and a trusted adult to call if he or she is feeling unsafe can be an important part of a plan.
   3. Parents can make a difference: simple things such as advising parents to eat dinner together and having open communication can decrease substance use.
   4. Many adolescents who use substances may also experience depression. Provide treatment for both substance use and depression *simultaneously* when they co-occur. Treatment of either one alone is unlikely to be successful.
   5. For patients with both ADHD and SUD, it is important to treat both conditions, including the use of stimulant medications as appropriate, even despite the potential risk for diversion. To prevent diversion or nonmedical use, we recommend that parents retain control of the prescription bottle.
   6. Chronic use of opioid analgesics leads to development of physiological tolerance and withdrawal, but these two alone do not define an addictive disorder. *Physiological dependence* on opioid analgesics should not be confused with an *OUD*.
   7. Although a smaller number of youth have OUD, having naloxone rescue kit in the home is recommended for those with OUD or parents with OUD.

Bibliography

PARENTS AND TEENS
Keeping Youth Drug Free. https://store.samhsa.gov/product/Keeping-Youth-Drug-Free/SMA17–3772.
NIDA for Teens (National Institute on Drug Abuse). http://www.teens.drugabuse.gov/.
Partnership for a Drug Free America. http://www.drugfree.org/.

WEB SITES
Monitoring the Future. www.monitoringthefuture.org.
National Survey on Drug Use and Health. http://oas.samhsa.gov/nhsda.htm.
Substance Abuse and Mental Health Services Administration. www.samhsa.gov.
Youth Risk Behavior Surveillance. http://www.cdc.gov/HealthyYouth/yrbs/index.htm.

TOOLS
BSTAD. https://www.drugabuse.gov/ast/bstad/#/.
Clinical guidelines for use of buprenorphine in the treatment of opioid addiction. http://buprenorphine.samhsa.gov/Bup_Guidelines.pdf.
S2BI. https://www.drugabuse.gov/ast/s2bi/#/.

PUBLICATIONS
Centers for Disease Control and Prevention. *Alcohol-Related Disease Impact - Home Page.* https://nccd.cdc.gov/DPH_ARDI/default/default.aspx.

Committee on Substance Abuse. Substance use screening, brief intervention, and referral to treatment for pediatricians. *Pediatrics*. 2011;128(5):e1330-e1340. doi:10.1542/peds.2011-1754.

Harstad E, Levy S, Committee on Substance Abuse. Attention-deficit/hyperactivity disorder and substance abuse. *Pediatrics*. 2014;134(1):e293-e301. doi:10.1542/peds.2014-0992.

RESOURCES FOR TEENS AND FAMILIES

7 Ways to Protect Your Teen from Alcohol and Other Drugs [Educational Brochure]. Boston, MA: Bureau of Substance Abuse Services, Massachusetts Department of Public Health; 2004.

National Institute on Drug Abuse. https://teens.drugabuse.gov/.

CHAPTER 79

Suicide

Michael H. Tang

I. DESCRIPTION OF THE PROBLEM

A. **Suicide.** The suicide rate in the United States is increasing and is now the second leading cause of death in children ages 1–19 years. A pediatric clinician's ability to assess a child's risk and protective factors, provide an appropriate intervention, and advocate for prevention has the potential to save a child's life.

Suicide lies on a spectrum, from thoughts of wanting to be dead (passive suicidal ideation); thoughts about actions to end one's life (active suicidal ideation), thoughts on methodologies (suicidal plan); an intent to act (suicidal intent); a self-injurious behavior with some intent to die (suicide attempt), to a death (suicide completion). Self-injurious behaviors with no intent to die (nonsuicidal self-injury or NSSI), such as cutting or burning, can be driven by an intent to relieve distress, "feel something", get attention, escape, or punish oneself.

B. **Epidemiology.** Although likely an underestimation, according to the Centers for Disease Control and Prevention 2014 Vital Statistics, suicide is the second leading cause of death in children less than 19 years of age, translating to 2265 deaths a year, 12.1% of all childhood deaths, and a rate of 2.9 per 100,000. Suicide is rare in young children but increases in frequency with age, becoming the second leading cause of death in ages 10–14 years (2.1 per 100,000), 15–19 years (8.7 per 100,000), and among adolescents and young adults ages 15–24 years (11.6 per 100,000) and 25–34 years (15.1 per 100,000).

Suicidal ideation and attempts are twice more common among American high school girls than boys, but suicide completions are three times greater among 15- to 19-year-old boys than girls. This gap is caused by males being more likely to choose firearms (with a 92% mortality rate), compared with females being more likely to choose less lethal methods such as overdosing on pills (with a 2% mortality rate). Suicide rates are higher among American Indian/Alaska Native and non-Hispanic white youth compared with Asian, non-Hispanic black, or Hispanic youth. Suicide attempts are more common among Hispanic girls. Adolescents who identify as lesbian, gay, bisexual, or transgendered (LGBT) have at least twice the rate of suicidal ideation. It is estimated there are 50–100 attempted suicides for every completed suicide.

Suicidal ideation is common in teenagers, whereas suicidal plans and attempts are less prevalent; for example, the estimated lifetime prevalence among adolescents for suicidal ideation is 12.1%, suicidal plans 4.0%, and suicide attempts 4.1%. NSSI has been estimated at 17.2% among adolescents.

C. **Developmental considerations.** As part of a risk assessment, it is important for a pediatric clinician to understand suicidal intent within a developmental context. A young child may say, "I just want to kill myself" because he hears this phrase at home, without having any intent to harm himself. A preadolescent who self-harms should still be taken seriously, even if she does not fully understand that death is final. An impulsive teenager has attempted suicide if she takes three tablets of acetaminophen—despite negligible risk of medical harm—if she intended to kill herself and she (inaccurately) believed the dose would have been lethal.

D. **Risk factors.** A suicide risk assessment is based on clinical judgment; there is no tool that reliably predicts suicide. Therefore, the clinician must understand suicide risk and protective factors, including the following:

1. **Predisposing and mediating risk factors.** These traits are fixed or only gradually modifiable.

Prior attempts, plans, ideation, or NSSI: The greatest risk factor for completing suicide is a prior suicide attempt (odds ratio [OR] = 67). Any prior nonsuicidal or suicidal thought, plan, or attempt is also strongly associated with completed suicide (OR = 23). Despite this link, 68% of all youth who completed suicide had no prior suicide attempt.

Psychiatric illness: Among adolescents who completed suicide, 90% had a history of at least one psychiatric diagnosis (and 70% with multiple diagnoses), showing the strong association between mental illness and suicide (OR = 9.4). Among diagnoses, mood disorders such as bipolar disorder and depression are closely associated (OR = 9.8), followed by substance use disorders (OR = 7.2), conduct disorders (OR = 4.6), and anxiety disorders (OR = 2.8). Other disorders including schizophrenia, eating disorders, and posttraumatic stress disorder also have elevated risks. However, among suicide completers younger than 16 years, about 40% had no apparent diagnosable psychiatric disorder.

Personality traits, including personality disorders, neuroticism, and perfectionism may all increase risk. A history of *sexual abuse* has an estimated 16.6%–19.5% population attributable risk for adolescent suicide attempts, suggesting eliminating sexual abuse could prevent at least one in six suicide attempts. As noted above, identifying as a *male, Native American, white,* or *sexual minority (LGBT)* youth increases risk. A *family history of suicide* increases risk two to six times. Having *physical illness, chronic pain,* or a *traumatic brain injury* is also associated with suicide. Beyond this individual-level risk, there are also population-level factors, including societal upheaval, economic turmoil, and social isolation.

2. **Precipitating factors.** These states are at, or recently before, the time of assessment and are potentially modifiable targets for treatment. The final common pathway to a completed suicide is current *suicidal and/or self-harm thoughts, plans, and intent*. Greater severity and sophistication at each step increases the risk. *Access to means* (especially firearms) raises the risk of both attempting and successfully completing suicide.

   Active psychiatric symptoms, including *depressed mood, hopelessness, impulsivity, anxiety, insomnia,* and *psychosis*, increase risk. Behavioral disinhibition is also needed to attempt suicide; this may come from *substance intoxication* and/or *withdrawal*. An at-risk youth may feel *media coverage* of a cluster of suicides or social media commentary gives "permission" to attempt suicide. *Recent discharge from a psychiatric unit* is a known major risk. A precipitant can be a *life stressor*, including being the victim of bullying, family discord, legal difficulties, and other perceived losses.

3. **Protective factors.** Balanced against these risks are several characteristics that can lower the chance of suicide. These include religious beliefs, a strong social network, healthy coping skills, a reason for living, and a sense of optimism.

II. **ASSESSING THE RISK.** The pediatric clinician should assess for suicide at every well-child visit. Knowledge about predisposing and mediating factors allows for baseline risk stratification, even before asking the patient about current precipitating states.

As part of routine care, the adolescent and his or her caregiver should be educated about confidentiality and its limits, saying for example, *"Everything you tell me is confidential, but if there is a concern about your safety or someone else's, we will have to decide who to tell next."* To promote open communication, the caregiver should always be asked to leave the room. The clinician should also be reassured by randomized clinical trials showing that suicide screening does not increase the risk for suicide.

A suicide screen should be part of a provider's routine questions on adolescent health, along with inquiries about depression (including using a standardized instrument such as the PHQ-9), substance use, school performance, and relationships with family and peers. An American Academy of Pediatrics Clinical Report offers two potential questions to always ask (with the target domain):

- *"Have you ever thought about killing yourself or wished you were dead?"* (history of suicidal ideation)
- *"Have you ever done anything on purpose to hurt or kill yourself?"* (history of suicide or self-harm attempts)

If the response to either of these questions is positive, and/or with other risk factors or clinical concerns, then further questioning must occur. Using the Columbia Suicide Severity Rating Scale as an example:

- *"When was the last time you actually had any thoughts of killing yourself?"* (current ideation)
- *"Have you been thinking about how you might do this?"* (ideation without specific plan or intent)
- *"Have you started to work out or worked out the details of how to kill yourself?* (plans)
- *"Do you intend to carry out this plan?"* (intent)
- *"Have you ever done anything, started to do anything, or prepared to do anything to end your life?"* (intent with suicidal behaviors, including preparation or preventing discovery)
- *"Have you told anyone about this plan?"* (intent with communication)

- *"Do you have access to a gun? Prescription or over-the-counter pills?"* (access to means)
- *"Are there things—anyone or anything—that stopped you from wanting to die or acting on thoughts of suicide?"* (protective factors)

Based on this information, the pediatric clinician should stratify the patient as being at high, moderate, or low risk for suicide. Although this decision is ultimately a subjective clinical judgment, examples include:

- *High risk:* Active or recent suicidal intent or behaviors; plans to use a firearm; recent suicide or self-harm attempts; serious precipitating factors such as active depression, hopelessness, and substance use.
- *Moderate risk:* Active suicidal ideation, but without intent; presence of predisposing, mediating, and precipitating risk factors; few protective factors.
- *Low risk:* Passive suicidal ideation; fewer risk factors and more protective factors

III. **MANAGEMENT.** For moderate-to-high-risk patients, the pediatric clinician should involve a behavioral health (BH) professional. For those at the highest risk, this likely includes calling a BH emergency services team or transferring to an emergency room, with subsequent psychiatric hospitalization; staying with the patient until a higher level of care is obtained; and following up after the visit to ensure a smooth transition in care. For moderate-risk patients, this may include (depending on local availability) an in-person or virtual consultation with a BH clinician; breaking confidentiality to speak with a parent; referral to outpatient BH care; reducing access to means (including locking up guns, knives, and medications), and developing a safety plan to call emergency services with worsening symptoms. For lower-risk patients, referrals to outpatient BH care are still recommended to address any underlying psychiatric illness.

Talk therapies are evidenced-based, especially dialectical behavior therapy (DBT), cognitive behavioral therapy (CBT), and mentalization-based therapy, with 14 adolescents needed to be treated to prevent one incident of self-harm. A recent randomized trial also suggested a DBT- and CBT-informed family-based treatment was effective at reducing suicide attempts among high-risk youth.

Although antidepressants are associated with increased odds of suicidality (OR = 2.39) in the months after initiating treatment, they can be appropriate to treat depression—even in suicidal youth—after weighing with the patient and family the risks, benefits, and alternatives.

IV. **PREVENTION.** The pediatric clinician can help reduce the risk factors that can contribute to suicide. On an individual level, early identification through universal depression screening in primary care and early treatment through strategies such as BH integration can lower the burden of depression. Early referral to treatment for other youth—such as those with substance use disorders or traumatized by a history of sexual abuse—can also be beneficial.

On a population level, pediatric clinicians can play an important advocacy role because reducing the availability of guns has lowered suicide rates in countries outside of the United States. Initiatives such as restraining orders, smart gun technologies, and gun safety campaigns (including using safety locks, gun lockers, and separating ammunition and the firearm) are promising, although there have been few studies. There is preliminary evidence that indicated prevention programs for high-risk populations (such as youth with a history of self-harm or depression) may be beneficial. A recent multinational cluster randomization trial suggested a universal school-based suicide program that used a "gatekeeper" training model for teachers, mental health awareness for students and indicated screening for higher-risk youth, reduced suicide attempts, and severe suicidal ideation. Clearly, more research is needed to identify effective suicide prevention efforts.

Bibliography

Calear AL, Christensen H, Freeman A, et al. A systematic review of psychosocial suicide prevention interventions for youth. *Eur Child Adolesc Psychiatry*. 2016;25(5):467-482.

Ougrin D, Tranah T, Stahl D, et al. Therapeutic interventions for suicide attempts and self-harm in adolescents: systematic review and meta-analysis. *J Am Acad Child Adolesc Psychiatry*. 2015;54(2):97-107.e2.

https://store.samhsa.gov/product/SAMHSA-Suicide-Safe-Mobile-App/PEP15-SAFEAPP1.

Shain B, Committee on Adolescence. Suicide and suicide attempts in adolescents. *Pediatrics*. 2016;138(1):e20161420.

Turecki G, Brent DA. Suicide and suicidal behaviour. *Lancet*. 2016;387(10024):1227-1239.

CHAPTER **80**

Temper Tantrums

Robert Needlman

I. **DESCRIPTION OF THE PROBLEM.** When parents complain of "anger outbursts" or "fits," they may be referring to normal temper tantrums or to symptoms associated with a wide range of behavioral, emotional, and medical diagnoses. Tantrums typically include expressions of frustration and anger (yelling, crying, swearing); self-injury (falling to the floor, hitting oneself, breath holding); breaking objects; and attacking others physically or verbally. In younger children, they often begin with anger and progress to sadness or distress. Tantrums overlap with oppositional or coercive child behaviors. "Meltdowns," although similar in appearance, may be expressions of extreme anxiety or panic. In sorting out normative from symptomatic tantrums, clinicians need to consider both incident-specific and contextual features.

A. **Epidemiology**
   - 50%–80% of 2- to 3-year-old children have tantrums at least weekly.
   - 20% have at least daily tantrums.
   - 60% of 2-year-olds with frequent tantrums will continue to have them at 3 years. Of these, 60% will continue at 4 years.
   - The prevalence of explosive "tempers" remains approximately 5% throughout childhood.
   - Severe tantrums are often accompanied by other significant behavior problems, such as disturbed sleep, anxiety, irritability, or hyperactivity.

B. **Etiology/contributing factors.** Speech and language deficits may predispose to tantrums, by limiting children's ability to understand the reasons for prohibitions and demands, as well as their ability to express themselves verbally and self-regulate using words.

   1. **Normal development.** Tantrums are communicative acts that serve to convey emotional states (anger, frustration) to an audience, typically the parents. They occur when emotional distress exceeds self-regulatory ability. They increase in response to short-term stressors (e.g., hunger, tiredness) and long-term ones (e.g. family discord), that undermine this ability. They often arise when the normal drive for autonomy conflicts with parental prohibitions or demands; or when the child's drive for mastery is frustrated by his or her limited competence. Transitions (having to stop a desired activity to do something else) are a common trigger. Tantrums appear *toward the end of the first year, peak in the third year, and recede substantially by the fifth year.*

   2. **Medical problems.** Look for chronic/recurrent minor illnesses that increase stress (eczema, allergies, recurrent serous otitis, constipation, irritable bowel); sleep disturbances (insomnia, sleep apnea); medications (e.g., anticonvulsants, antihistamines, steroids); and medical or developmental conditions that can predispose to parental overprotection (Chapter 87).

   3. **Disabilities.** Consider autism spectrum disorders (ASDs); cognitive disability; attention-deficit/hyperactivity disorder; traumatic brain injury (especially frontal lobe); and unrecognized impairments of hearing or vision. Tantrums in the face of ASD may require a functional behavioral analysis to define relevant triggers and inhibitors.

   4. **Temperament.** Predisposing traits include high intensity and activity; persistence; predominantly negative mood; low sensory threshold; and high sensitivity to novel stimuli. Irregular patterns of sleep and hunger make it difficult for parents to anticipate the child's needs.

   5. **Environment.** Physical factors include overcrowding; limited access to outdoor play; and non-childproofed homes that make frequent parental prohibitions necessary. Social factors include martial stress and verbal or physical violence; tensions arising from siblings or grandparents with behavioral problems or medical illness; parental depression, and alcohol and/or drug abuse.

6. **Parenting.** Tantrums may be unintentionally reinforced either by parents' giving in or, paradoxically, by the intense albeit negative attention they elicit. Hand-held electronic games also worsen the problem because children may tantrum whenever "their games" are taken away, while parents resort to the games to pacify restless or obnoxious children, inadvertently reinforcing the tantrums and other negative behaviors.

7. **Interacting factors.** Tantrum persistence is predicted by either (1) high tendency to frustration plus high parental intrusiveness or (b) low emotional self-regulation plus low parental control.

C. Recognizing the issue

1. **Signs and symptoms.** Concerning features include the following:

   a. Children aged less than 12 months or greater than 48. Tantrums are normally mild and infrequent in these age ranges.

   b. Tantrums occur more than three times a day and last 15 minutes or longer. Frequent, prolonged tantrums are associated with multiple behavior problems, for example, problems with sleeping, eating, or peer interactions.

   c. A high degree of parental concern, anger, guilt, anxiety, or sadness, perhaps out of proportion to the severity of the child's actual behavior.

   d. Parents who seem unable to identify positive things about the child and see the child as antagonistic and controlling. (This pattern may arise after the child witnesses domestic violence and subsequently acts out his or her identification with the aggressor.)

   e. Aggressive tantrums that seem to be unrelated to any apparent trigger, driven by intrinsic mood instability; particularly in the presence of general irritability and a family history of depression, consider disruptive mood dysregulation; with extreme tantrums, consider bipolar disorder.

   f. Tantrums in school. These are concerning because children typically "pull it together" in front of peers. Tantrums in school may be due to social, academic, or emotional problems. Consider bullying, ostracism, dyslexia, or other learning disability with consequent shame and also meltdowns as a symptom of separation anxiety.

2. **History: key clinical questions**

   a. *"What exactly happened the last time your child had a tantrum? What set it off? What did your child do first? How did you respond? Was that a typical episode?"* Try to get a moment-by-moment account of a recent episode. Focus on the ABCs: antecedents, behaviors, and consequences. Look for triggers (hunger, tiredness, sources of frustration); unintentional reinforcement (e.g., increased attention); and delayed consequences, such as special treats the parents may offer to atone for their own feelings of anger.

   b. *"What feelings do your child's tantrums bring out in you?"* If parents report strong anger, shame, or guilt, these feelings need to be addressed.

   c. *"How often do tantrums result in your child's getting what he/she wants?"* Behaviors maintained by intermittent reinforcement (the child gets what he or she wants or escapes an unwanted task) are particularly resistant to extinction.

   d. *"What do other adults in the family say about the tantrums? How do they respond? What do they think you should do?"* Family dynamics often plays a role in maintaining tantrums. If tantrums occur more frequently with, say, the mother, it may be that she is more ambivalent about limit setting; or the other parent may be subtly undercutting her authority, for example, by acting overly solicitous to the child after a tantrum.

   e. *"Does your child have other behavior problems, such as hyperactivity, aggressiveness, food refusal, clinginess, or sleep problems?"* A pattern of multiple behavior problems suggests the need for a more comprehensive evaluation. Consider developmental delay as well.

   f. *"When your child is happy, how does he/she show it? Are all emotions expressed intensely? Does he/she tend to stick with a challenge until he/she masters it?"* In the absence of other concerning features, long and loud tantrums in an intense, persistent child may be normal.

   g. *"How was your pregnancy with this child? What about the delivery, newborn period, first year of life, etc.? Any significant illnesses or injury?"* A special pregnancy (e.g., unplanned, or long-awaited) may fuel parental guilt and poor limit setting. A past life-threatening event and continued perceived vulnerability suggests vulnerable child syndrome (see Chapter 107).

3. Office evaluation

a. **Physical examination.** Look for signs of allergies, recurrent otitis, dental caries (a source of pain), scars suggestive of abuse, evidence of an endocrinopathy (e.g., genital enlargement, striae), and obesity (consider Prader–Willi). Subtle dysconjugate gaze may be an overlooked sign of visual disturbance that makes children feel on edge.

b. **Observations.** Crayons and paper may elicit themes of anger or threat (e.g., a burning house, a shark that attacks), indicating that the child understands that gaining some control over such feelings is the purpose of the visit. Provision of a few age-appropriate toys allows observation of the child's play skills, an indication of cognitive development, and the child's response to the request to clean up.

c. **Written data and tests.** A tantrum log, listing the antecedents, behaviors, and consequences of each tantrum, as well as the times of onset and resolution, can help identify patterns and document improvement with therapy. Standardized questionnaires such as the Pediatric Symptom Checklist can detect relevant patterns of behavior and may suggest the need for psychiatric evaluation.

D. Management

1. Primary goals

a. **Clarify the diagnosis.** Differentiate between tantrums due to developmentally appropriate stresses or challenging temperament and tantrums due to underlying delays, disorders, or familial dysfunction.

b. **Address contributing factors.** For example, refer for speech and language therapy; adjust medications for asthma or allergies; advocate for improved housing; refer parents for marital counseling or treatment of depression.

c. **Educate parents.** Reduce parental distress by correcting unrealistic expectations and fears and explaining the developmental forces driving the tantrums; help parents to problem-solve (e.g., providing a small snack before going to the grocery store).

2. Specific strategies. Tantrums respond well to parent counseling/training individually and in groups.

a. **Childproof the home.** Reducing hazards and temptations minimizes how often the child must hear "no." Regardless of such efforts, there are always plenty of opportunities for children to learn to accept limits.

b. **Allow limited choices.** Children comply better when they feel in control. For a young child, it is best to offer two alternatives, both acceptable (e.g., red shirt or blue shirt.) Small children need to make small choices.

c. **Provide routines.** Predictability increases a small child's sense of control, reducing frustrations; for example, before going to the store, make a list of what you will buy.

d. **Adjust to temperament.** A very active child needs space to run around; a slow-to-warm-up child needs time to adjust to new situations and people; a highly persistent child may need five- and one-minute warnings to prepare to end a pleasurable activity.

e. **Pick battles and win them.** Parents often say "no" when they really mean, "I'd rather you didn't." If the issue really isn't very important, the parents are more likely to reverse themselves in the face of a tantrum. For such issues, it's better for parents to state their preference ("I'd rather you didn't have a cookie right now"), offer alternatives ("How about a carrot stick?), or simply say "yes" right off the bat. When parents do say "no," they should not give in. "No" needs to be absolute and nonnegotiable.

f. **Offer comfort.** Young children may need to be held, to help contain their out-of-control emotions. Older children need to know that a parent is nearby and attentive so that they don't feel abandoned in their time of upset. After the tantrum, offer a hug and return to the task or activity that was interrupted.

g. **Prevent harm.** The parent may have to move the child to a rug or away from hard furniture. A child intent on hurting himself or herself or anyone else needs to be stopped, even if that means physical restraint. Parents should not allow a child to hit, pinch, or bite them.

h. **Use helpful language.** How parents talk about a child's tantrums matters. Tantrums are about "losing control" rather than "being bad." It is not helpful to dwell in detail on tantrums past, but it may help to remind a child to, "Tell me when you're mad; use your words." Later, in quiet moments, parents can make up stories about children who are furious but triumph by controlling themselves, or stories about how they (the parents) have needed to take three deep breaths to avoid "losing it."

i. **Celebrate successes.** Parents need to pay attention whenever their child uses words to express frustration or to protest a perceived injustice. A warm "good job!" and a hug powerfully reinforce the child's accomplishment.

j. **Skillful communication.** Specific skills, such as reflective listening, naming the child's emotions, and granting wishes in fantasy, can enhance communication and reduce tantrums (see Ginott, in parent references).

3. **Criteria for referral.** The following features should suggest referral for subspecialist care for tantrums.

a. **Developmental disability.** Severe tantrums arising in the context of cognitive disability, ASDs, deafness, or other developmental disabilities may benefit from intensive behavioral approaches.

b. **Emotional disturbance.** Consider among others: parental depression or other mental illness; traumatic separations or recurrent hospitalizations; presence of a sibling with special health care needs; domestic violence; associated internalizing or externalizing behaviors.

c. **Failure to improve.** In the absence of more specific indications, failure for tantrums to show improvement after two or three visits may trigger referral for more extensive evaluation and protracted management.

Bibliography

FOR PARENTS

Ginott H. *Between Parent and Child*. New York: Macmillan; 1965. (Still one of the best guides for talking with children, giving clear messages and effective feedback.)

Lieberman A. *The Emotional Life of the Toddler*. New York: Free Press; 1993. (A remarkably clear, insightful, readable explanation of toddlers and their feelings.)

Turecki S, Tonner L. *The Difficult Child*. New York: Bantam Doubleday; 1989. (Practical and sensitive advice, with an emphasis on temperament as a major determinant of children's behavior.)

WEB SITES

KidsHealth. http://kidshealth.org/parent/emotions/behavior/tantrums.html (Conversational, solid information). Accessed June 1, 2018.

Iowa State University Extension—www.extension.iastate.edu/publications/PM1529J.pdf (Clear, low literacy, includes a helpful worksheet). Accessed June 1, 2018.

FOR PROFESSIONALS

Belden AC, Thomson NR, Luby JL. Temper tantrums in healthy versus depressed and disruptive preschoolers: defining tantrum behaviors associated with clinical problems. *J Pediatr*. 2008;152(1):117-122. (Describes tantrums associated with behavioral disorders.)

Degnan KA, Calkins SD, Keane SP, et al. Profiles of disruptive behavior across early childhood: contributions of frustration reactivity, physiological regulation, and maternal behavior. *Child Dev*. 2008;79(5):1357-1376. (A developmental psychopathology analysis explaining tantrums that persist past the toddler years.)

Goodenough F. *Anger in Young Children*. Minneapolis, MD: University of Minnesota Press; 1931. (A classic monograph.)

Needlman R, Stevenson J, Zuckerman B. Psychosocial correlates of severe temper tantrums. *J Dev Behav Pediatr*. 1991;12:77-83. (An analysis of a large, community-based sample.)

CHAPTER 81

Temperamentally Difficult Children

Stanley Turecki

I. **DESCRIPTION OF THE PROBLEM.** A "difficult child" is a normal young child whose innate temperament makes him or her hard to raise. Inherent in this definition is a view of normality that is broad: children are different and do not have to be average to be normal. For a child to be considered temperamentally difficult, a basic criterion must be met: the child's constitutionally determined personality traits—their very nature—must cause significant problems in child-rearing.

A. **Epidemiology**
- About 15% of young children are temperamentally difficult according to this definition.
- Difficult children are not alike. Some are impulsive, distractible, and highly active; others are shy and clingy. Some throw loud tantrums; others whine and complain. Some can hit, kick, or even bite; others are verbally defiant. Some are unpredictable in their eating or sleeping habits; others are sensitive to noise, textures, or tastes. Most difficult children have trouble dealing with transition and change, and almost all are strong-willed and extremely stubborn.
- Highly active, impulsive, difficult children are more likely to be boys. All other temperamentally difficult traits are as likely to be seen in girls as in boys.
- There is no correlation with birth order, intelligence, or socioeconomic status.

B. **Etiology**
- Temperament refers to dimensions of personality that are largely constitutional in origin. Genetic factors contribute. Pregnancy and delivery complications may be somewhat more common in the histories of difficult children. Some of these children are allergic, with a propensity to develop ear infections. Uneven language and development of learning skills are not uncommon. Many difficult children are intelligent but socially immature. These factors suggest a biologic basis for a difficult temperament.

C. **The concept of temperament.** Temperament is the *how* of behavior, rather than the *why* (motivation) or the *what* (ability). For example, three equally motivated and able children may approach a homework assignment quite differently, depending on their behavioral style. One will begin on time and work steadily to completion, the second will delay and procrastinate but then work very persistently, and the third will jump in immediately and quickly lose patience. Inherent in the temperamental perspective is a broad view of normality and a bias toward seeing atypical behavior as different rather than abnormal.

   Temperament may also be defined as the behavioral expression, evident early in life, of those dimensions of personality that are constitutional in origin. Family, twin, and adoption studies point to a 50% multigenetic heritability. The stability of temperament is detectable at 18 months, substantial at 3 years, and most evident in middle childhood. As development proceeds, temperamental qualities are neither rigidly fixed nor completely malleable—like cartilage rather than bone or muscle. A range exists for each category. Table 81-1 lists the categories of temperament.

   1. **The child and the environment: a transactional model.** The concept of a difficult temperament should always be combined with that of *goodness of fit*—the match or compatibility between a child and his or her environment. Behavior that presents a problem to one family may be readily accepted by another. For example, a child's idiosyncratic and strongly held tastes in clothing and food would only trouble a fashion- and nutrition-conscious parent. The context of the behavior is always important. A highly active boy who has some problems with self-control and concentration, if placed in a class of 25 children (of whom another 5 are "challenging") with one somewhat inexperienced teacher, would undoubtedly meet all the criteria for attention-deficit/hyperactivity disorder (ADHD). However, if the following year he is in a class of 15 children with a high ratio of girls to boys and the teacher has an assistant, the child would still be a handful, but a clinical diagnosis of disorder would be inappropriate.

Table 81-1 • CATEGORIES OF TEMPERAMENT

Trait	Description	Easy	Difficult
Activity level	General statement about level of motor activity; actual amount of physical motion during play, eating, sleep etc.	Low to moderate	Very active, restless, fidgety; always into things; makes you tired; "ran before they walked"; easily overstimulated; gets wild or "revved up"; impulsive, loses control, can be aggressive, hates to be confined
Self-control	Ability to delay action or demands	Good, patient	Poor, impulsive
Concentration	Ability to maintain focus in the face of distractions	Good, stays with task	Poor, distractible, has trouble concentrating and paying attention especially if not really interested; doesn't listen, tunes you out; daydreams, forgets instructions
Intensity	Energy level of responses; how forcefully or loudly reactions are expressed, whether positive or negative	Low, mild, low-keyed	High, loud, forceful whether miserable, angry, or happy
Regularity	Predictability of physical functions such as appetite, sleep–wake cycle, and elimination	Regular, predictable	Irregular, erratic, can't tell when they'll be hungry or tired; has conflicts over meals and bedtime; wakes up at night; moods are changeable; has good or bad days for no obvious reason
Persistence	Single-mindedness, "stick-to-itiveness"; may be positive (focused when involved) or negative (stubborn and doesn't give up)	Low, easily diverted	High, stubborn, won't give up, goes on and on nagging, whining, or negotiating if wants something; gets "locked in"; has long tantrums
Sensory threshold	Sensitivity to physical stimuli—sound, light, smell, taste, touch, pain, temperature	High, unbothered	Low, physically sensitive, "sensitive"—physically not emotionally; highly aware of color, light, appearance, texture, sound, smell, taste, or temperature; "creative" but with strong and unusual preferences that can be embarrassing; clothes have to feel and look right; picky eater; refuses to dress warmly when weather is cold
Initial response	Characteristic initial reaction to new persons or new situations	Approach, goes forward	Withdrawal, holds back, doesn't like new situations; may tantrum if forced to go forward
Adaptability	Tolerance of change; ease with which gets used to new or altered situations	Good, flexible	Poor, rigid, has trouble with change of activity or routine; inflexible, very particular, notices minor changes; can want the same food or clothes over and over
Predominant mood	General quality of mood; basic disposition	Positive, cheerful	Negative, serious, or cranky; doesn't show pleasure openly; not a "sunny" disposition

2. **Difficult children are, above all, hard to understand**
    Their behavior confuses and upsets the most experienced parent or teacher. The tried-and-true methods of child-rearing simply do not work so that effective discipline is replaced by inconsistency, power struggles, excessive punishment, or over-indulgence. Parents will say that "nothing works" or that the child controls the family. A vicious cycle develops wherein the child's trying behavior and the erratic overreactions of the parent augment each other.
    The primary caregiver of such a difficult child (usually the mother) may also be bewildered, overinvolved, and exhausted. She may feel guilty, inadequate, and victimized. Often such children are somewhat easier with their fathers, who may become increasingly critical of the mothers. Marital strain is common. A fragile but potentially viable marriage may be ruptured by the stress of a difficult child. In addition, individual vulnerabilities of adult personality may be accentuated, resulting in parental syndromes of anxiety, depression, or substance abuse. The siblings are often expected to behave in an excessively adult manner, and their needs can be neglected as the household increasingly revolves around the difficult child. The child is also affected by the vicious cycle. Behavior problems are accentuated and secondary manifestations, such as fears and feelings of being "bad," are quite often evident.

II. **MAKING THE DIAGNOSIS.** A pathology-oriented model is limiting and often counterproductive. There is no "difficult child syndrome," just as there is not a definitive "test for ADHD." Much more valid in dealing with problem behaviors in young children is a **model that focuses on individual differences and goodness of fit.** The aim is to describe the child's behavior, temperamental profile, and strengths, as well as areas of vulnerability.
  A. **History.** Questioning the parent about the manifestations of a child's difficult temperament and its impact on the family is the key to identification. The clinician should inquire about the parents' approach to discipline, the child's school functioning, and the presence of secondary manifestations, such as fearfulness, nightmares, excessive anger, and emotional oversensitivity. Impaired self-image is seen in poorly managed difficult children.
  B. **Temperamental questionnaire.** These may be used as part of well-child examinations or to determine areas of difficulty with a view to temperament-based parent guidance. Research-based questionnaires tend to be lengthy with 75–100 parent responses. It is often acceptable for a busy primary care clinician to devise his or her own brief questionnaire, provided it is used as an aid in conjunction with other information and not as a "diagnostic instrument."
  C. **Behavioral observations.** Some problem behaviors are clear in the office visit: impulsivity, hyperactivity, disruptiveness, clinging and withdrawal, tantrums, aggressiveness, or undue sensitivity to pain. However, a child may be stubborn, irregular, negative and cranky, intense, sensitive to light and taste, or poorly adaptable. When a parent reports such "nonvisible" difficult behavior that is not apparent during the office visit, the clinician should not assume that the parent is inventing or causing the problem.
  D. **Differential diagnosis.** A difficult temperament is evident from an early age and is relatively stable and consistent over time. A child, 3 years or older, whose behavior has become difficult may be going through a developmental stage or reacting to stress. An example is a youngster who begins to misbehave after parents separate. When does the clinical picture go beyond a very difficult temperament and become indicative of a psychiatric disorder? The distinction is not only problematic but it is actually often irrelevant to treatment decisions as well. A "brain disorder," such as ADHD, is essentially a behavioral syndrome based on descriptive criteria subject to some extent of observer bias. There is no "test" for ADHD. Although it is now generally accepted that ADHD is neurobiologically based, the same can be said for temperament. Adopting a continuum-based, rather than a categorical approach to diagnosis, allows a clinician much greater flexibility.

III. **MANAGEMENT: THE ROLE OF THE PEDIATRIC CLINICIAN—HELPING THE CHILD AND FAMILY.** The difficult child's adjustment can be greatly enhanced by the ongoing involvement of the primary care clinician. The central therapeutic goals are to improve the compatibility between a child and the significant persons in his or her life, relieve the child's suffering, and improve adaptation.
  A. **General issues**
    1. **Erroneous perceptions can be corrected.** The parents of very difficult children invariably feel victimized and often assume that the child's behavior is intentional. Parents need to understand that their children are not enemies who are "out to get

them." Seeing the problem behavior as temperamentally determined rather than willful disobedience allows the parent to deal with it far more neutrally. Many parents are confused and made anxious by pressures to have their child "diagnosed" and placed on medication.

2. **The caregivers need support and understanding.** Especially so when the child's behavior is very difficult at home but unremarkable at school or in the clinician's office.

3. **Practical advice can be offered.** Parents can be guided on issues such as school selection and communication with teachers. The parents may need guidance on how to share responsibility more evenly, how to deal with other family members, and how to respond to the often plentiful advice offered from several quarters that tends to make parents (particularly single parents) feel defensive and inadequate.

B. **Principles of adult authority.** The fundamental goal for the parents of a difficult child is to replace the power struggles, frustration, and wear-and-tear of an ineffective disciplinary system with an educated, rational, kind, accepting, yet firm attitude of adult authority. Inevitably, habitual patterns of negative interaction have developed. It is the parents' job to initiate the necessary changes to improve the fit between their child-rearing style and expectations and their child's temperament. To begin the process, a key shift in attitude is needed. It should be clear to everyone that the parents are in charge. Certainly, the child's opinion should be solicited when appropriate, but the ultimate decision lies with the parents. The model is that of the excellent supervisor at work: approachable, supportive, clear in expectations, and very much in charge. Key ingredients of this model are as follows:

1. **Strategic planning and planned discussions.** The automatic, often excessively punitive reactions to the child's behavior must be replaced with a system that emphasizes structure and predictability. Decisions about rules, new procedures or routines, and consequences should be made privately by the adults and then presented to the child. Such a planned discussion always takes place away from the heat of the moment. The child is calmly, clearly, and deliberately told what will be expected from now on. Both parents, if possible, should be present at such a meeting. The attitude is kind but serious. The parents should be concise and avoid moralizing, lest they lose the child's attention. The child should be viewed to some extent as a junior collaborator in the planning to improve the family atmosphere and input elicited. At the end of a planned discussion, the child needs to repeat the key points to make sure he or she understood them and is then encouraged to "do your best." Asking a young child, at a calm time, to try hard to meet a specific and reasonable expectation is a very powerful statement. Generally planned discussions can be used with children as young as age 3 years.

2. **Active acceptance.** The parent makes the deliberate choice, based on understanding his or her child and the child's temperament, to accept the youngster for the person he or she truly are, vulnerabilities as well as strengths. The practical consequence of this conscious decision is that parental expectations become more consistent with the genuine capacities of the child.

3. **Rational punishment.** Going hand in hand with planned discussions is the clear and firm enforcement of consequences for unacceptable behaviors that are within the child's control and important enough to warrant taking a stand. In a typical vicious cycle, a mother may find herself punishing and saying "no" repeatedly, but no parent can possibly be effective in such circumstances. Most difficult children need less punishment, rather than more, and this can be achieved through consistency, structure, and routines in everyday life.

   The important first step for parents is to recognize and address major unacceptable behaviors and ignore the myriad minor irritations that take place every day with a very difficult child. Whenever possible, punishment should contain a natural consequence. For example, a child who continues to act too roughly with the family pet should be prohibited contact for a day, rather than being given a time-out. Ideally, a punishment should be administered briefly and without anger. Its main objective is to show the child that the parents are serious about stopping the behavior. Simplicity and predictability are important; a variety of punishments are unnecessary. With a younger child, parents can show seriousness by facial expression, direct action, and tone of voice.

C. **Management strategies.** Management, as distinct from punishment, is used when the adult decides that the misbehavior is temperamentally based; the child, in effect, "can't help it." The parent's attitude, while still firm, is much more sympathetic and kind. The basic message is, "I understand what's happening. I know you can't really control yourself, and I am going to help you with this." Sometimes behavior falls into a gray area, where it is not clear whether it is deliberate. In such instances, it is best for the parent to make the emotionally generous decision and help rather than punish the child.

Management suggestions designed to promote the child's success can be geared to temperamental characteristics. Strategies should be explained to the youngster during a planned discussion.

1. **The impulsive child.** A child who is easily excited can lose control in an overly stimulating environment and misbehave or become aggressive. The most common mistake parents and teachers make is to wait for the youngster to strike out and then lecture or punish, instead of intervening early.

   If the child is easily excited, it is important to recognize the signs of escalation—for example, moving more rapidly, talking in a louder voice, or laughing excessively. The adult should try to step in before the child gets out of hand. This technique is called **early intervention.** Some youngsters can be distracted. Others need a **time-out** (not as punishment, but as a cool-down period away from the action). A parent can say, "You're getting too excited. Let's do something quiet until you calm down."

2. **The highly active child.** High-energy children can become restless when they are confined to the dinner table or a classroom seat. They may begin to fidget or have difficulty paying attention. This behavior can be managed once the adults in charge **recognize the signs.** A restless youngster can be permitted to leave the dinner table and walk around between courses; a sympathetic teacher could ask the child to run an errand. Building vigorous physical activity into their daily routine is also helpful.

3. **The irregular child.** Most people fall easily into a regular rhythm of sleeping and eating, but some are naturally irregular. Battles can result when parents insist that a child who is not hungry must eat or that a youngster who is not tired must sleep. One strategy is to **differentiate between bedtime and sleep time, mealtime and eating time.** It is reasonable to require a child to be in bed by a certain hour or to join parents and siblings at dinner. However, parents should not force a youngster to sleep when he or she is not tired or to eat when he or she is not hungry. To avoid overburdening the family chef, a child with an irregular appetite can be taught to fix simple snacks, such as fruit, cold cereal, or yogurt.

4. **The poorly focused child.** Some children are easily distracted by their environment or even by their own thoughts. As a result, they appear to not "listen" or, if they miss instructions, to be willfully disobedient. Parents and teachers can manage the problem by **making eye contact** in a friendly way before giving such a child directions. Instructions are kept brief and simple. Set up, with the child, a system of reminders. Begin to teach organizational skills early.

5. **The child who resists change.** Some youngsters have difficulty with transitions. A poorly adaptable or shy child may be distressed by anything new. Other children focus so intently that they are locked into one activity and refuse to move to another. When they are asked to shift gears, they may cling, have a tantrum, or otherwise react negatively. If the issue is poor adaptability, parents can help by **preparing the child for change.** Even a simple warning, such as, "Finish playing with your trains, because we have to go shopping in 10 minutes," can be effective.

6. **The shy child.** Shy children require time and sympathetic understanding. A parent might say, "I know it's hard for you to get accustomed to new things, so I won't leave until you're used to being here." At the same time encourage a time-limited trial of an activity the youngster has previously shown he or she enjoys.

7. **The stubborn child.** Persistent, stubborn children can be extremely frustrating for parents and teachers. With these children, adults can take a stand early and terminate the confrontation. This technique is called **bringing it to an end.** A parent should not try to reason with a stubborn expert negotiator. Instead, the discussion should be ended. However, it is common for parents of a stubborn child to engage in a constant battle of wills and say "no" all the time. They should be encouraged to say "yes" more often, especially when the issue at hand is not really important.

8. **The finicky child.** Certain children are particular because they have heightened sensitivity to touch, taste, smell, sound, temperature, and colors (not necessarily all of these). Parents may get into arguments because a youngster insists on wearing the same comfortable green corduroy pants day after day or refuses to eat the inexpensive brand of frozen pizza that the rest of the family enjoys. Parents should be advised to **respect a child's preferences** when possible and to seek compromises that avoid unnecessary power struggles.

9. **The cranky child.** Parents can be distressed and angered by a child who is generally negative, somber, or pessimistic. Treats that would delight most children scarcely rate a smile from this youngster. The harder the parent tries (and fails) to make the child happy, the greater the tension becomes. A suggestion for parents is to **accept the child's nature** and not to expect a level of enthusiasm that they cannot give. The parent should not feel guilty; the child's negative mood is not the parent's fault.

D. **The use of medication.** If one aims for the relief of suffering rather than the cure of illness, target symptoms can be greatly reduced by the judicious and often temporary use of psychotropic medications. According to this view, the use of a stimulant would be completely appropriate for the balance of the school year in the child described earlier who was in an unfortunate but unavoidable classroom situation. A referral to the parent's clinician may be appropriate for the parent who is tense and caught up in the "vicious cycle."

E. **Criteria for referral.** The decision to refer to a mental health professional is often determined by the primary care clinician's interest in behavioral issues, expertise in parent guidance, and time availability. Assuming the presence of all these, a referral would still be needed in the case of an extremely difficult child, when the vicious cycle of ineffective discipline is long-standing, or when a clinical syndrome is suspected or can be identified in the child or other family members.

Bibliography

FOR PARENTS

BOOKS

Brazelton T. *Touchpoints: Emotional and Behavioral Development*. Reading, MA: Addison-Wesley; 1992.

Carey WB. *Understanding Your Child's Temperament*. New York: MacMillan; 1997.

Chess S, Thomas A. *Know Your Child*. New York: Basic Books; 1987.

Turecki S. *The Difficult Child*. New York: Bantam; 1989.

WEB SITES

http://www.stanleyturecki.com

FOR PROFESSIONALS

Chess S, Thomas A. *Temperament in Clinical Practice*. New York: The Guilford Press; 1986.

Conture EG, Kelly EM, Walden TA. Temperament, speech and language: an overview. *J Commun Disord*. 2013;46(2):125-142.

Turecki S. *The Emotional Problems of Normal Children*. New York: Bantam; 1994.

CHAPTER 82

Thumb-Sucking

Stephanie Blenner

I. DESCRIPTION OF THE PROBLEM. Most infants engage in nonnutritive sucking. In some children, this behavior persists into early or middle childhood.

A. Epidemiology
- Seen in the fetus on ultrasound as early as 16–18 weeks.
- Infants commonly suck their fingers or toes.
- 30%–45% of preschool children and 5%–15% of children older than 5 years continue to engage in thumb-sucking.
- 30%–55% of children who suck their thumb or fingers also use an attachment object, blanket, or twirl or caress their own hair when thumb-sucking.

B. Etiology. Historically, psychoanalysts *conceptualized thumb-sucking as an expression* of infantile drives and felt it could reflect emotional disturbance if it persisted beyond infancy. Some believe thumb-sucking is a learned habit. Most view thumb-sucking as a sensory-based activity and means of self-comforting. It may help relieve stress and calm a child in the face of environmental challenges. Thumb-sucking is often seen when a child is relaxing, falling asleep, tired, bored, hungry, or anxious. It is not associated with emotional disturbance in most cases.

C. Negative sequelae
1. **Dental.** The most common consequences of thumb-sucking are dental, in particular, malocclusion of both primary and permanent dentition. It may also lead to temporomandibular problems, anterior overbite, posterior cross bite, atypical root resorption, mucosal trauma, narrowing of the maxillary arch, and abnormal facial growth. The risk is highest among children who suck continuously and persist beyond age 4 years.
2. **Digit abnormalities.** Callous formation, paronychia, irritant eczema, and herpetic whitlow can be seen. With chronic thumb-sucking, a digital hyperextension deformity can occur that may require surgical correction.
3. **Accidental poisoning.** Children who thumb suck are at increased risk of accidental poisoning (e.g., lead poisoning).
4. **Psychological effects.** Thumb-sucking can contribute to impaired parental and peer relationships. It is often viewed as immature and socially undesirable. Parents and peers may criticize, tease, or punish the child for engaging in thumb-sucking. These reactions may, in turn, adversely affect a child's self-esteem.

II. MAKING THE DIAGNOSIS. Thumb-sucking becomes a problem at any age when it interferes with normal developmental achievements, physical health, social interactions, or self-esteem.
- **History**: Thumb-sucking will typically be brought to a clinician's attention by a concerned parent/caregiver or, in school-age, sometimes by the child.
- **Physical examination.** Examination may reveal a wrinkled, red digit with or without callous formation. Oral examination should be performed looking for malocclusion or other dental complications.

III. MANAGEMENT
A. Primary goals. The goals of treating thumb-sucking are to prevent dental complications and potential adverse effects on the child's social interactions and self-esteem. In general, targeted intervention is not necessary until after age 4 years, when adverse sequelae become more common. Most children will spontaneously stop thumb-sucking as they develop other self-regulatory strategies.

B. Treatment principles
1. **Identify triggers and reinforcers.** Emotional and situational triggers should be identified. Thumb-sucking often occurs at particular times of day, during certain activities, or accompanying specific emotional states. Some children only thumb suck while twirling their hair or holding a blanket. As a child gets older, thumb-sucking may provide secondary gain through attention paid to the behavior. Intervention should not be considered during a time of unusual stress for the child. For example, it would not be ideal to begin an intervention program at the start of school or during a family move.

2. **Empower the child.** For successful treatment, the child must be actively involved, cooperative, and motivated to stop. Parents should be counseled not to use threats or aversive punishment, as these may increase resistance, paradoxically prolonging the behavior. Parents should remain patient and provide support without criticism. They need to realize it is the child's, not their, task to overcome the habit.
3. **Specific interventions**
   a. **Before age 4 years.** Thumb-sucking is normal if it does not interfere with social or developmental functioning. The behavior should be ignored and given no special attention lest it accrue secondary gain. When thumb-sucking is noted, the child should be distracted without mentioning the behavior. The child should be praised when not sucking their thumb.
   b. **After age 4 years.** Infrequent thumb-sucking is still not usually a significant issue. If thumb-sucking is persistent and problematic, however, several behavior modification and habit reversal techniques can be used:
      (1) **Modifying associations** by changing the bedtime routine for a child who sucks while falling asleep or encouraging giving up attachment objects, such as a blanket used while sucking.
      (2) **Praise**, given when the child is not thumb-sucking.
      (3) **Rewards** such as stickers, treats, extra story time, or special outings with parents for specified periods without thumb-sucking. These can be given on a differential schedule, i.e., giving an increasing reward (for example, redeemable tokens) for greater time spent without thumb-sucking.
      (4) **Replacing** thumb-sucking with a socially acceptable habit that occupies the thumb, such as squeezing a sensory ball or holding the thumb with the other hand. Children can be instructed to do the replacement behavior for 1–3 minutes (i.e., while counting to 100) when they have the urge to suck.
      (5) **Display of** a chart or calendar the child uses to keep track of progress.
      (6) **A bitter-tasting, nontoxic liquid** (available over the counter) can be applied to the thumb during times the child is known to thumb suck. If after 1 week, the child does not thumb suck, the application is discontinued. Should thumb-sucking recur, the application schedule is resumed. This approach is useful with children who want to stop but put their thumb in their mouth without thinking. It should be emphasized the liquid is a reminder to help the child stop, not a punishment.
      (7) If thumb-sucking occurs at night, **thumb splints, gloves, or socks** can be tried. Thumb splints specifically designed for children who thumb suck are available for purchase (see below). An elastic bandage can also be wrapped around a straightened elbow. When the child raises hand to mouth, gentle pressure is exerted reminding the child not to thumb suck. The child should be responsible for putting on the splint or bandage and should not be reminded.
      (8) **Referral to a pediatric dentist** for placement of an intraoral device may be considered with an older motivated child who has been unsuccessful using other measures and is developing malocclusion as a consequence of thumb-sucking. A palatal bar or crib interferes with placement of the thumb in the palatal vault and often can be removed once the habit has extinguished.

IV. CLINICAL PEARLS AND PITFALLS

- Do not worry about thumb-sucking until a child is older than 4 years.
- Keep the child actively involved in management and treatment choice.
- Ensure the solution is not worse than the problem and doesn't become the focus of parent–child interactions.

Bibliography

FOR CLINICIANS
Davidson L. Thumb and finger sucking. *Pediatr Rev*. 2008;29:207-208.

FOR PARENTS
Mayer CA. *My Thumb and I: A Proven Approach to Stop a Thumb or Finger Sucking Habit, For Ages 6–10*. Chicago: Chicago Spectrum Press; 1997.
Van Norman RM. *Helping the Thumb-Sucking Child: A Practical Guide for Parents*. Vonore, TN: Avery Publishing Group; 1999.

FOR CHILDREN
AGES 4 TO 8

Dionne W. *Little Thumb*. Grenta, LA: Pelican Publishing Company; 2001.

Heitler S. *David Decides About Thumbsucking*. Denver, CO: Reading Matters; 1996.

Sonnenschein H. *Harold's Hideaway Thumb*. New York: Simon & Schuster Books For Young Readers; 1991.

Wulfing Van Ness A. *Thumbuddy to Love: Fireman Fred (or Ballerina Sue Version for Girls)*. Denver, CO: LLC; 2008.

CHAPTER 83

Tic Disorders and Tourette Syndrome

Adrian D. Sandler

I. DESCRIPTION OF THE PROBLEM

A. Definitional issues

1. Tourette syndrome
- Tourette syndrome (TS) is a disorder with multiple motor tics and one or more vocal tics (not necessarily concurrently), lasting a period of at least 1 year, in which the individual is never tic-free more than three consecutive months.
- The tics may change in nature and severity and are associated with distress or impairment in function.
- Onset is before age 18 years, with peak onset around 5–8 years.
- Although there is wide variability in symptoms and clinical course, there is a tendency for severity to peak around 9–11 years, with improvement or even resolution during puberty.

2. The tic disorder spectrum
- *Transient tic disorders* include single or multiple motor and/or vocal tics, lasting at least 4 weeks up to 12 months.
- Most transient tics are simple rather than complex and they do not usually cause great distress. A child with complex and distressing motor and vocal tics lasting a few months is at risk for developing TS.
- *Chronic tic disorders* are single or multiple motor *or* vocal tics that last more than a year. It is thought that these disorders share the same pathogenesis and occur on a spectrum.

B. Epidemiology

1. Prevalence of tic disorder spectrum
- Simple tics are very common in childhood. The 3-month prevalence is 4.3% in boys and 2.7% in girls, and 6%–13% of all children will experience a transient tic at some time during childhood.
- The childhood incidence of chronic tic disorder is around 1%–2%, with approximately 3:1 ratio of boys to girls.
- TS is less common, with prevalence around 3–6 per 1000 in 6- to 17-year-olds, based on the 2007 NSCH (National Survey of Children's Health) survey and other epidemiologic data. TS was twice as likely for teenagers than for preteens, and the ratio of boys to girls was 3:1.
- White children were twice as likely as black and Hispanic children to have TS, but there were no differences by parental education or household income.

2. Comorbidity of TS with obsessive–compulsive disorder and attention-deficit/hyperactivity disorder (ADHD)
- More than 50% of children with TS have extensive obsessions and/or compulsions, and 40% meet criteria for obsessive–compulsive disorder (OCD). More than 20% of all children with tic disorders have OCD. Conversely, 18% of children with OCD also have a concurrent tic disorder.
- Among all children previously diagnosed with TS, 64% had been diagnosed in the past with attention-deficit/hyperactivity disorder (ADHD). Fifty percent of all children with tic disorders have ADHD.
- Children with TS are 3–4 times as likely to have ADHD and 11 times as likely to have OCD as children without tic disorders.
- Among all children with TS, clinical depression (36%), anxiety (40%), developmental problems (28%), and learning difficulties (80%) are common.
- Sixty percent of children with mild high functioning autism spectrum disorder (ASD) have a tic disorder at some time during childhood.

C. Etiology/contributing factors

1. The genetics of tic disorders and TS. Twin studies show fairly high heritability, but there are clearly nongenetic factors influencing phenotypic expression. Linkage studies and genome-wide association studies have indicated signals on chromosomes 2p21, 17p, 3q, 8q, 9q, and 11q, but to date no single candidate gene has been identified. Other lines of evidence suggest several vulnerable genes plus environmental stressors causing increased fetal sensitivity in regions of the developing brain. Similar genetic and nongenetic factors appear to be operating in OCD.

2. **The neurobiology of tic disorders and TS.** Specific cortico-striato-thalamo-cortical circuits have been implicated because of their role in initiating and inhibiting psychomotor activity and in harm detection/avoidance. Emotional (limbic), cognitive, and motor circuits function in integrated ways to suppress behaviors triggered by internal and external stimuli. In patients with TS, fast-spiking inhibitory interneurons in caudate and putamen are decreased, and inhibitory striatal GABAergic (gamma-aminobutyric acid) networks may be deficient. Cortical disinhibition may be related to hypersensitivity of dopamine D2 striatal receptors.

II. MAKING THE DIAGNOSIS
A. Signs and symptoms
1. **What is a tic?**
   - Tics are more easily recognized than precisely defined. They can be described as rapid, coordinated, isolated fragments of normal motor or vocal behaviors. Tics can be easily mimicked and sometimes are confused with normal behavior.
   - Motor tics are typically brief, nonrhythmic, repetitive movements of the eyes, face, neck, and shoulders, with eye blinking, facial grimacing, and head jerking the most common. Vocal or phonic tics may commonly include repetitive throat clearing, sniffing, grunting, or barking.
   - Tics may be described in terms of location, number, frequency, and duration. They may also be characterized by their intensity, forcefulness, and complexity. Although tics are most commonly *simple* (brief and meaningless), they may be *complex* (longer and more elaborate). A few specific terms have been used to describe particular recognizable kinds of tic, such as palilalia (repeating others), coprolalia (uttering obscenities), and copropraxia (making obscene gestures).
   - Tics may increase with fatigue or stress. They may be temporarily suppressed, followed by a temporary increase in frequency or intensity. They may be more common in winter.
   - Children as young as 6 years describe premonitory sensory urges, a feeling of pressure or a kind of "itch." These distracting urges may contribute to attentional problems. Tics are not entirely involuntary and may be experienced as intentional surrender to virtually irresistible sensory urges, usually accompanied by a fleeting and incomplete sense of relief.

2. **Differential diagnosis: what isn't a tic?**
   - Children with allergies often have recurrent throat clearing and sniffing, but tics are more repetitive and less variable.
   - Habits such as hair-twirling, nose-touching, and skin-picking lack the repetitive uniformity of tics. Repetitive habits such as rocking and thumb-sucking are more rhythmic and continuous than tics.
   - Stereotypies are usually voluntary, bilateral, continuous, self-stimulatory rhythmic movements ("flapping," hand movements, jumping/stepping), associated with excitement, that may be present in children with or without ASD.
   - Brief epileptic seizures and movement disorders (such as chorea, athetosis, dystonia and myoclonic jerks) are more clearly *abnormal* movement patterns than tics.
   - There is no definitive test for tics, and so there are gray areas between habits and simple tics, and between the compulsions of OCD and complex tics.

3. **Evaluation of tic disorders**
   - Evaluation of tic disorders includes detailed medical and developmental history, child interview, and careful neurologic examination. It is important to ask the child and family about the time course of tics, relationship to medication use, and possible exacerbating factors. The child's subjective experience of the tics and their social or emotional consequences should be explored. Specific inquiry about recent or previous streptococcal exposures or infections should be made. The history should include screening questions regarding OCD, ADHD, learning problems, anxiety, and depression. In addition, the pediatrician should take a family history regarding tic disorders and the associated conditions.
   - **Physical and neurologic examination** is important to rule out other movement disorders. Other than tics, children with TS usually have a normal examination. Many children effectively suppress tics during the clinic visit, and the absence of tics does not preclude a diagnosis of tic disorders.

- **Neurodevelopmental examination** can be helpful in providing opportunities to observe attention deficits and other processing problems. Also, many children begin to have tics when stressed in this way.
- There are no specific diagnostic tests. Electroencephalogram and imaging studies are not routinely indicated. Standardized rating scales and checklists may be very helpful regarding ADHD symptoms and general functional impairment at home and school. Other self-report or clinician-rated measures of tics and obsessive–compulsive symptoms may be useful both for clinical and research purposes, for example, Yale Global Tic Severity Scale.

B. Pediatric autoimmune neuropsychiatric disorders associated with group A Streptococcus

- Pediatric autoimmune neuropsychiatric disorders associated with group A *Streptococcus* (PANDAS) are closely related to Sydenham chorea of rheumatic fever. Circumstantial evidence suggests antineuronal antibodies are affecting basal ganglia function.
- Some children appear susceptible to abrupt onset of tics, compulsions, emotional lability, and anxiety during or following streptococcal pharyngitis. This condition may be episodic and recurrences are common. Other bacterial and viral infections have been implicated.
- Children usually, but not always, have clinical evidence of tonsillopharyngitis. Anti-DNAase B titers are very high, but there is no clear relationship between titers and clinical course. If there are clinical indications, including sudden onset of symptoms or known exposure to *Streptococcus*, most clinicians obtain streptococcal culture, antistreptolysin O titers, and anti-DNAase B. If there is confirmation of streptococcal infection, treatment with penicillin often leads to improvement in tics and obsessive–compulsive symptoms.
- Antibiotic prophylaxis with penicillin or azithromycin may help to prevent recurrences and exacerbations of neuropsychiatric symptoms.

III. MANAGEMENT

A. Treatment goals and modalities. The goals of management of tic disorders are to **minimize stress, social isolation, and functional impairment.** Education and demystification for the affected child, his or her family, and school personnel help to promote support and tolerance.

1. If available, behavioral techniques may be considered as first-line treatment.
   - **Habit reversal** involves training the individual in awareness, relaxation, and establishment of a competing response. An NIMH (National Institute of Mental Health)-funded study of **Comprehensive Behavioral Intervention for Tics (CBIT)** demonstrated 53% positive response, with 40% reduction in tics after an eight-session, 10-week, randomized controlled intervention (RCT).
   - **Cognitive behavior therapy** involving repeated exposures and response prevention is of benefit in OCD, sometimes enhancing medication response or allowing responders to discontinue medications. Similar techniques may be effective treatments in tic disorders and TS.

2. **Pharmacotherapy** is also an effective treatment for tic disorders, but tics should not be treated too aggressively if they are not causing major functional impairment. The presence, scope, and severity of comorbid diagnoses (ADHD, OCD, depression) should be assessed in planning pharmacotherapy.
   - **Alpha-2 norepinephrine agonists:** Clonidine and guanfacine may be useful first-line medications in tic disorders and TS. These agents tend to decrease hyperactivity, impulsivity, hyperarousal, exaggerated stress responses, and aggression, in addition to decreasing tics. Both are approved by FDA (Food and Drug Administration) for treatment of ADHD. An adequate trial may be 2 months. Sedation is the major side effect, especially for clonidine.
   - **Stimulant therapy in children with ADHD and tic disorders:** Guanfacine may be helpful in treating ADHD symptoms in children with ADHD and tics, but a combination of stimulant plus alpha agonist may be necessary. In children with tic disorders, a trial of stimulant therapy may increase tics in one-third, have no effect in one-third, and lead to improvement in tics in one-third. The combination of methylphenidate and clonidine in children with TS and ADHD was more effective than either medication alone (Treatment of ADHD in Children with Tic Disorder [TACT] study). Children with tic disorders and ADHD who have side effects on stimulants may respond to atomoxetine, which does not affect tic frequency.
   - **Antipsychotics/neuroleptics:** Older dopamine receptor blockers such as haloperidol and pimozide can be very effective in treating severe tic disorders but are

associated with weight gain, drowsiness, and hyperprolactinemia, and long-term use may cause tardive dyskinesia (TD) and other extrapyramidal side effects (EPS). Pimozide may have fewer EPS but can cause QT prolongation. The atypical antipsychotics are associated with a lower risk of TD and EPS. Risperidone, a potent D2 antagonist, has proven effective (mean daily doses 1.5–2.5 mg) in short-term clinical trials in children and adults with TS, and pilot data with aripiprazole and other atypical antipsychotics are encouraging.
- **SSRI antidepressants:** The selective serotonin reuptake inhibitors (SSRIs) are of proven effectiveness in the treatment of OCD, and they may also help to decrease compulsions in children with tics and TS. In children with TS, OCD, and ADHD, a combination of SSRI and stimulant may be helpful.
- **Other medications:** Topiramate was found to be safe and effective in RCTs. Clonazepam, levetiracetam, topiramate, tetrabenazine, nicotine, and cannabinoids (THC) have been effective in uncontrolled studies, and vitamin B_6, magnesium, and omega-3 fatty acids have been used with anecdotal success.
3. **Invasive and emerging treatments** have been used in preliminary studies to treat severe, treatment refractory patients in some centers. These include botulinum toxin injections, deep brain stimulation (DBS), electroconvulsive therapy, and repetitive transcranial magnetic stimulation. DBS of the thalamus or globus pallidus has been especially promising.

B. Clinical pearls and pitfalls
- Demystification is critical: Although tics are involuntary, it may be helpful for children to become more aware of their tics and to use behavioral strategies to decrease tic frequency.
- Tic disorders and TS may respond well to behavioral interventions alone.
- Tics should not be treated too aggressively with medications unless they are causing stress, social rejection, or other functional impairment.
- The presence of tics does not preclude the use of stimulants in children with ADHD.
- Think of PANDAS when there is a sudden emergence or dramatic increase in tic frequency/severity or obsessive–compulsive symptoms.

Bibliography

FOR PARENTS

Chansky TE. *Freeing Your Child From Obsessive-Compulsive Disorder. A Powerful, Practical Program for Parents of Children and Adolescents.* New York, NY: Three Rivers; 2001.

Dornbush MP, Pruitt SK. *Teaching the Tiger: A Handbook for Individuals Involved in the Education of Students With Attention Deficit Disorders, Tourette Syndrome or Obsessive-Compulsive Disorder.* Duarte, CA: Hope Press; 1995.

Eddy CM, Rickards HE, Cavanna AE. Treatment strategies for tics in Tourette syndrome. *Ther Adv Neurol Disord.* 2011;4:25-45.

Haerle T. *Children With Tourette Syndrome: A Parent's Guide.* Rockville, MD: Woodbine; 2003.

Himle MB, Woods DW, Piacentini JC, Walkup JT. Brief review of habit reversal training for Tourette syndrome. *J Child Neurol.* 2006;21:719-725.

WEB SITES/DVD

OC Foundation. www.ocfoundation.org.

Tourette Syndrome Assocation. www.tsa-usa.org. Available from TSA: "I have Tourette's, but Tourette's Doesn't Have Me," Emmy award winning HBO documentary DVD.

FOR PROFESSIONALS

Leckman JF, Cohen DJ, eds. *Tourette's Syndrome—Tics, Obsessions, Compulsions: Developmental Psychopathology and Clinical Care.* New York, NY: Wiley; 1999.

Leckman JF, Zhang H, Vitale A. Course of tic severity in Tourette syndrome: the first two decades. *Pediatrics.* 1998;102:14-19.

Singer HS. Tourette's syndrome: from behaviour to biology. *Lancet Neurol.* 2005;4:149-159.

Swain J, Scahill L, Lombroso PJ, King RA, Leckman JF, et al. Tourette syndrome and tic disorders: a decade of progress. *J Am Acad Child Adolesc Psychiatry.* 2007;46(8):947-968.

Tourette Syndrome Association. Diagnosing and Treating Tourette Syndrome, a comprehensive CD/DVD set.

Tourette Syndrome Study Group. Treatment of ADHD in children with tics: a randomized controlled trial. *Neurology.* 2002;58:527-536.

Woods D, Piacentini J, Walkup J. *Treating Tourette Syndrome and Tic Disorders: A Guide for Practitioners.* New York, NY: Guilford Press; 2007.

Woods D, Piacentini J, Chang S, et al. *Managing Tourette Syndrome: A Behavioral Intervention for Children and Adults.* New York, NY: Oxford University Press; 2008.

CHAPTER 84

Toilet Training

Alison Schonwald | Arda Hotz

I. DESCRIPTION OF THE PROBLEM. Toilet training is one of the great developmental challenges of early childhood. Although there are a variety of cultural differences and caregiver preferences that influence timing and technique of toilet training, the most commonly used technique is currently the "child-oriented approach". This approach, first described by Brazelton in 1962, is still supported by the American Academy of Pediatrics and generally has been found to be effective. Other techniques, such as the "toilet training in less than a day" method or the "assisted infant toileting training" method (also called "elimination communication technique"), are less popular.

In his seminal paper on the child-oriented approach, Brazelton encouraged parents not to pressure their children into toilet training before they had achieved the developmental skills to do so. Table 84-1 lists 15 readiness skills necessary for children to toilet train.

A. Epidemiology

- The average age to complete toilet training in the United States has increased over the last few decades.
- Girls tend to complete toilet training before boys (32–35 months vs. 35–39 months).
- Nighttime control usually occurs within a few months after daytime control is achieved, but may take longer.
- The average time to successful toilet training is 3 months.
- Differences exist in expectations for timing of toilet training among racial and ethnic groups in the United States.

II. MANAGEMENT. Suggestions for caregivers on toilet training strategies are listed in Table 84-2.

Some families may prefer alternative approaches to the child-oriented method. "Assisted infant toilet training" requires close attention to the body signals of an infant who lacks the vocabulary and mobility to use the toilet independently. This may not be viable for infants in childcare settings.

Rapid toilet training methods take place over 24–48 hours and include frequent reminders and checks for soiled pants. Children are usually given large amounts of liquid for frequent urination to occur. Although healthy children can successfully train using this method, we recommend avoiding reprimands for accidents and keeping the experience positive to encourage the child's sense of mastery.

A. Information for parents. The issue of toilet training is best discussed as part of anticipatory guidance during well-child visits. Table 84-3 addresses how and when a pediatric clinician can address this.

A number of key principles should be discussed with the parents:

1. **There is no benefit to expect a child to become toilet trained before the child is developmentally ready.** Although the process is sometimes initiated in response to outside pressures (e.g., daycare requirements), there are good reasons to try to wait until the child is developmentally prepared. **If for any reason the timing is wrong, it can always be postponed.**

2. Like many developmental challenges of childhood, **caregivers can empower the child to take responsibility for achieving the milestone of continence.** Rather than engaging in a battle of the wills, leverage a child's desire to achieve mastery of his or her environment with encouragement.

3. The process of toilet training for any one child typically has both successes and relapses; **anticipate regression as an opportunity to learn and progress.**

4. **Caregivers should not transmit a sense of disgust toward the stool,** even when it may be a natural response. Attaching negativity to the task of toileting can inadvertently repel the child from embracing the task.

B. Resistance to toilet training. Some children resist toilet training, regardless of parental technique. Difficulty toilet training has been associated with more difficult temperament traits and constipation.

Table 84-1 • SIGNS OF DEVELOPMENTAL READINESS FOR TOILET TRAINING

Language skills

- Able to follow two-step independent commands (e.g., "Take off your pants and go to the bathroom")
- Uses two-word phrases (e.g., "bye-bye poop," "go potty")

Cognitive skills

- Imitates actions of caregivers (e.g., sweeps the floor)
- Understands cause and effect (i.e., is capable of understanding the reasons for mastering the actions involved in toilet training)

Emotional skills

- Desires to please parents/caregivers by complying with their requests
- Desire to become independent
- Shows diminishing oppositional behaviors and power struggles
- Shows drive for independence and autonomy in self-care activities (e.g., insists on feeding self, tries to take off own clothes)
- Evinces pride and possessiveness toward belongings ("my car" and eventually "my poop")

Motor skills

- Ambulates with ease
- Pulls pants off independently
- Sits still for 5 min without help
- Possesses some control over urinary/anal sphincter (e.g., urinates large amounts sporadically, rather than constant wetting)

Body awareness

- Shows awareness of wet or soiled diaper
- Manifests signs of urge to void or defecate (e.g., facial expression, goes off into a corner)

Table 84-2 • TEN STEPS TO SUCCESSFUL TOILET TRAINING

1. Buy a potty chair, and place it in a conspicuous, convenient place in a bathroom. Tell the child, "This is your potty chair. This is where you will [use child's terms for urination and defecation]." Be sure to stress what a special and wonderful chair it is.
2. Allow the child to get used to the chair by sitting on it, fully clothed, for about 5 min a few times a day for about a week. Have the child wear loose-fitting pants such as sweat pants that he or she can pull off easily, quickly, and independently when he or she starts using the potty. Try to choose times when the child is more likely to have a bowel movement (e.g., after meals). Never force the child to sit on it.
3. Encourage the child to watch parents or siblings use the bathroom. Explain, "This is where we go potty." Let the child watch the excreta being flushed down the toilet and wave "bye-bye" to it (skip this if the flushing frightens the child).
4. Have the child sit on the potty bare-bottom. Do not urge or expect results, but if it happens, praise the child.
5. With the child, throw the stool from the soiled diaper into the potty. Tell the child that this is where the stool and urine should go. Then take the pail and dump the stool down the toilet. Wave "bye-bye poop" with the child.
6. Ask the child during the day, "Do you have to go potty?" to help the child recognize bodily sensations. Observe the child for signs of impending urination or defecation. Say, "Let's take off your pants and go potty." Assist the child in disrobing and going to the potty chair. Sit for as long as the child wants. Praise success, but do not criticize failure ("Oh, you don't want to go. Okay. Maybe next time").
7. Reinforce positive features of potty training to child (e.g., "just like a big boy," "just like Mommy does," "You did it by yourself!"), and praise successes as they occur.
8. Once a semiconsistent pattern of voiding/stooling on the potty is established, ask the child if he or she wants to give up the diaper "like a big boy or girl" during the day. If yes, make a show of throwing them all away in the garbage and wave "bye-bye" to them. Admire the child for putting on training "big boy or girl" pants.
9. Once training is well established, try an over-the-toilet-seat chair.
10. Nighttime continence may take a few months or longer to acquire after daytime dryness is achieved. No special strategy is typically needed, as children will wake up dry.

Table 84-3 • HEALTH SUPERVISION VISITS AND TOILET TRAINING

9–12 mo Visit

- Assess parent expectations.
- Address readiness criteria conceptually and discourage active toilet training.

15–18 mo Visit

- Discuss readiness criteria.
- Start to discuss process of toilet training/consider giving handout on child-oriented approach.

24–30 mo Visit

- Assess readiness criteria (Table 84-1).
- Review the child-oriented approach to toilet training.
- Discuss current status/troubleshoot problems (constipation, battles) if process is under way.

36 mo Visit

- Assess toileting plan and progress; troubleshoot problems (constipation, battles).

48 mo Visit

- Assess toileting plan and progress; troubleshoot problems.
- If continued issues with daytime toilet training or toileting refusing, consider referral to a specialist in child behavior, consider the ceremony (see point 11 in section "B. Resistance to toilet training"), consider broad picture for other developmental or medical concerns.

The primary care clinician can make these suggestions to caregivers:

1. **Do not fight, punish, shame, or nag the child about using the toilet.** Keep the efforts positive; recognize the child's developmental need to master his or her world, with the consequent frustration that emerges when tasks are difficult.
2. **Discontinue training for a few weeks or months if the child is emphatically negative and battles are developing.**
3. **Encourage the child to imitate parents and siblings** by inviting the child into the bathroom. Keep it positive without overstating its importance, or the task becomes overwhelming.
4. Read potty training books or view potty training videos together.
5. Remind the child that this task is his or her responsibility when he or she is ready to do it.
6. **Encourage the child to participate in changing soiled diapers or pants.** This task is part of being in charge of your own body.
7. **Matter-of-factly remind the child at the first sign of impending defecation to use the potty.**
8. **At any sign of painful stools, treat constipation.** Start with prune juice or added fiber to the diet, but if constipation persists then consider medical treatment. Postpone toilet training until stooling is comfortable.
9. **Offer small rewards in response to successful toilet training.** Try star charts to reinforce successful sit-down times, periods of clean pants, wiping, and flushing.
10. Take the child to settings where other same-aged children use the toilet.
11. **Consider a ceremony for recalcitrant cases.** In situations where lack of toilet training is becoming a problem for the family and the child has been obstinately unable to be trained despite breaks, the child may benefit from a solemn ceremony transitioning him or her out of diapers to be a big boy or girl. This should only be considered in situations where the child is older than 3 years, is emotionally healthy, and is developmentally capable of mastering toilet training. During the ceremony, parents and child will throw away the diapers, announce that the child is a big boy or girl now, and allow maturational urges to work in conjunction with the drive for autonomy.

Bibliography

FOR PARENTS

Azrin NF, Foxx RM. *Toilet Training in Less Than a Day*. New York: Pocket Books; 1989.

Gomi T. *Everyone Poops*. San Diego, CA: Kane/Miller Book Publishers; 2001.

Sparrow JD, Brazelton TB. *Toilet Training the Brazelton Way*. Cambridge, MA: Da Capo Press; 2004.

WEB SITES
WebMD. http://children.webmd.com/tc/toilet-training-topic-overview.

FOR PROFESSIONALS
Blum N, Taubman B, Nemeth N. Why is toilet training occurring at older ages? A study of factors associated with later training. *J Pediatr*. 2004;145:107-111.
Brazelton TB. A child-oriented approach to toilet training. *Pediatrics*. 1962;29:121-128.
Michel RS. Toilet training. *Pediatr Rev*. 1999;20:240-245.
Schonwald A, Sherritt L, Stadtler A, Bridgemohan C. Factors associated with difficult toilet training. *Pediatrics*. 2004;113(6):1753-1757.
Stadtler AC, Gorski PA, Brazelton TB. Toilet training methods, clinical interventions, and recommendations. *Pediatrics*. 1999;103(6):1359-1368.

CHAPTER 85

Unpopularity

Melvin D. Levine (deceased)

I. DESCRIPTION OF THE PROBLEM. Chronic rejection by peers condemns a child to a life of isolation, extreme self-doubt, and perpetual anxiety. The unpopular schoolchild is susceptible to daily embarrassment through both passive and active exclusion by classmates. Such a child must endure the inevitable painful refrain, "Sorry, this seat is saved." In many cases, exclusionary comments and actions may be augmented by bullying and verbal abuse. It is regrettably true that many of the most popular children can boost their status among peers by being especially creative and demonstrative in their predatory acts against unpopular children. The victim's imposed isolation and constant fear of further humiliation is likely to take its toll on development and behavior.

  A. Contributing factors. There are multiple pathways that may culminate in a state of unpopularity during the school years. In many instances, more than one factor may predispose a child to peer rejection. The following are among the common predisposing factors:

   1. **Intrinsic social cognitive dysfunction**, such as a "learning disability," impairing social awareness, practice, and skill. Social cognitive dysfunction, probably the most common source of unpopularity, may mediate or interact with other factors to yield unpopularity in a child. Table 85-1 contains 18 of the most important subcomponents of social cognitive dysfunction. A clinician assessing a patient's social cognition can make use of such a list to pinpoint a child's troubles in specific subcomponents. This process may ultimately provide a basis for coaching the child in the social domain.
   2. **Attention deficits.** Traits such as impulsivity, insatiability, and verbal disinhibition associated with attentional dysfunction engender unpopularity.
   3. **Physical unattractiveness.** Children whose physical appearance is somehow displeasing to their peers have been shown to be vulnerable to social isolation.
   4. **Poor gross motor skills.** Inferior athletic abilities may potentiate unpopularity.
   5. **Language disability.** Children with expressive language problems may not be able to use verbal communication to control relationships and keep pace with the banter and lingo of peers.
   6. **Autism spectrum disorders.** Children who show signs of an autism spectrum disorder display varying degrees of social cognitive dysfunction, which commonly incites peer rejection.
   7. **Shyness.** Some youngsters who are chronically shy in their temperament and therefore avoid social contact may fail to gain the experience needed in the quest for popularity.
   8. **Poor coping skills.** A lack of adaptability and problem-solving skills may cause some children to react to daily stresses and conflicts with maladaptive behaviors, such as aggression. Such behaviors alienate others and promote rejection by classmates.
   9. **Eccentricity.** Children who are nonconformists or have unusual interests, speech patterns, tastes, or values may be rejected by their more conventional peers who feel more comfortable with close replicas of themselves and harbor fears of contamination with "weirdness." Thus, a child who loves to learn about spiders or enjoys listening to Handel oratorios may be ostracized by more conventional classmates.
   10. **Family patterns.** There exist self-contained families that do not value generalized popularity, or the family unit itself remains isolated, either voluntarily or of necessity (perhaps due to genetic social cognitive dysfunctions).

  B. Secondary phenomena. The clinical picture of an unpopular child is likely to be complicated by a chain of secondary phenomena, which may include extreme anxiety (or even depression), low self-esteem, and a repertoire of maladaptive defense tactics, such as excessive and inappropriate clowning, extreme controlling behaviors, or outright withdrawal. Often, these children seek relationships with adults or with much younger children because they are unable to form alliances within their own age group.

Table 85-1 • SOCIAL COGNITIVE DYSFUNCTION: THE TROUBLED SUBCOMPONENTS

Subcomponent	Description
Weak greeting skills	Trouble initiating a social contact with a peer skillfully
Poor social predicting	Trouble estimating peer reactions before acting/talking
Deficient self-marketing	Trouble projecting an image acceptable to peers
Problematic conflict resolution	Trouble settling social disputes without aggression
Reduced affective matching	Trouble sensing and fitting in with others' moods
Social self-monitoring failure	Trouble knowing when one is in social trouble
Low reciprocity	Trouble sharing and trouble supporting/reinforcing others
Misguided timing/staging	Trouble knowing how to nurture a relationship over time
Poor verbalization of feelings	Trouble using language to communicate true feelings
Inaccurate inference of feelings	Trouble reading others' feelings through language
Failure of code switching	Trouble matching language style to current audience
Lingo dysfluency	Trouble using the parlance of peers credibly
Poorly regulated humor	Trouble using humor effectively for current context/audience
Inappropriate topic choice/maintenance	Trouble knowing what to talk about and for how long
Weak requesting skill	Trouble knowing how to ask for something inoffensively
Poor social memory	Trouble learning from previous social experience
Assertiveness gaps	Trouble exerting right level of influence over group actions
Social discomfort	Trouble feeling relaxed while relating to peers

In some cases, school phobic behaviors or somatic symptoms may be encountered. Finally, it is not unusual for children who experience social difficulties at school to become aggressive, oppositional, and/or excessively demanding and dependent at home.

II. **MAKING THE DIAGNOSIS.** Unpopular children merit careful clinical assessment. Their social difficulties may in fact represent the tip of an iceberg with respect to behavioral and developmental health. The causal factors and potential complications of unpopularity need to be sought through direct history taking, direct observations of the child's image and manner of relating, physical and neurodevelopmental examinations, and reports from teachers. Especially difficult cases may necessitate investigation by a multidisciplinary team.

Information can be gathered from several sources to detect the presence of subcomponents of social cognitive dysfunction listed in Table 85-1.

The unpopular child should be interviewed alone to elicit their perspective. Nonthreatening questions may be posed to acquire insight into traumatic social scenarios at school. The most common interpersonal "hot spots" are the bus stop, the school bus, the playground, the bathroom, the gymnasium, and the area around lockers. Children can often recreate vividly the stressful scenes that unfold daily against these backdrops. The patient should be reassured that many other children have such difficulties and that it is safe and important to talk about them with an adult.

III. **MANAGEMENT.** The management of the unpopular child must take into consideration the multiplicity of factors operating to engender peer rejection. Associated neurodevelopmental problems (such as a language disability or an attention deficit) require appropriate treatment. The complications, such as somatic symptoms or depression, also demand targeted intervention. In addition, the child's individual social cognitive dysfunction must be addressed. Some possible management approaches to deal directly with a child's unpopularity are summarized below.

A. Explain the social skill problems carefully to the child.

These may require multiple sessions; not all affected children can process such information readily.

B. Have the parent of the child who needs social improvement accompany the child to an activity with other children.

Then, during a calm and private interlude, the parent can discuss the social interactions (especially the *faux pas* and transgressions) that occurred.

C. Help the child locate one or two companions with whom to relate and begin to build skills.

It can be helpful if such peers share interests and perhaps some traits with the unpopular child.

D. Inform the classroom teacher or building principal if a child is victimized by peer abuse in school.

It is the school's responsibility to make every effort to contain this activity. A strongly worded note from a primary health care provider may be vital in such cases.

E. Help the rejected child to develop skills, hobbies, or areas of expertise that can enhance self-esteem and be impressive to other children.

The management of such a child should always include the diligent quest for and development of such specialties. Ideally, such pursuits should have the potential for generating collaborative activities with other children.

F. Never force these children into potentially embarrassing situations before their peers.

For example, an unpopular child with poor gross motor skills needs some protection from humiliation in physical education classes.

G. Manage any family problems or medical conditions through counseling, specific therapies (e.g., language intervention or help with motor skills), and/or medication (e.g., for attention deficits or depression).

H. Identify social skills training programs within schools and in clinical settings.

Clinicians should be aware of local resources that offer social skills training to youngsters with social cognitive deficits. Most commonly this training makes use of specific curricula that are used in small group settings in a school or in the community.

I. Reassure these children that it is appropriate for them to be themselves, that they need not act and talk like everyone else in school, and that there is true heroism in individuality.

Clinicians, teachers, and parents need to tread the fine line between helping with social skills and coercing a child into blind conformity with peer pressures, expectations, and models.

Bibliography

FOR PARENTS AND CHILDREN

Levine MD. *All Kinds of Minds*. Cambridge, MA: Educators Publishing Service; 1993.

Osman B. *No One to Play With: The Social Side of Learning Disabilities*. New York: Random House; 1982.

WEB SITES FOR PARENTS AND PROFESSIONALS

All Kinds of Minds. http://www.allkindsofminds.org/index.aspx.

FOR PROFESSIONALS

Asher SR, Coie JD, eds. *Peer Rejection in Childhood*. Cambridge, MA: Cambridge Press; 1990.

Cartledge G, Milburn JF, eds. *Teaching Social Skills to Children*. New York: Pergamon Press; 1980.

Coleman WL, Lindsay RL. Interpersonal disabilities: social skill deficits in older children and adolescents—their description, assessment, and management. *Pediatr Clin North Am*. 1992; 39(3):551-568.

Kafer NF. Interpersonal strategies of unpopular children: some implications for social skills training. *Psychol Sch*. 2006;9(2):255-259.

CHAPTER 86

Visual Disability: Developmental and Behavioral Consequences

Michael E. Msall

I. DESCRIPTION OF THE PROBLEM. Legal blindness is defined as central visual acuity in the best eye with corrective lenses of 20/200 or worse or a restriction in the visual field so that the widest diameter of vision subtends an angle of 20°. The term legal blindness is a misnomer as approximately 75% of individuals with legal blindness have some residual visual function. In addition, most adults with legal blindness can read large print. For children with vision worse than 20/400, ophthalmologists use functional descriptors such as child's ability to count fingers or detect hand motion, recognize nearby large objects, or detect the direction of a light source. Students can be classified as educationally visually impaired if their corrected vision is 20/70 or worse.

The 2010 World Health Organization (WHO) ICD-10 classifies visual disabilities into five categories with three levels of visual function described in Table 86-1. These categories describe vision in the better eye with the best possible glasses correction. Categories 3, 4, and 5 are classified as blindness. Categories 1 and 2 are often referred to as low vision.

A. Epidemiology. Worldwide, approximately 14 million children are blind. In developing countries the rate of childhood blindness is estimated to be 12–15 per 10,000 children <16 years old. The rate in developed countries is 3–4 per 10,000. Blind children are more likely to live in socioeconomically deprived situations, be hospitalized as children, not attend school, and die early than children who are not blind. The most prevalent causes of childhood blindness in lower-income settings have been moving to resemble patterns in higher-income settings. Previously, the most prevalent causes in lower-income settings were related to nutritional and infective corneal opacities as well as congenital anomalies. Researchers postulate that this changing epidemiology is due to the establishment of national vitamin A supplementation programming as well as improvements in vaccination and sanitation programs over the past 20 years.

Across developing and developed countries there have been increases in visual morbidity due to ROP (retinopathy of prematurity) and CVI (cerebral or cortical visual impairment). These increases reflect improved survival of preterm births, infants with malformations and term infants with encephalopathy Children who are diagnosed with severe visual impairment and blindness in the first year of life—most blind children in many populations—always display clinical signs consistent with very poor vision.

The United States does not keep a registry for children with severe visual disability, but 50,000 children are considered visually impaired by school systems of which 20,000 require Braille as a reading medium. Children with combined deafness and blindness number 500 per year and include 10,000 children from birth to age 21 years.

B. Etiology. Table 86-2 describes the major known etiologies of severe visual impairment in childhood. The timing of these etiologies is prenatal in 43%, perinatal in 27%, postnatal in 8%, and unknown in 22%. Several multiple malformation syndromes involve visual impairment and include chromosomopathies, CHARGE association (coloboma, heart disease, choanal atresia, intellectual disability, growth and genital anomalies, ear anomalies), Lowe syndrome (intellectual disability, cataracts, renal tubular dysfunction), neurocutaneous disorders (tuberous sclerosis complex, optic gliomas in neurofibromatosis-1), metabolic (homocystinuria) and neurodegenerative disorders (leukodystrophies and optic atrophy, gangliosidosis and cherry red macula, Batten disease).

1. Many syndromes affect both vision and hearing. These include Alport, Usher, Cockayne, Stickler, and Refsum syndromes as well as congenital infections, lysosomal storage disease, and leukodystrophies. Children with several of these disorders have benefitted from cochlear implants.

Table 86-1 • WHO ICD-10 CLASSIFICATION OF VISUAL DISABILITY

Category 1	Moderate Impairment	20/70 to 20/160
Category 2	Severe impairment	20/200 to 20/400
Category 3	Blind	20/500 to 20/1000
Category 4	Blind (near total)	<20/1000 and light perception
Category 5	Blind (total)	No light perception

Table 86-2 • THE MAJOR KNOWN ETIOLOGIES OF SEVERE VISUAL IMPAIRMENT IN CHILDHOOD

Retina	Optic Nerve	Lens	Posterior Visual Pathways
Severe retinopathy of prematurity	Optic nerve atrophy Optic nerve hypoplasia	Cataract	Periventricular leukomalacia
Retinitis pigmentosa	Leber congenital amaurosis	Corneal dystrophies	Occipital malformations

2. Postnatal causes of blindness account for 8%–11% of all childhood blindness. Etiologies include infections, trauma, complicated hydrocephalus, retinoblastoma, craniopharyngioma, demyelinating diseases, and leukemia ·with central nervous system (CNS) involvement.

3. Blindness and associated developmental disabilities: It is important to recognize that in more than 50% of children with visual disability, there are additional major disorders including cerebral palsy, intellectual disability, autism spectrum disorders, recurrent seizures, hearing impairments, and learning disabilities. Among children with visual disability in a comprehensive community registry, 65% had additional disabilities. Of the children with multiple disabilities, CVI occurred in 50%.

   Some infectious diseases causing blindness are on the rise. For example, one-third of Brazilian children with suspected Zika-associated microcephaly also have ocular abnormalities.

   One study found that, among the US participants, blindness was primarily caused by CVI (18%), optic nerve hypoplasia (15%), and ROP (14%). These three primary causes have not changed over two decades. Other causes included optic atrophy, albinism, coloboma, glaucoma, non-ROP retinal detachment, Leber congenital amaurosis, retinitis pigmentosa, microphthalmia/anophthalmia, cataract, and nystagmus.

   Understanding of ROP's pathogenesis has been recently advanced. Retinal vessels grow under the control of mediators that are regulated by oxygen levels. These include hypoxia inducible factor and vascular endothelial growth factor (VEGF). In addition, insulin-like growth factor 1, which is not regulated by oxygen, is essential for VEGF signaling, and thus vessel growth and survival. There are some studies suggesting that the concentration of intravitreal bevacizumab needed to neutralize VEGF in eyes with ROP is dramatically less than dosages currently in use

C. **Developmental aspects of vision.** Pupillary light reactions and lid closure to bright light are present at 30 weeks' gestation. Brief visual fixation is present at birth including brief saccades to a moving person, moving face, and dangling ring. At birth, acuity has been assessed as approximately 20/400 by optokinetic nystagmus, forced preferential looking, and visual evoked potentials. By 3 weeks, watching a mother speak occurs. The presence of strabismus is easily identified by an off-center asymmetry of reflected corneal light, the Hirschberg reflex. Eyes that do not see well tend to deviate or drift, and this along with nystagmus may be the first indication of poor vision. Pupillary responses, an intact red reflex, and the ability of a child to track 360° are indicators of globally adequate vision. Developmental consequences of these core visual skills affect motor, manipulative, communicative, social, and adaptive skills and are shown in Table 86-3.

Table 86-3 • VISUAL SKILLS AND DEVELOPMENTAL MILESTONES

Age of Child	Visual Milestone Present	Formal Visual Testing
Birth	Alertness to visual stimulus presented 8–10 inches from eyes	20/400 FPL = VEP = OKN
1 mo	Follows red ring 90°, smiles in response to faces	
2 mo	Follows red ring 180°, chest up in prone	20/200 FPL = OKN, 20/60 VEP
3 mo	Tracks red ring 360°, begins midline hand play	
4 mo	Bats at ring, on wrists in prone, holds bottle, turns to voice	
5 mo	Attains ring, crumples paper, looks for source of sound, rolls	
6 mo	Early sitting balance, transfers blocks, lifts cup	20/150 FPL, 20/100 OKN, 20/40 VEP
9 mo	Crawls, pulls to stand, mature pincer, finger feeds, gesture language	
12 mo	Cruises, walks with support, puts cube in cup, removes socks, points	20/60 OKN, 20/50 FPL, 20/20 VEP

FPL, forced preferential looking; OKN, optokinetic nystagmus; VEP, visual evoked potentials.

II. MAKING THE DIAGNOSIS
   A. Clinical Presentation. Infants with visual disability present in one of three clinical scenarios.
1. In the first scenario, **parents are concerned that their child is not seeing**. At 6–10 weeks, the child is not smiling reciprocally and does not follow faces or rings but does have a normal papillary response, red reflex, and intact globe. These children either have CVI, delayed visual maturation (DVM), or evolving intellectual disability. Both CVI and DVM have high rates of motor, intellectual, and communicative disability. However, in DVM, functional visual recovery occurs, whereas in CVI, some visual improvement may occur but low vision is a common sequela. In children with severe evolving developmental disability, the children stare and are inattentive because of disorders of nonvisual higher cortical function affecting learning, perception, communicating, and social skills. CVI is visual impairment caused by a varied group of disorders that affect the optic radiations, visual cortex, or associated visual areas. It can be potentially caused by periventricular leukomalacia, hydrocephalus, hypoglycemia, stroke, infection, CNS malformations, or neoplasia.
2. In the second scenario, **children present in infancy with nystagmus, sluggish pupils, and visual inattention**. Ophthalmologic findings reveal anterior segment or optic nerve disorders such as cataract, corneal opacities, glaucoma, and microphthalmia. The posterior segment abnormalities include colobomas of the optic nerve or retina, optic nerve hypoplasia or atrophy, retinal dystrophy, ROP, or retinoblastoma.
3. In the third scenario, **infants show visual inattention, nystagmus, and variable pupillary responses**. Ophthalmologic evaluation reveals a normal globe and intact red reflex. Strabismus may be present. Electroretinogram (ERG) testing is most helpful in revealing the nature of these disorders. The most common is Leber congenital amaurosis, a recessively inherited retinal dystrophy with an extinguished ERG. This disorder currently accounts for 10% of childhood blindness with a range of visual function from legal blindness to no light perception. Associated findings may include renal and skeletal anomalies and cataracts, strabismus, and keratoconus. Major advances in molecular genetics have led to ongoing and anticipated gene and pharmacologic therapies. Additional differential diagnoses in this scenario are rod monochromatism, an autosomal recessive disorder with missing cone photoreceptors, congenital stationery night blindness, and retinitis pigmentosa.
   B. Acuity testing. Teller acuity cards use preferential looking at standardized cards with varying width of black and white stripes. They can be used in preverbal children and have been widely used in children with ROP and in children with motor or developmental disability. By age 3 years, many children can cooperate with a variety of tasks

such as Allen Cards, Multiple E Charts, and HOTV cards. If there are parent concerns, presence of any developmental or neurologic disability, or clinician concern about vision screening, then referral to an ophthalmologist is warranted.

The **differential diagnosis** of the infant who demonstrates a reduced visual response from birth includes the following:

1. **Persistent neurodevelopmental abnormalities** such as evolving cerebral palsy, intellectual disability, or autism spectrum disorders.
2. The presence of **perinatal problems** including inborn errors of metabolism, sequelae of hypoxic–ischemic encephalopathy, perinatal stroke, or an evolving seizure disorder.
3. **Severe visual impairment** due to significant ocular problems.
4. **Visual impairment of unknown cause.**

C. **Developmental assessment of blind children**
1. **Cognitive development.** A key area to monitor in children with severe visual impairment is communicative milestones. Children who are ocularly blind and who do not have associated neurologic abnormalities achieve developmental milestones at a slower pace but should not be considered motor or cognitively disabled. The slower developmental milestones are the result of different experiences of nonverbal skills, motor exploration, and understanding spatial relations. For example, the infant is unable to see details of facial expression, lip movements, gestures, object position in space, use of utensils, indoor and outdoor activities. As a result, different tactile, verbal, and orientation experiences are required to help the child construct knowledge of both immediate and distant environments.
2. **Motor development.** Fraiberg's classic longitudinal study involved 10 children with congenital blindness and demonstrated both the differences in the learning of gross motor and hand skills and the value of developmental interventions and family supports. The median age of sitting balance was 8 months, pulling to stand 13 months, walking alone 15 months, and walking across a room 19 months. Over 30 years later, we are in a different era of visual disability and premature infants who develop severe ROP. Even among children with legal blindness, those whose residual vision is between 20/500 and 20/800 make better developmental progress than if their vision is 20/800 or worse.

III. **MANAGEMENT**
A. **Primary goals.** The responsibility of the clinician is to interpret and facilitate the infant's behavior and development, to coordinate diagnostic evaluations, and to understand their child's strengths, challenges, and ways of learning. In addition, referral to early intervention programs, provision of supplementary security income, visual aids, parent groups, family supports, and advocacy are required.
B. **Emotional supports: Normal grieving, parental fears, and hope.** It is the clinician's task to support parents through the stages of normal grieving, allow them to express their sadness and anger, and clarify sources of confusion. Except in neurodegenerative disorders, all children with visual disability continue to learn. It is important to also help parents understand the importance of residual functional vision. Families are highly sensitive to feelings of isolation and abandonment by clinicians, especially if they perceive discomfort with the disability. Clinicians can also assist with anticipating some of the challenges, especially if they include behavior supports for day-to-day management. This strategy includes supports for addressing sleep difficulties, feeding skills, hygiene, toileting, and demanding behaviors. Recognition of parental stress, anxiety, depression, and feelings of being overwhelmed requires empathy, appropriate counseling, and referral and advocacy for mental health services. Supports to siblings should include discussion of etiology, contagiousness, stigma, dealing with peers, and family crisis.
C. **Developmental interventions.** It is critical to remember that children with blindness are children first and benefit from proactive biopsychosocial interventions that promote use of residual vision if possible, and optimize communicative, cognitive, behavioral, and social competencies. **Several model curricula** are available to early intervention teams:
1. **Infancy.** Family supports, communicating and recognizing infants' cues, mobility, manipulation, and orientation should be the major themes. Touching, labeling, smelling, and exploring people, toys, and objects encourage the infant to learn about their surroundings. Participation in small group experiences with visually impaired and nonvisually impaired peers is important.
   • Fraiberg and colleagues used auditory–tactile paired cues to stimulate interactions and taught parents to recognize infant's tactile gestures for communicating basic needs.

- Joffee program is a home-based model for orientation and mobility. Parents learn how to enrich their home environment by auditory toys that are brightly colored and have tactual cues, interactive paired verbal and tactile activities, singing, guided touch, and describing daily activities.
- In Erwin parent-centered approach, parents are trained to teach toddlers how to ask questions, describe objects by using modifiers (e.g., hot, warm, and cold water), and use personal social labels in speech.
- Klein's Parent and Toddler Training emphasizes social responsiveness. Target training themes include understanding early childhood development, social development, family reactions, behavior management, enhancing infant development, family communication, and problem-solving.
- Philip and Dutton have elegantly summarized practical suggestions for managing the complexity of CVI. They highlight adaptive behaviors and management strategies addressing low vision for near and far, impaired perception of movement, visual field defects, dorsal stream dysfunction, impaired visual guidance of upper or lower limb, and ventral stream dysfunction. Martin and colleagues emphasize the opportunities for neuroplasticity in CVI with elegant illustrations of critical role of dorsal–ventral stream, and its complex connectome. They used high angular resolution diffusion tensor imaging to elegantly illustrate the superior longitudinal fasciculus (the neural anatomical correlate of the dorsal visual processing stream), the inferior longitudinal fasciculus (the neuroanatomical correlate of the ventral visual processing stream), and the inferior fronto-occipital fasciculus, which mediates visual attention and orienting.

2. **Preschoolers.** Preschoolers can have small-group, quality, early childhood educational experiences as well as receiving extensive consultation from a teacher of the visually impaired. A functional and developmental approach can emphasize communication, rich sensory experiences exploration, and learning through play, music, adaptive, and social skills. All state educational systems receive funds to ensure appropriate educational supports and visual aids.

3. **School age.** A comprehensive individualized curriculum is essential. Both talking books and specialized computer screens are important. Clinicians in partnership with families can set goals that allow the child to learn appropriate academic, social, and extracurricular skills. The school-aged child should participate in community-based classroom activities that will allow preparation for higher education, as well as for independent living. Children with visual disability and multiple additional disabilities require strategies that do not leave them and their families isolated and in only part day learning activities.

4. **Adaptations and technology:** Braille continues to be the mainstay of nonvisual communication. The use of records and tapes are critical sources for reading and information about the world. The OPTACON (Optical to Tactile Converter) was developed by the Stanford Research Institute to convert printed text to a tactual dot figuration. In many public libraries, there are print to speech converters (Kurzweil devices) that allowed printed material to be read aloud. A variety of computerized technology systems in conjunction with video camera technology have been developed to translate environmental information to tactile or optic nerve stimuli. It is important for professionals to understand that adults with adventitious blindness (i.e., individuals with some experience of sight before they became blind) have been the initial users of these prototypes.

5. **Orientation and mobility skills (peripatology)**
   a. **Orientation** requires that a child know present position and space, their destination, and the pathway for travel.
   b. **Mobility** refers to the technique for safely and efficiently traveling to a predetermined indoor or outdoor destination. These skills can be enhanced with long canes. Guide dogs are widely used with adults. The Canterbury Child's Aid is based on sonar wave emissions that are converted to audible stimuli.
   c. There remain major gaps in the knowledge base for understanding in children both quantifiable positive outcomes and challenges with current devices, for developmentally appropriate independence, vocational opportunities, and community participation. However a recent review highlights the potential of new technologies to enhance orientation and mobility.

Bibliography

FOR PARENTS

American Foundation for the Blind. Louisville, KY, www.afb.org also includes Family Connect for parents of children who are blind or visually impaired.

Educational Booklets and Videos in English and Spanish: The Blind Children's Center. Los Angeles, CA. http://www.blindchildrenscenter.org/.

Fraiberg S. *Insights from the Blind*. New York: Basic Books; 1977.

Holbrook C. *Children with Visual Impairments: A Parent's Guide*. 2nd ed. Bethesda, MD: Woodbine House Inc.; 2006.

Little Bear Sees, a foundation which provides families with information, products, and tools for their children with CVI. www.LittleBearSees.com.

Lueck AH, Dutton GN, eds. *Vision and the Brain: Understanding Cerebral Visual Impairment in Children*. AFB Press; 2015.

National Library Services for Blind and Physically Handicapped. http://www.loc.gov/nls/.

Resources on Cortical Vision Impairment (CVI) in Children by Shannon Carollo posted on 4/17/2017 on Family Connect.

WonderBaby.org is a website sponsored by the Perkins School for the Blind. It is dedicated to helping families with children who have vision impairments and multiple disabilities.

FOR PROFESSIONALS

Blencowe H, Lawn JE, Vazquez T, Fielder A, Gilbert C. Preterm-associated visual impairment and estimates of retinopathy of prematurity at regional and global levels for 2010. *Pediatr Res*. 2013;74(suppl 1):35-49. doi:10.1038/pr.2013.205 [PMID:24366462].

Cuturi LF, Aggius-Vella E, Campus C, Parmiggiani A, Gori M. From science to technology: orientation and mobility in blind children and adults. *Neurosci Biobehav Rev*. 2016;71:240-251 [PMID:27608959].

Dammeyer J. Deafblindness: a review of the literature. *Scand J Public Health*. 2014;42:554-562.

Dammeyer J. Development and characteristics of children with Usher syndrome and CHARGE syndrome. *Int J Pediatr Otorhinolaryngol*. 2012;76(9):1292-1296 [PMID:22721527].

Darlow B Retinopathy of prematurity. new developments bring concern and hope. *J Paediatr Child Health*. 2015;51:765-770.

Philip SS, Dutton GN. Identifying and characterizing cerebral visual impairment in children: a review. *Clin Exp Optom*. 2014;97:196-208.

Solebo AL, Teoh L, Rahi J. Epidemiology of blindness in children. *Arch Dis Child*. 2017;102(9): 853-857.

Ventura LO, Ventura CV, Lawrence L, et al. Visual impairment in children with congenital Zika syndrome. *J AAPOS*. 2017;21(4):295-299.e2.

CHAPTER 87

Vulnerable Children

Carol C. Weitzman

I. DESCRIPTION OF THE PROBLEM. The term *vulnerable child* is used to refer to children who have an increased, atypical, or exaggerated susceptibility to disease or disorder due to medical, socioeconomic, psychological, biological, genetic, and environmental risk factors. The term *vulnerable child syndrome* (VCS) was coined by Green and Solnit (1964) to describe children who have often experienced a real or imagined life-threatening incident or illness and are now viewed by their parents as being at greater risk for behavioral, developmental, or medical problems. Although these children appear to have recovered from their initial illness, their parents continue to view them as especially prone to illnesses and death. Perceiving both an essentially healthy child and a chronically ill child as *exceedingly vulnerable has been shown* to adversely influence many aspects of children's health, development, and adaptation. The VCS represents a transactional relationship between child and parent factors.

- The VCS represents the extreme end of a spectrum. The severity of any individual contributing factor will influence how fully the syndrome is expressed and how fixed the beliefs of the family system will be. The term *VCS* should be reserved only for cases meeting the criteria in Table 87-1.

A. Epidemiology. The percentage of parents who perceive their child as vulnerable is unknown, as is the extent to which the VCS underpins a child's problems. The literature on outcomes related to perceptions of child vulnerability is limited but suggests that children's development may be adversely influenced in a number of ways.

- In a community-wide study of 1095 children aged 4–8 years, 10% of children were categorized as "perceived vulnerable." In that study, 21% of all the mothers reported that they had had prior fears that their child might die.
- Studies have shown that 64% of infants born prematurely continued to be viewed as vulnerable by their parents when they were preschoolers.
- In a cohort of 116 premature infants, those children whose parents had high perceptions of child vulnerability were more likely to have lower adaptive development at 1-year adjusted age.
- In a cohort of 69 children with chronic rheumatologic and pulmonary diseases, those children whose parents had increased perceptions of child vulnerability had greater social anxiety.
- A number of studies have demonstrated an increased sense of vulnerability among mothers who are unmarried, of younger age, and of lower socioeconomic status. The influence of maternal education has been less clear on the development of VCS across different studies.
- The persistence of parental perception of child vulnerability remains unclear. In some studies, it has been shown to decrease over time as the child's health improves and parents are able to reshape their views of their child's health and resilience. Other studies have shown that early perceptions continue to predict later perceptions.
- Children with chronic and serious illnesses, such as diabetes, cancer, and asthma, and whose parents perceive them as vulnerable have been shown to have poorer behavioral and social adjustment and greater uncertainty about their illness, than children whose parents do not hold these beliefs.

B. Etiology. Child, parent, and sociodemographic factors can all contribute to a parent perceiving his or her child as vulnerable. Parent risk factors may relate to problems with fertility, pregnancy, or birth, as well as parental psychopathology or mental health (Table 87-2). In general, the earlier that an event occurs in a child's life, the more likely it is to enhance the parent's perception of the child as vulnerable. The transformation of parental fears into childhood problems is a complex process that is transactional in nature. Perceptions of vulnerability reflect parents' cognitions, attitudes, and beliefs related to their child's health and well-being. These perceptions may lead to a pattern of parents' behaviors including overprotection, reluctance to allow the child to have typical separation and individuation experiences, and a need to maintain control. The child, in turn, sensing parents' concerns and their need or desire to keep the child close may begin to

Table 87-1 • DIAGNOSTIC CRITERIA OF THE VULNERABLE CHILD SYNDROME

1. A real or imagined event in the child's life that the parent considered to be life-threatening.
2. The parent's continuing unrealistic or disproportionate belief that the child is especially susceptible to illness or death (often associated with a high frequency of health care use).
3. The presence of symptoms in the child that appear disproportionate to the apparent level of illness or impairment.

Table 87-2 • ANTECEDENTS OF THE VULNERABLE CHILD

Child Factors
- Newborn period
  - Prematurity
  - Neonatal illness or complications
  - Congenital abnormalities
  - Hyperbilirubinemia
  - False-positive results of screening (e.g., phenylketonuria)
- Early childhood
  - Excessive crying, colic, spitting up
  - Any serious illness
  - Admission to hospital for things such as "to rule out sepsis"
  - Self-limited infectious illnesses (e.g., croup, gastroenteritis)

Parent Factors
- Fertility related
  - Difficulty getting pregnant
  - Recurring stillbirths or miscarriages
  - Concern for fetal loss during the pregnancy
- Pregnancy related
  - Pregnancy complications such as vaginal bleeding
  - Abnormal screening results (e.g., abnormal alpha-fetoprotein)
  - Delivery complications
- Death of a relative or a previous child early in life
- Parent psychopathology and mental health
  - Depression
  - Negative portrait of child
  - Anxiety
  - Displacement of intense emotions onto the child
- High levels of parental stress

behave in ways that reinforce these beliefs, such as acting frailer and having more illness complaints. Conversely, children may act out in ways to defy these perceptions.

II. MAKING THE DIAGNOSIS

A. **Presentation.** The hallmark of VCS is in the high health care utilization rates seen in these children and what frequently seems to be the misperception by parents of the severity of the child's illnesses and risks. In addition, many parents who experience VCS will be refractory to standard pediatric interventions such as reassurance. These features may be among the most important clues to identifying a family system grappling with VCS. VCS can also present with a number of both specific and nonspecific parent and/ or child behaviors (Table 87-3). VCS is to be distinguished from factitious disorder imposed on another (formerly known as Munchausen syndrome by proxy). In factitious disorder imposed on another, a caretaker voluntarily and consciously induces or simulates symptoms of an illness and then seeks medical attention for that problem.

B. **History: key clinical questions.** Sensitive history taking begins the therapeutic process by conveying support and empathy to the parents. The clinician should ask questions that lead to an understanding of the parent's sense of vulnerability.
   1. *"To understand your child better, I need to know more. Let's go back to the beginning. Let's start with your getting pregnant."* This allows a more complete history that can focus on factors contributing to perceptions of vulnerability.
   2. *"What did the doctors tell you might happen? Did you at any time fear that the child might not make it or worry that this was more serious than what was being told to you?"* This type of question should be asked whenever a parent reports a problem, particularly during the pregnancy, delivery, and childhood, no matter how minor it might appear and allows the clinician to understand more about parents' cognitions and beliefs.

Table 87-3 • ANTECEDENTS OF THE VULNERABLE CHILD

- Parental attitudes and behaviors
  - Reluctance to separate from the child
  - Difficulty setting appropriate limits
  - Tolerance of physical aggression by the child toward them
  - Overvigilant toward the child
  - Overdirective toward the child
  - Overindulgence of the child
  - Disproportionate concern for seemingly minor illnesses or health risks
  - Description of the child as less developmentally competent than other children
  - Frequent visits to the pediatrics clinician for seemingly minor illness
- Child behaviors
  - Recurring symptoms of minor illness such as stomachache and headache
  - Regulatory problems including sleep and eating difficulties
  - Dysregulation of attention
  - School underachievement
  - Reluctance to separate from parents
  - Learning challenges

3. *"That must have been very frightening for you."* Whenever parents report something that might have been particularly worrisome to them, an empathic response will encourage them to talk further about their fears.

4. *"How often are you and your child apart? How does that typically go?"* Try to assess the parents' level of comfort in separating from their child by asking questions about the use of babysitters and their level of worry when separated from the child. Other questions should include information about other separation difficulties (e.g., when the child first started childcare or school).

5. *"Overall, how stressful has it felt to parent this child particularly in light of his/her earlier or current difficulties?"* Parental stress has been shown to moderate the relationship between perceptions of child vulnerability and child-reported symptoms of depression and adjustment.

6. *"Tell me more about your discipline strategies and how easy or hard it is to enforce them?"* Parents who perceive their child as vulnerable may have more difficulty in setting and enforcing appropriate limits and have also been reported to be overindulgent.

7. *"Have you ever experienced symptoms of worry or depression unrelated to your child's health?"* Questions such as these may help the clinician to understand a parent's mental health profile and risks for psychopathology. Parents with high levels of anxiety have been linked in some studies to having a higher likelihood of VCS.

    C. Assessment. A number of standardized measures exist that can provide a fuller understanding of the complex beliefs and attitudes of parents that may accompany the VCS. The Vulnerable Child Scale and the Child Vulnerability Scale are brief measures with cut points above which VCS should be suspected. The Vulnerable Baby Scale is a 10-item measure that is a modification of the Child Vulnerability Scale and may be more suitable in detecting parent perceptions of vulnerability in infants and young children.

III. MANAGEMENT

    A. Prevention. The clinician must realize that any event or illness, even one considered to be medically insignificant, may have a very different meaning and implications for the parent. The clinician needs to take time to understand parents' beliefs and fears and address these appropriately. This may occur, for example, when a colicky infant's formula is changed. Some parents might interpret the change as implying that the child has a gastrointestinal abnormality. By explaining that colic is a self-limited condition affecting normal infants and by reinforcing this concept by changing back to the original formula within a few weeks, the clinician can help to prevent the development of perceptions of vulnerability. When a child who is hospitalized for an acute but treatable illness is ready for discharge, the clinician should emphasize to the parents that recovery is or will be complete, that no special precautions will be necessary after a certain time, and that the child is no more vulnerable to illness than other children. For some children, such as preterm infants, who have had life-threatening illness and/or children with chronic illness, the clinical course may remain unclear. Clinicians must be honest with parents and be clear about current risks and a predicted time course for symptoms if known. It is helpful for pediatricians to explore episodically parents' worries, beliefs, and attitudes about the health risks they perceive for their child. Clinicians need to be attentive to signs of parental anxiety and stress or the presence of other risk factors that may place this child at greater risk of being seen as vulnerable.

B. Treatment. Once it is recognized that parental perceptions of vulnerability are affecting a child's behavior or development, the following approach should be taken:

1. **After taking a complete history and performing a conspicuously meticulous physical examination, if the child is well, the clinician should give a clear statement that the child is physically sound.** He or she should not use equivocal comments, such as "He doesn't look too bad" or "I can't find anything wrong."

2. **Assist parents by explaining that it is a natural tendency to worry about a child after a serious illness or event.** This explanation may begin a discussion of the adverse effects of viewing the child as vulnerable and the effects this can have on everyone in the family.

3. **Allow parents of chronically ill children to express their worries and help them to identify a child's coping skills and resilience.** These types of conversations can help parents not only articulate their worries but also construct a more robust profile of their child.

4. **Support the parents in dealing with the child more appropriately** by setting consistent limits, discontinuing patterns of infantilization and overprotectiveness, dealing more effectively with problems of separation, and being less panicked about the child's somatic complaints. It may be necessary to schedule additional visits to reinforce parents' efforts, provide reassurance, and address anxious worries before they escalate. It needs to be emphasized to parents, however, that these extra visits are not due to the child's illness or the clinician's worries.

5. Although these problems can usually be managed by the primary care clinician, a mental health referral may be necessary if the parents are unable to make the link between past events and current beliefs and attitudes and are unable to adjust their current perceptions of the child.

Bibliography

Chambers PL, Mahabee-Gittens EM, Leonard AC. Vulnerable child syndrome, parental perception of child vulnerability, and emergency department usage. *Pediatr Emerg Care*. 2011;27(11):1009-1013.

Forsyth BW, Horwitz SM, Leventhal JM, et al. The child vulnerability scale: an instrument to measure parental perceptions of child vulnerability. *J Pediatr Psychol*. 1996;21(1):89-101.

Green M, Solnit A. The threatened loss of a child: a vulnerable child syndrome. *Pediatrics*. 1964;34:58-66.

Kerruish NJ, Settle K, Campbell-Stokes P, et al. Vulnerable baby scale: development and piloting of a questionnaire to measure maternal perceptions of their baby's vulnerability. *J Paediatr Child Health*. 2005;41(8):419-423.

Kokotos F. The vulnerable child syndrome. *Pediatr Rev*. 2009;30(5):193-194.

Pearson SR, Boyce WT. Consultation with the specialist: the vulnerable child syndrome. *Pediatr Rev*. 2004;25(10):345-349.

Index

Note: Page numbers followed by "f" indicate figures and "t" indicate tables.